A Colour Atlas of

Chest Trauma

and Associated Injuries

Volume two

Augustin Besson
MD, Dr Med, Chirurgien FMH, FACS, FCCP, FICS
Privat-docent and Agrégé at the
Faculty of Medicine, University of Lausanne,
Médecin-adjoint, Service de chirurgie générale et
thoracique 'A', Centre Hospitalier Universitaire
Vaudois, Lausanne, Switzerland.

Frédéric Saegesser
MD, Dr Med, FACS, FCCP, FICS
Foreign member of the Academy of Surgery,
(Paris), Professor of Surgery at the
University of Lausanne School of Medicine,
Directeur du Service de chirurgie générale
et thoracique 'A', Centre Hospitalier
Universitaire Vaudois, Lausanne, Switzerland.

Wolfe Medical Publications Ltd

With contribution from

Marcel Savary, MD, Dr Med,
Professor of ENT at the University of Lausanne School of Medicine, Directeur du Service d'Oto-rhino-laryngologie, et de chirurgie cervicofaciale, Centre Hospitalier Universitaire Vaudois, Lausanne, Switzerland

Translated by

Marcus D Hellyer, BA(Cantab)

Contents

Detailed contents precede each chapter

Volume II

Volume I (published 1982)

Acknowledgements

Most of the photographs in this Atlas were produced by the Audio-visual centre for Medical Teaching of the Centre Hospitalier Universitaire Vaudois (Director, Dr P. Gygax) or by Dr A. Besson. We thank Mr and Mrs S. Daldoss, Mrs N. Mattille, Mrs E. Mayor (Kodak Ltd, Lausanne), Mrs M. Nater, Mr Y. Delaunay, Mr P. Gallay, Mr F. Schaeffer and the photography departments of the Lausanne Police (Commander, Major M. Emery; Chief of the ambulance department, Adj. J.-Cl. Francfort), and the Cantonal Police (Commander, Lt. Col. R. Mingard).

A number of colleagues kindly put at our disposal original photographs (each of which is individually credited in the text). We thank:
in Lausanne – Dr M. Boumghar, Dr Z. Bozič, Prof. G. Candardjis, Dr P.-G. Chassot, Prof. P. Desbaillets, Prof. L. Freedman, Prof. Cl. Gailloud, Dr A. Jost, Prof. J.-J. Livio, Dr H. Loosli, Dr P. Mavrothalassitis, Prof. Th. Rabinovicz, Prof. J.-L. Rivier, Prof. H. Sadeghi, Dr D. Schwander P.-D., Mrs H. Weber;
in Switzerland – Dr P. Babaiantz (Morges), Prof. G. Chapuis (Morges), Prof. Ch. Hessler (Pompaples), Dr W. Hilan, Prof. St. Kubik (Zurich), Dr P. Loup (Yverdon), Prof. R. Mégevand (Geneva), Dr G. Miller (Soleure), Dr M. Rigo (Monthey), Dr S. Schneider P.-D. (La Chaux-de-Fonds), Prof. A. Senn (Bern), the late Prof. U. E. Uehlinger (Zurich);
abroad – Prof. M. O. Cantor (Bloomfield Hills, Michigan), Dr R. Carter (Washington DC), Dr E. T. Gelfand (Edmonton, Alberta), Dr Ph. Levasseur (Centre chirurgical Marie Lannelongue, Paris), Prof. K. G. Swan (Newark, New York).

Most of the artwork was drawn by Dr A. Besson; for the rest, we thank Mrs C. Niemeyer.

We are grateful to the following companies and their representatives:
ASIF (Association for the Study of Internal Fixation); Boehringer; Ethicon (Johnson & Johnson); GASS (Garde Aérienne Suisse de Sauvetage); Heurtey-Bergeon; Hoechst USA; Hoffmann-La Roche; Hospal; Merck, Sharp & Dohme; Opopharma (Argyle, Lederle); Ricker, Rhône-Poulenc Pharma (Switzerland); Smith, Kline & French; Upjohn; Zyma.

The collaboration of the School of Engineering in Bienne, General Motors Research Laboratories, Volvo and IBM was much appreciated.

We thank also Dr M. Bonard and Dr D. Waridel who co-operated in the establishment of our card file, Dr S. Mazzoni who reviewed the ECGs, Prof. A. Roch and Dr J.-M. Peiry who checked our physics, and Dr Ph. Eisner, who checked ballistics data.

Mrs M. Besson (iconographic classification, typing, manuscript checking, indexing, proof reading), Mr J. Besson (manuscript and proof reading), Mrs D. Besson (bibliographical research and audiovisual programmes), Mr F. Cunéo (manuscript photographs), and our secretaries Mrs S. Bovard (supervisor), Mrs R. Vaucher, Mrs Ch. Volkart and Mrs G. Wütrich each gave sustained and invaluable support.

We thank Mr M. Hellyer, B.A.(Cantab.) for the English translation, Mrs S. J. Callander (Windsor) for typing this manuscript with great attention to detail, Prof. Ph. Sandblom (Lund) for checking some chapters and offering useful criticisms.

Finally, we are indebted to the Directors of the Centre Hospitalier Universitaire Vaudois and the Canton de Vaud Authorities for making our enterprise possible.

Preface

It is a privilege and honour to preface this work, for CHEST TRAUMA constitutes a unique reference book which sums up current knowledge on this important subject.

The Atlas sets out in great detail the diagnosis and management of chest injuries but always – from the first chapter onwards – in the general perspective of traumatology. Emphasis is placed on associated injuries of the trunk as well as of more distant anatomical areas and on the frequency of multiple injuries. Therefore, the authors demonstrate precisely to what extent the prognosis of each injury depends upon associated trauma to other structures or systems.

It is clearly shown that the general prognosis of trauma of the chest – whether open or closed – has improved significantly over the last decades. Of course, despite evident progress in management, a number of patients still die more or less rapidly after injury because some situations constitute real therapeutic deadlocks – for instance, severe lung contusion with deep refractory hypoxia, bilateral flail chest, associated brain injuries.

Life-threatening chest trauma is still a common problem and its frequency does not decrease. On the contrary, there are today more victims who die soon after admission to hospital, since the speed and quality of first aid and care during transportation have improved in most countries.

CHEST TRAUMA is of considerable value since it encompasses all aspects of the diagnosis of various injuries and displays a remarkably complete and rich iconography to illustrate each lesion, frequent as well as rare, but life-threatening or potentially incapacitating. Management is described in precise manner, often step-by-step, in a way that every surgeon ought to be familiar with. The chapter (in Volume II) on oesophageal injuries is particularly didactic. The management of chest injuries is almost codified or, at least, the principles of management have been defined with such precision that most indications for treatment are now quite clear, even if some cases remain delicate to appreciate. Arguments, such as the one concerning the best treatment for flail chest – artificial ventilation versus internal fixation of ribs – are now out-of-date.

This Atlas will be useful to all who are involved in the treatment of patients with chest injuries or multiple injuries, even when they are not specialists in this field. The aim is to save life in the early phase, or at least to keep patients alive until specialists are at hand. CHEST TRAUMA should help to decrease the number of erroneous decisions, and of useless or dangerous procedures which sometimes produce superimposed iatrogenic pathology.

Nevertheless, the management of chest injuries requires concentrated teamwork and unfailing attention to details. Emphasis should be placed on the sequelae of such injuries, and of their elaborate treatment, some of which were unknown previously. Appreciation of these can constitute a difficult problem of forensic medicine. A number of severe sequelae can be prevented by the energetic use of physiotherapeutic procedures.

Having maintained a special interest in the field of chest trauma throughout the past twenty-five years, I can measure the progress that has been made recently. Assuming that such progress continues, I consider that this essential book will remain a true classic, a bible for all those – whether specialised or not in chest surgery – who are involved in the caring for patients with chest injuries.

Henri Le Brigand, M.D.
Member of the Academy of Surgery (Paris),
Chief of Surgery at the Centre Chirurgical
Marie Lannelongue, Paris.

Introduction

Injuries to the thoracic wall, vessels and viscera – whether severe or seemingly slight – often give rise to elusive symptoms and signs that are overshadowed by those of associated injuries.

The objectives of this Atlas are to *familiarise the reader with the symptoms and signs* of (common and rare) chest injuries and associated damage, to *codify the indications for surgical treatment*, to *evaluate the risks and assess the prognosis* of each injury and combination of injuries, and to *illustrate possible complications*.

The origins and forms of chest trauma are by definition protean; while endeavouring to do full justice to the complexity of our subject, we have attempted in each case to interpret clearly the *causal mechanism(s)* and the *physiopathological consequences*.

From time to time we have been faced with terminological problems; for the sake of simplicity, we have developed a number of neologisms whose sense we trust will be clear, even though their form may be unorthodox.

The Atlas contains a large number of illustrations: series of photographs and/or X-rays, graphs, diagrams and drawings. In the linking passages and tables, we have tried to present facts rather than chimerical personal interpretations. Throughout, we have made ample use of iconography to illustrate both specific aspects of individual cases and the general characteristics of each type of injury. Since many patients present multiple chest injuries, the same case has sometimes been used to illustrate a number of different points in different chapters.

We have adopted this approach in the belief that X-rays and photographs give a more faithful and concrete account of the dynamics of physiopathological processes than the written word.

We have not omitted *disappointing or fatal evolutions*, whatever the cause, and we have paid close attention to failed treatments and iatrogenic complications; we feel that these cases are particularly instructive.

The Atlas is planned as a reference work in which each subdivision forms a whole. The detailed table of contents at the beginning of each chapter, the index and, above all, the numerous cross-references from one photograph/X-ray to another are designed for swift orientation on precise problems.

We have had to select our material to some extent, because many photographs and X-rays of emergency cases are inevitably snatched in dramatic circumstances when there is no time for technical nicety.

Our overall aim has been not only to present ideas or examples of how to deal with critical situations – whether classic or rare – but also to induce reflection, the prelude to all action.

7 Trauma of the trachea and major bronchi

Incidences

Although injuries to the cervical trachea occur outside the chest, they are included in this chapter because of the fundamental kinship between the symptoms, signs and surgical treatment of all tracheal injuries.

Among the many different types of accident responsible for the rare tracheobronchial rupture, the common denominator is violence. Taking 205 cases from the literature, Dor and Le Brigand offer the following figures:

Crush-injury (by the buffer or wheel of a railway carriage or truck, under a tractor, under a mechanical shovel or crane, under a tree trunk or pylon, or by accidental burial): 48%

Road accidents:

– Driver	12%	
– Passenger	24%	52%
– Pedestrian, motorcyclist	16%	

702

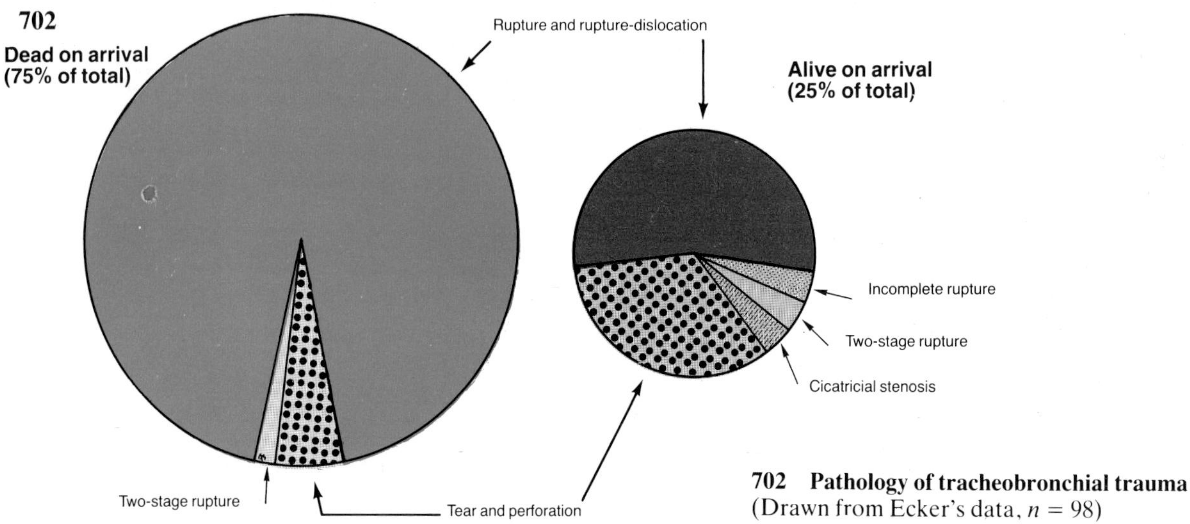

702 Pathology of tracheobronchial trauma (Drawn from Ecker's data, $n = 98$)

The incidence of tracheobronchial rupture is highest among children and young people. The average age of patients is 31 years (compared with an average of 46 years for all chest trauma casualties).

The average age of those who are dead on arrival is 33 years, and of those alive on arrival, 25 years.

703

703 Age distribution of tracheobronchial injuries (Drawn from Ecker's data, $n = 105$)

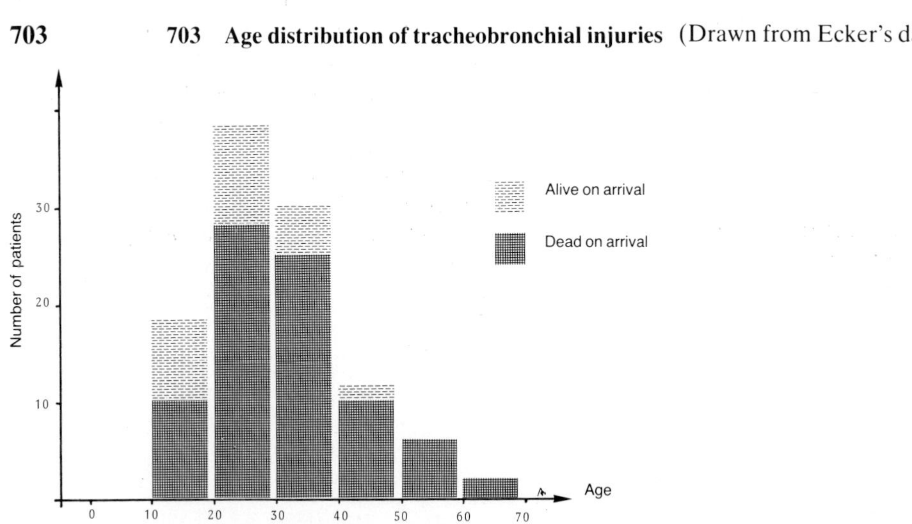

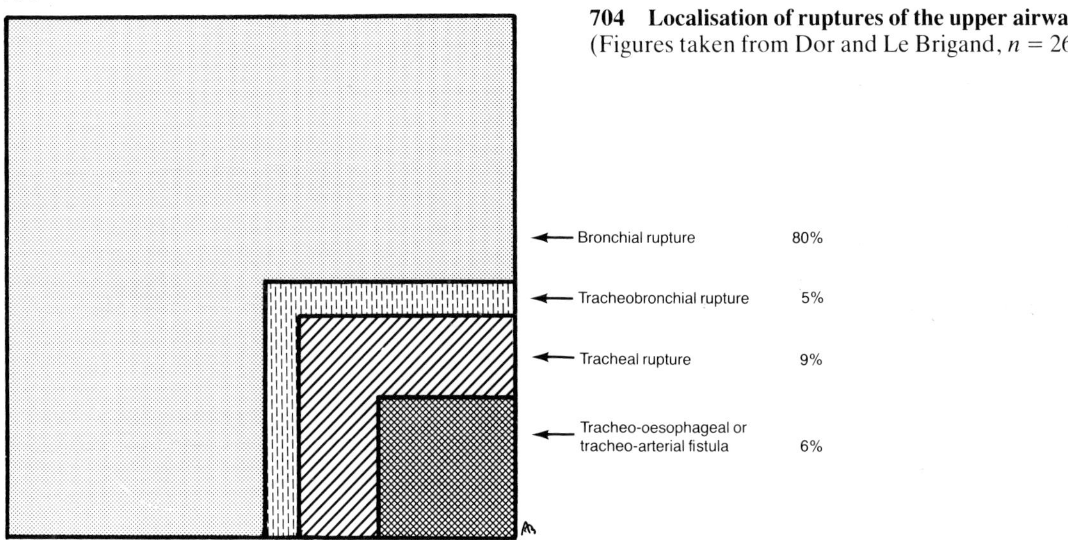

704 Localisation of ruptures of the upper airways (Figures taken from Dor and Le Brigand, $n = 264$)

Symptoms and signs

In 75% of cases, tracheobronchial rupture is *fatal*, either on the scene of the accident, or in the ambulance (see **702**).

At the other extreme, some ruptures of the trachea and major bronchi pass *unnoticed* until cicatricial stenosis has developed.

Rupture is sometimes discovered when an *intubation* tube deflects off course into the subcutaneous tissue of the neck, or when positive pressure ventilation *suddenly produces a compressive gaseous syndrome* (pneumothorax with mediastinal and subcutaneous emphysema). The latter situation is particularly dangerous.

An immediately symptomatic rupture (with a compressive gaseous syndrome, or an irreducible pneumothorax) is rarely overlooked during initial examination. Diagnosis is confirmed through an emergency *tracheobronchoscopy*. However, in labile patients with respiratory difficulties, tracheobronchoscopy can cause cardiac arrest; in such cases, endoscopy should be followed by immediate repair.

A tracheobronchial rupture that evolves in *two stages* poses further difficulties. The typical patient initially shows nothing more than slight and easily allayed symptoms and signs; up to four days later, he suddenly develops a compressive gaseous syndrome or emphysema. Swift diagnosis and treatment are then imperative.

Rupture of the upper airways results in one or more of the following syndromes:

- *a gaseous syndrome:*
  - mediastinal and subcutaneous emphysema: *90% of cases*
  - ipsilateral pneumothorax (rarely contralateral, sometimes compressive): *50% of cases*
  - persistent pleural air leak.
- *a haemorrhagic syndrome* with haemoptysis (or aspiration of blood through an intratracheal or tracheostomy tube): *10% of cases.* Haemoptysis can be due to the drainage of a bloody pleural effusion through the breach in the airways.
- *respiratory exclusion syndrome* with pulmonary atelectasis due as much to occlusion of the bronchi by blood and secretions as to the loss of continuity (one lung often completely collapses): *5% – 10% of cases seen early.*

In practice, significant *subcutaneous emphysema* initially cervical strongly suggests a compressive gaseous syndrome (mediastinal emphysema and/or tension pneumothorax); in turn, a compressive gaseous syndrome often signals an *injury of the upper airways.* The injury should be suspected also in any patient with early haemoptysis or atelectasis.

705a

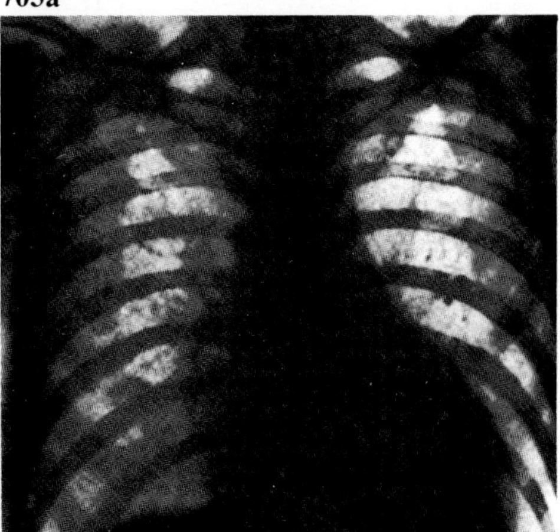

E.I. ♀ 41 yrs. Dec. 1957

705b

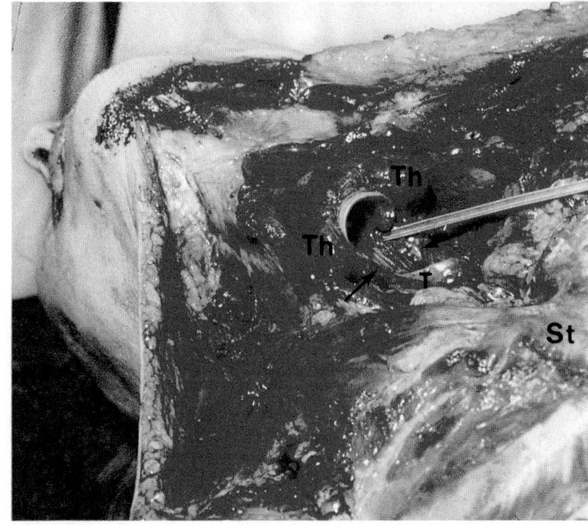

Dec. 1957

705a An initially asymptomatic tracheal rupture can prove fatal. This woman's neck was dashed against the steering wheel when she drove into a lorry at 100 km/h. She walked alone to the hospital, holding her head. There was no subcutaneous emphysema, and her chest X-ray was normal. **705b** Two hours later, the patient suffocated when her head was tilted to take a Towne's projection X-ray of the skull. Tracheal intubation was attempted but the tube repeatedly deviated out of the trachea. This autopsy photograph reveals a rupture-dislocation of the trachea, between the 2nd and 3rd rings (probe), immediately above the thyroid gland (Th). Only the membranous part of the trachea (→) is intact. The distal part (T) has withdrawn about 4 cm, to a position almost behind the sternum (St).

706

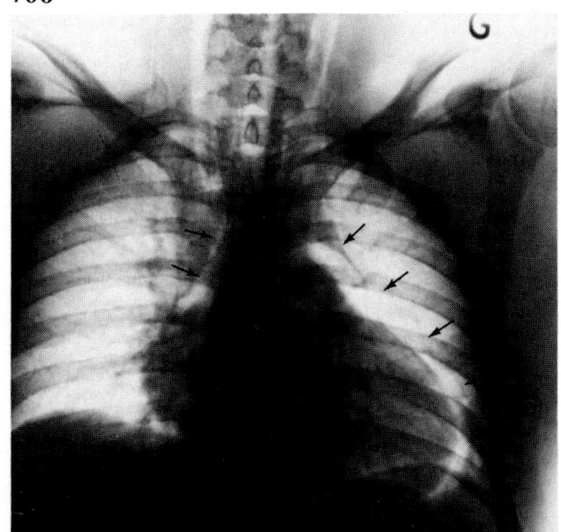

M.F. ♂ 22 yrs. 8 Nov. 1970

706 Mediastinal emphysema is often a sign of tracheobronchial rupture. Tracheal rupture can give rise to mediastinal and cervical emphysema. So too can oesophageal rupture and certain pulmonary injuries. The sign, therefore, is not pathognomic.

707a Mediastinal emphysema does not necessarily appear early even when the upper airways are severely injured. This admission X-ray shows slight subcutaneous emphysema in the neck.

707b Nine hours later, the cervical emphysema is more pronounced and there is suggestion of mediastinal emphysema. Despite the insignificance of her signs, the patient nevertheless was found to have a complete and almost total rupture of the trachea (see **767d**).

707a

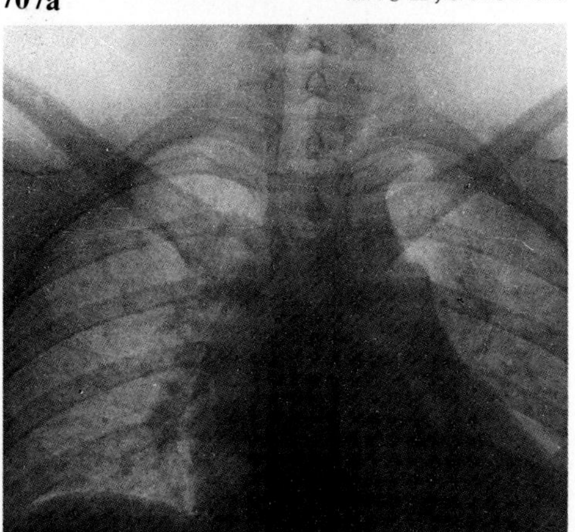

W.C. ♀ 19 yrs. 1 Oct. 1969. 23hrs.

707b

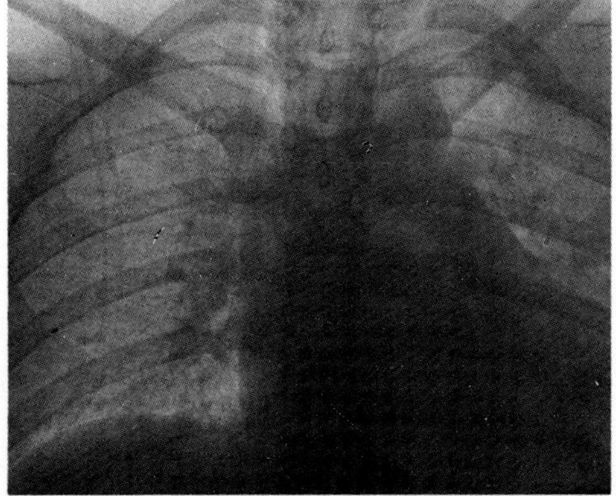

2 Oct. 1969. 08 hrs.

708a

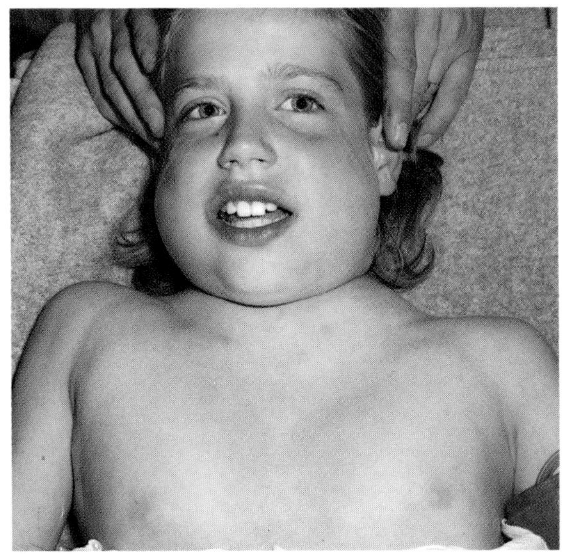

D.P. ♀ 10 yrs. 1 June 1966

708a Mediastinal emphysema can spread immediately and induce massive subcutaneous emphysema of the trunk, neck and face. This young girl sustained a small tear of the lower trachea when she contused the anterior region of her neck in a fall against the handle-bars of her scooter.

708b The admission X-ray shows massive subcutaneous emphysema of the face, neck . . .

708c . . . and chest wall.

708d Retrosternal mediastinal emphysema separates the structures of the superior and anterior mediastinum.

708b

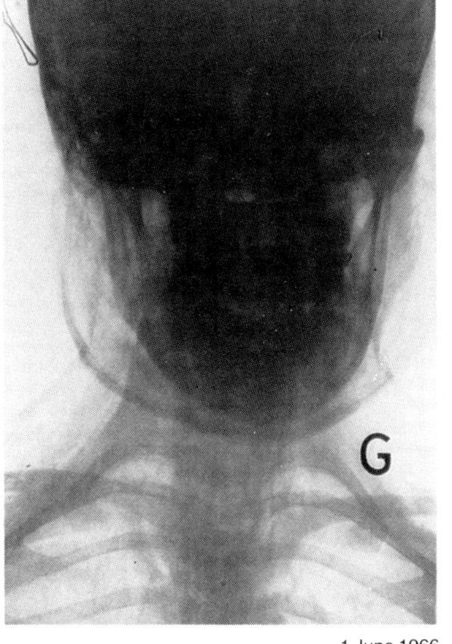

1 June 1966

708c

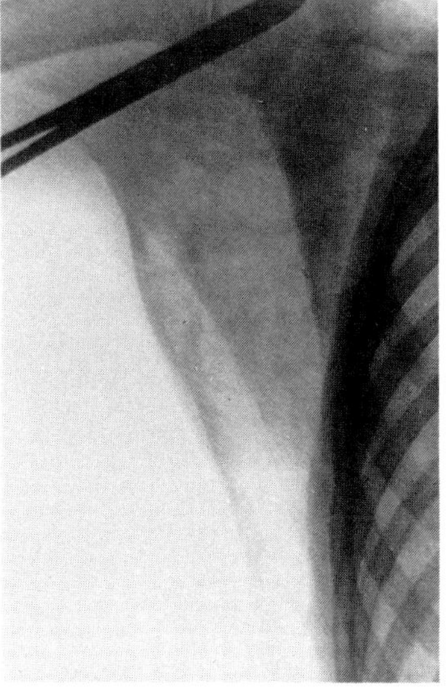

1 June 1966

708d

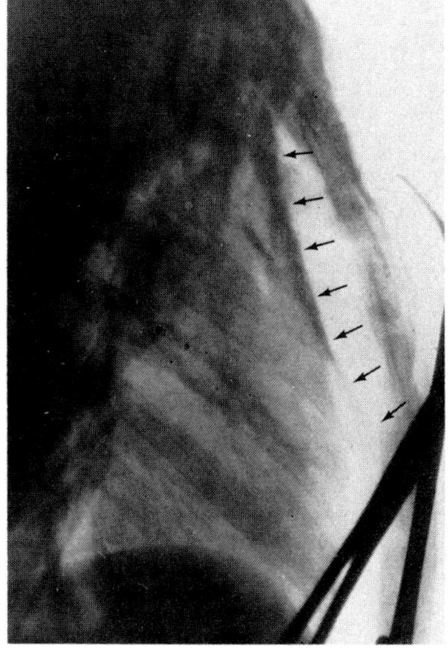

1 June 1966

709

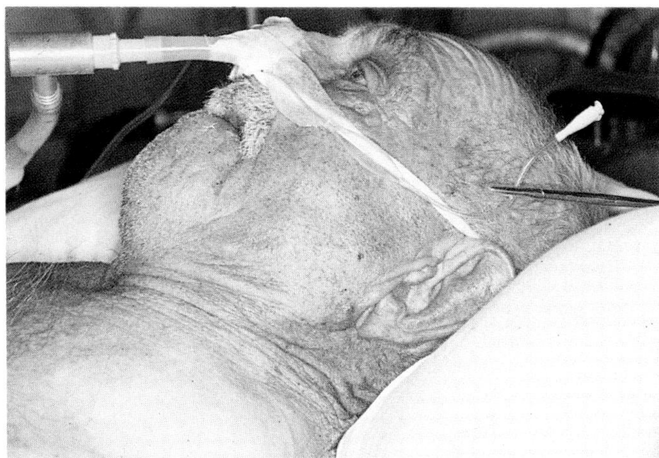

J.R. ♂ 80 yrs. 15 Sep. 1976

709 Mediastinal emphysema followed by cervical emphysema is an unspecific sign. This elderly patient's fall from a tree led not to a rupture of the upper airways, but to contusion – laceration of the lungs (see Volume I, **494**). The previous obliteration of the pleural cavity allowed air to spread directly to the subcutaneous tissues and mediastinum. Conservative treatment. Recovery.

710

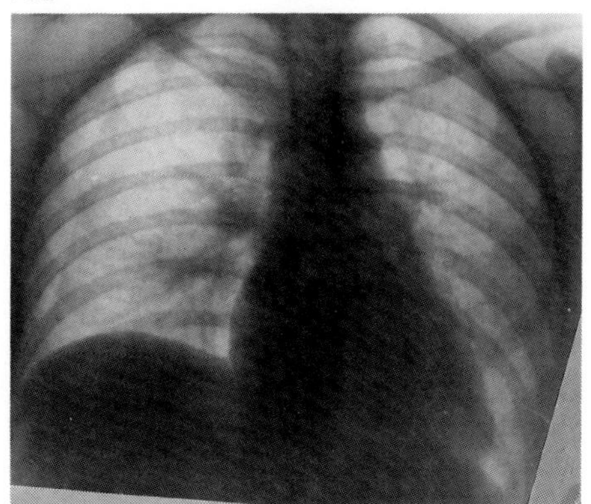

M.B. ♀ 22 yrs. 28 Nov. 1971

710 Tracheobronchial injuries often cause simple pneumothorax; in this case, a 20% right pneumothorax.

711a

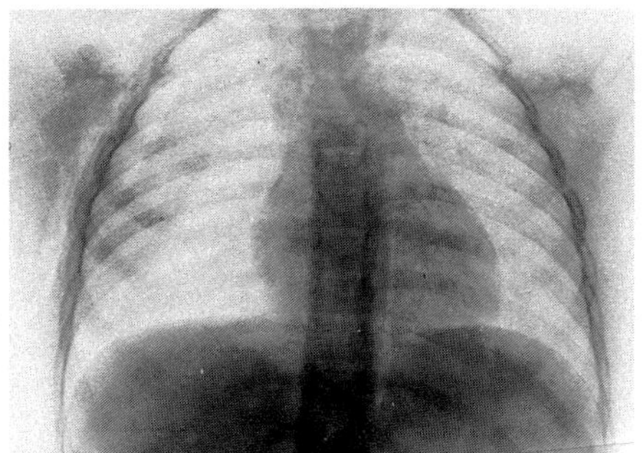

V.M. ♀ 7 yrs. 13 June 1965

711b

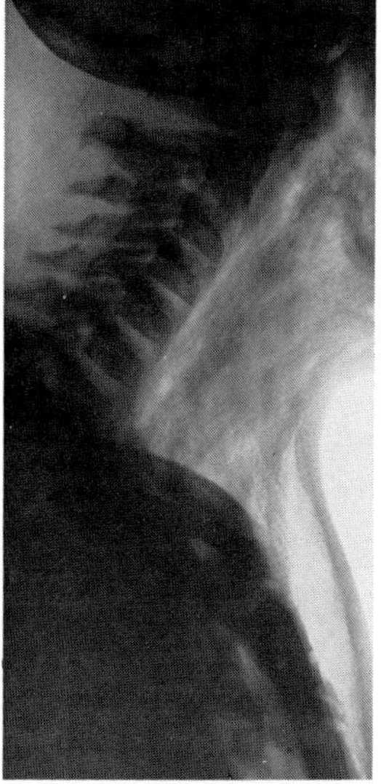

19 June 1965

711c

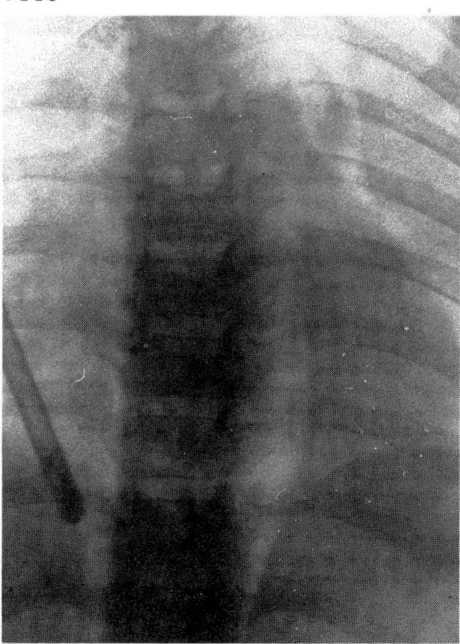

19 June 1965

711d

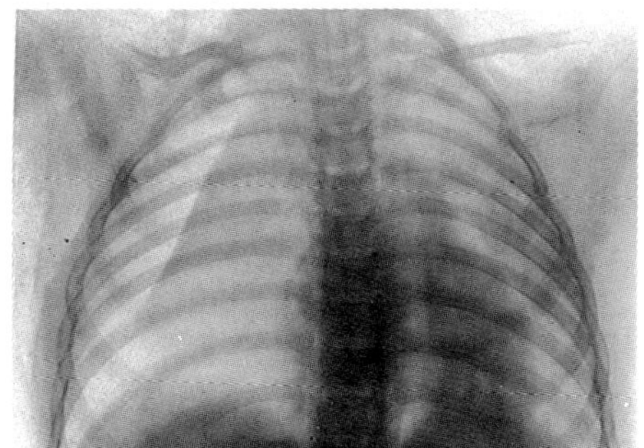

19 June 1965

711e

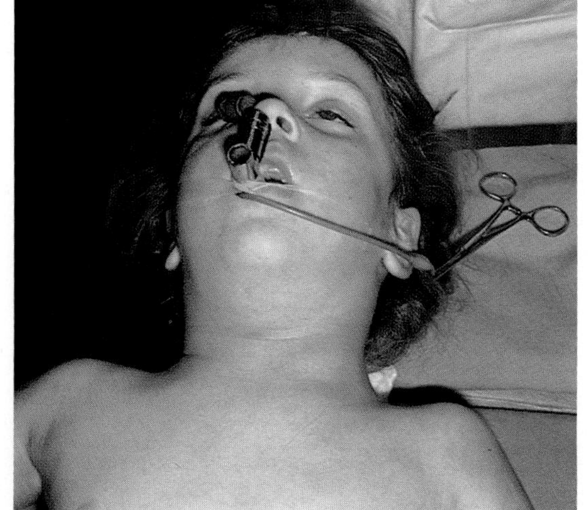

19 June 1965

711a Tracheal rupture sometimes leads to tension pneumothorax. Under these circumstances, positive pressure ventilation is risky. This child rapidly developed significant subcutaneous emphysema after falling against the handle-bars of her scooter.

711b Respiratory insufficiency develops despite intubation, due to secondary mediastinal emphysema and a right pneumothorax, both under tension.

711c The mediastinal emphysema spreads upwards to the neck and chest wall . . .

711d . . . and downwards along the descending aorta as far as the diaphragmatic crura. The right pleura has been drained.

711e Notice that immediately before surgery (consisting of a cervical incision for repair and a mediastinotomy for decompression) *ventilation is not assisted, but spontaneous.* In this way, aggravation of the gaseous syndrome – by coughing or by Valsalva's manoeuvre – is forestalled. Recovery in a fortnight.

712a

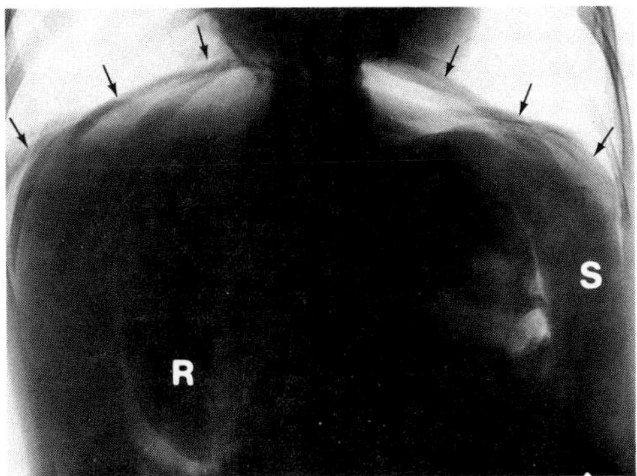

K.J.–D. ♂ 7 yrs. 17 Sep. 1972

712b

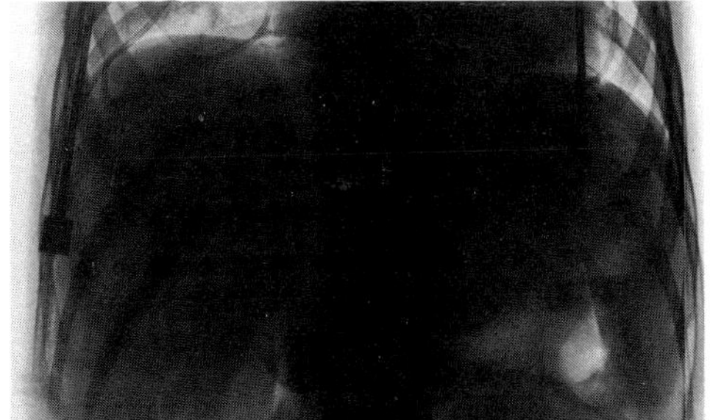

17 Sep. 1972

712c

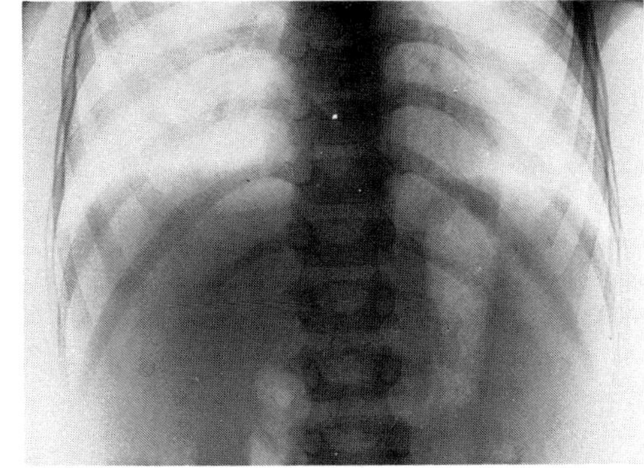

Sept. 1972

712a Tracheal perforation can cause bilateral tension pneumothorax, and even pneumoperitoneum (see **738**). This supine X-ray shows retroperitoneal emphysema around the right kidney (R) and the spleen (S), and a significant pneumoperitoneum along the diaphragm (→).

712b The lungs have re-expanded after pleural drainage, but the pneumoperitoneum is more significant.

712c Recovery.

General Management

Anaesthesia

Injuries to the trachea and major bronchi invariably make resuscitation and anaesthesia difficult, if not harmful. For example:

- *the tube may deflect* through the rupture and never reach the distal trachea.
- intubation may directly *aggravate* the damage.
- positive pressure ventilation may *increase the pressure* of a gaseous syndrome. If there is a pneumothorax, it is likely to become compressive and to displace the mediastinum (see **815** and Volume I, **478**); if there is mediastinal emphysema, venous return may be obstructed.
- the *escape of large volumes of air* through the chest tubes can make it impossible to ventilate the remaining lung.

Hence it is crucial that an anesthetist, an endoscopist and a surgeon co-operate in the investigation of every suspected rupture of the upper airways.

Once the pleural cavity has been drained and evacuated, endoscopy can provide a precise evaluation of the damage. The dangers of blind intubation are thus avoided. Meanwhile, of course, the preparatory steps for cervical or thoracic exploration should be taken.

Approaches

713 **Approaches to injuries of trachea and major bronchi.**

713

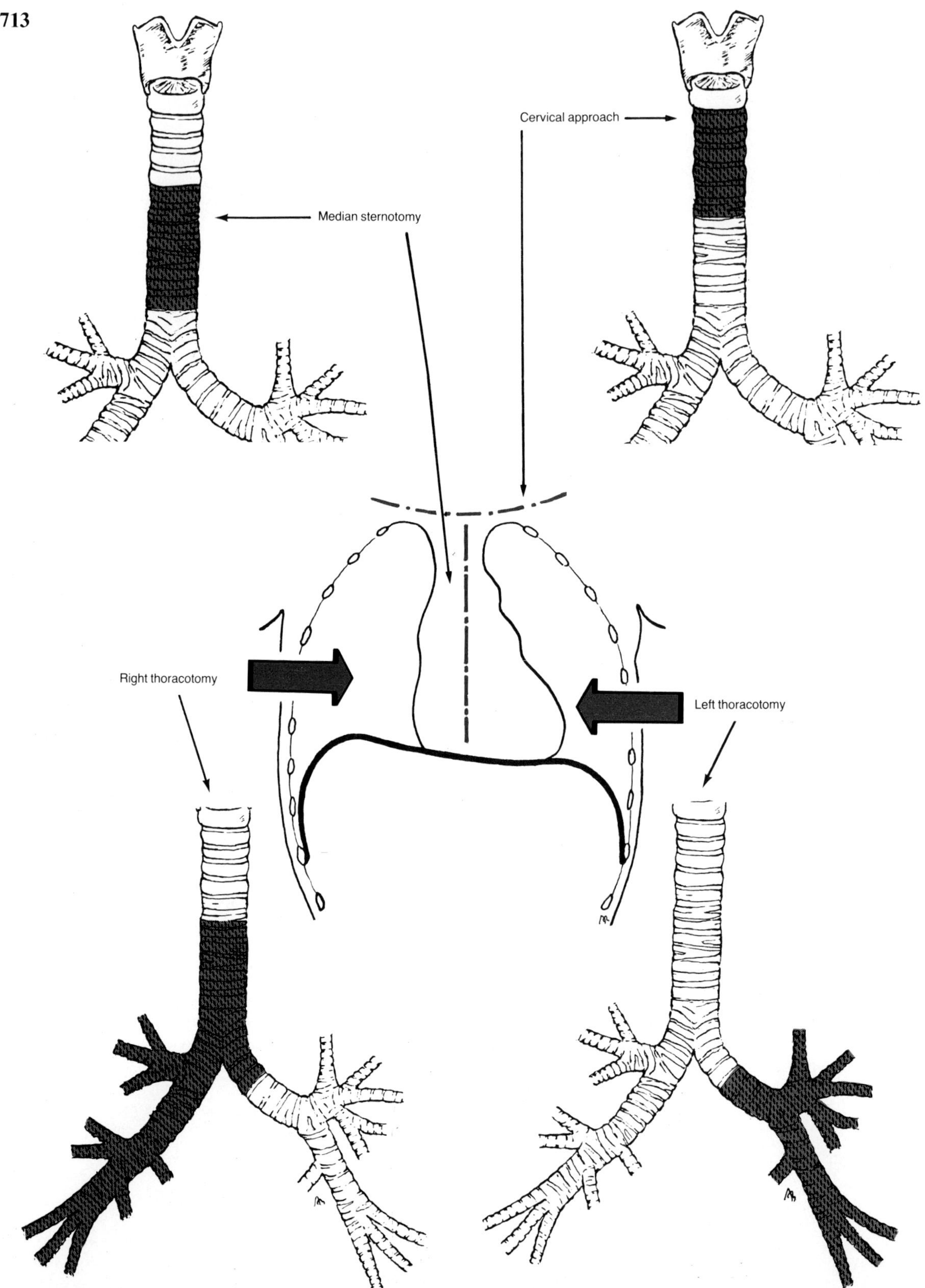

Tracheal Intubation

Tracheal intubation as a method of resuscitation dates at least from Vesalius (16th century). However, it was not until the 19th century that it became a widely used anaesthetic and therapeutic procedure in humans.

714

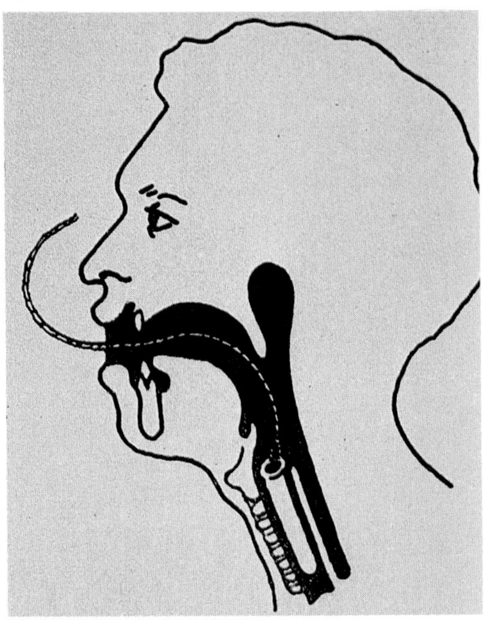

714 Bouchut's pharyngo-tracheal intubation technique (1858) for the treatment of respiratory distress in diphtheria patients.

715

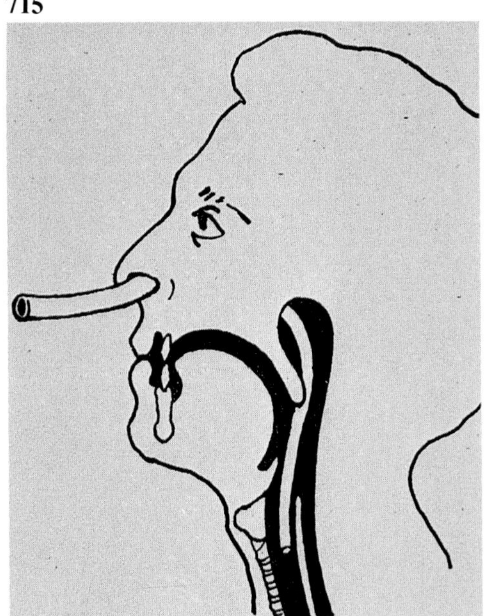

715 Desault's naso-tracheal technique.

716

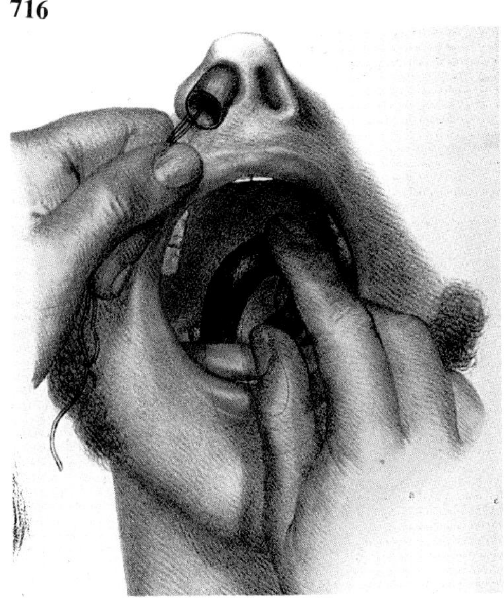

716 Oro-tracheal intubation can be switched to naso-tracheal intubation. (*Médecine opératoire*, Bourgery and Claude Bernard, 1867.)

717

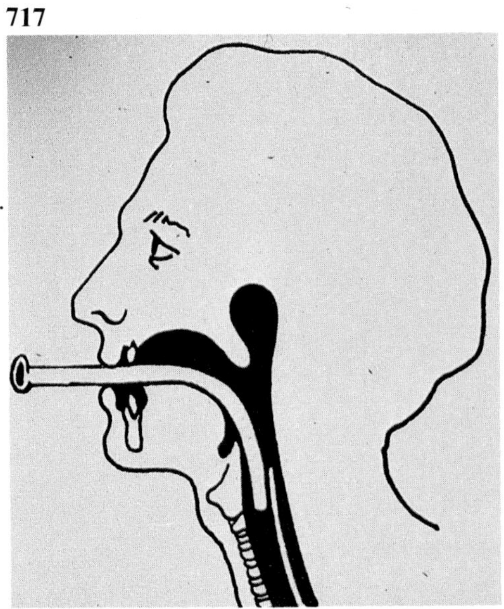

717 Arab, rigid tube technique.

718a

côtés de la canule avec le pouce et l'indicateur de chaque m:
tandis que les deux médius relevés servent à boucher le nez
comprimant les narines. On aspire alors les mucosités qui eng
gent les bronches en exerçant la succion à l'autre extrémité du tu

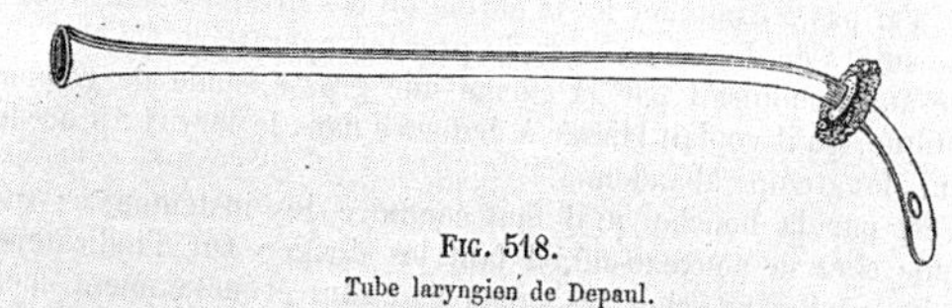

puis on pratique l'insufflation avec la bouche, en imitant les tem
égaux de la respiration. On peut faire dix, douze et jusqu'à quin
insufflations par minute; après chacune d'elles, on laisse lib

718b

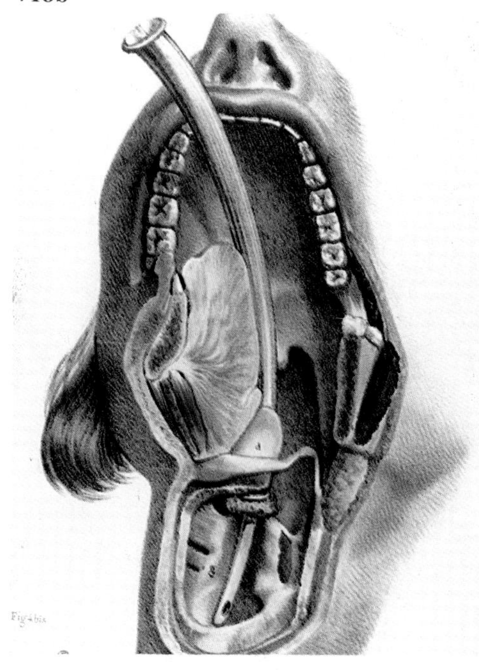

718c

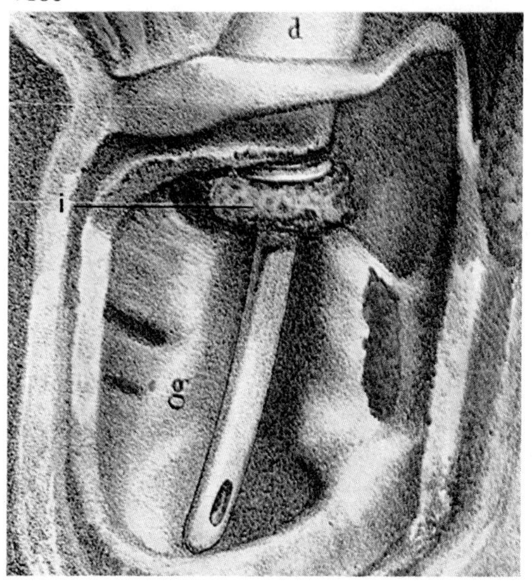

718a Metal intubation tube. (*Manuel de médecine opératoire*, J.F. Malgaigne, Baillière, Paris 1877.)

718b Depaul's oro-tracheal technique. (*Médeine opératoire*, Bourgery et Claude Bernard, 1867.)

718c A hundred years ago, inflatable cuffs did not exist. Instead, a slice of sponge (i) was placed manually over the glottis.

Tracheal intubation is now in widespread use, but the act of intubating a patient can be difficult.

With careful monitoring and adequate local care, intubation can be prolonged for several weeks (see page 20).

719a

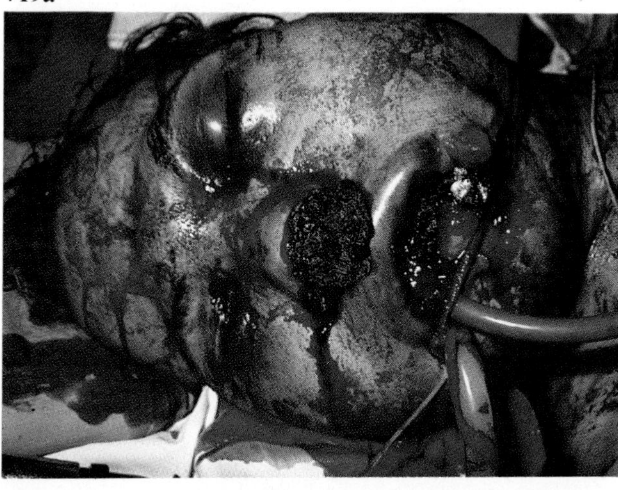

719b

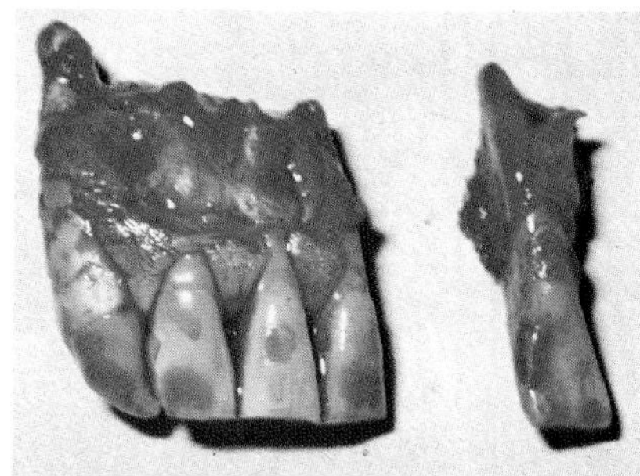

719b Fragments of the maxilla were removed from the pharynx before intubation (see **719a**). Such fragments sometimes have to be removed from the trachea or bronchi (see **753** and page 31, and Volume I, **65**).

719a Road accident casualties with **facial and cranial injuries** are often **difficult to intubate**. The trachea and bronchi must be cleared first of aspirated blood. This patient has a bilateral palpebral haematoma due to a fracture at the base of the skull. Massive epistaxis has been controlled. (Prof. J. Freeman, Lausanne.)

720

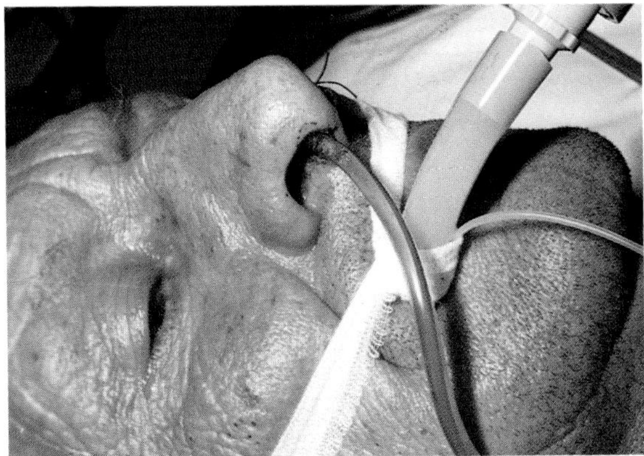

720 Provided the patient co-operates, **oro-tracheal intubation** can be maintained for several weeks without undue hazard.

721

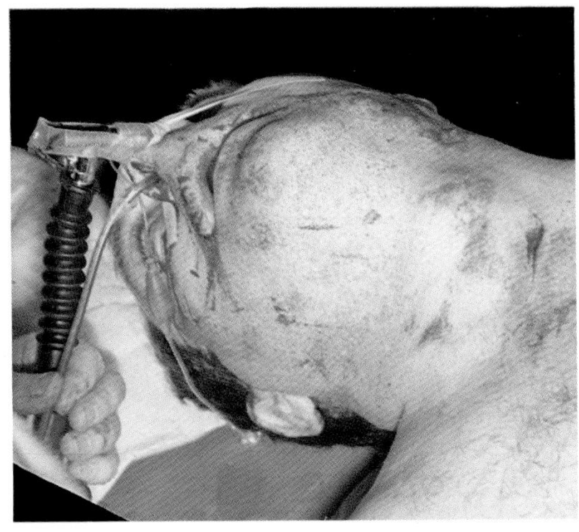

B.C. ♂ 44 yrs. 12 Feb. 1974

721 Immediate naso-tracheal intubation can obviate the necessity for transtubation in a dangerously hypoxic patient.

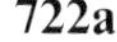

722a

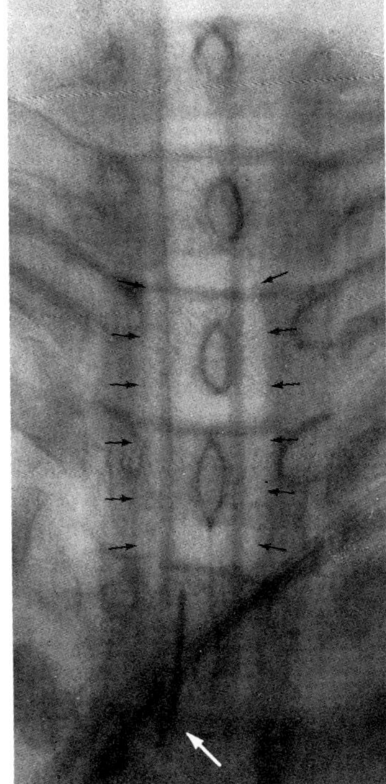

L.F. ♀ 60 yrs. Oct. 1976

722a Correct position (the large arrow indicates an X-ray marker in the tube); the long, low pressure cuff is hardly inflated (→).

722b

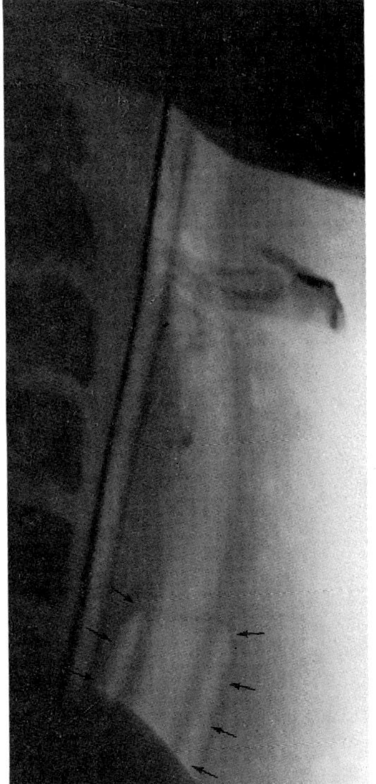

Oct. 1976

722b Lateral view: the cuff is located at the thoracic outlet. The oesophageal lumen contains a marked Levin tube.

723

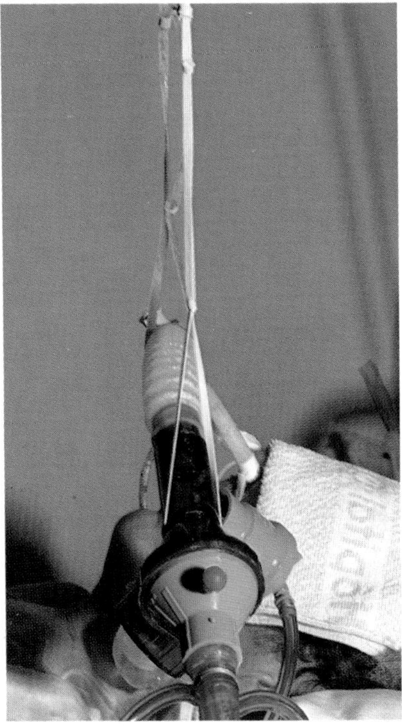

723 If the tubing is suspended on rubber bands, the likelihood of damage to the trachea is greatly reduced.

Prolonged tracheal intubation can result in various complications. Complications have become less frequent, however, since the development of new tubing materials and large, low pressure cuffs. Damage to the larynx and trachea during prolonged intubation consists of erosion, ulceration and sometimes tracheal necrosis (see page 45).

724

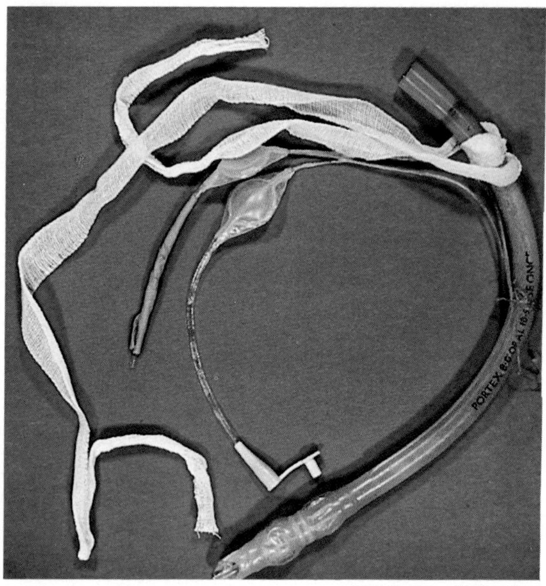

M.H. ♀ 44 yrs. 25 Jan. 1975

724 This tube with two cuffs remained in place for 92 days (see **1173**) without damaging either the larynx or the trachea. (Dr. D. Schwander, P.-D., Fribourg.)

725

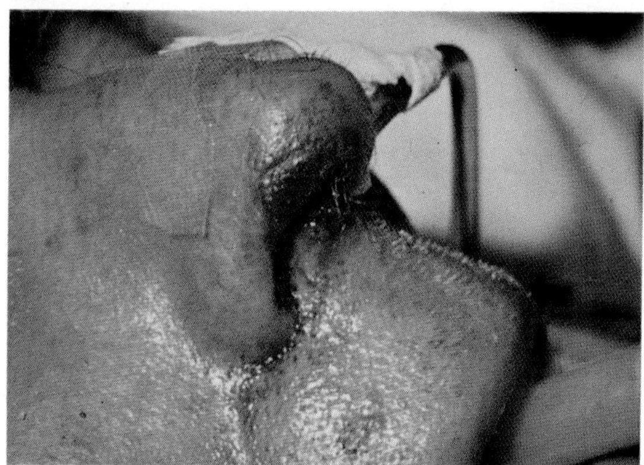

725 Nostril pressure-sore after prolonged naso-tracheal intubation. The photograph was taken after the naso-tracheal tube had been replaced by an oro-tracheal tube. (Dr. D. Schwander, P.-D., Fribourg.)

726

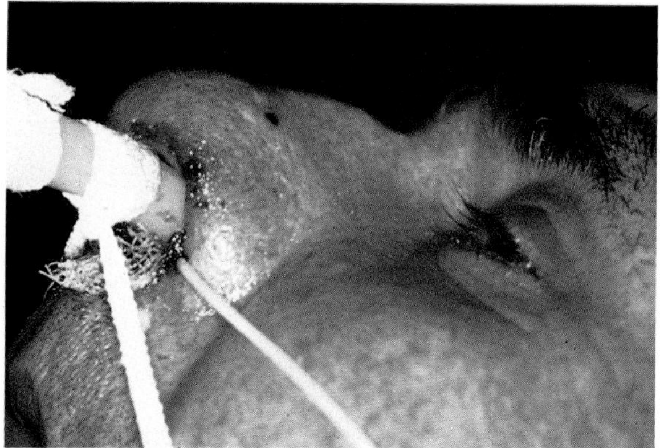

726 Pressure from a tracheal tube can quickly irritate the nostril. The fragment of green gauze is also partly responsible. (Dr. D. Schwander, P.-D., Fribourg.)

Endobronchial intubation is sometimes required. The procedure requires a tube with two canals and two cuffs; its effect is to ventilate the lungs separately and to prevent communication between them. There are two varieties: the Carlens tube for left endobronchial intubation and the White tube for right endobronchial intubation. The White tube also has a small lateral aperture to ventilate the right upper lobe.

Endobronchial tubes have specific indications and advantages. Their position always should be carefully checked by auscultation and X-ray before surgery.

727a

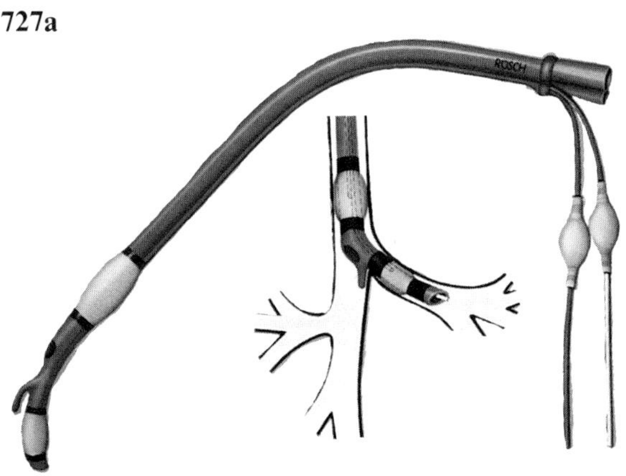

727a Carlens . . .

727b

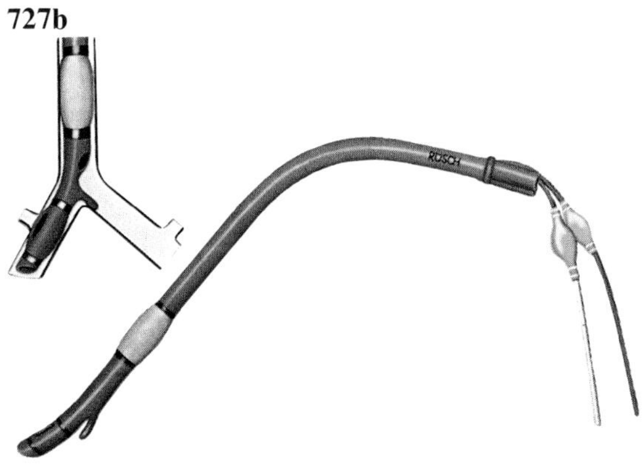

727b . . . and White endobronchial tubes. The position of the tube should be checked by X-ray. The limits on the cuffs are radio-opaque.

728

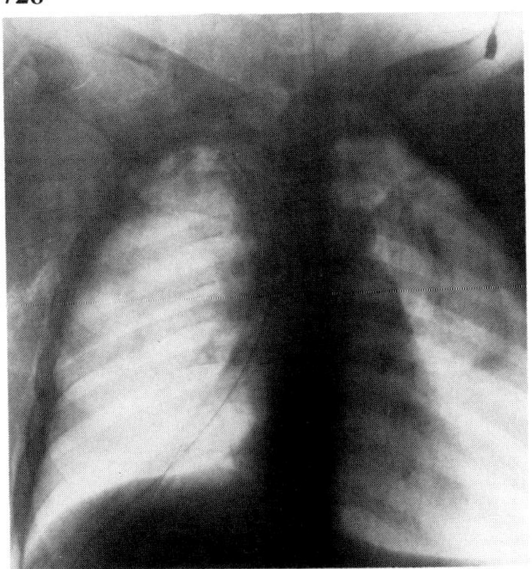

F.R. ♂ 21 yrs. 3 Dec. 1973

729

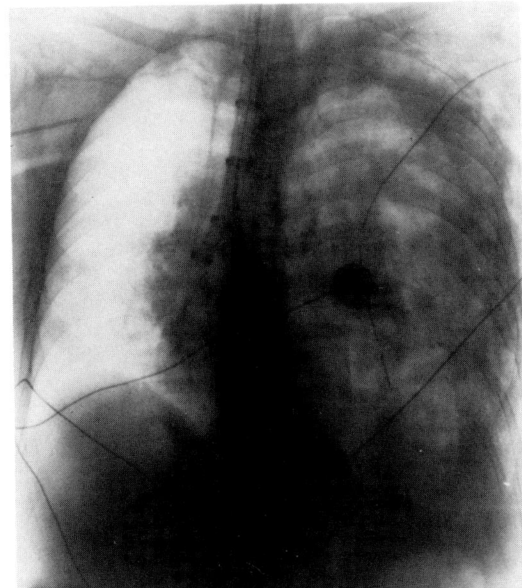

D.A. ♂ 79 yrs. 5 May 1975

728 Carlens tube used to control massive right bronchopleural air leak (with tension pneumothorax). In this patient with multiple ruptures of the segmental bronchi and a pneumothorax under massive tension, a Carlens tube has controlled the air leak by excluding the right lung. Upper right lobectomy. Recovery.

729 Blood-filled left bronchi are excluded by White tube. This patient has a laceration of the lower left lobe and a tension haemopneumothorax. A White endobronchial tube has been introduced into the right mainstem bronchus to prevent the massive haemorrhage in the left bronchial tree from flooding the right lung. Lobectomy.

730 The diameter of suction cannula that can be passed through each canal of an endobronchial tube is 3 times smaller than in an ordinary endotracheal tube of equal external diameter; the functional calibre of the suction cannula is therefore *9 times smaller*. Bronchial suction may then be impossible, especially in a case of massive haemoptysis.

730

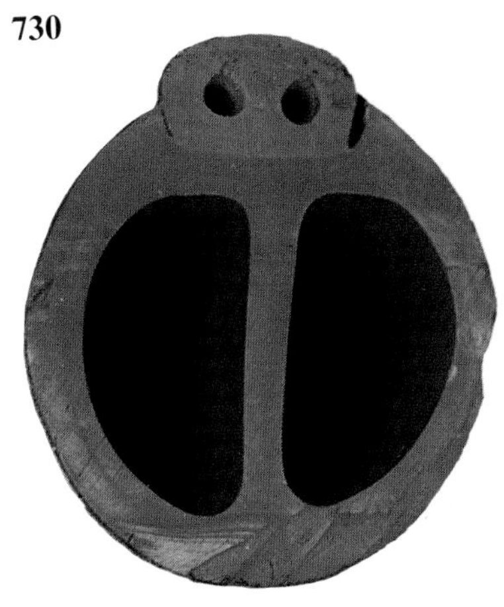

731a

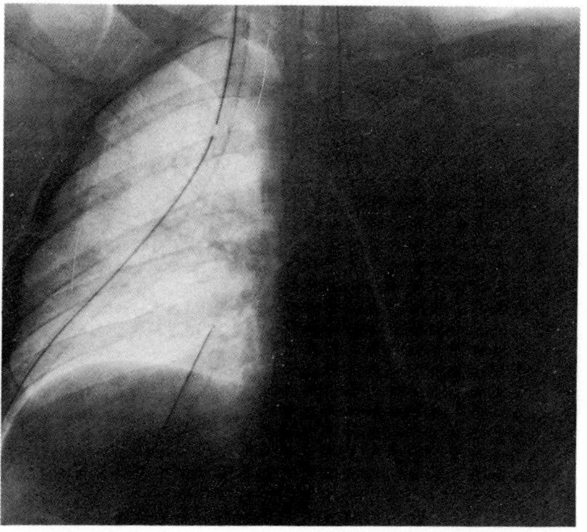

731b

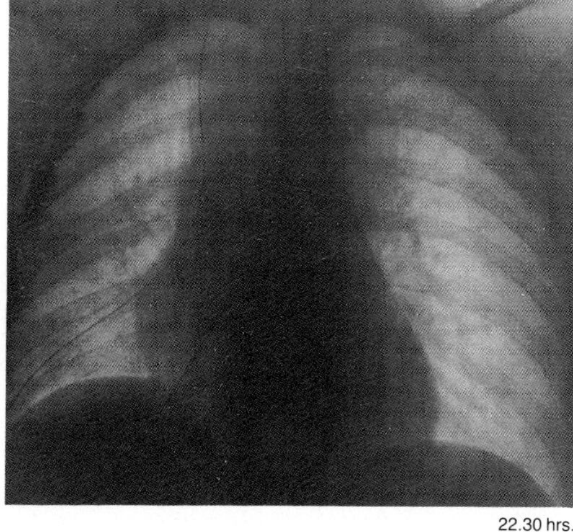

731a The use of an endobronchial tube can have dangerous consequences. A Carlens tube was introduced into the left main-stem bronchus for a right thoracotomy indicated by repeated episodes of massive haemoptysis. During the operation, the patient developed complete atelectasis of the left lung and severe hypoxia: the calibre of the tube was too fine to allow evacuation of the blood clots occluding the entire left bronchial tree. Postoperative X-ray. **731b** The Carlens tube has been replaced by an ordinary tube. A 5ml clot is extracted by intensive physiotherapy: hypoxia recedes and ventilation is restored. Recovery without sequelae after temporary neurological disturbances.

Inadequate ventilation and atelectasis are often attributable to the state or position of the intubation tube.

732

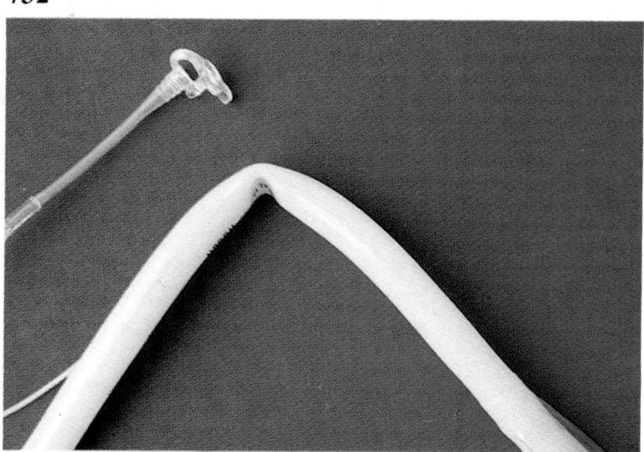

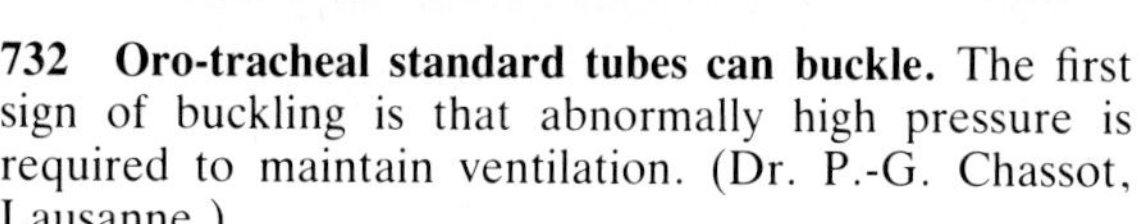

732 Oro-tracheal standard tubes can buckle. The first sign of buckling is that abnormally high pressure is required to maintain ventilation. (Dr. P.-G. Chassot, Lausanne.)

733

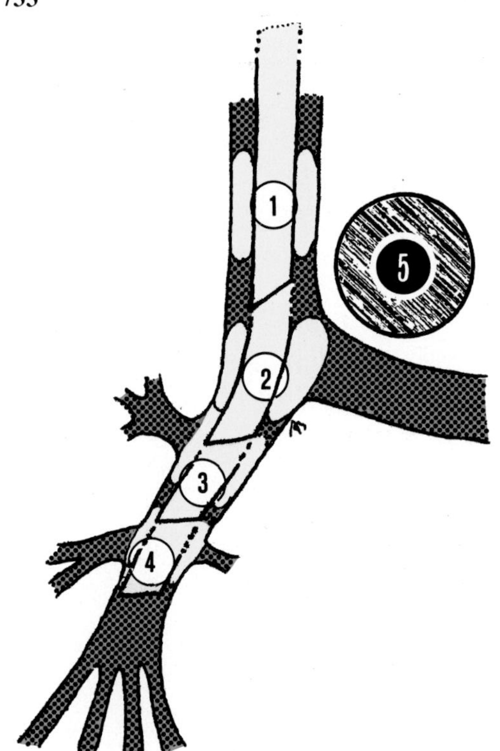

733 When a standard intubation tube is inserted too far, it can terminate *in the right main-stem bronchus* (2), the *intermediate bronchus* (3), or the *right lower lobe bronchus* (4). These three structures lie more or less along the vertical axis of the trachea; the left main-stem bronchus, on the other hand, has a more horizontal course as it goes under the aortic arch (5). There are several possible consequences: (1) adequate symmetrical ventilation, (2) exclusion of the left lung, (3) exclusion of the left lung and right upper lobe, or (4) exclusion of the left lung and right upper and middle lobes. Since most tubes are bevelled to the left, slight displacement in the trachea is rarely harmful.

734

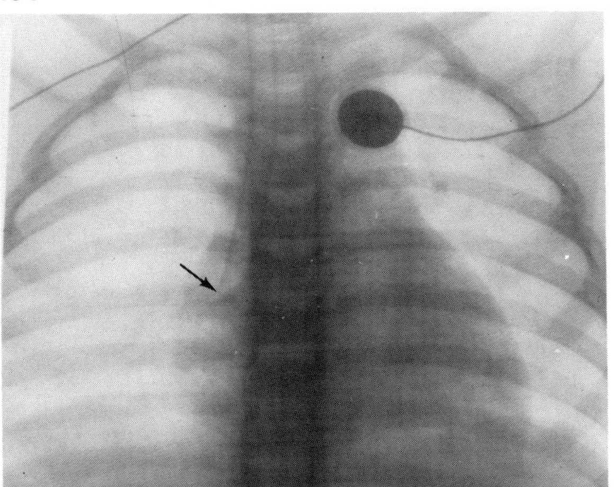

W.N. ♀ 3 yrs. 3 June 1970

734 In this child, an ordinary intubation tube has been inserted *as far as the right main-stem* bronchus or even, perhaps, as far as the intermediate bronchus.

735a

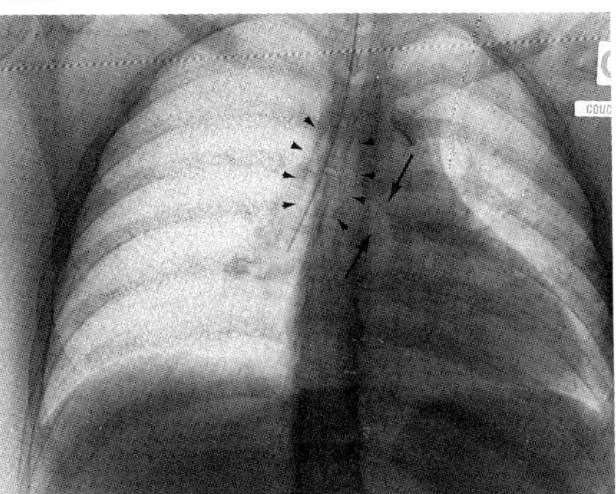

M.P.-J. ♂ 21 yrs. 6 Nov. 1977

735b

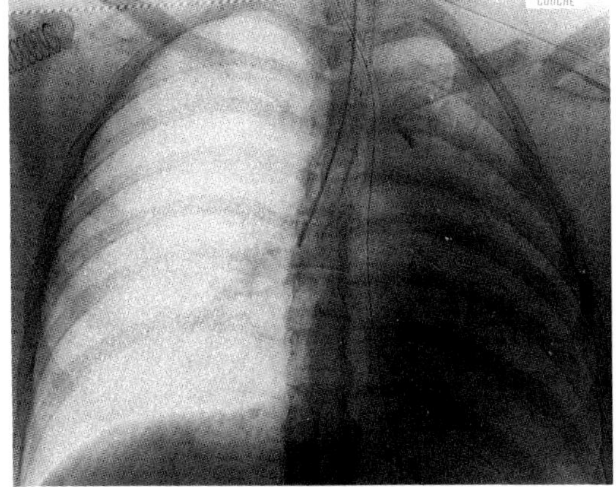

6 Nov. 1977

735c

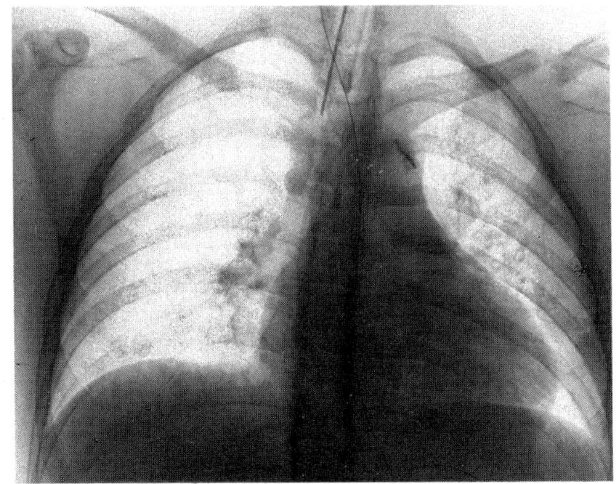

6 Nov. 1977

735a Atelectasis of the left lung after an oro-tracheal tube was pushed as far as the right main-stem bronchus. The cuff (→) can be seen to obstruct the left main-stem bronchus (**→**).

735b The tube has been withdrawn, but insufficiently. The atelectatic left lung attracts the mediastinum, causing a right pulmonary hernia. The result is a severe pulmonary arterial shunt.

735c Ventilation returns to normal and the lung re-expands as soon as the tube is withdrawn sufficiently.

736

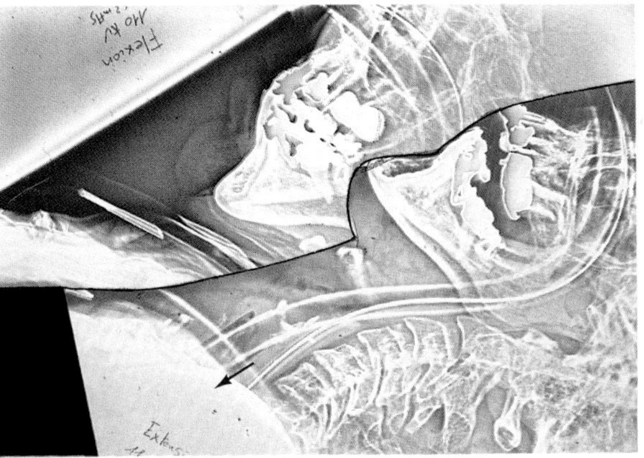

736 When **the head** of a patient wearing a naso-tracheal tube is **flexed**, the tube and cuff are forced some 4cm deeper (see **776**).

737a

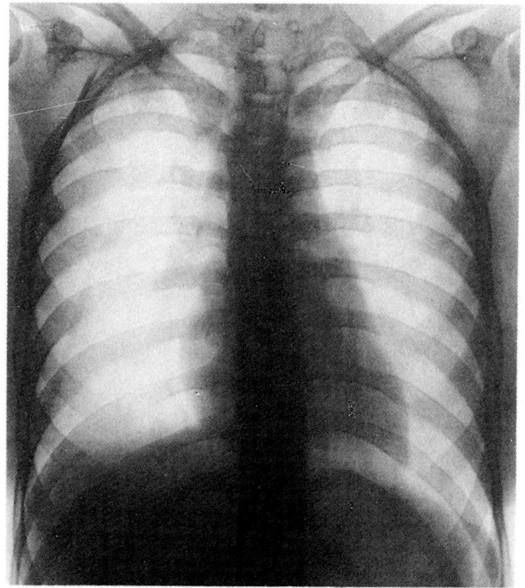

N.C. ♀ 16 yrs. 4 Nov. 1977

737b

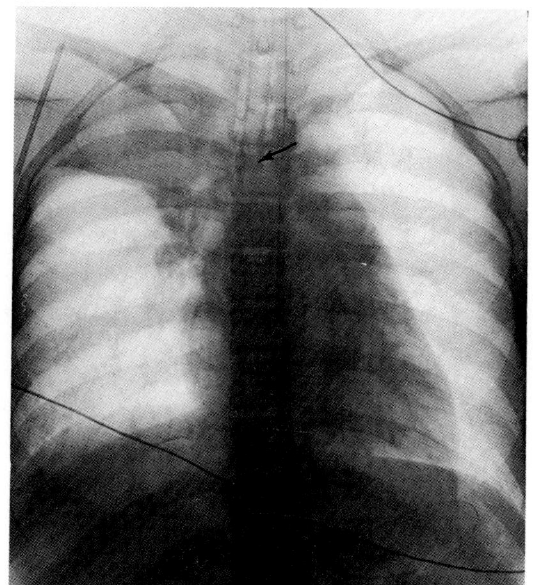

4 Nov. 1977. 19 hrs.

737c

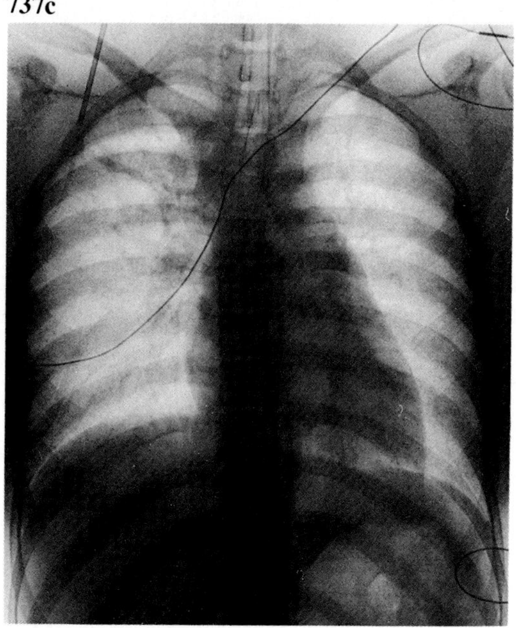

20 hrs.

737a **Flexion of the head** of an intubated patient can cause **atelectasis of the right upper lobe**. Head-on car accident; coma. Film taken before intubation.

737b The admission X-ray, taken after a 60 km helicopter transfer shows atelectasis of the right upper lobe. According to the position of the radiological marker (→) and the cuff, the tube is correctly placed. This picture could be due to **occlusion of a tracheal bronchus**.

737c Partial withdrawal of the tube followed by positive pressure ventilation leads to the immediate re-expansion of the atelectatic lobe. It was later learned that the patient's head had been flexed for half an hour during the helicopter flight. As a result the tube had plunged temporarily as far as the intermediate bronchus. Bronchoscopy reveals no bronchial damage.

Intubation can be hazardous: several types of accident and complication can occur.

738a

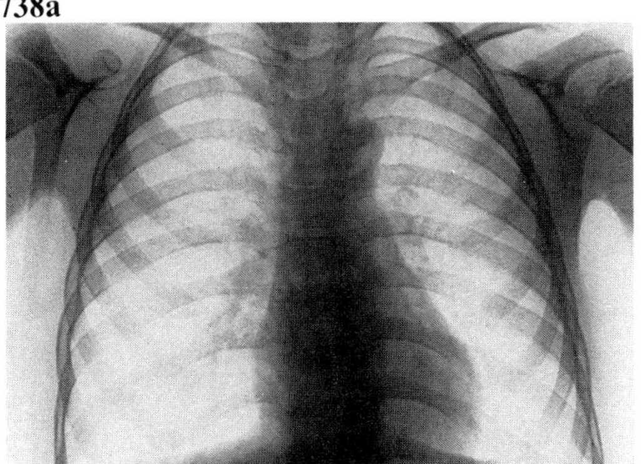

K.J.-D. ♂ 7 yrs. 17 Sep. 1972

738b

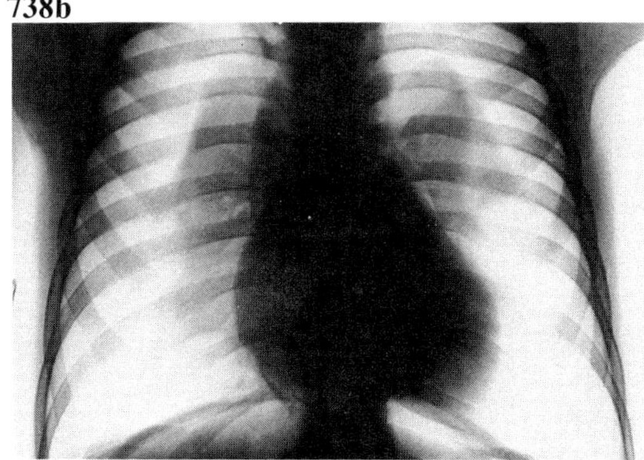

17 Sep. 1972

738c

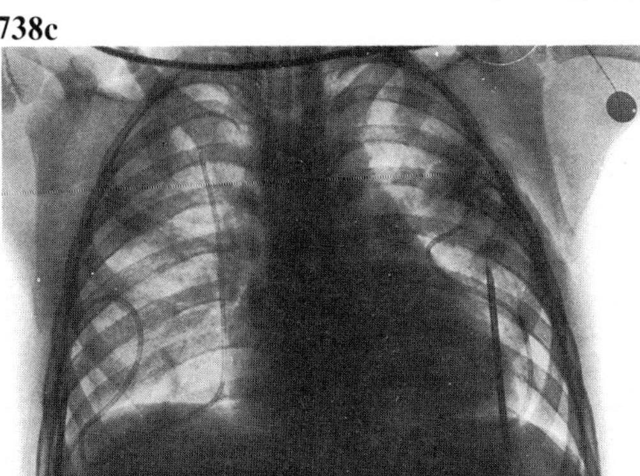

17 Sep. 1972

738d

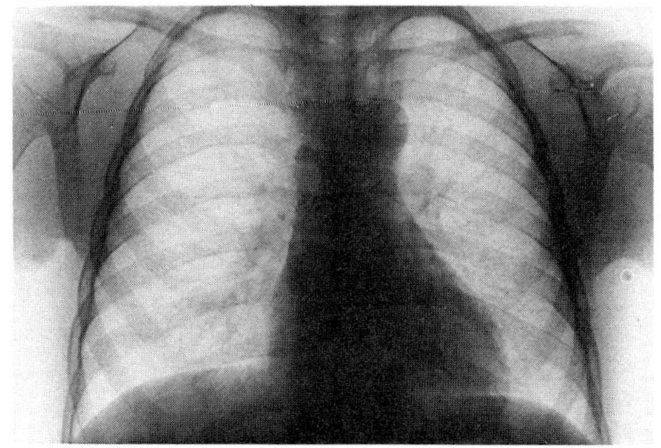

25 Sep. 1972

738a Perforation of trachea during intubation. Chest X-ray before anaesthetisation for an appendectomy.

738b During a difficult intubation, the introducer perforated the trachea and lacerated the pharynx. The result is a bilateral tension pneumothorax and a pneumoperitoneum (see **712**).

738c The pleuras and neck have been drained; the peritoneum was drained through the laparotomy.

738d Recovery in 8 days.

739a

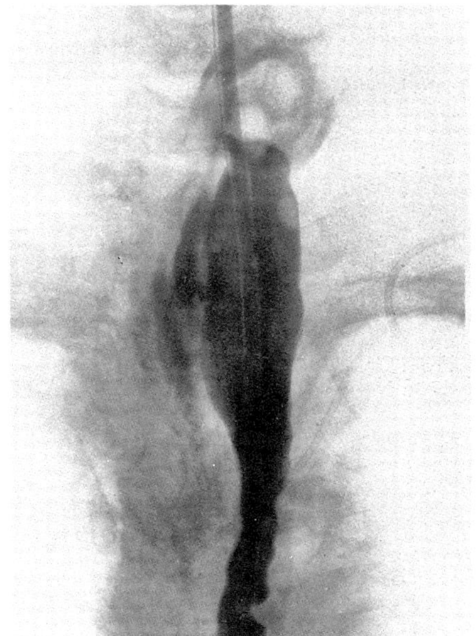

B.L. ♀ 75 yrs. 3 Jan. 1979

739b

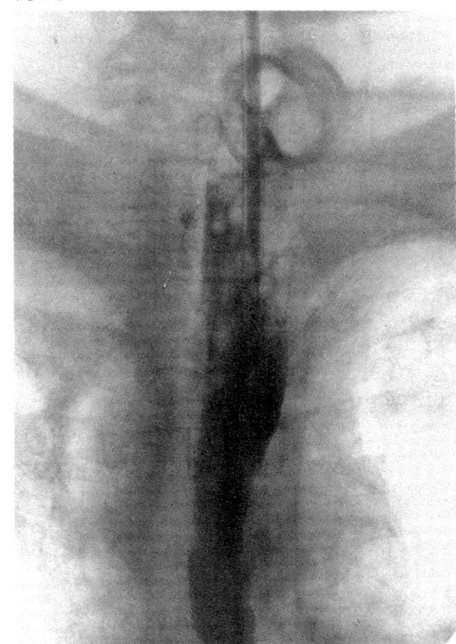

3 Jan. 1979

739a Perforation of oesophagus during intubation attempt. A tracheostomy has already been performed when a gastrografin oesophageal study documents the perforation.

739b The oesophagus heals after 10 days of conservative treatment. There is no mediastinitis. Death from late pulmonary embolism.

740

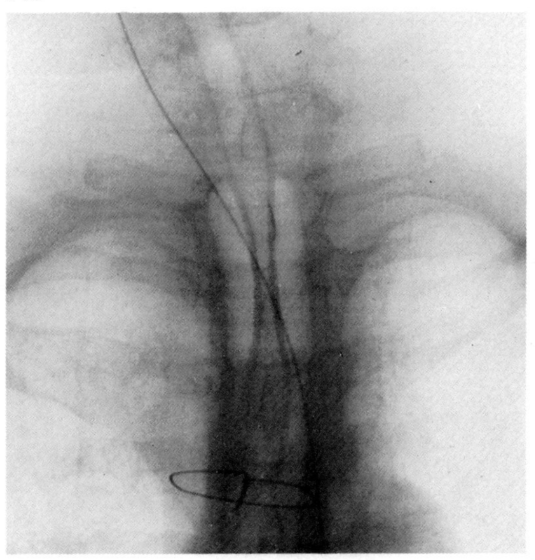

S.R. ♀ 63 yrs. 18 March 1978

740 When the tracheal wall is particularly resistant, **over-inflation of the cuff can almost occlude the endotracheal tube**.

741a When the tracheal wall is more fragile, **over-inflation of the cuff can result in tracheal rupture**. The high pressure cuff of an ordinary tube is already heavily inflated in this very old lady who is recovering from anaesthesia. (X-ray measurement: 2.5 × 4cm.)

741b Half an hour later, the cuff is further over-inflated. (X-ray measurement: 3.5 × 5cm – a 2.5 increase in volume over **741a**.)

741c The over-inflated cuff avulsed the membranous wall from the cartilages.

741d The longitudinal rupture extends the full length of the cuff (6cm) and only stops shortly before the carina (C).

741a

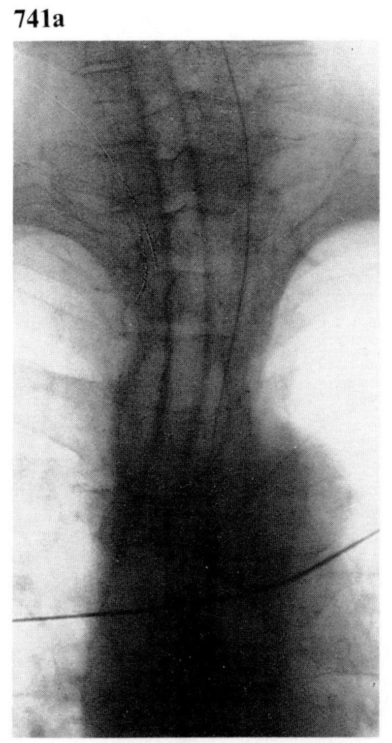

J.L. ♀ 87 yrs. 26 Feb. 1976. 20 hrs.

741b

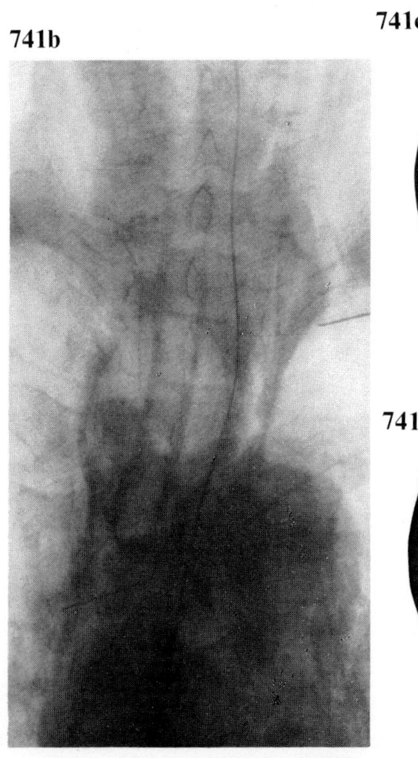

20.30 hrs.

741c

741d

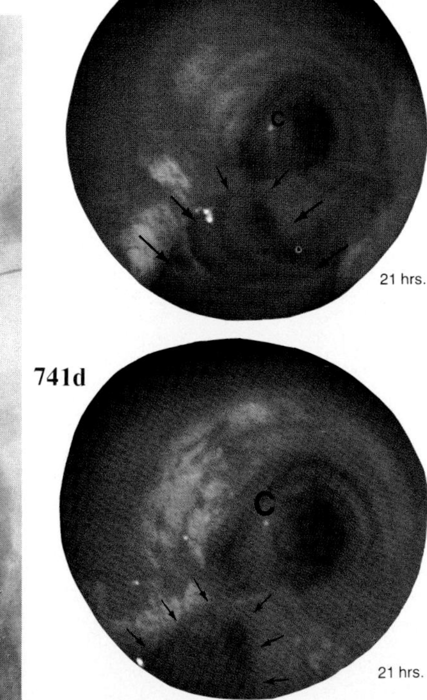

741e

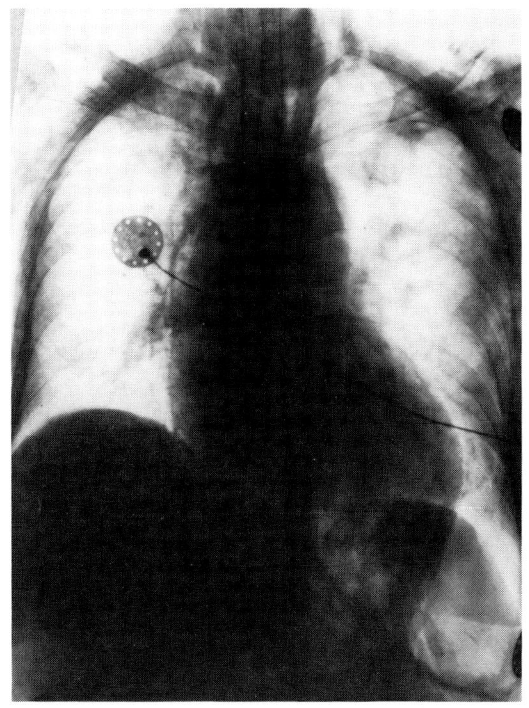

21 hrs.

741f

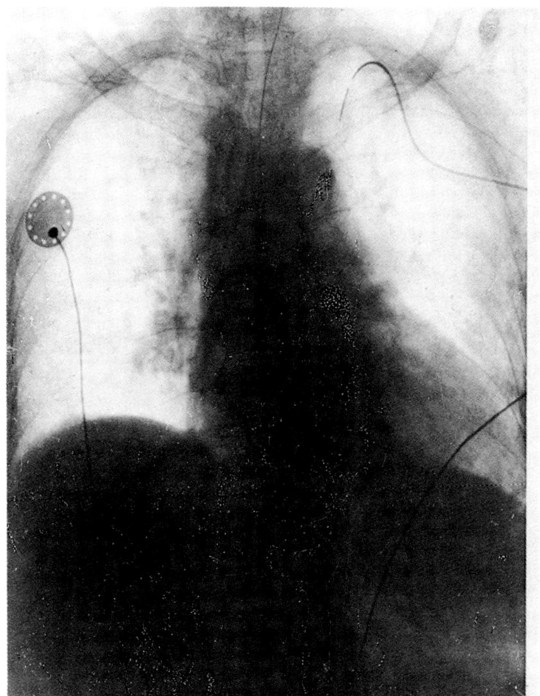

21.30 hrs.

741e The rupture causes a left tension pneumothorax (with inversion of the left hemidiaphragm) and massive mediastinal emphysema that subsequently spreads to the subcutaneous tissues.

741f The left pleura is drained and the patient left in spontaneous respiration for 10 days through an intubation tube with an uninflated cuff. Sudden death on the 16th day from massive pulmonary embolism.

741g Anterior incision of the trachea at autopsy exposes the healed rupture. It measures 6cm. (Institute of Pathology, Lausanne.)

741g

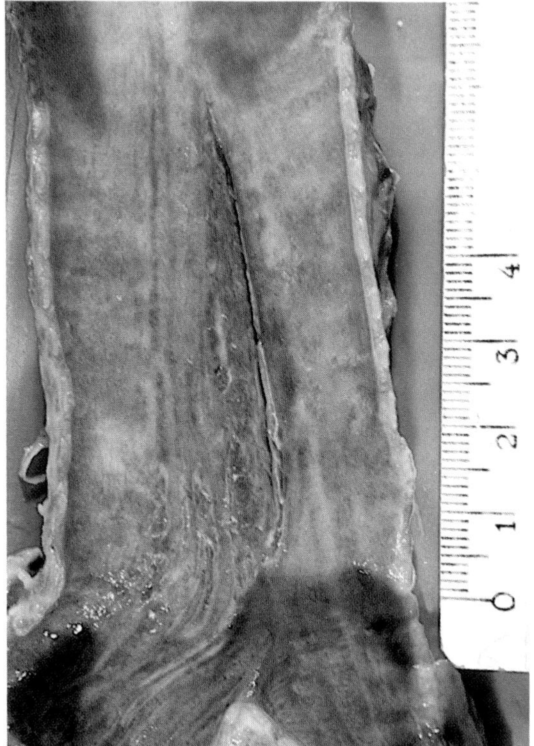

5 Mar. 1976

Tracheostomy

Björk's tracheostomy technique is to be recommended: a horizontal incision along the second tracheal ring terminates at either end in a short vertical contra-incision; the fiberated distal flap of the tracheal wall is then sutured to the skin. This technique facilitates the exchange of the tube and largely obviates late local complications.

Tracheostomy is now rarely necessary; the indications are discussed in Volume I, page 189.

742

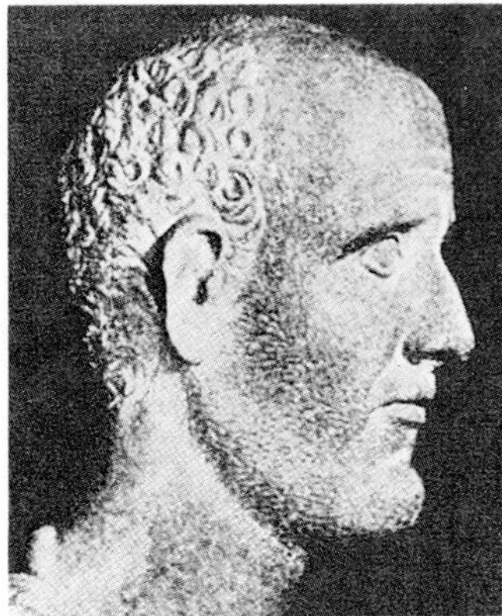

742 Asclepiades proposed and first performed a tracheostomy in the first century A.D.

743

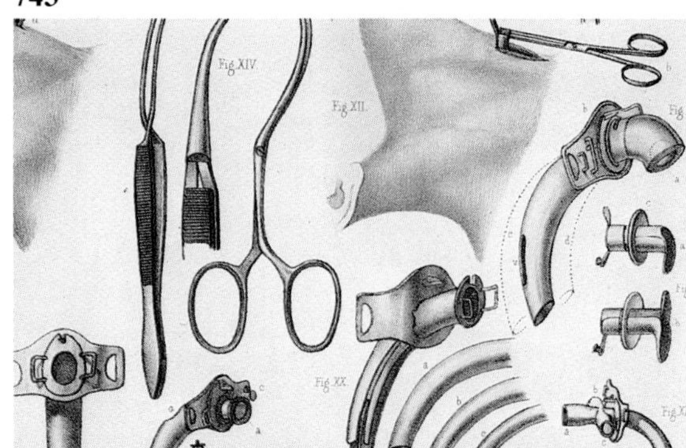

743 Some 19th century instruments are still in use. (Bourgery, 1867.)

744

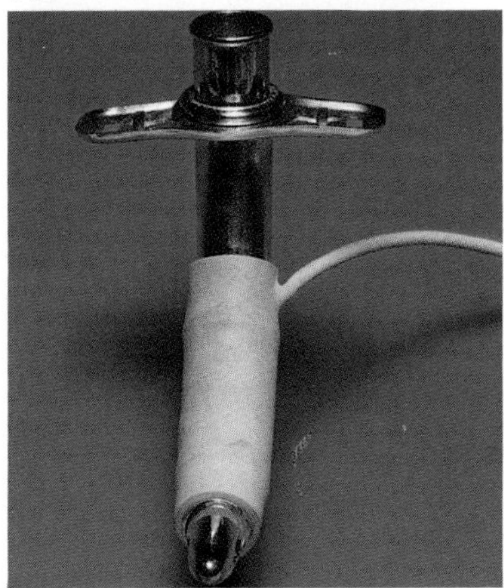

745

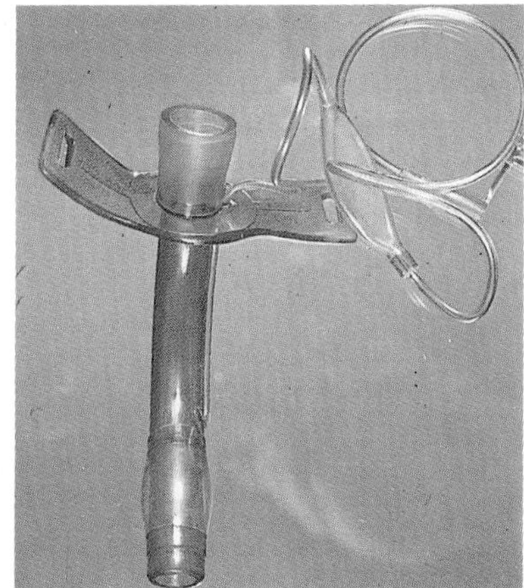

744 Silver tracheostomy tube with removable cuff.

745 Plastic tracheostomy tube with high-pressure cuff.

746a

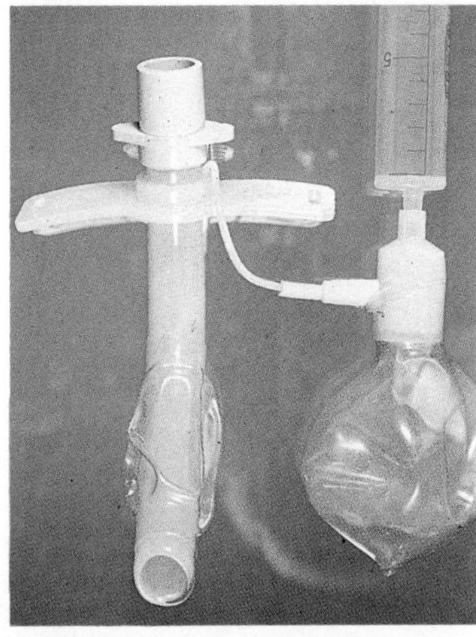

746b

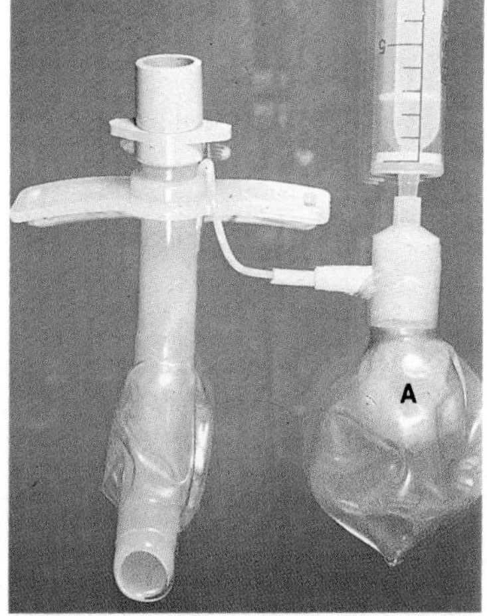

746c

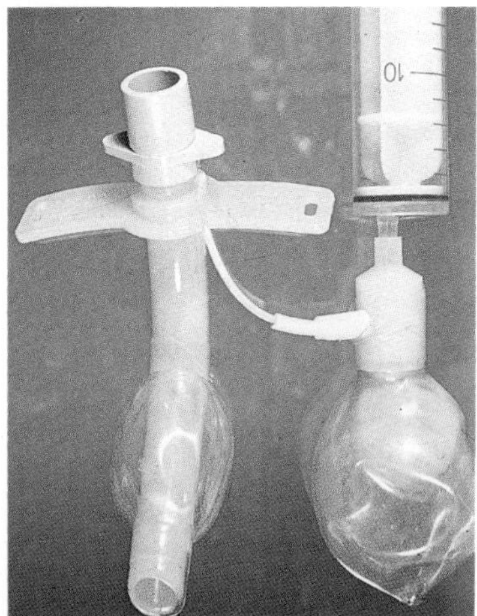

746a Modern tracheostomy tube with low-pressure cuff: the long cuff is here deflated.

746b Inflation with **10 ml** of air: the control balloon and security valve (A) are inflated, but little air has so far reached the cuff.

746c Inflation with **20 ml**: the cuff is slightly inflated at low pressure.

747

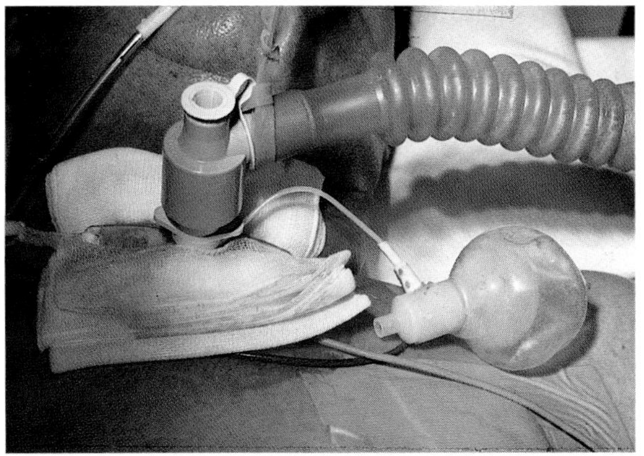

747 Tracheostomy tube in place.

748

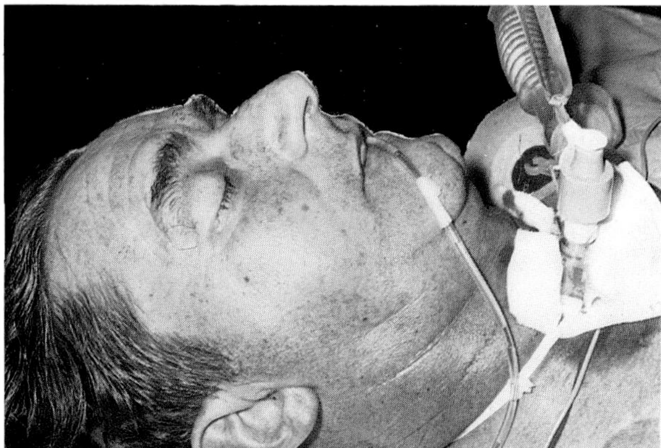

B.M. ♂ 49 yrs. 17 April 1976

748 Tracheostomy has now largely been replaced by long-term intubation. In this flail chest patient, nevertheless, a fracture of the base of the skull has indicated a tracheostomy; notice that a Levin tube has also been inserted through the mouth. In this way, meningitis is less likely.

749

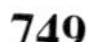

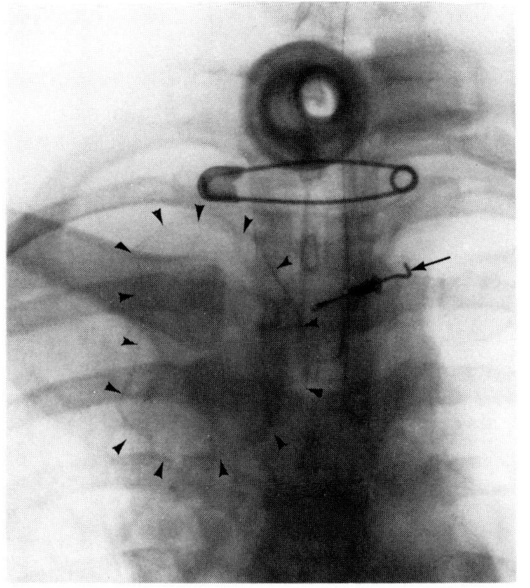

G.G. ♀ 19 yrs. 18 Dec. 1974

749 Tracheostomy cannula in position. Its low pressure cuff cannot be seen on the X-ray; the shadow (→) is that of the control balloon and its safety valve (→).

Tracheostomy patients are prone to certain accidents and complications: the cannula is sometimes incorrectly positioned; it can become plugged (see page 38); it can cause ulceration (see page 41) or even tracheal necrosis (see pages 45, 47) or cicatricial stenosis (see page 52); and in some instances, a fistula develops between the trachea and the innominate artery (see page 48, **996**) or between the trachea and the oesophagus (see page 272).

750a

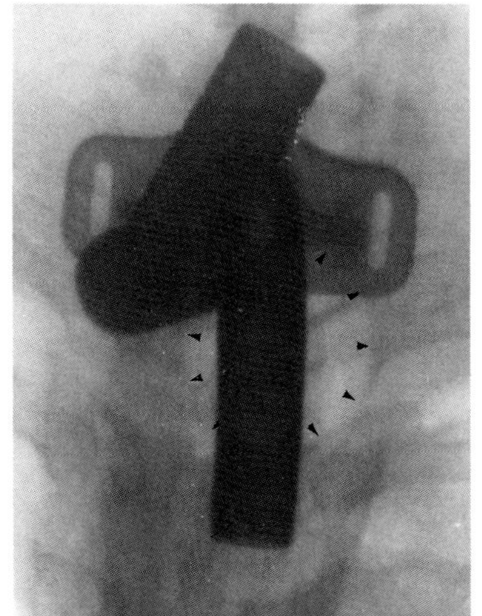

V.R. ♂ 52 yrs. 28 June 1971

750b

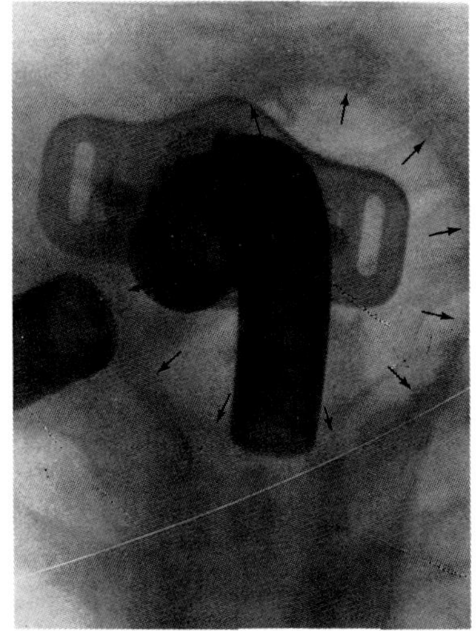

7 July 1971

750a Fatal tracheostomy complication (18th day). Farmer crushed under his tractor. A tracheostomy was performed 7 days previously for internal stabilisation of a flail chest. On this film the dimensions of the cuff (→) are moderate.

750b Progressive over-inflation of the cuff during intensive care over the next 9 days results in tracheal necrosis. Death 2 days later due to obstruction of the cannula.

Inhalation trauma

Inhalation burns

Inhalation burns were thought rare, but routine fiberoptic tracheobronchoscopies have shown that about a third of all burn victims are affected. They are as common in the pulmonary parenchyma as in the upper airways.

Inhalation burns vary in their gravity. Damage to the mucosa can be (1) erythematous (2) oedematous or (3) ulcerous. Damage usually lies between the larynx and the segmental bronchi.

Even if only a small area of the body has been burned, the airways still may be affected. Facial burns in particular almost invariably are accompanied by inhalation burns. As a rule, the admission X-ray is normal.

Serious complications develop quickly. Particularly common are oedema with asphyxia, pulmonary oedema and bronchopneumonia. Mortality is 33%, and in three-quarters of cases, death is due specifically to the respiratory burns.

751

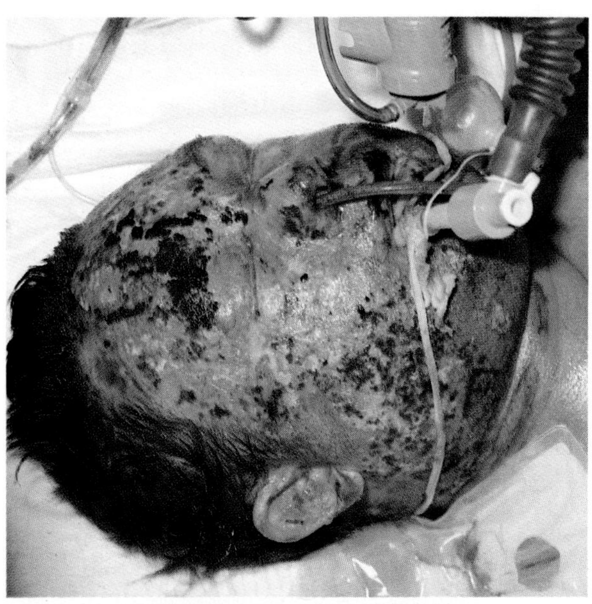

R.M. ♂ 66 yrs. 14 April 1975

751 Facial burns are almost invariably accompanied by inhalation burns.

752a

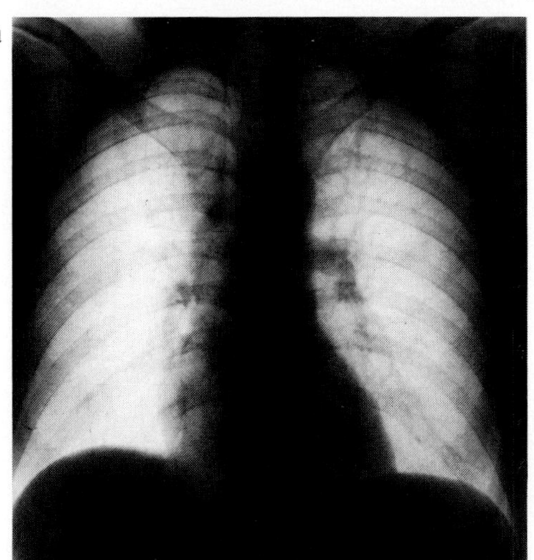

J.M. ♂ 26 yrs. 18 Aug. 1979

752b

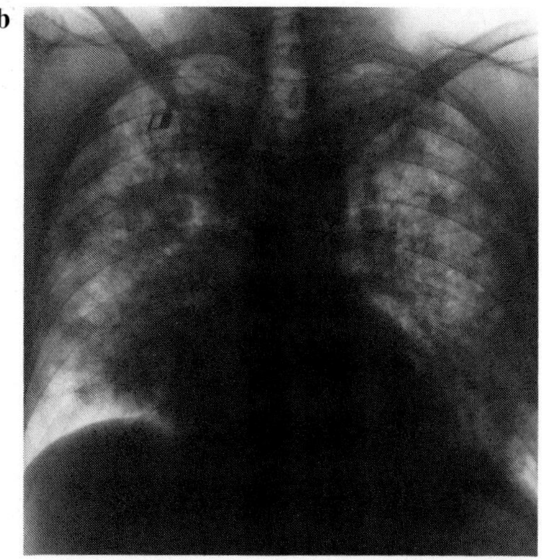

22 Aug. 1979

752a Laryngeal, tracheal and bronchial burns after a garage explosion. Burns encompass the face, scalp, and 70% of the body's surface (third degree). Admission X-ray is normal.

752b A combination of rapidly worsening dyspnoea, pulmonary oedema, respiratory insufficiency, hypoxaemia and bronchopneumonia proves fatal 8 days after the accident.

Aspiration of foreign bodies

In a **conscious** subject, the aspiration of a foreign body immediately provokes several reactions: suffocation with gasping, cyanosis and violent coughing. This is a common condition and is well handled in E.N.T. manuals.

However, when a **partially conscious or unconscious** patient aspirates a small foreign body, the event often passes unnoticed. The foreign body usually becomes lodged in a segmental bronchus.

Patients with facial damage – for example, victims of the windscreen syndrome – are particularly prone to this type of injury. The aspirated fragment – be it a piece of glass or a broken tooth – is often difficult to detect on an X-ray (see **719**, **753** and Volume I, **65**).

753a

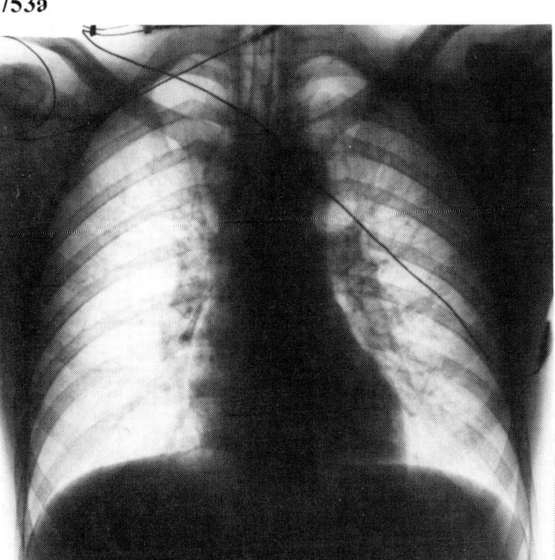

Z.P. ♂ 22 yrs. 2 July 1978

753a X-ray detection of foreign bodies in the bronchi is dificult. Admission X-ray of a driver who sustained very severe cranial and facial injuries in a head-on collision.

753b

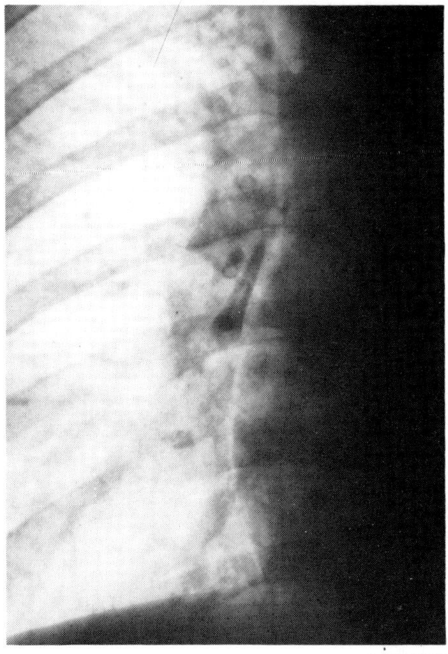

2 July 1978

753b Close examination reveals a filled tooth in the right lower lobe bronchus.

753c

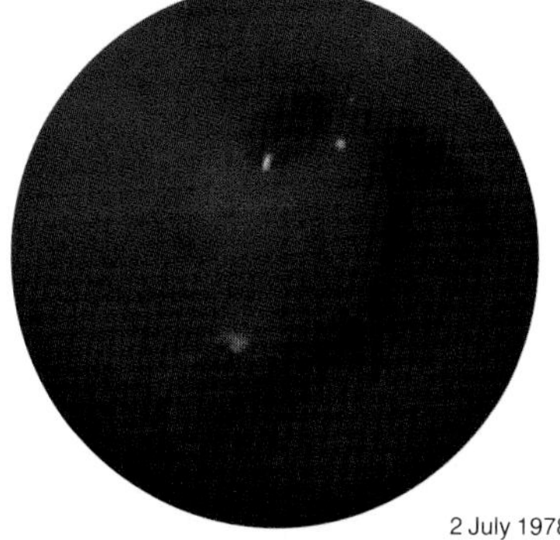

2 July 1978

753c Preoperative endoscopy clearly shows the blood-covered apex of the tooth canal. (E.N.T. Clinic, Lausanne.)

753d

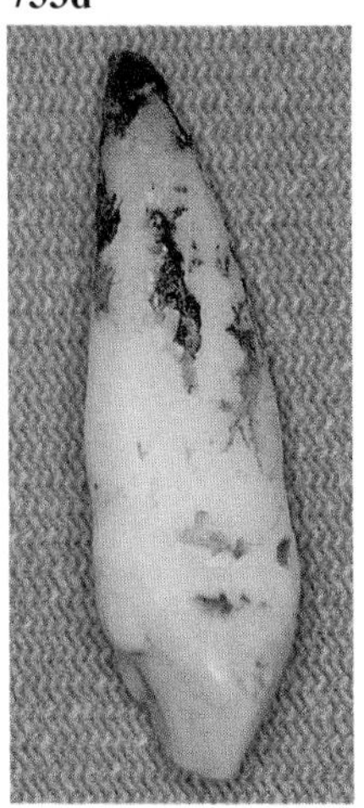

753d The tooth.

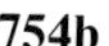

754a

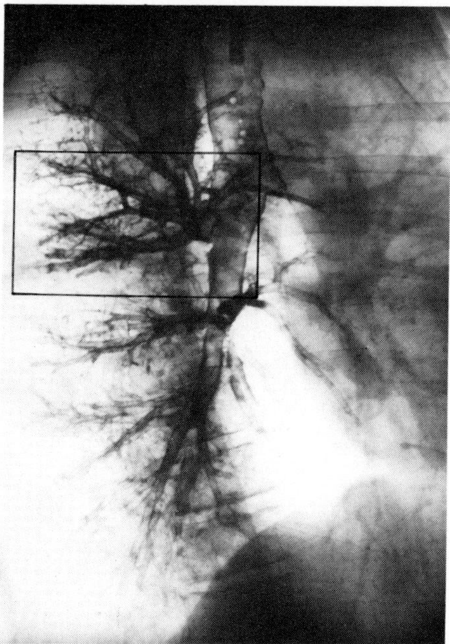

M.P. ♂ 55 yrs. 1 Feb. 1963

754b

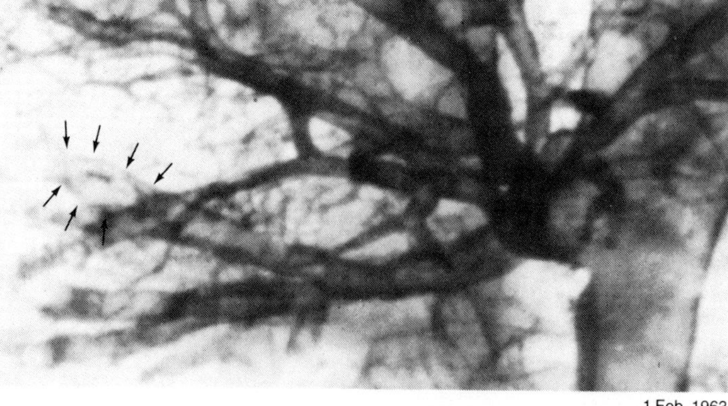

1 Feb. 1963

754a Segmental bronchiectasis after aspiration of foreign body. Four years after a small twig of pine was removed from the superior lobe bronchus, a bronchogram reveals bronchiectasis of the dorsal segment of the right upper lobe. In the intervening period, the patient experienced repeated episodes of haemoptysis and pulmonary infection.

754b The bronchiectasis in detail. The arrows point to what was thought afterwards to be a foreign body.

754c The segment is removed and opened. Part of the offending twig had remained in the bronchial tree, but was too distal to be observed endoscopically.

754c

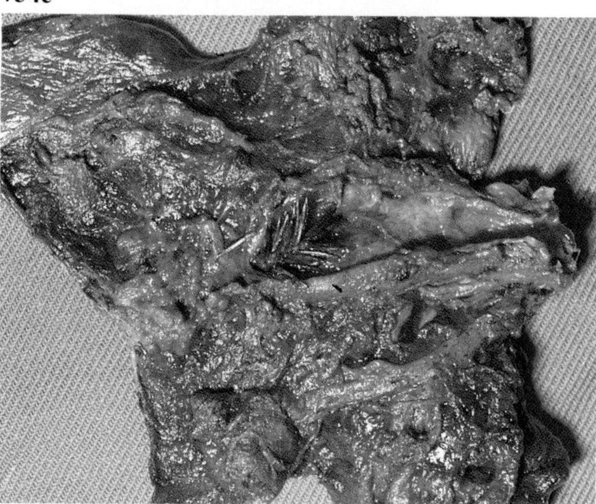

18 June 1963

Endoscopic removal of an incarcerated foreign body can be dangerous. The inflamed oedematous bronchus surrounding the foreign body is easily ruptured, especially in children.

Bronchotomy is therefore often preferable, particularly if diagnosis and treatment are delayed.

755

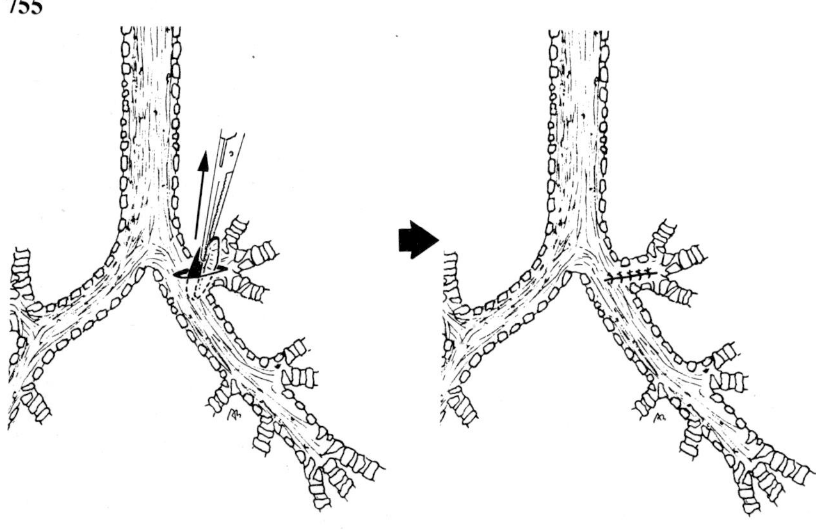

755 Removal of incarcerated foreign body (here a peanut): bronchotomy obviates the danger of perforation that attends endoscopic extraction.

Trauma of the trachea

Tracheal injuries are rare. They represent only 3% of all severe thoracic injuries.

The following types can be distinguished:

- **direct** or **indirect** rupture of the trachea,
- **rupture from within** (by the cuff of an intubation tube or by an explosion, for example),
- tracheal or tracheobronchial **perforation** from within, usually arising during endoscopy,
- exposure of cartilages by **erosion** and **ulceration**,
- tracheal **necrosis**,
- **tracheomalacia**,
- **fistulisation** into the oesophagus or into the great vessels at the thoracic outlet,
- tracheal **stenosis**, usually arising either from an unrepaired injury or from iatrogenic damage.

Each type of injury has a different causal mechanism.

Localisation and extent of tracheal injuries (in our material, $n = 57$)

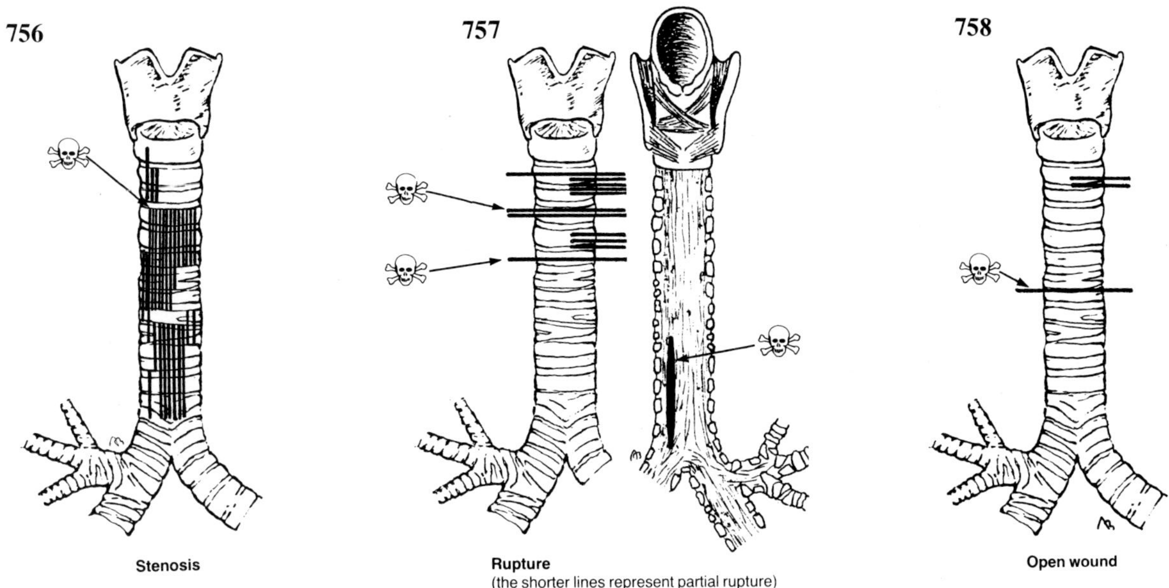

756 Stenosis

757 Rupture
(the shorter lines represent partial rupture)

758 Open wound

Each line represents an injury, and each skull a fatality.

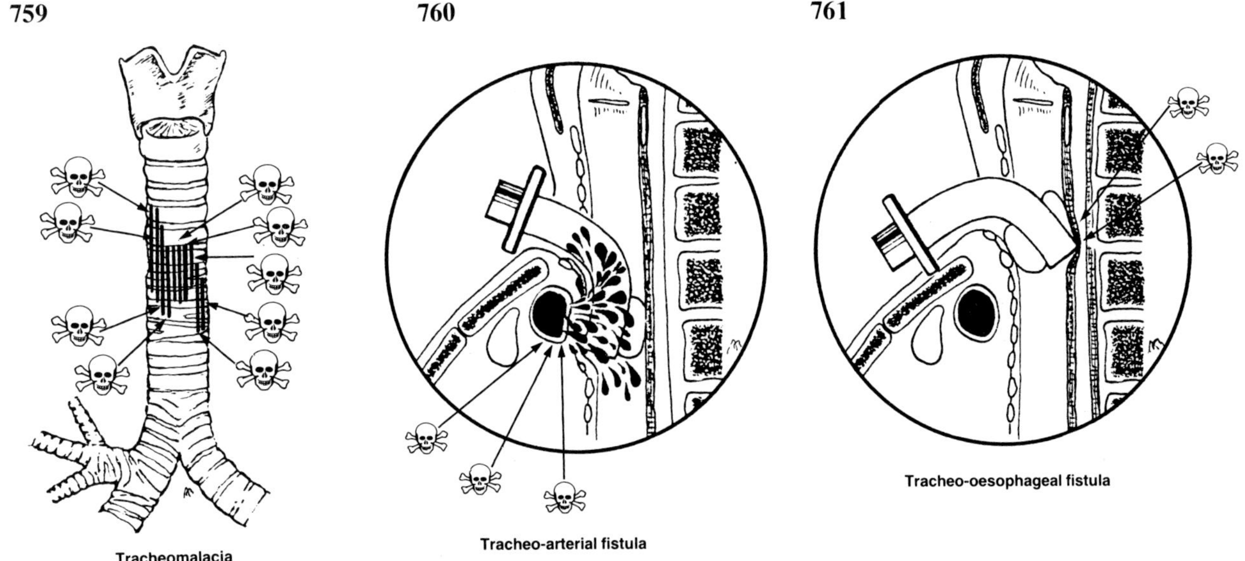

759 Tracheomalacia

760 Tracheo-arterial fistula

761 Tracheo-oesophageal fistula

762a

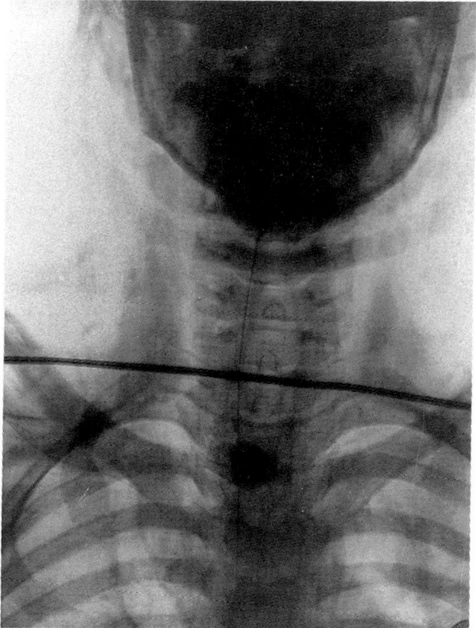

M.V. ♀ 9 yrs. 11 June 1974

762a Partial tracheal rupture with massive subcutaneous and mediastinal emphysema in a child who fell on to a chair.

762b

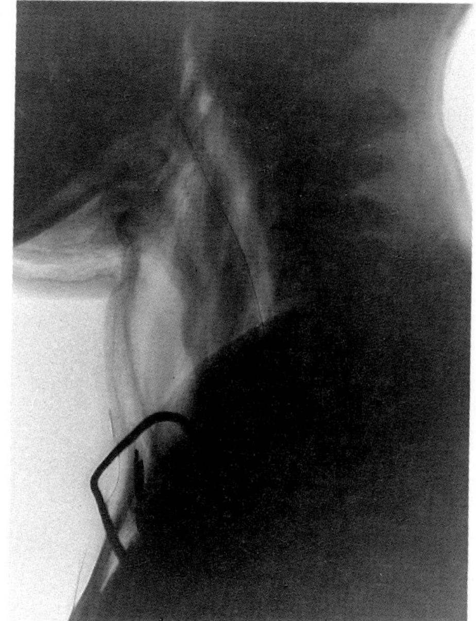

11 June 1974

762b Recovery after cervical exploration and mediastinal decompression.

763

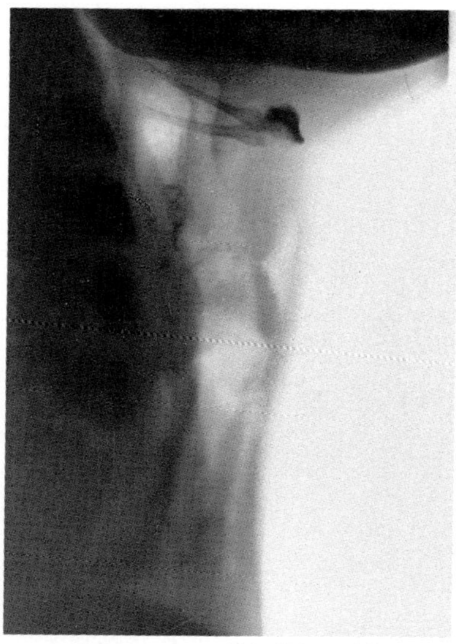

H.J. ♂ 32 yrs. 13 Dec. 1961

763 Subtotal tracheal rupture without emphysema on X-ray (car accident). The trachea is almost totally ruptured at the first ring. Slight subcutaneous emphysema can be palpated. Emergency repair. Recovery.

764

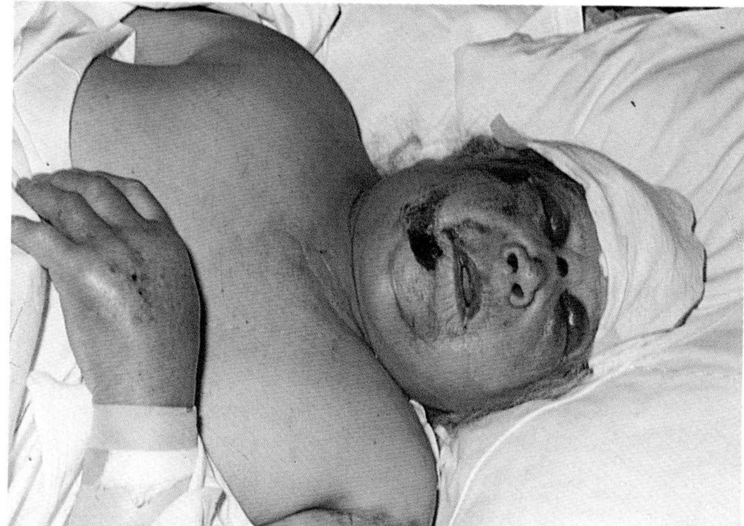

D.L. ♀ 88 yrs. 10 Nov. 1966

764 Unrecognised total rupture of trachea. This old lady sustained fractures to the ribs, face and base of the skull when knocked over by a car. Massive subcutaneous emphysema of the face, neck and upper thorax (without pneumothorax) was thought likely to impair venous return, so a mediastinotomy was performed for decompression; the trachea, however, was not explored. The patient died suddenly a week after the accident. Autopsy revealed a total rupture of the trachea at the 5th ring. (Dr. S. Schneider, P.-D., La Chaux-de-Fonds.)

Tracheal rupture

Tracheal rupture accounts for 15% of all ruptures of the upper airways.

The trachea can rupture either longitudinally or transversely. **Longitudinal rupture** is the rarer of the two types: it usually gives rise to a gaseous syndrome with a massive air leak and intermittent episodes of haemoptysis. The characteristics of **incomplete transverse rupture** are not significantly different from those of longitudinal rupture. But when **transverse rupture is complete and total**, the entire lower portion of the trachea is likely to dislocate, causing immediate asphyxia. In some cases, dislocation occurs even when the membranous wall remains intact (see **705**).

765

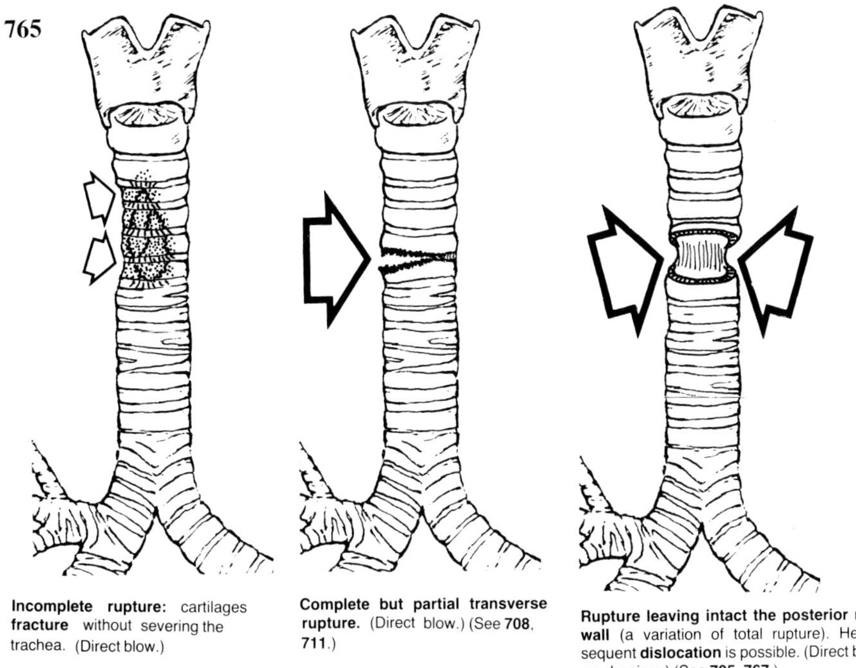

Incomplete rupture: cartilages **fracture** without severing the trachea. (Direct blow.)

Complete but partial transverse rupture. (Direct blow.) (See **708**, **711**.)

Rupture leaving intact the posterior membranous wall (a variation of total rupture). Here, too, subsequent **dislocation** is possible. (Direct blow or tearing mechanism.) (See **705**, **767**.)

Total rupture at the thoracic outlet. Subsequent **dislocation** is possible. (Tearing mechanism.) (See **764**.)

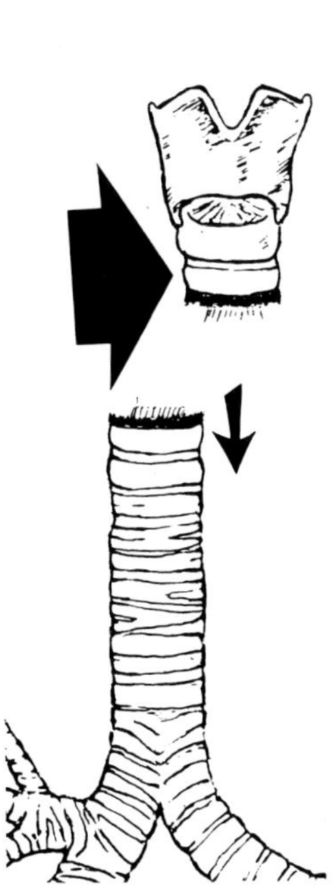

Transverse **upper cervical rupture-dislocation**. (Direct blow.)

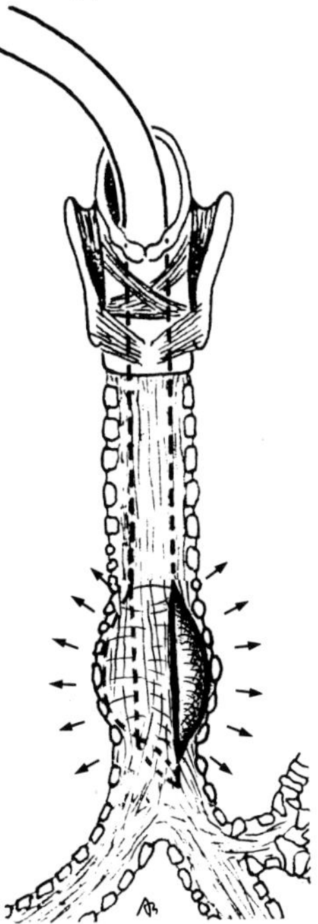

Longitudinal avulsion of the posterior membranous wall. (Over-inflation of an intubation tube cuff.) (See **741**.)

765 Pathology and biomechanics of tracheal rupture.

766

Immediate or early: 53%

Mid-term (1 to 6 weeks): 11%

Late: 18%

Only detected at autopsy: 18%

766 Early, mid-term and late diagnosis of tracheal rupture (According to Dor & Le Brigand's historical survey, 1964. $n = 38$)

Biomechanics

Rupture of the **cervical portion** of the trachea is caused by one of two mechanisms.

It can be due to a *direct blow* to the neck. This type of injury is common in children who fall against the handle-bars of a scooter or bicycle, and in car occupants who are thrown against the steering wheel or dashboard.

Alternatively, rupture of the cervical trachea can arise indirectly *when the head is thrown violently backwards*; injury is then the result of a whiplash mechanism. The resultant tear of the trachea usually occurs between two cartilaginous rings; the membranous wall often remains intact. A small fragment of the anterior face of an upper cervical vertebra is often torn away simultaneously by the vertebral ligament. The possibility of such an *avulsion fracture* should be investigated in every case of indirect tracheal rupture by the whiplash mechanism.

Rupture of the **thoracic portion of the trachea** can result from (1) an *accident during anaesthesia*, (2) a *bronchoscopy accident*, (3) *so-called spontaneous* rupture during a tetanus spasm or during labour, or (4) a serious *crush-injury*.

767a

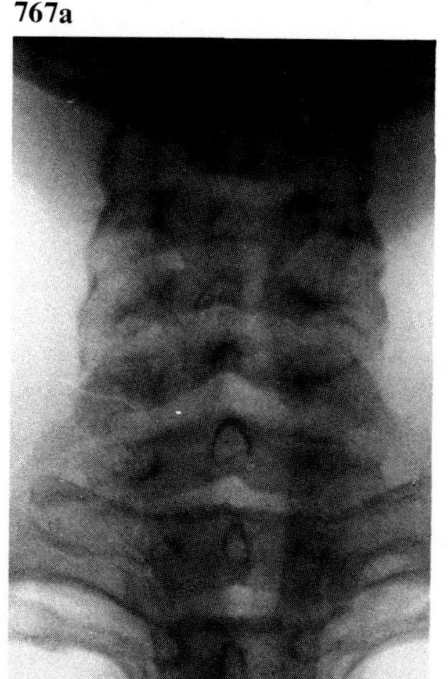

W.C. ♀ 19 yrs. 2 Oct. 1969. 0.50 hrs.

767b

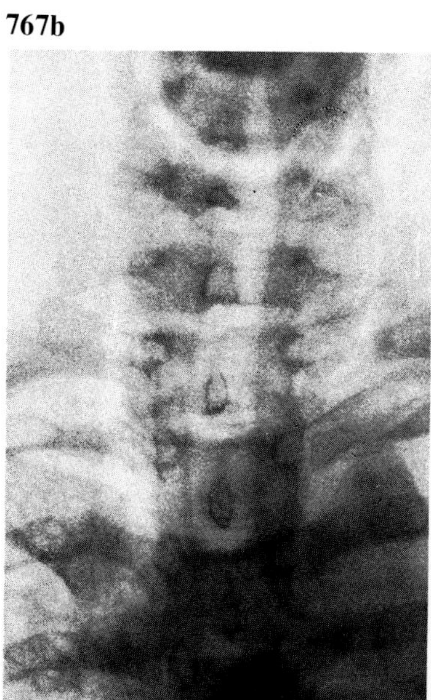

2 Oct. 1969, 8 hrs.

767c

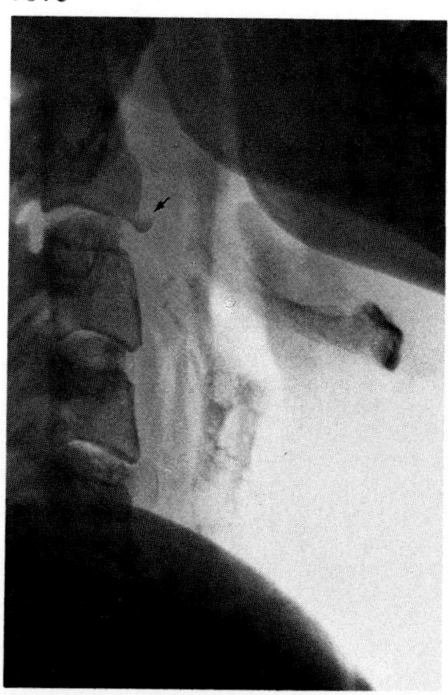

2 Oct. 1969. 8 hrs.

767d

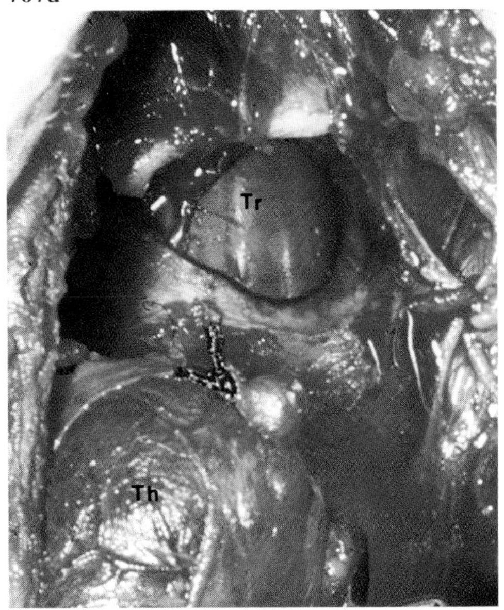

2 Oct. 1969. 9.30 hrs.

767a Subtotal tracheal rupture with fracture of axis in a car passenger whose head was whipped violently backwards and then hurled forwards on to the dashboard. No injury is visible on the anterior view admission X-ray.

767b Eight hours after the accident, slight subcutaneous emphysema appears in the neck.

767c The emphysema later spreads around the oesophagus. Here, as so often, tracheal rupture is accompanied by an avulsion fracture of the axis (→). In this case, however, the fracture passed unrecognised.

767d Immediate cervical exploration reveals a total rupture of the trachea at the 1st ring, just above the thyroid gland (Th): only the membranous wall remains intact. The tracheal tube (Tr) is exposed. Because of the attendant risk of suffocation, **intubation should always be carried out in the operating theatre. In this way, ventilation can be restored quickly surgically if the trachea dislocates** (see **705**).
(Pr. G. Chapuis, Lausanne.)

767e

2 Oct. 1969. 11.30 hrs.

767f

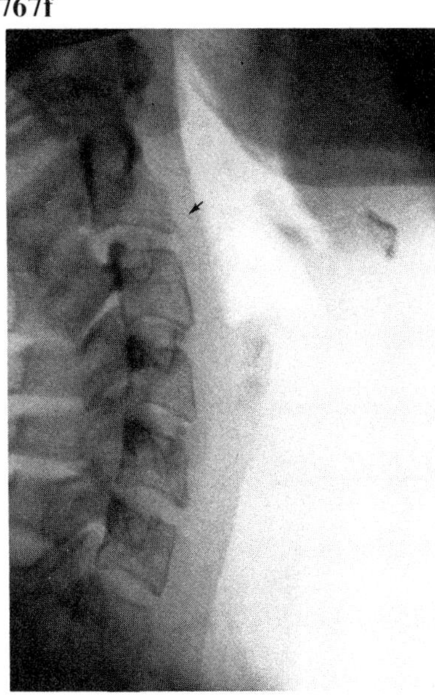

10 Feb. 1970

767g

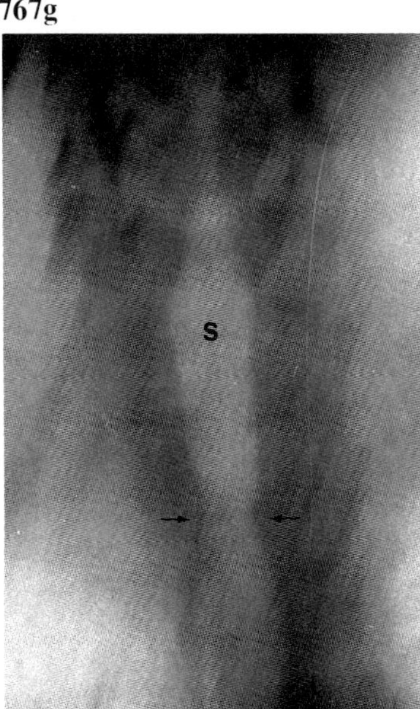

11 Feb. 1970

767e Emergency repair is effected under cover of a tracheostomy. Mediastinal emphysema can be seen around the heart.

767f Recovery. Lateral view: the axis has consolidated without treatment.

767g Anterior view: the sutured portion of the trachea (S) has healed completely, but the tracheostomy has produced slight stenosis.

Management

As soon as tracheal rupture is suspected, a careful tracheobronchoscopy should be carried out while the operating theatre is prepared.

If rupture is confirmed, it should be closed immediately with direct sutures. It is sometimes advisable to freshen the edges before suturing.

The approach depends on the level of the rupture and on the accompanying injuries. A minor rupture can be treated by prolonged intubation or by tracheostomy. The goal here is to prevent closed-glottis coughing and so to avoid high pressure in the bronchial tree.

Tracheobronchial trauma from within

Tracheobronchial injuries of intraluminal origin are invariably iatrogenic. Their incidence has risen steadily with the development of new instruments and new resuscitative techniques.

They can be categorised as follows: (1) sudden asphyxiating **obstruction** during intubation, (2) **rupture** due to over-inflation of the cuff of an intubation or tracheostomy tube, or to distension of the airways during manual bag ventilation, (3) **perforation**, (4) **erosion and ulceration**, (5) **tracheal necrosis**, (6) **tracheomalacia** and (7) **tracheal fistulas**.

Obstruction

Tracheobronchial obstruction of an intubated patient can be **progressive** or **sudden**, **incomplete** or **complete**. Obstruction is sometimes **limited** to certain pulmonary segments or lobes. In most instances, the result is potentially fatal asphyxia. As soon as asphyxia is noticed, the cause should be elucidated as quickly as possible. *Intraluminal aspiration* can suffice to clear certain types of obstruction; *X-ray* sometimes reveals misplacement or deflection of the tube; and *tracheobronchoscopy* allows direct observation of the contents of the airways.

Tracheostomy and intubation tubes become obstructed for different reasons. Here are some examples of tube obstruction (see also **732**).

768

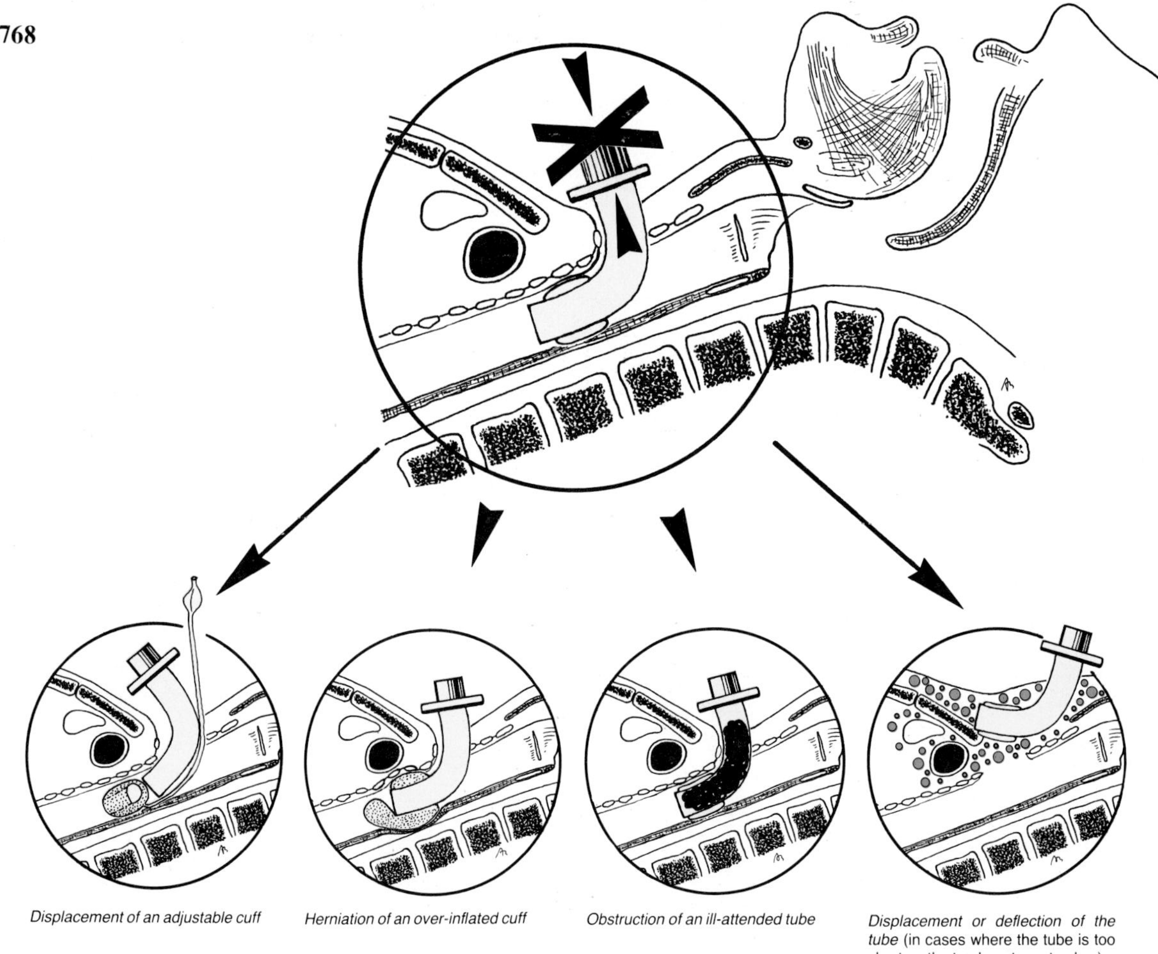

768 Causes of asphyxia in tracheostomy patients.

769a

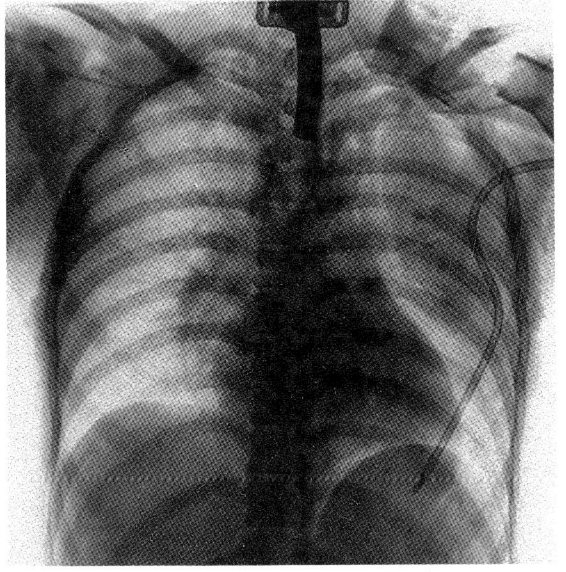

M.M. ♂ 19 yrs. 17 Oct. 1966

769a Obstruction of trachea and bronchi after tracheostomy. The patient sustained multiple injuries – coma, bilateral lung contusion and a bilateral pneumothorax – when thrown from his car at high speed. Tracheostomy is followed by moderate atelectasis of the left upper lobe.

769b

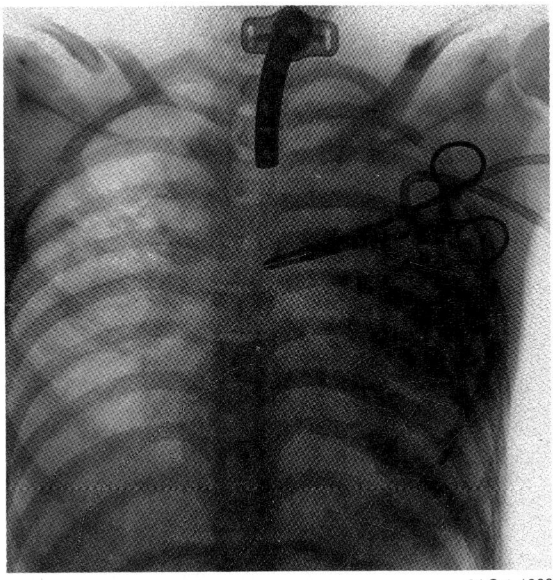

24 Oct. 1966

769b Seven days later, most of the left lung and part of the right are affected. Death.

769c

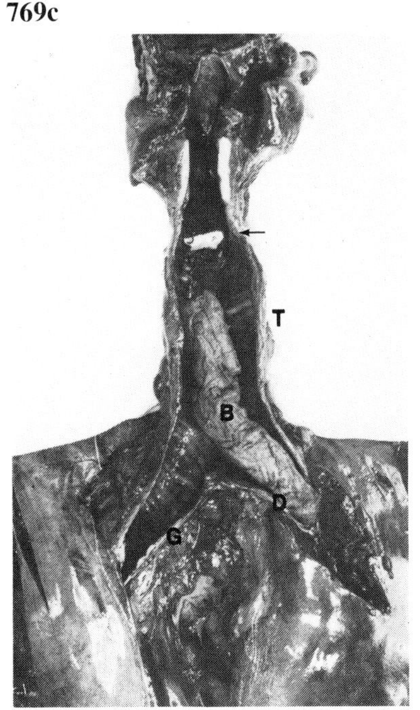

Oct. 1966

769d

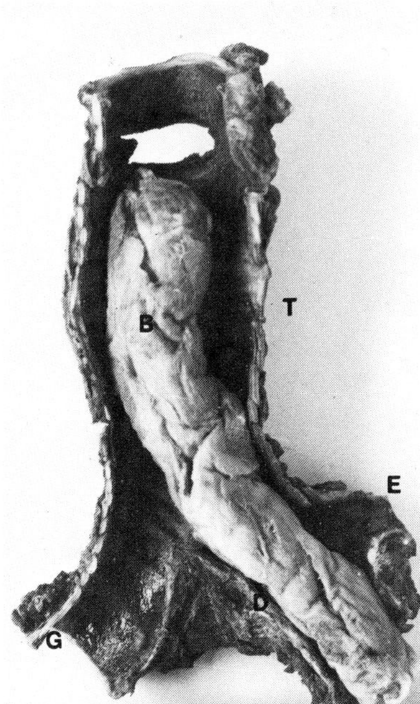

Oct. 1966

769c Autopsy reveals an occlusive cotton-wool wad (B) in the trachea (T) and right main-stem bronchus (D). (The specimen is viewed from behind.) The tracheostome (→) is visible. Both lungs are atelectatic.

769d The huge wad almost completely obstructs the left main-stem bronchus (G) and the right upper lobe bronchus (E). No explanation of its origin was found.

770

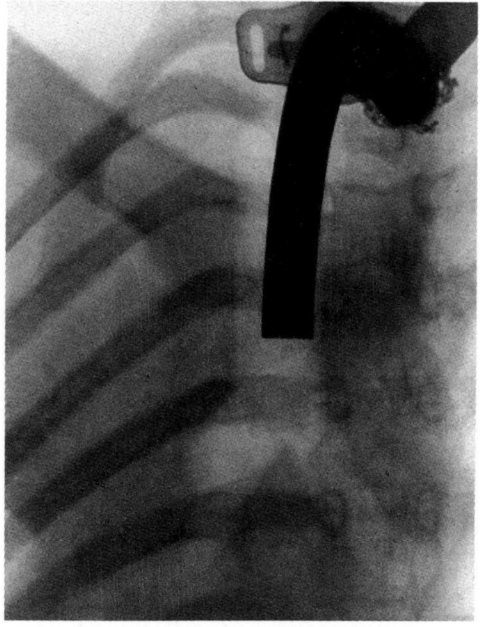

770 Complete **right pulmonary atelectasis** following inadequate bronchial toilet. The obstruction in the right main-stem bronchus is clearly visible.

771

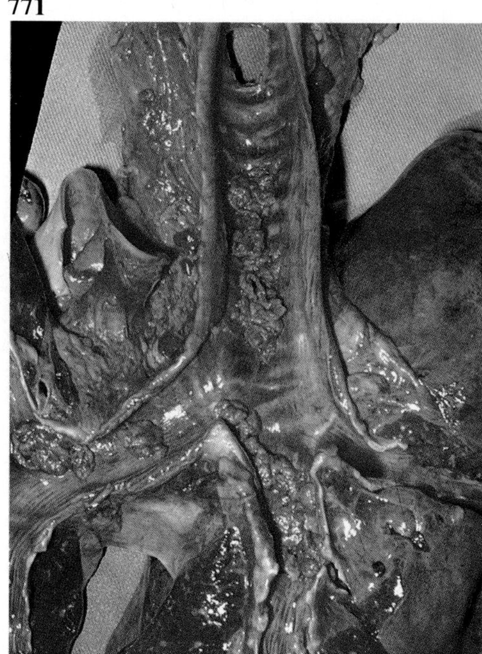

771 Bilateral pulmonary atelectasis due to aspiration of cellulose. The tracheobronchial tree of a multiple injury casualty opened from behind at autopsy. Most of the segmental bronchi are obstructed with fragments of cellulose; attempts to establish whether the fragments entered through the glottis or through the tracheostomy tube were inconclusive.

Rupture

When the trachea is ruptured from within, it is usually in an intubated patient. The commonest cause is cuff over-inflation during reanimation or anaesthesia. Whether rupture is gradual or sudden (see **741**, **772**) depends upon how slowly or violently the cuff is over-inflated (see **750**, **788**, **790**, **996**, **997** and **1175**).

In most instances, the posterior membranous wall ruptures longitudinally at its junction with the cartilages. The length of the rupture corresponds to the length of the cuff (4 to 5 cm). The symptoms and signs are the same as for any other type of tracheal injury.

Age and hypoproteinaemia are common predisposing factors.

As a rule, surgical repair is required through a cervical or cervicothoracic incision; under certain circumstances, however, intubation may suffice. For the latter treatment there are two important provisos: first, the cuff must not be inflated; second, the patient must be left in spontaneous respiration for at least ten days. In this way, endotracheal pressure is minimised and the danger of air leakage avoided.

772

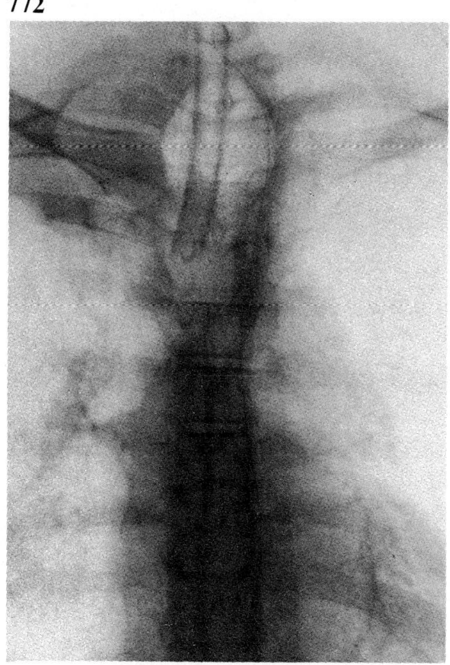

772 Tracheal laceration due to over-inflation of cuff of endotracheal tube during resuscitation. A subsequent tracheostomy precluded the possibility of air leakage (see Volume I, **650**).

Perforation

Perforation is usually inflicted by the tip of an endotracheal tube or its introducer. The accident commonly occurs during anaesthesia or tracheobronchoscopy.

On occasion, however, a perforation can be inflicted during the extraction of an incarcerated foreign body (see **755**). When this happens, thoracotomy is indicated.

773a

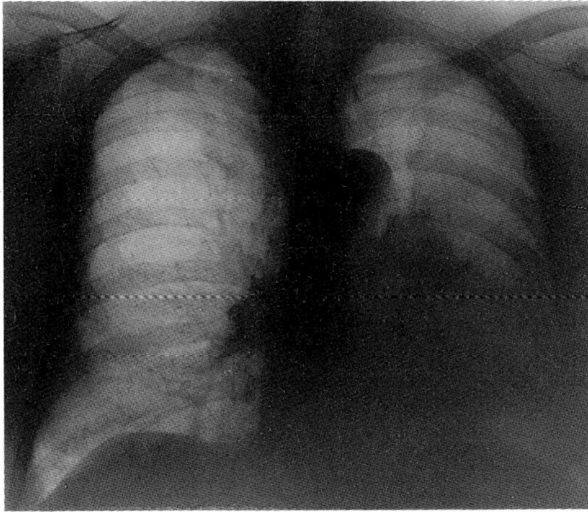

A.P. ♂ 60 yrs. 28 Nov. 1974

773b

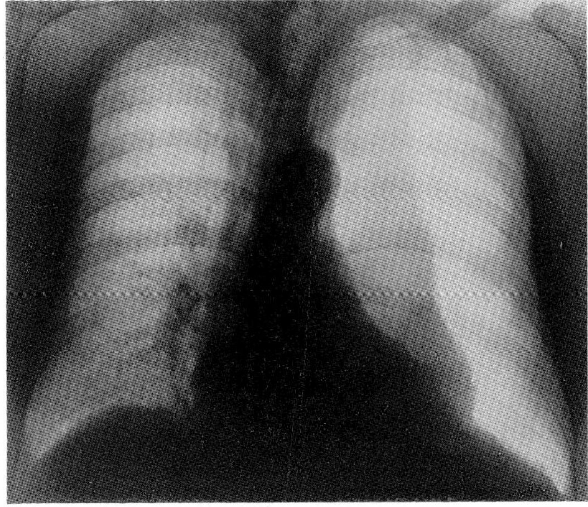

30 Nov. 1974

773c

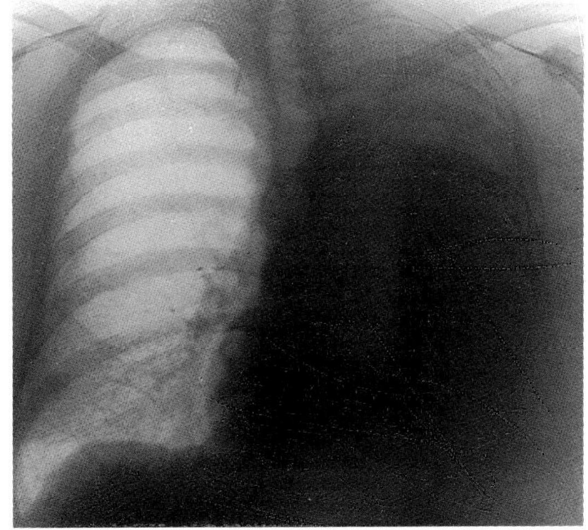

11 Dec. 1974

773a Bronchial perforation during rigid bronchoscopy. A squamous-cell carcinoma of the left lower lobe is accompanied by pulmonary atelectasis.

773b During bronchoscopy, the endoscope was accidentally pushed through the left main-stem bronchus. The result is a 50% pneumothorax.

773c Recovery after an emergency pneumonectomy. Postoperative X-ray. Total survival of about 4 years.

Erosion and ulceration

The incidence of tracheal erosion and ulceration has greatly diminished since the introduction of modern materials and of low pressure cuffs in particular. When intubation and tracheostomy patients are correctly supervised, damage is exceptional.

774 Localisation of laryngotracheal injury during prolonged intubation

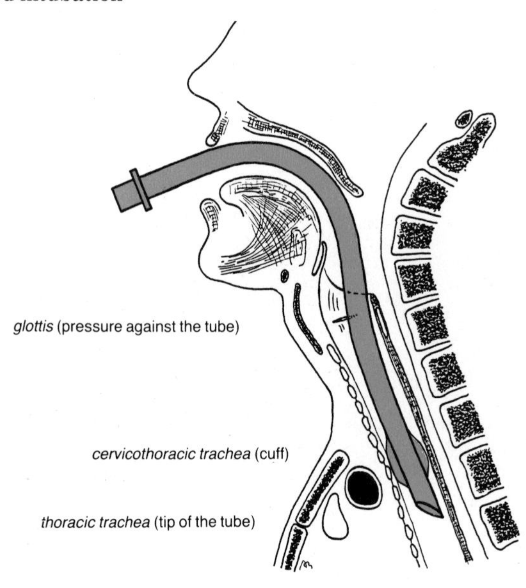

775 Tracheal injuries in tracheostomy patients

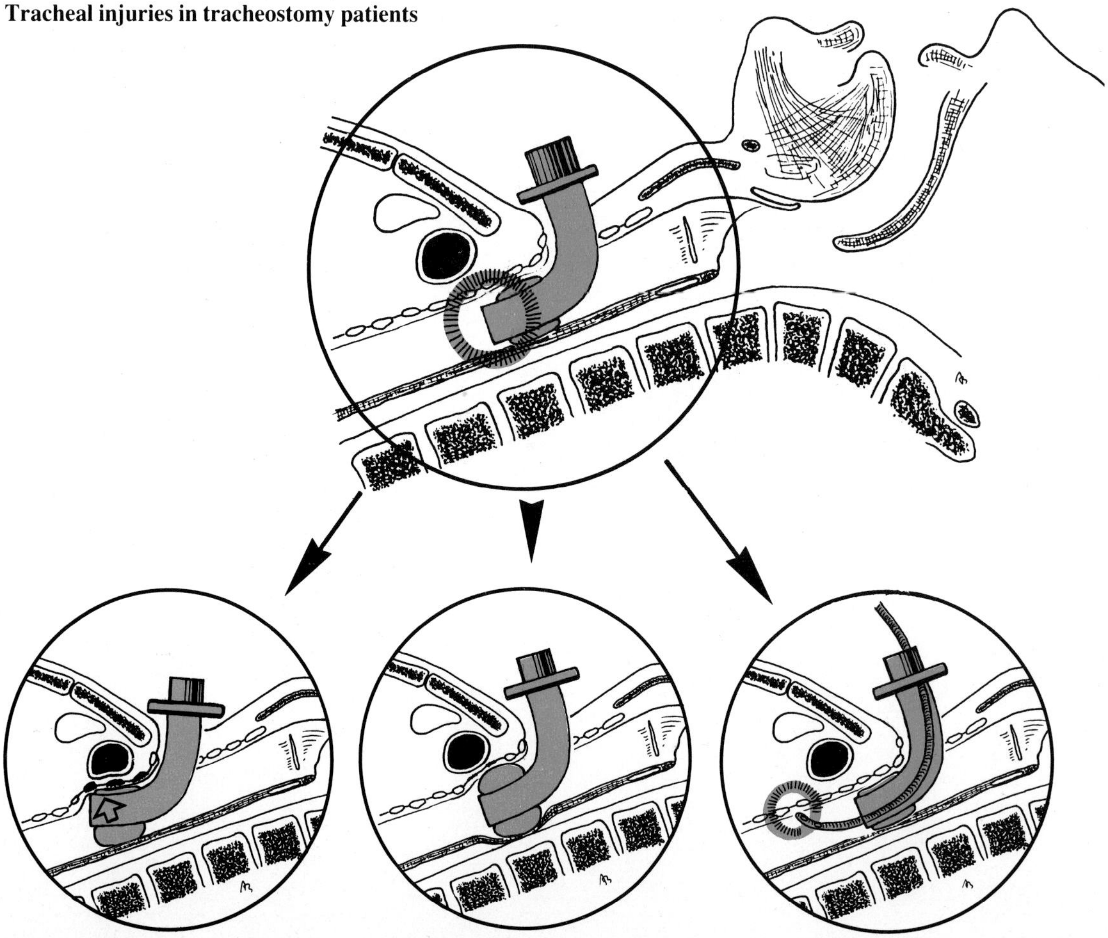

Laceration or necrosis of the anterior wall (cannula inserted too deep)

Circumferential tracheomalacia or tracheal necrosis (over-inflated cuff). (See **750, 788, 790, 997 and 1175**)

Repeated aspiration injuries (insufficiently flexible tube)

Tracheal erosion is generally the result of friction with the inflated cuff during resuscitation or intensive care.

Friction can be produced variously. Many patients restlessly move their heads and cough violently when their bronchial secretions are aspirated. In some cases, irritation is increased during displacement of the ventilator or even by the mere weight of the ventilator tubings; in others, over-inflation of the cuff is the major source of aggravation.

776a

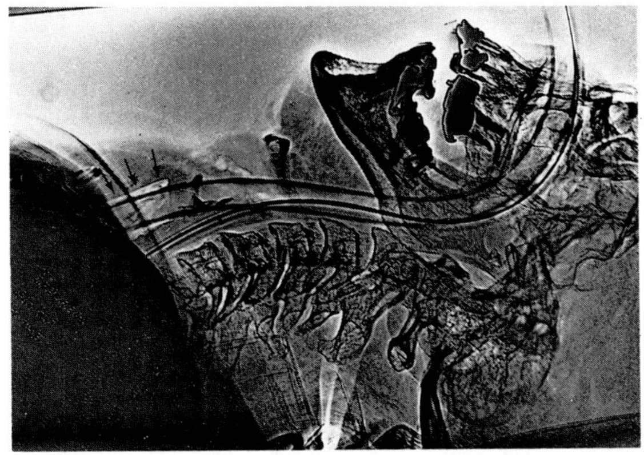

May 1978

776a Friction by displacement of intubation tube and its cuff during head movements. The nasotracheal tube and its low pressure cuff (→) are clearly visible at the cervicothoracic outlet.

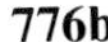

776b

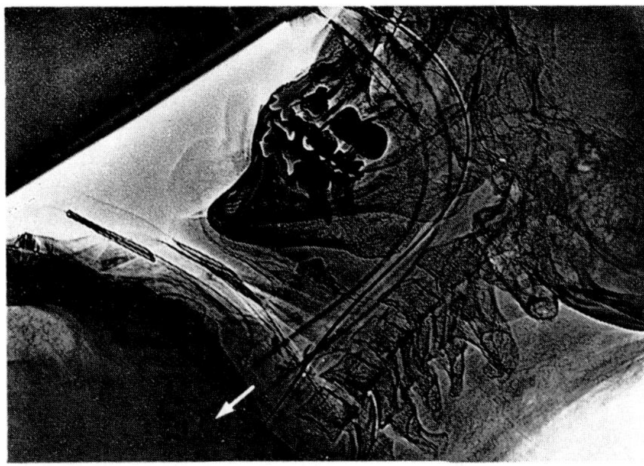

May 1978

776b When the neck is flexed, the whole cuff slides into the thorax, completely disappearing from the cervical xerography. In these circumstances, it is not unusual for occlusion of the right upper lobe bronchus to lead to atelectasis of the upper lobe (see **737**).

Cases **777 – 782** show where an intratracheal tube has been variously, if not poorly tolerated.

777

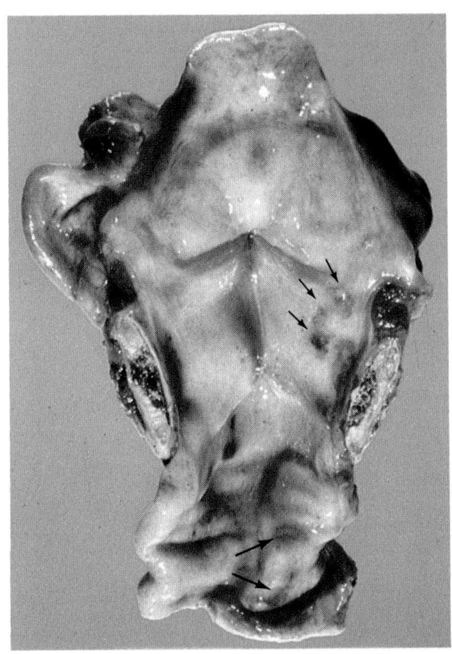

B.E. ♂ 1977

777 The patient was intubated with a Portex tube **for 12 hours** before death. The autopsy specimen shows petechiae on the right vocal cord (→) and at the level of the cuff (→). (Dr. W Hilan, Lausanne.)

778

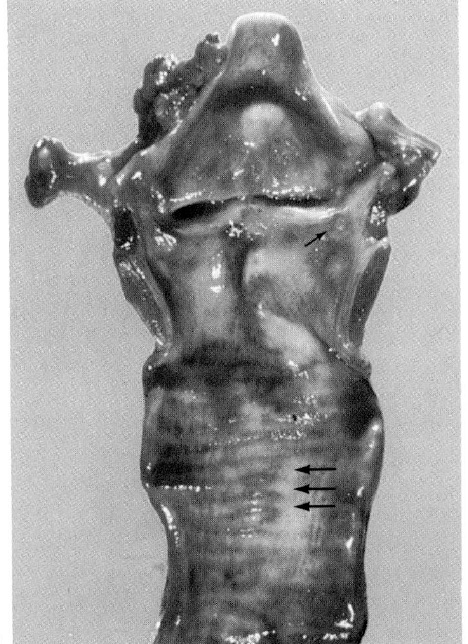

W.G. ♀ 1977

778 Portex intubation **for 24 hours** has resulted in superficial ulceration of the vocal cords (→) and erosion of the 3rd tracheal ring (→). (Dr. W. Hilan, Lausanne.)

779

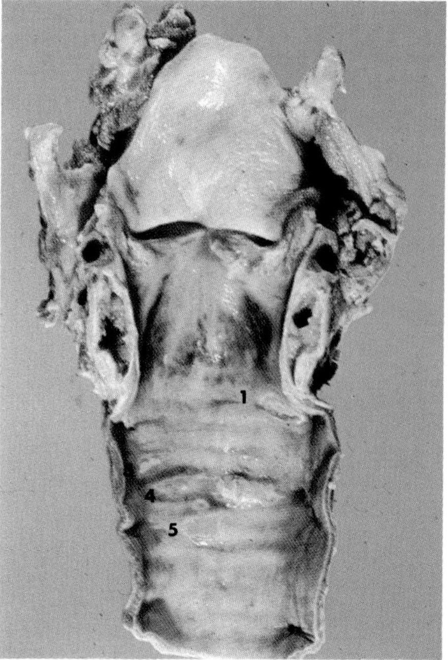

S. 1977

779 Portex intubation **for 14 days** has resulted in partial exposure of the 1st, 3rd and 4th cartilages and erosion of the 5th. Injuries of this gravity can cicatrize without stenosis. (Dr. W. Hilan, Lausanne.)

780

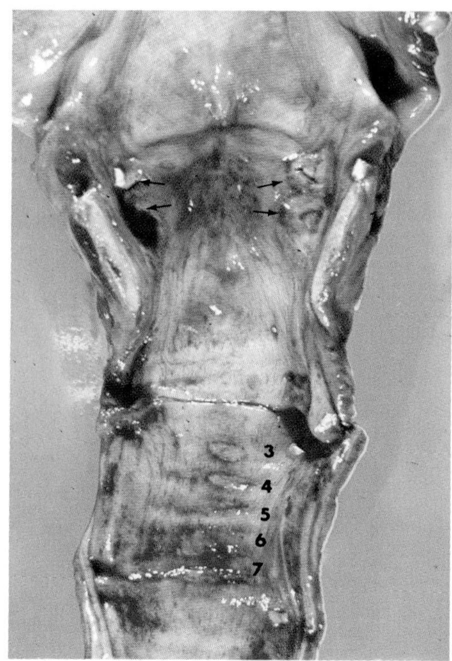

B. 1977

780 Lanz intubation **for 10 days** has led to severe bilateral necrotic ulceration of the vocal cords (→) and erosion by the cuff of the mucosa from the 3rd, 4th, 5th, 6th and 7th cartilages. (Dr. W. Hilan, Lausanne.)

781

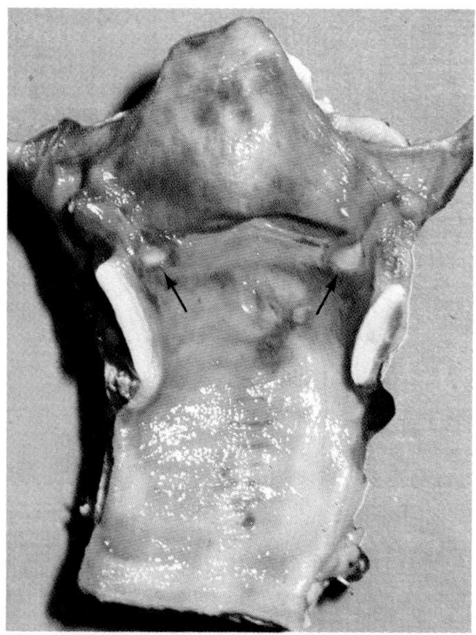

A.R. ♂ 20 yrs. 1977

781 Lanz intubation for **10 days** has led to extensive bilateral ulceration of the vocal cords. The tracheal mucosa, however, is almost intact. The epiglottis is hyperaemic and petechial. (Dr. W. Hilan, Lausanne.)

782

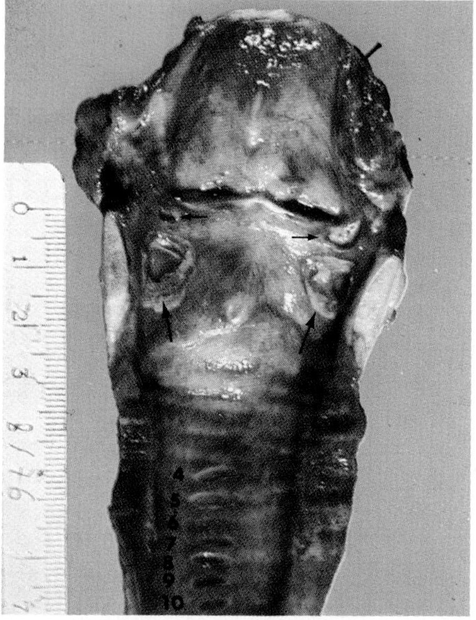

F. 1977

782 Orotracheal Lanz intubation **for 18 days** has led to severe necrotic ulceration of the glottic (→) and subglottic regions (**→**). The arytenoid cartilages and the 4th, 5th, 6th, 7th, 8th, 9th and 10th tracheal rings are exposed. (Dr. W. Hilan, Lausanne.)

Erosion or ulceration only become dangerous when they lead to the complete disappearance of several cartilages with tracheal necrosis or, later, to tracheomalacia. When this happens, extubation is often impossible.

Slight or limited erosion or ulceration usually heals by itself. Extensive damage, on the other hand, usually leads to tracheal stenosis. At this point, surgery is mandatory.

Tracheal necrosis

Transmural necrosis during long-term tracheal cannulation is the result of ischaemia. It is most common in seriously injured patients who have wasted. Localised abscesses often attend.

Surgery is the only possible treatment but there is often little hope of success.

783a

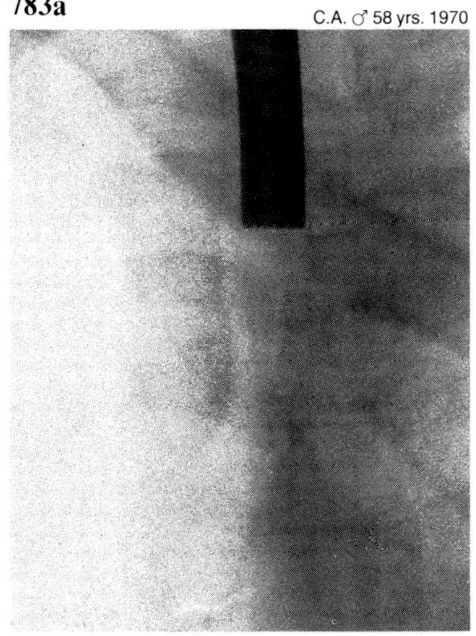

783a A tracheostomy tube can damage the trachea under the weight of the ventilator tubings. The tube is correctly positioned with the cuff deflated.

783b

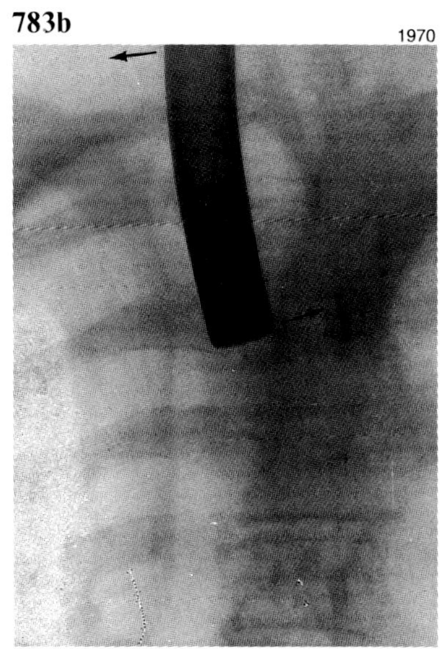

783b The tube twists under the weight of the ventilator tubings and the tip injures the tracheal wall. The cuff is inflated well beyond the usual diameter of the trachea.

784

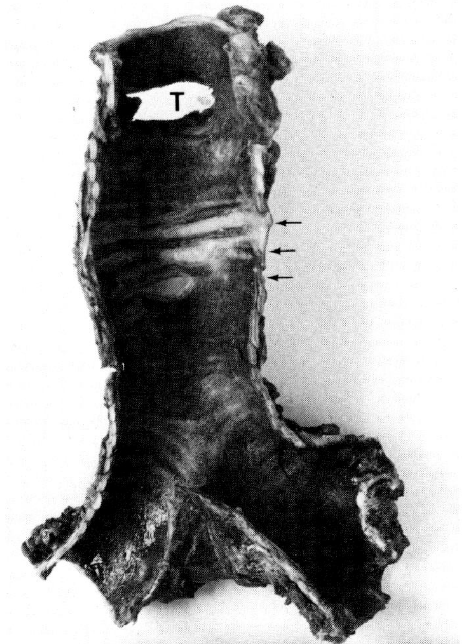

784 Early stages of tracheal necrosis caused by cuff of tracheostomy tube. This autopsy specimen was taken from a victim of severe multiple injuries who spent 7 days under controlled ventilation through a tracheostomy (T). Three tracheal cartilages (→) are exposed at the level of the cuff. (See also **769**). The tracheobronchial tree is seen from behind. (Institute of Pathology, Lausanne.)

785a

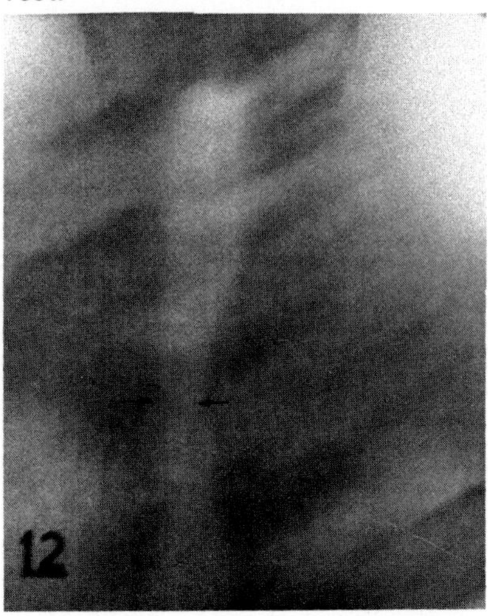

D.L. ♂ 23 yrs. 18 Aug. 1969

785b

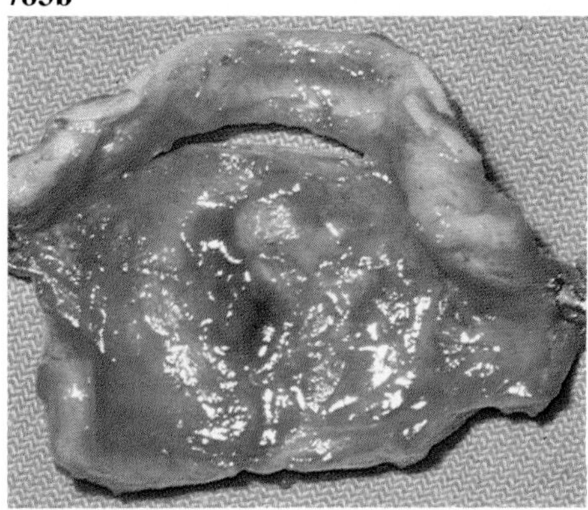

5 Sep. 1969

785a Tracheal necrosis caused by tip of orotracheal tube in position for 5 days. This X-ray was taken one month after extubation.

785b The anterior wall of the 4cm operative specimen of cervical trachea displays a transmural necrotic ulcer.

786a

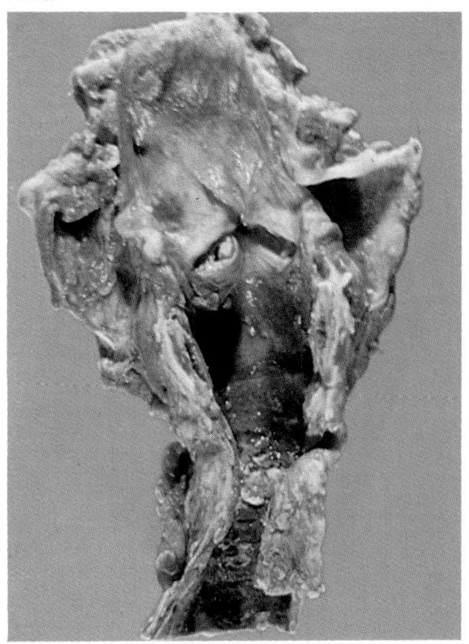

M.E.♂ 69 yrs. 9 Feb. 1975

786a Tracheal necrosis caused by high pressure cuff of orotracheal tube. A plain rubber tube in position for 8 days has caused transmural, necrotic tracheitis. (Institute of Pathology, Lausanne.)

786b

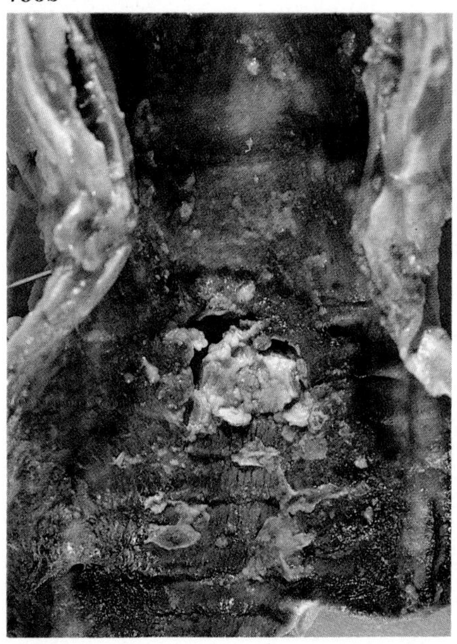

9 Feb. 1975

786b Close-up of the section of trachea in contact with the rubber cuff. Necrosis is transmural, and the surrounding mucosa has sloughed off. Death was due to a massive gastrointestinal haemorrhage from a stress ulcer probably caused by hypoxia. (Institute of Pathology, Lausanne.)

Tracheomalacia

Tracheomalacia results from the destruction of several tracheal cartilages – after the healing of localised tracheal necrosis, for example. The disappearance of a number of cartilages softens the tracheal walls; they then expand and collapse according to the phase of respiration. The result is severe inspiratory dyspnoea and sometimes even suffocation.

When the cause is an over-inflated cuff, decannulation is often impossible.

The affected segment usually has to be excised (see page 54). Tracheoplasty is often required (see page 60).

787

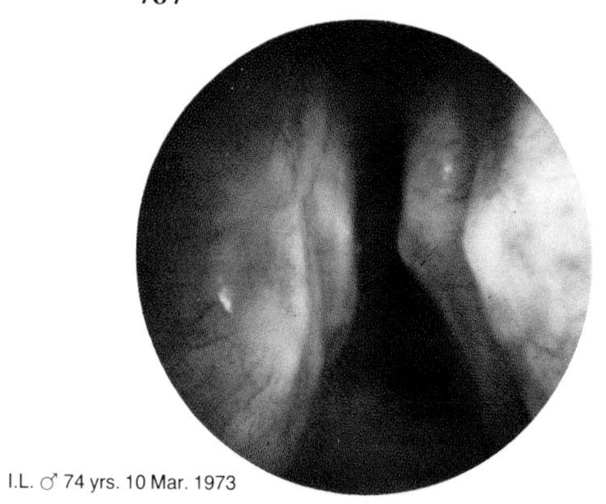

I.L. ♂ 74 yrs. 10 Mar. 1973

787 Tracheomalacia: The walls of the trachea collapse on inspiration. The patient died from suffocation 6 months later.

788a

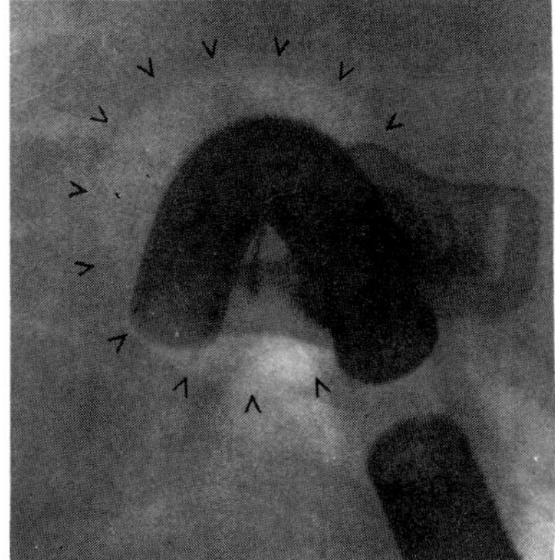

de B.E. ♀ 61 yrs. 27 May 1971

788b

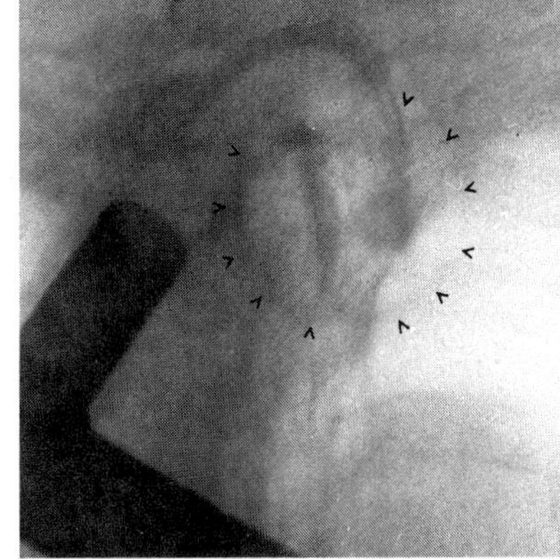

2 Oct. 1971

788c

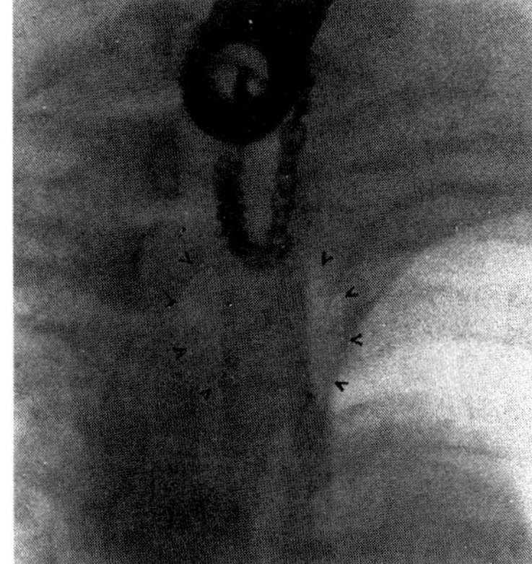

10 Oct. 1971

788d

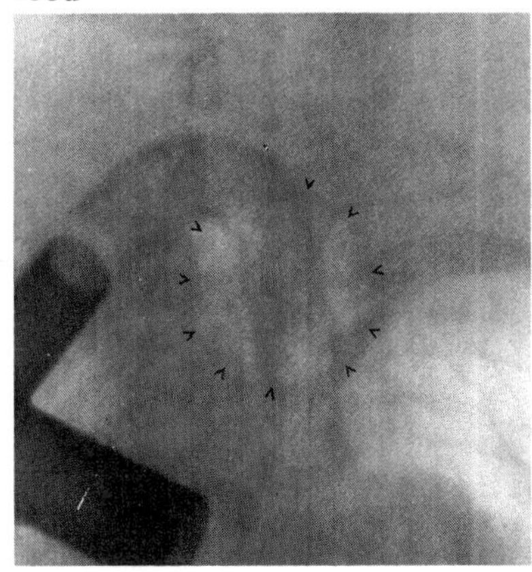

30 Oct. 1971

788e

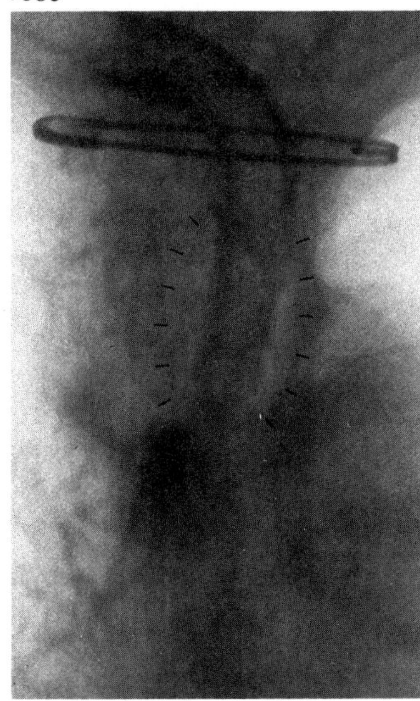

2 Nov. 1971

788a Tracheomalacia can make extubation impossible. After sustaining serious multiple injuries, the patient is under controlled ventilation for deep hypoxia due to fat embolism.

788b Over the next months, the short high-pressure cuff of the tracheostomy tube is inflated to various sizes.

788e Recovered from her multiple injuries, the patient has been able to come off the ventilator. However, tracheomalacia is such that a permanent tracheal tube is necessary. Stenosis subsequently develops and, 2 years later, resection is indicated. Postoperative death. (Dr. R. Meyer, P.-D., Lausanne.)

Tracheal fistulas

Tracheo-arterial fistulisation is one of the most life-threatening complications of tracheostomy. Until the advent of the low-pressure cuff, arterial fistulisation complicated 0.5 to 4% of all tracheostomies.

The tracheal damage nearly always consists of a necrotic eschar on the anterior wall due to pressure from the cuff (see **786**).

The *vascular damage* generally consists of a pressure perforation with necrosis over an area of 3 to 5 mm^2. The vessel can be the innominate artery (if it passes abnormally high between the sternum and trachea), the right carotid artery, the lower thyroid artery or even the aortic arch.

Patients with a tracheo-arterial fistula usually die immediately from a massive haemorrhage through the tracheostomy tube (94% of reported cases), (see **790, 997**).

However, temporary haemostasis can be obtained either by immediate over-inflation of the cuff, or by digital compression of the artery against the sternum after the removal of the cannula. If the finger compressing the artery is of smaller diameter than the tracheostome, there is a possibility that ventilation can be maintained long enough for the patient to be intubated.

If immediate haemostasis is successful, the artery should be ligated without delay. Vascular reconstruction is not always necessary. The incidence of postoperative infection is high, but some successes have been reported.

Whenever tracheal necrosis is suspected below the tracheostome, and especially if the tracheostomy tube is seen to be pulsating, a tracheoscopy should be performed immediately to check on the possibility of incipient fistulisation.

If a fistula is found to be developing, two palliative measures can be taken: a shorter or longer tube can be selected that does not interfere with the innominate or carotid arteries, or a section of pectoral muscle and skin can be interposed between the artery and the trachea.

789 **Causes of massive haemorrhage through tracheostomy tube** (Erosion of a major artery) (see **996 – 998**)

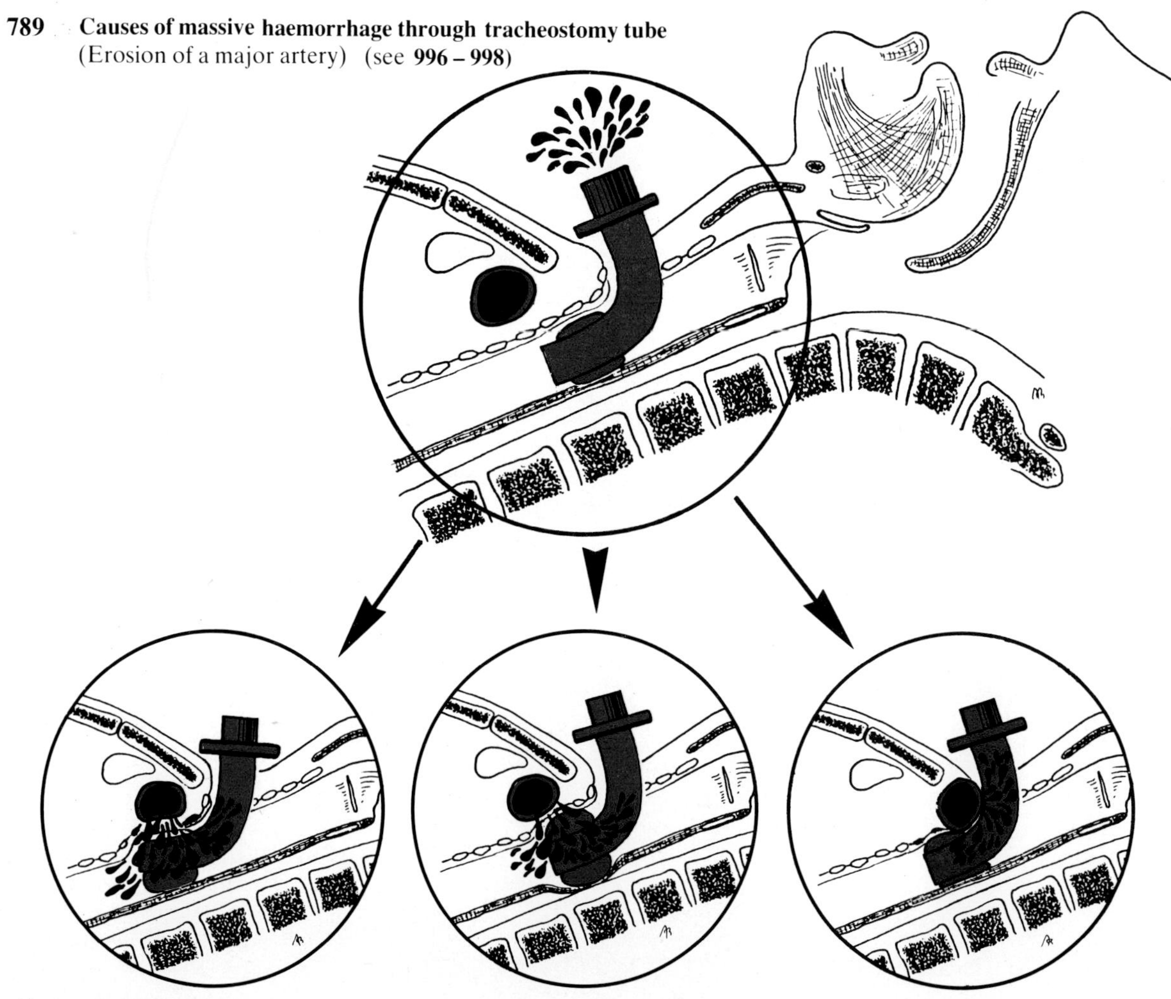

Tracheo-arterial laceration (tube inserted too deep or too low)

Tracheal and arterial pressure necrosi (over- inflation of the cuff) (see **788, 790, 997**)

Abnormally high innominate artery (or tracheostome that is too low)

790a

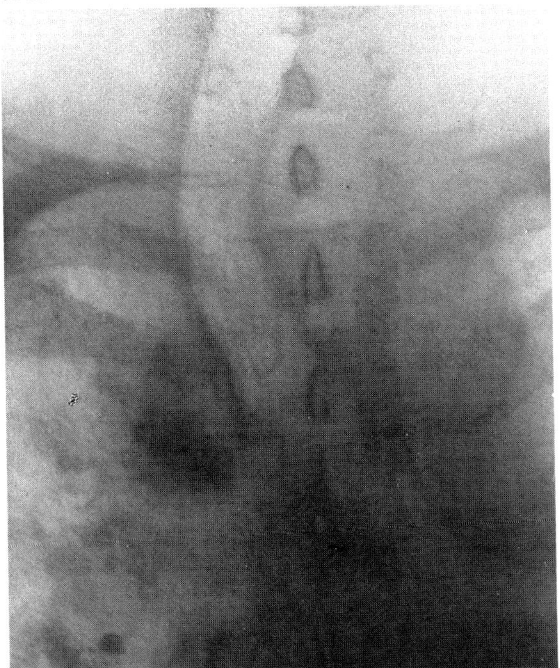

M.G. ♀ 66 yrs. 28 Aug. 1971

790a Tracheal necrosis by over-inflation of cuff. Fatal tracheo-arterial fistula. Admission X-ray of a multiple injury casualty. The trachea is sinuous.

790b

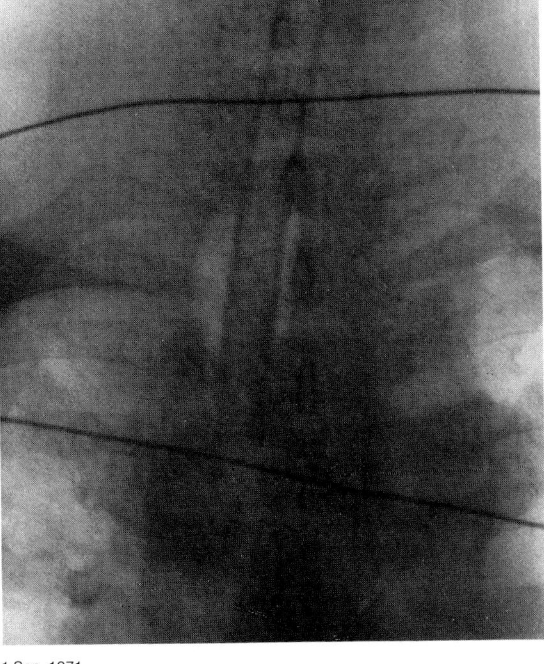

1 Sep. 1971

790b Four days later, an orotracheal tube is introduced to ease respiratory distress. The cuff is only slightly inflated.

790c

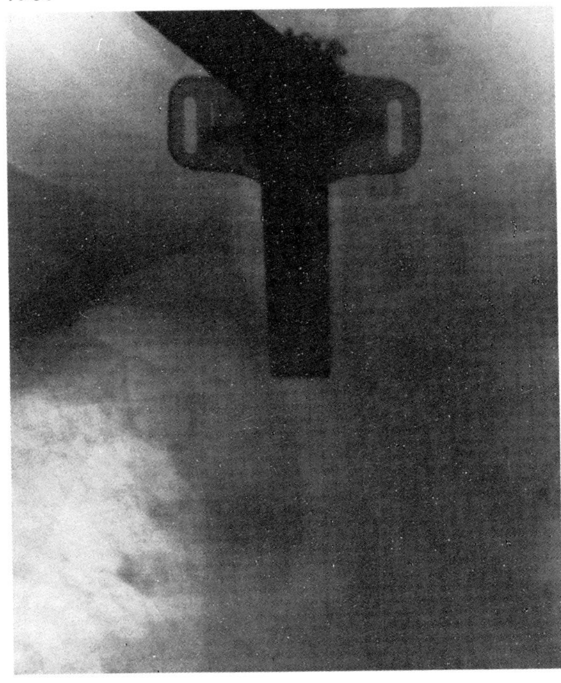

4 Sep. 1971

790c Respiratory distress worsens and a tracheostomy is performed. Initially, the cuff is correctly inflated . . .

790d

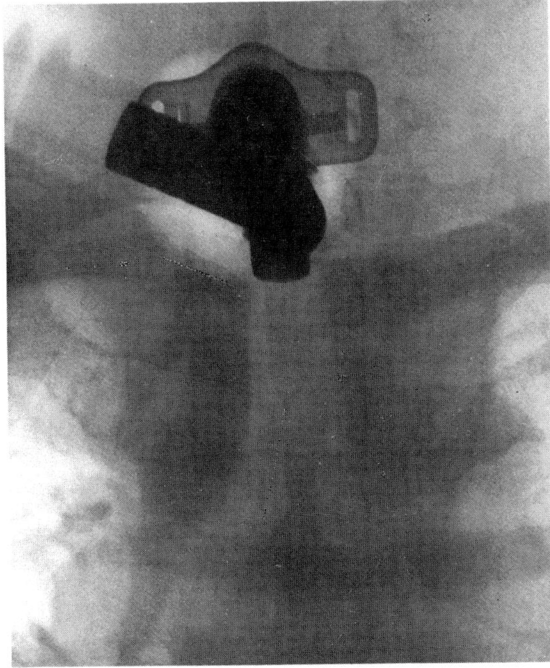

6 Sep. 1971

790d . . . but it is gradually dilated out of all proportion. Immediate death from erosion of the right carotid artery.

791

Prevention of tracheo-arterial fistulisation in tracheostomy patients.

Pulsating tube

Insertion of a *longer tube*

Interposition of a flap of pectoral muscle and skin

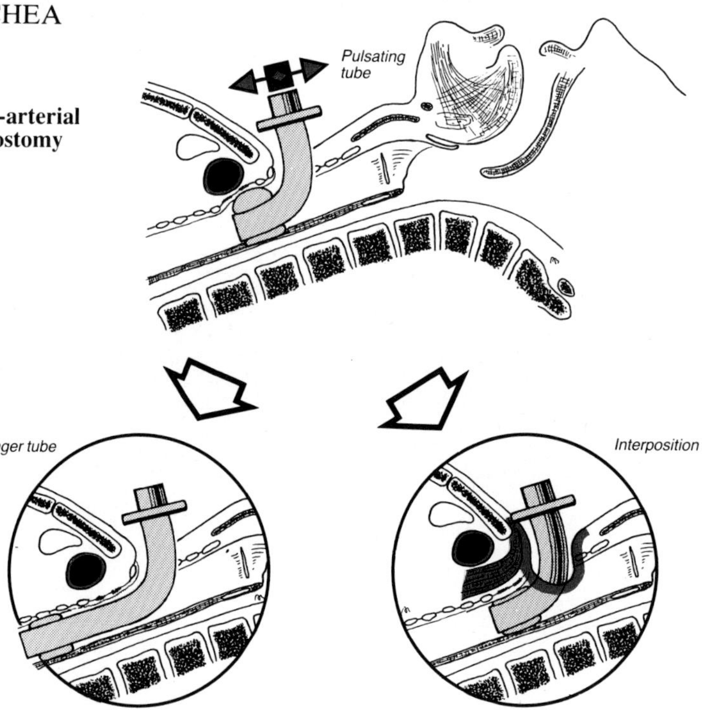

792

792 Haemostasis in cases of tracheo-arterial fistulisation in tracheostomy patients

Immediate *over-inflation of the cuff*

Digital compression while the tube is exchanged

Sudden massive *haemorrhage*

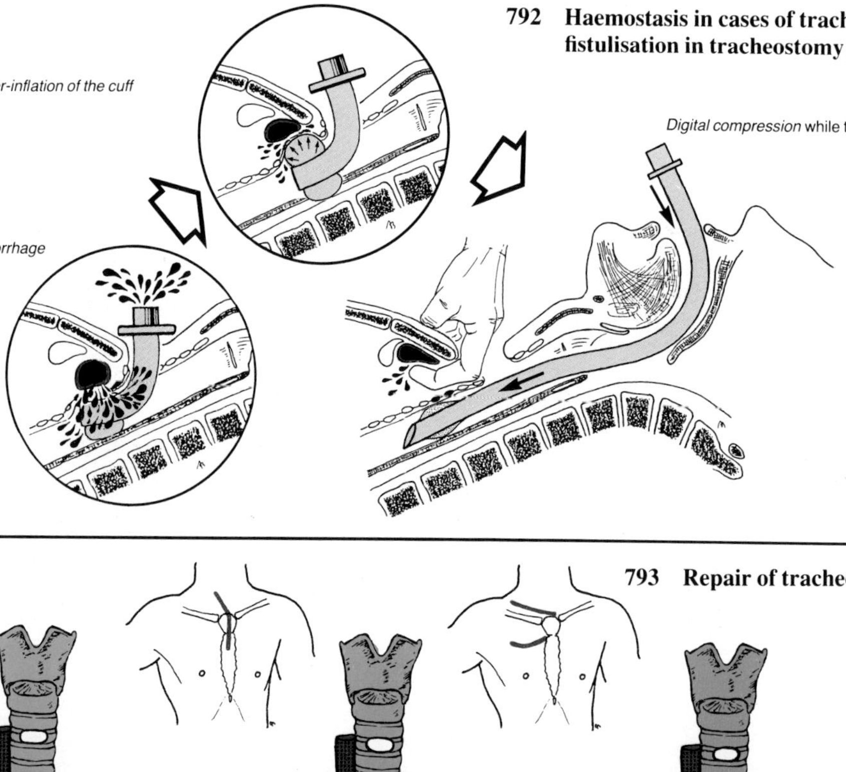

793

793 Repair of tracheo-arterial fistulas

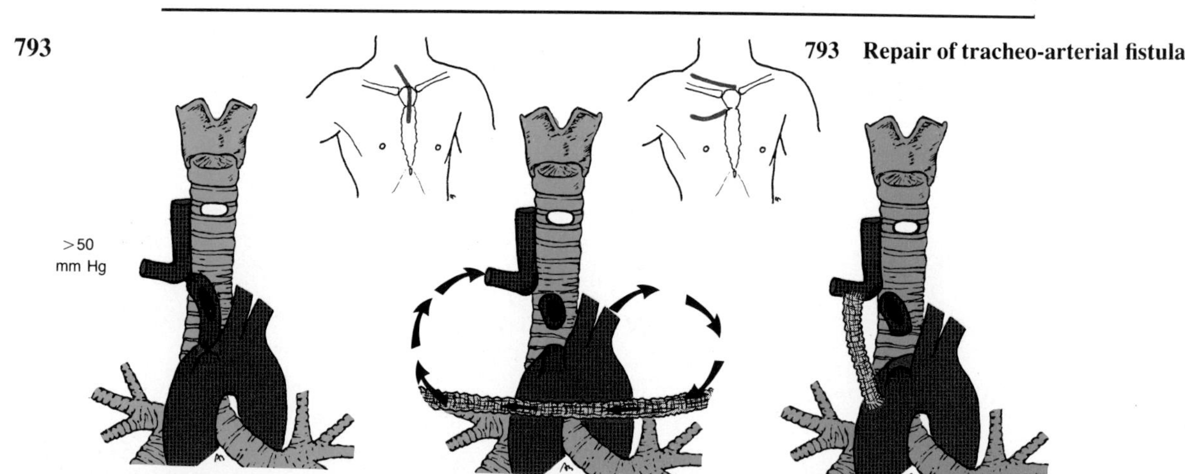

Simple Ligation
(provided pressure in the carotid artery remains high enough). This manoeuvre is not to be recommended.

Ligation with an axillo-axillary by-pass

By-pass, leaving a sliver of artery over the necrotic section of the trachea

794

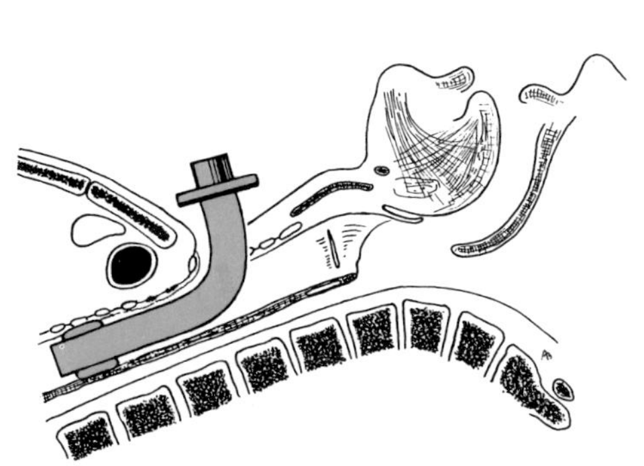

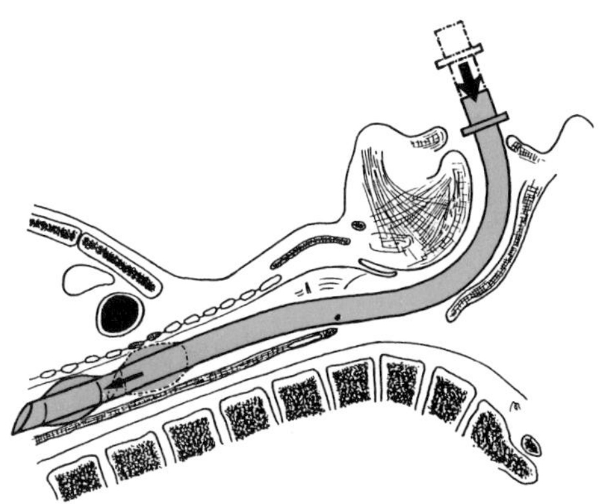

794 After the tracheo-arterial fistula has been repaired, **ventilation** is maintained through a long intubation or tracheostomy tube whose cuff should be positioned below the necrotic part of trachea. To minimise the risk of infection, repair should be delayed.

Tracheo-oesophageal fistulisation usually results from pressure between an oesophageal Levin tube and the cuff of a tracheostomy tube; the immediate cause is necrosis of the membranous wall of the trachea and of the anterior part of the oesophagus. Debility and nitrogen imbalance are common predisposing factors (see **1175**).

Tracheo-oesophageal fistulisation is rare (0.5%) and is probably becoming rarer since the advent of low pressure cuffs. Once established, a fistula is normally progressive and finally fatal. It will not cicatrize spontaneously even if the Levin tube and the tracheostomy tube can be removed.

If, however, a patient survives respiratory insufficiency, resection of the trachea and repair of the oesophagus can be envisaged. The method has been described by Grillo. Some successes have been reported.

In some cases, a tracheo-oesophageal fistula can be the direct result of a blunt thoracic trauma. The injury is rare, however, affecting only 6% of patients with trauma of the upper airways, or 0.36% of all chest trauma patients (in our material).

When a tracheo-oesophageal fistula of this type is located in the upper or mid-trachea, the oesophageal injury is usually detected when the trachea is explored: both injuries, therefore, are repaired at the same time. Fistulas in the lower trachea, on the other hand, are detected later, when the patient is observed to cough every time he swallows. In most cases, the fistula is readily located by a gastrografin oesophageal study. Repair, however, is difficult; the approach varies from case to case, but is always complex.

795 Causes of tracheo-oesophageal fistulas in tracheostomy patients

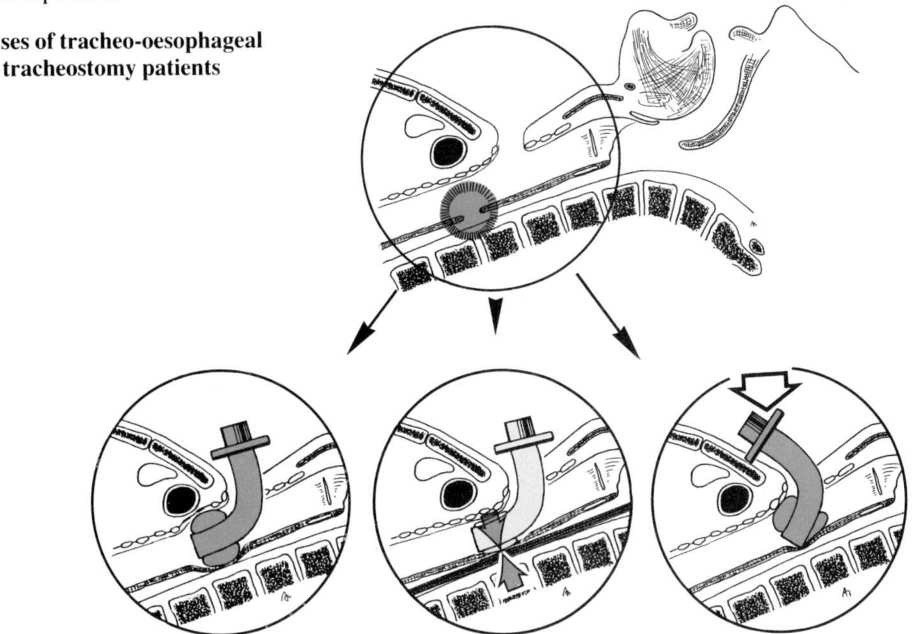

Circumferential tracheal necrosis (over-inflation of the cuff). (see **1175**)

Necrosis of the posterior membranous wall (compression between the cuff and the oesophageal Levin tube)

Laceration of the posterior wall of the trachea (weight of the ventilator tubings). (see **783**)

Tracheal stenosis

The preponderance of post-traumatic tracheal stenosis in the cervical trachea is explained by the fact that it usually results from one of the two causes:

- *direct traumatic rupture,* whether repaired or not in the preceding weeks/months/years;
- *iatrogenic injury* during long-term intubation and/or tracheostomy.

Tracheal stenosis is redoubtable; if it is not repaired adequately, death through gradual asphyxia is inevitable.

Various factors combine during long-term intubation or tracheostomy to produce the tracheomalacia that finally leads to tracheal stenosis.

Several different *mechanical* factors can play a part: friction caused by an inadequately secured tube, local injury from a deflected tube or from an over-inflated high pressure cuff, ischaemia through infrequent deflation of the cuff, torque exerted by ill-counterweighted ventilator tubings (see **783, 795).**

Infection of damaged mucosa rapidly produces an active granulation tissue that in turn causes hypertrophic cicatrisation and, later, stenosis.

The process of cicatrisation usually takes 3 to 6 weeks; stenosis develops most quickly after tracheal necrosis but it has been known to take up to 20 years to appear.

In most cases, tracheal stenosis is progressive; a patient's final condition cannot be assessed until at least six months after treatment has been completed.

Type, Localisation

After tracheostomy, stenosis can occur above, at, or below the tracheostome.

Stenosis that develops *above the tracheostome* is usually the result of a faulty operative technique.

Stenosis at the level of the tracheostome itself is likewise usually the result of a faulty technique (especially if tracheostomy is performed through a longitudinal tracheal incision). Björk's tracheostomy technique reduces the likelihood of this type of stenosis in the mid- and long-term.

Stenosis below the tracheostome, on the other hand, is produced either by the cuff, or by the tip of the tube, or by repeated damage during endotracheal aspiration.

Prolonged intubation rarely causes stenosis; when it does occur, it is usually in the lower portion of the cervical trachea, either around the cuff or at the tip of the tube. This type of stenosis, therefore, can be regarded as a variant of the subtracheostome type described above.

The development of low pressure, large diameter cuffs and the use of new types of tubing material, has meant that stenosis after tracheostomy or long-term intubation is becoming increasingly rare.

796

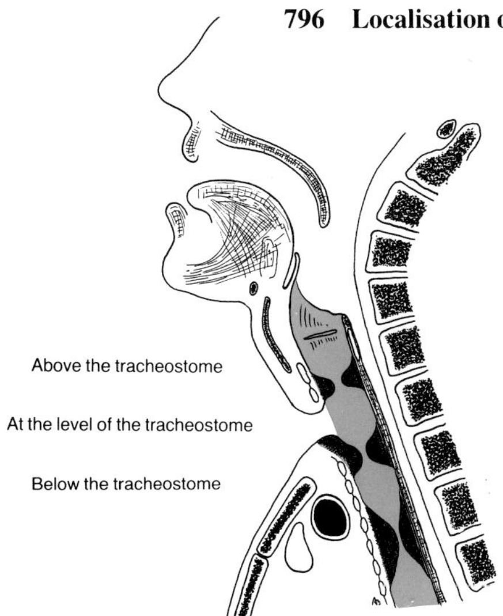

796 Localisation of tracheal stenosis after tracheostomy

Diagnosis

The symptoms of tracheal stenosis depend upon its gravity. A resting patient usually shows no symptoms until stenosis has reduced the cross-sectional area of the trachea by *70 to 80%*.

Thereafter, the likely symptoms are:

- an irritating and unproductive *cough* (often hoarse).
- *dyspnoea,* increasing on exertion. If respiration is rapid the accessory respiratory muscles are often brought into use.
- *wheezing,*
- *cyanosis.*

Before being brought to surgery, stenosis always should be examined endoscopically and radiologically.

Tracheobronchoscopy determines the length of resection required and *X-ray* (or preferably, *tomography*) establishes the approach. Sharper X-ray pictures are obtained if the patient inhales tantalum powder.

Management

797a

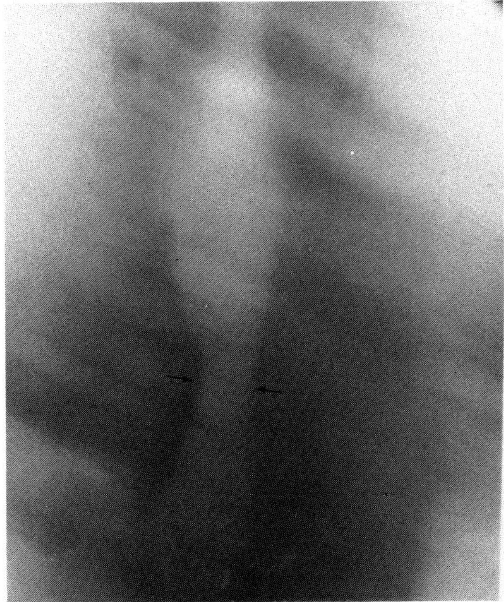

C.R. ♂ 53 yrs. 14 July 1971

797a No treatment for stable, 50% tracheal stenosis caused by the tip of a tracheostomy tube. The initial symptoms are slight . . .

797b

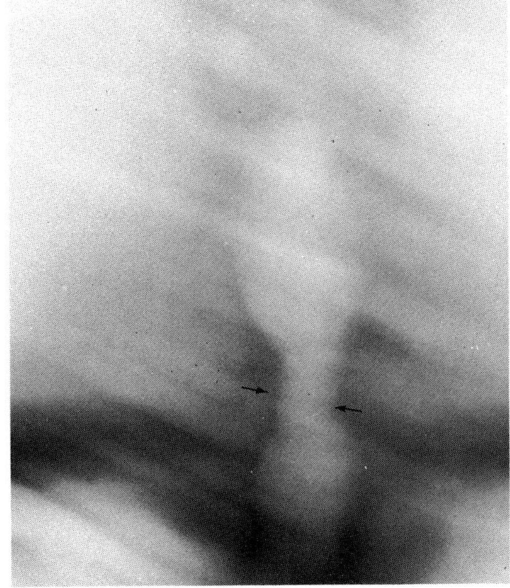

19 Mar. 1974

797b . . . and the patient's condition is unchanged 3 years later.

Tracheal resection is not too difficult a procedure if the correct approach is used (see **713**). If the head is flexed to diminish tension, as many as four or five cartilages (about 4 to 5 cm) can be resected with direct end-to-end anastomosis. Re-absorbable suture (vicryl) should be used. When the approach is appropriate, the thoracic part of the trachea and both main-stem bronchi can be freed and the triangular pulmonary ligaments sectioned to permit *longer resections* (see **798, 799**).

798 **Maximum resection of upper trachea** (Grillo, 1969).

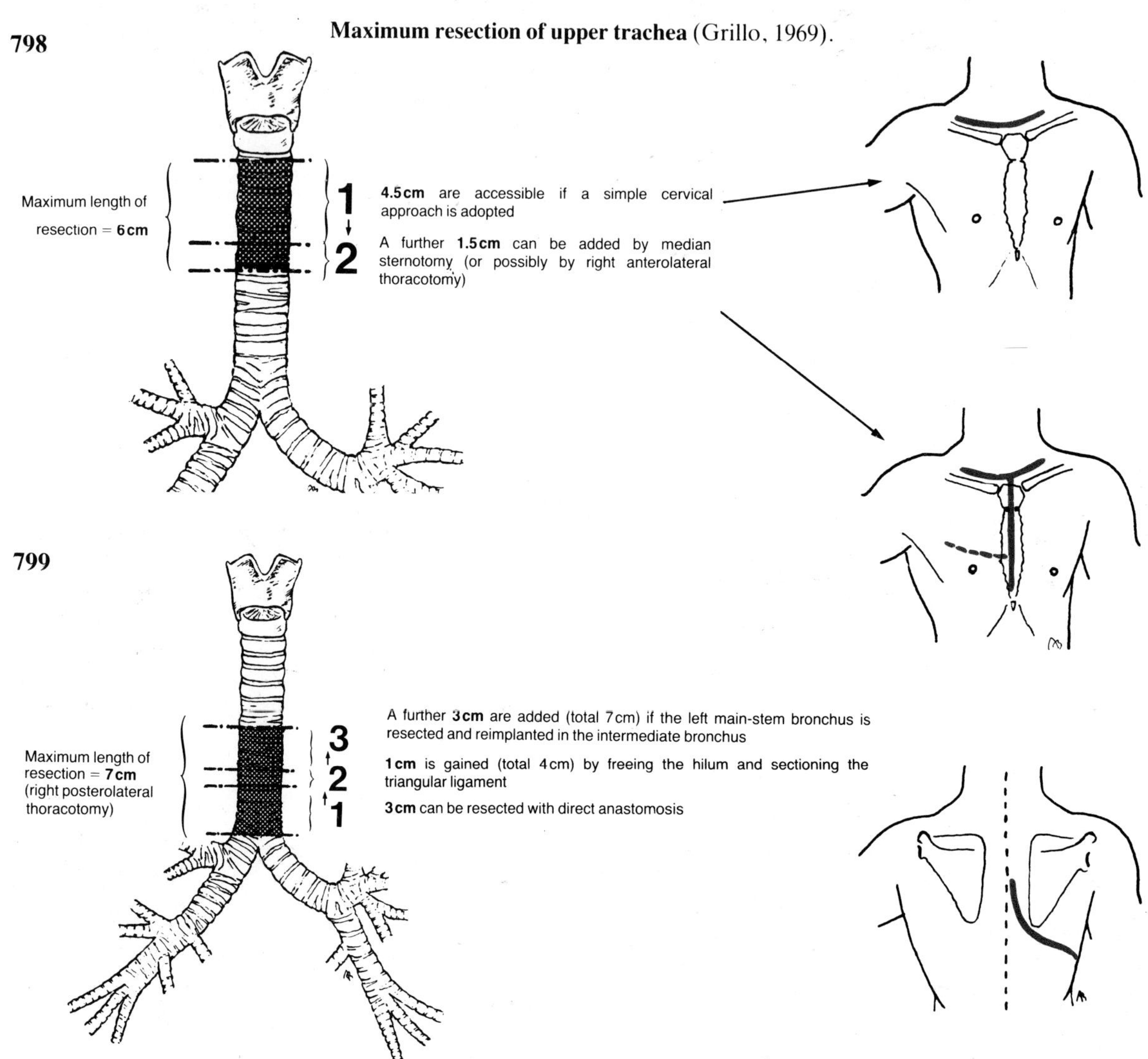

799

Maximum resection of lower trachea (Grillo, 1969).

800a

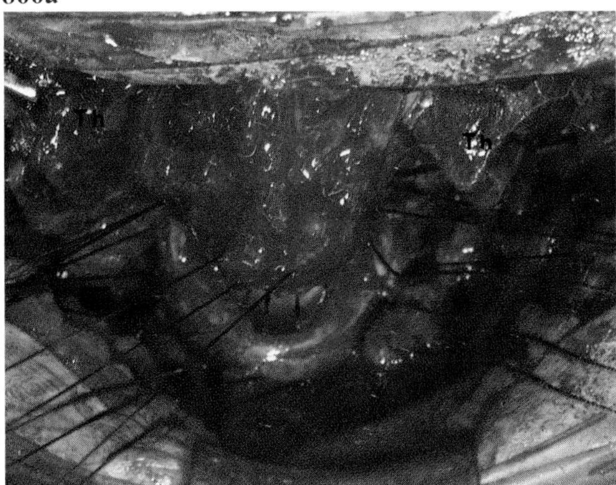

B.L. ♂ 46 yrs. 14 Feb. 1975

800a Late stenosis of mid-trachea following tracheostomy. Resection through cervical approach. The patient was ventilated for two weeks through a tracheostomy tube during a tetanus attack 20 years ago. Since then, stenosis (extending over two cartilages) has developed at the level of tip of cannula.

800b

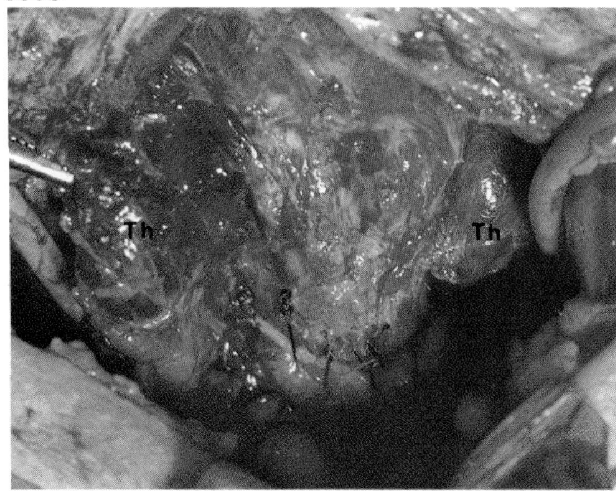

14 Feb. 1975

800b Cervical approach: segmental resection and end-to-end closure with interrupted sutures. The two lobes of the thyroid are marked (Th).

801a

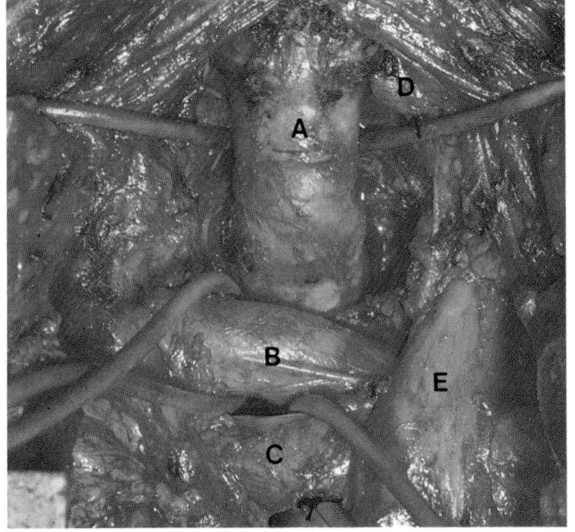

G.I. ♀ 69 yrs. 21 Feb. 1973

801a Stenosis of mid-trachea following tracheomalacia. Resection through combined cervical and trans-sternal approach. The external wall of the trachea gives no hint of the long fibrous stenosis. The trachea (A), the right innominate artery (B), the left innominate vein (C), the thyroid gland (D) and the thymus (E) are exposed.

801b

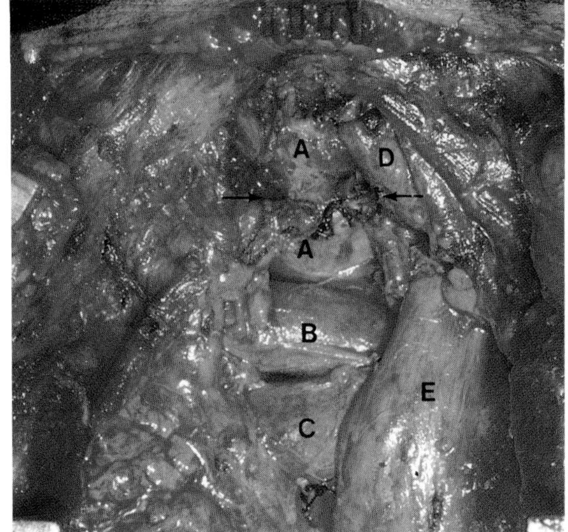

21 Feb. 1973

801b Four cartilages are resected and trachea repaired with end-to-end anastomosis. (→).

802a

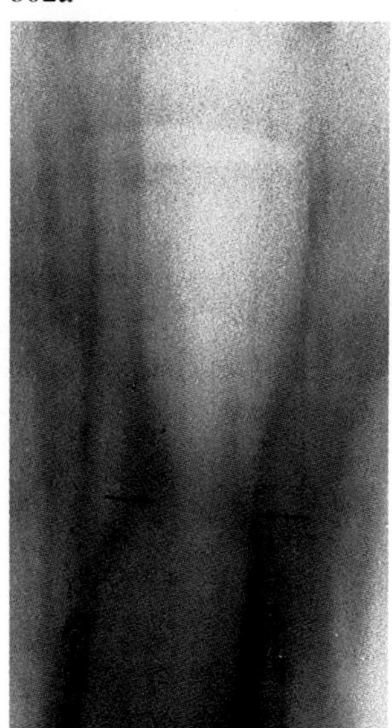

A.R. ♂ 60 yrs. 9 Dec. 1969

802b

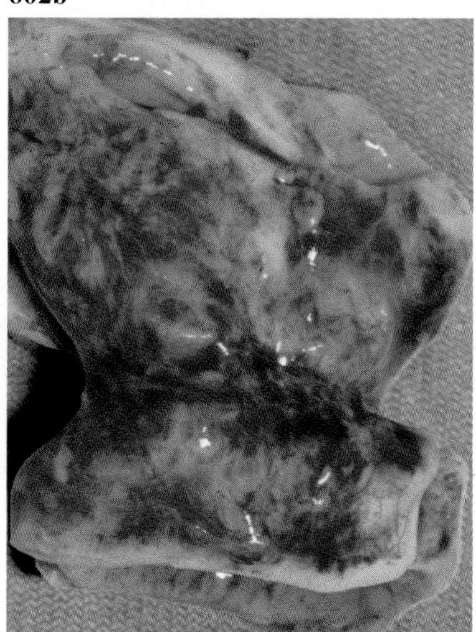

19 Dec. 1969

802c

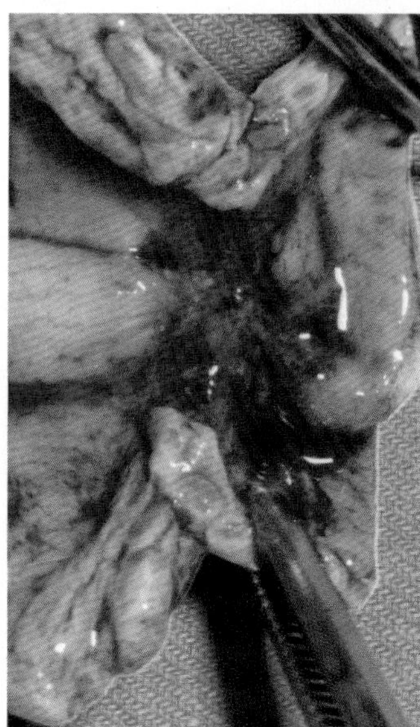

19 Dec. 1969

802a Ulcerated tracheal stenosis ten weeks after a tracheostomy. **Early resection through cervicothoracic approach.**

802c Recent, ulcerated stenosis 80% in diameter and 94% in cross-section. (Operative specimen.)

803a

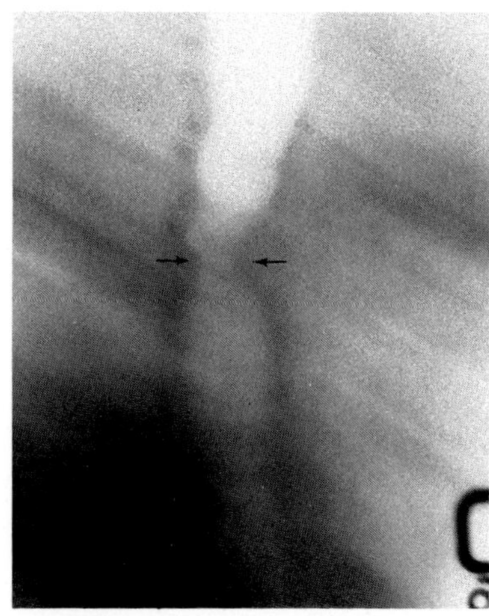

B.A. ♂ 53 yrs. 15 Oct. 1971

803b

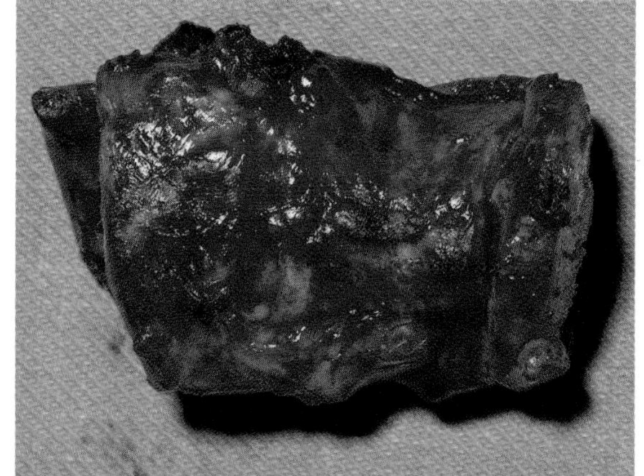

19 Nov. 1971

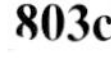

803c

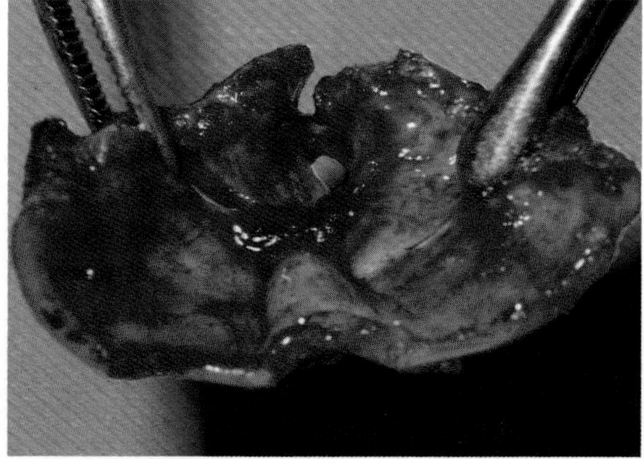

19 Nov. 1971

803a Severe stenosis of mid-trachea. Combined cervical and trans-sternal approach. Stenosis (→) has developed at the tip of the tube 6 months after a tracheostomy for ventilatory support.

803b The resected segment measures 4cm (4 cartilages).

803c Stenosis totals 84% in diameter and 97% in cross-section. Recovery.

804a

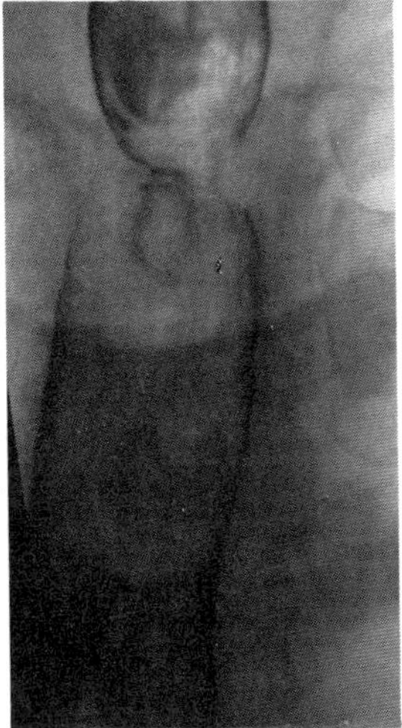

T.A. ♂ 47 yrs. 11 May 1966

804b

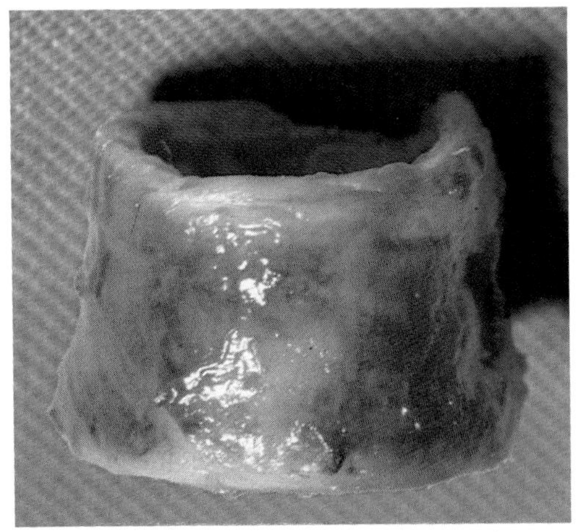

24 June 1966

804c

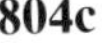

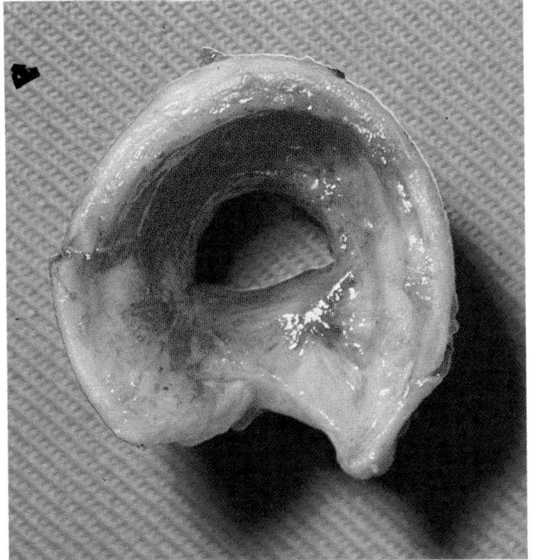

24 June 1966

804a Late stenosis of mid-trachea nine months after a tracheostomy performed for a prolonged coma. **Cervico-thoracic resection.** Endoscopic dilatations of the trachea have been attempted, without success. The patient remains dyspnoeic.

804b Three cartilages are resected through a combined cervical and trans-sternal approach.

804c Stenosis totals 60% in diameter and 83% in cross-section.

804d Tomogram of the restored trachea: the suture line is arrowed.

804d

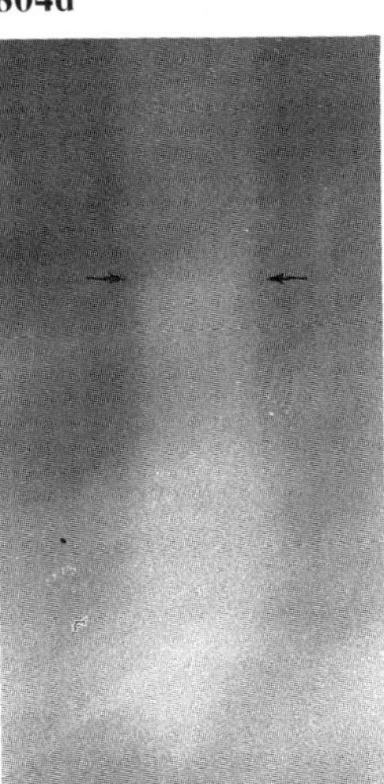

29 June 1966

804e

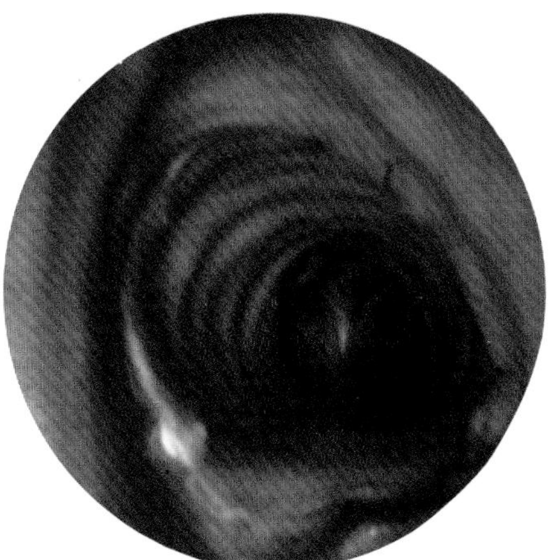

17 Jan. 1967

804f

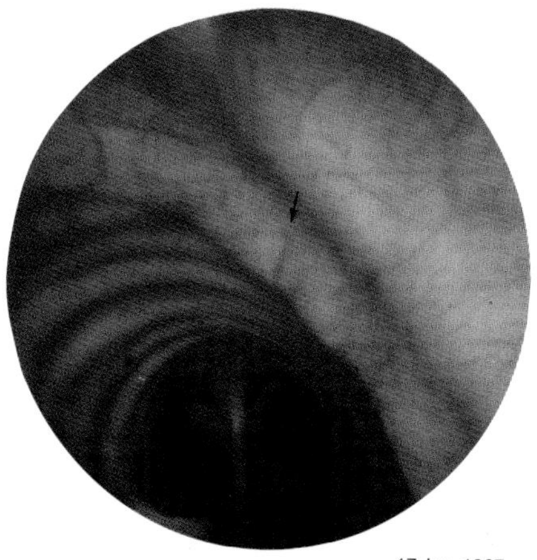

17 Jan. 1967

804e Long-term endoscopic follow-up. The diameter of trachea is normal.

804f Close-up of the anastomosis. One of the sutures is visible through the mucosa.

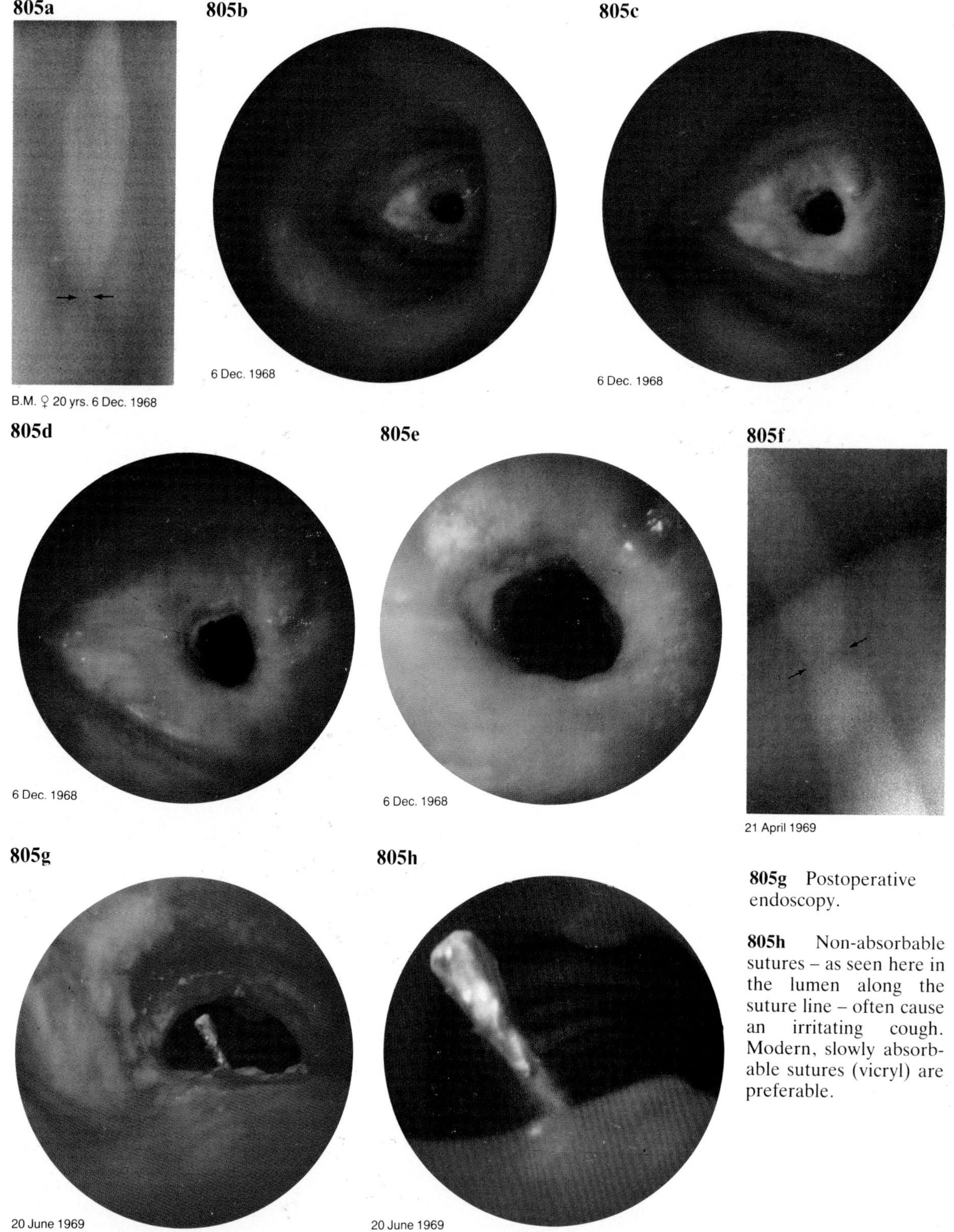

805g Postoperative endoscopy.

805h Non-absorbable sutures – as seen here in the lumen along the suture line – often cause an irritating cough. Modern, slowly absorbable sutures (vicryl) are preferable.

805a **Stenosis of mid-trachea** one year after intubation followed by a tracheostomy (maintained for three days only). **Resection through median sternotomy.**
805b The stenosis, measuring 5 mm in diameter, is here seen from the glottis . . .
805c . . . here from the trachea . . .
805d . . . and here from a distance of 1 cm.

805e Contact view. Stenosis totals 83% in diameter and 97% in cross-section. **Comparison of the 4 photographs 805b – 805e shows the extent to which an endoscope distorts the scale.**
805f This tomogram was obtained one month after resection. Stenosis persists – 45% in diameter and 70% in cross-section – but is asymptomatic.

806a

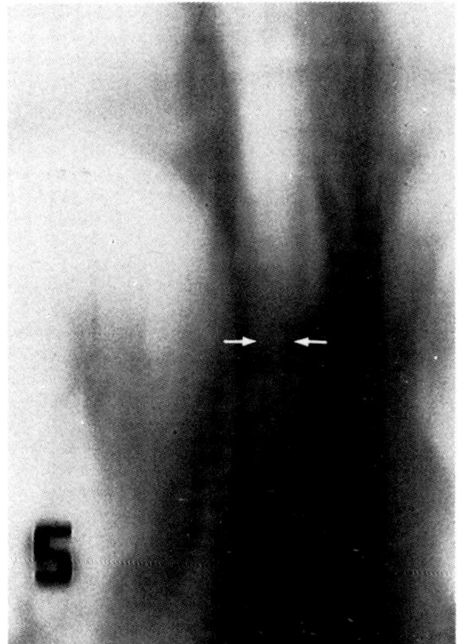

B.I. ♂ 24 yrs. 12 Mar. 1974

806b

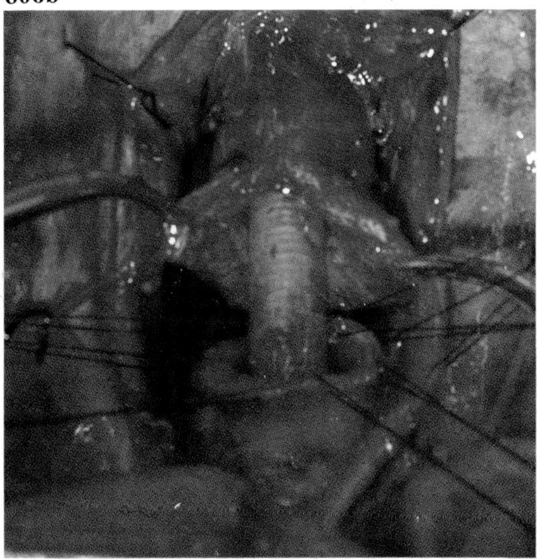

12 Mar. 1974

806c

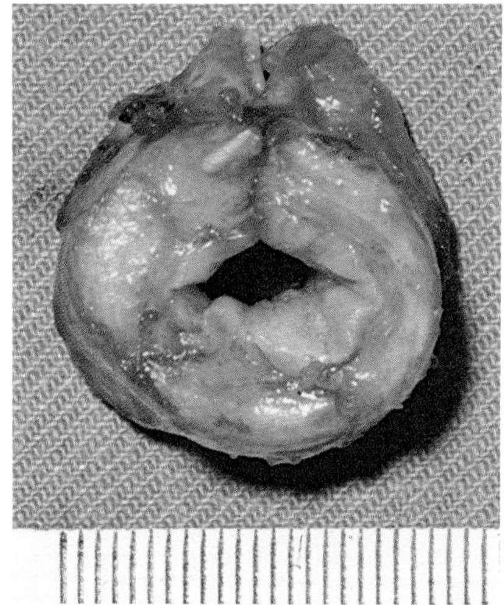

12 Mar. 1974

806d

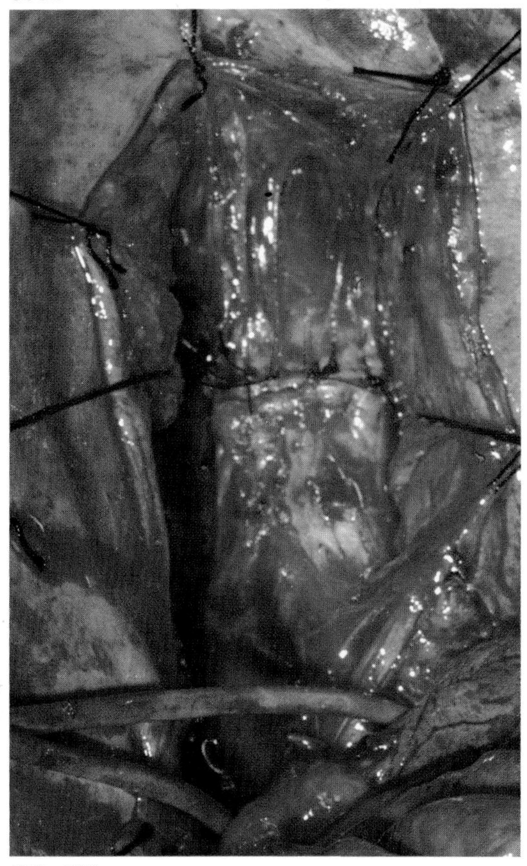

12 Mar. 1974

806a Late stenosis of lower trachea. Resection through right thoracotomy. A tomogram shows fibrous stenosis two years after a tracheostomy.

806b Right thoracotomy according to Grillo: the stenosis is seen here partially open. *N.B. A reinforced intubation tube has been chosen for safety.*

806c Stenosis totals 78% in diameter and 95% in cross-section.

806d Tracheal continuity is re-established after an excision of 2cm.

807a

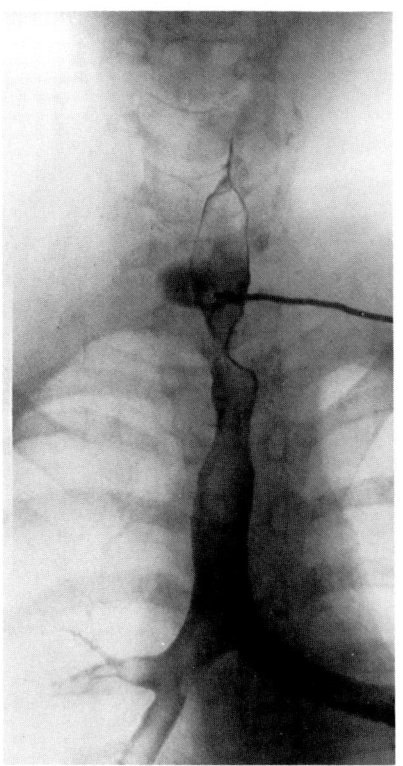

D.C. ♂ 30 yrs. 14 Aug. 1970

807b

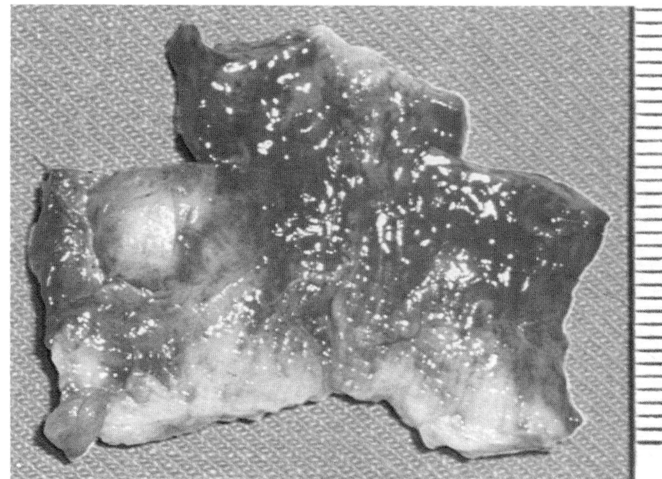

14 Aug. 1970

807c

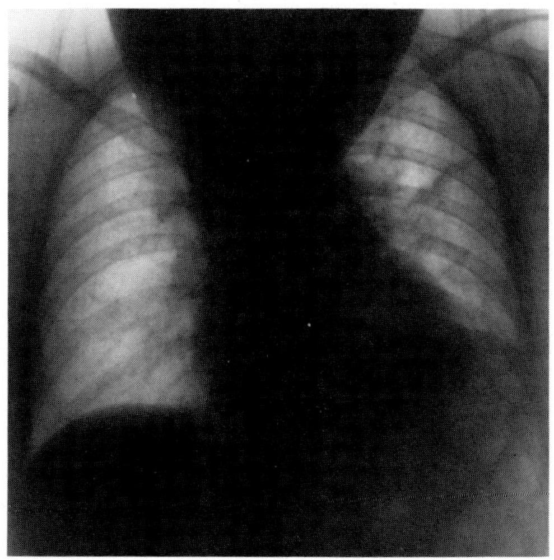

2 Sep. 1970

807a Postoperative flexion of the neck facilitates extended tracheal resection. Severe tracheal stenosis at the thoracic outlet.

807b Resection is performed through a combined approach.

807c Postoperative flexion of the neck relaxes the trachea and allows the suture line to cicatrize without tension. If this technique is used, up to five cartilages can be resected.

TRACHEOPLASTY

Extended tracheal resection generally requires tracheoplasty. None of the various tracheoplasty techniques is easy. Moreover, apparent success is often undermined by mid- and long-term complications.

808

Localisation and extent of resection and tracheoplasty for tracheal stenosis (in our material, $n = 23$).

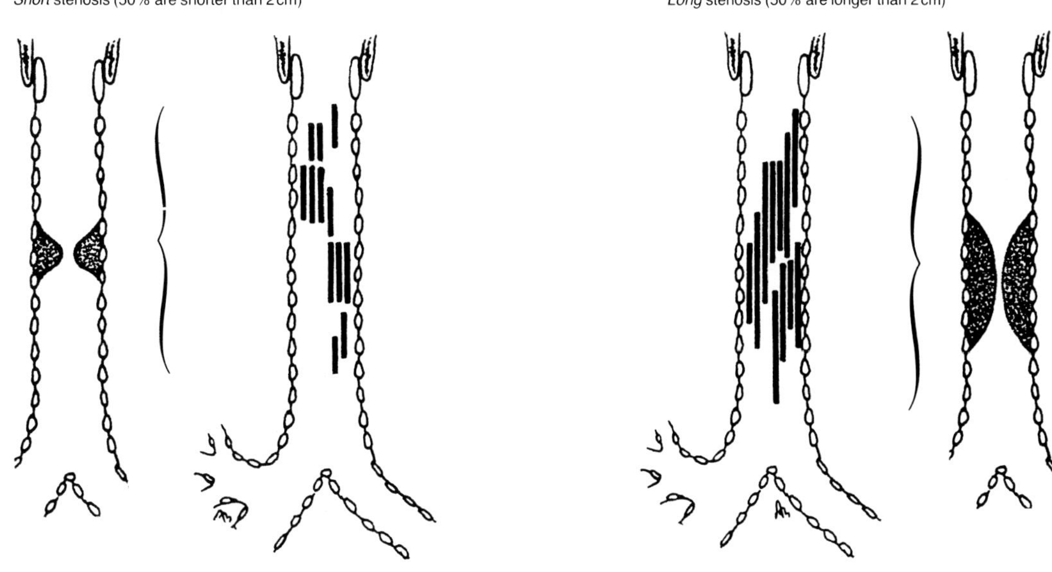

Each black line indicates the localisation and length of an excision.

Tracheoplasty for less than circumferential stenosis.

The *free graft* method requires a reinforced autologous fragment. It can be a fragment of pericardium, facia lata, skin or mucosa from the inside of the cheek. The reinforcing frame can be a mesh of plastic or metallic threads (silver, tantalum or stainless steel), or a sliver of plastic; some surgeons prefer a bony or cartilaginous rib fragment.

The alternative is a *pediculate graft,* which is taken from the chest wall and is composed of pleura, intercostal muscle and rib with periosteum. This type of graft is usually performed when the pleural activity is empty (after lobectomy or pneumonectomy) because, under these circumstances, a simple free graft would be likely to necrose.

Tracheoplasty for extended, circumferential stenosis.

In some cases, a *free reinforced graft* is still possible, but the procedure is delicate. An autologous fragment of mucosa from the inside of a cheek is sutured internally to the tracheal mucosa; a reinforcing section of rib cartilage is then sutured to the cartilaginous tracheal sheath.

Extensive *prosthetic reconstruction* is still at an experimental stage.

Over the years, different types of prosthesis have been tried:
- tubes of skin or mucosa,
- steel or plastic tubes,
- porous tubes,
- dacron meshes on metal frames.

So far, only temporary success has been achieved. Almost invariably, a fatal complication intervenes: for example, massive haemoptysis, or asphyxia due to the expulsion, displacement or obstruction of the prosthesis, or to late stenosis.

However, Björk (in animals) and Neville (in humans) have had patients who survived several years with long prostheses of siliconised rubber tubing.

Current animal experiments suggest that soon it may be possible to prepare *reinforced autologous grafts* in areas where blood vessels are abundant, and then to *transplant* them into the neck. The basis of this technique is microsurgical vascular anastomosis.

809 **Treatment of short tracheal stenosis**

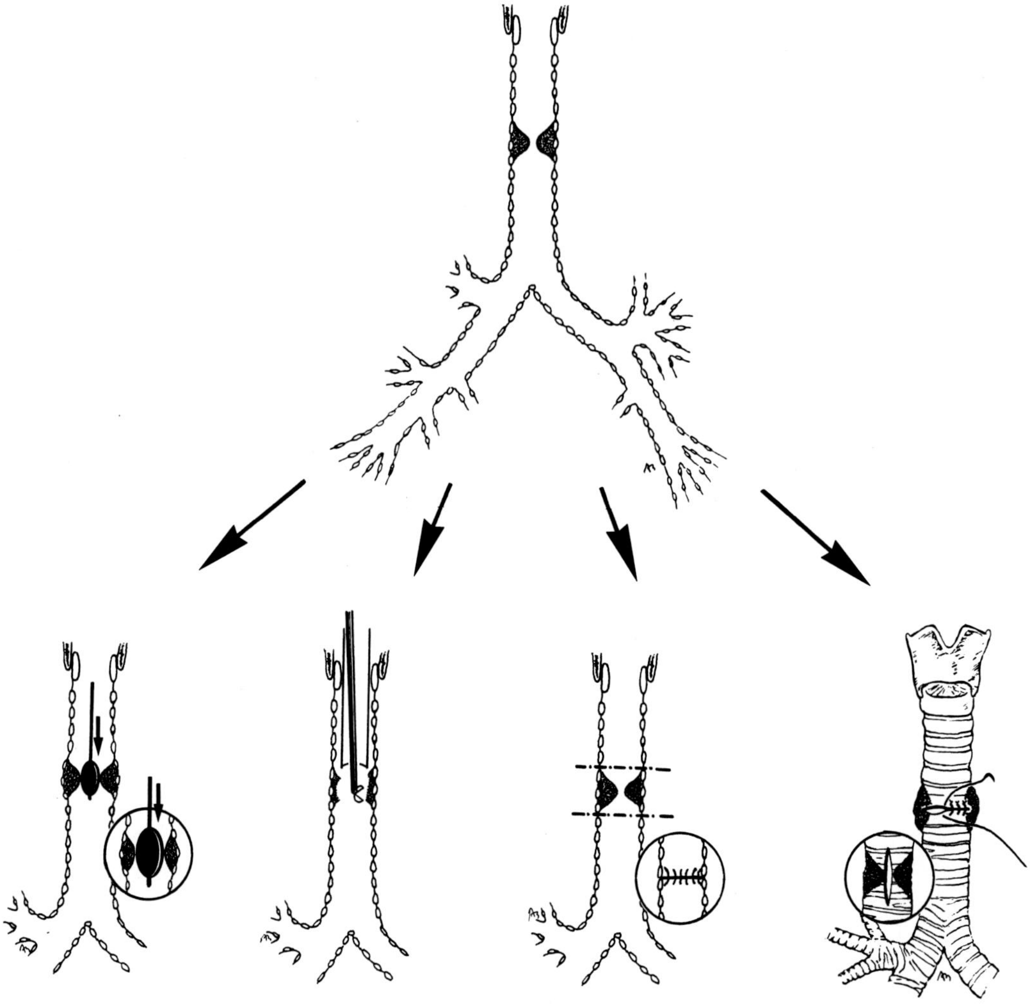

Endoscopic **bougienage**

Endoscopic resection

Surgical resection with direct end-to-end anastomosis

Longitudinal incision with **transverse** suturing

810 **Treatment of extensive tracheal stenosis**

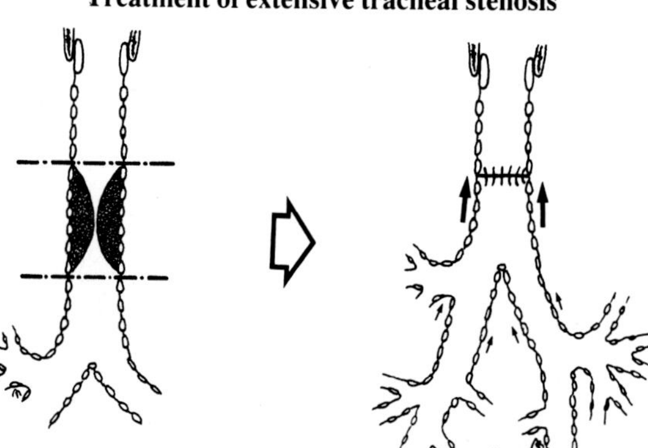

I. Extended resection (up to 7.cm depending on the approach)

Direct anastomosis after liberation of the tracheobronchial tree (according to Grillo)

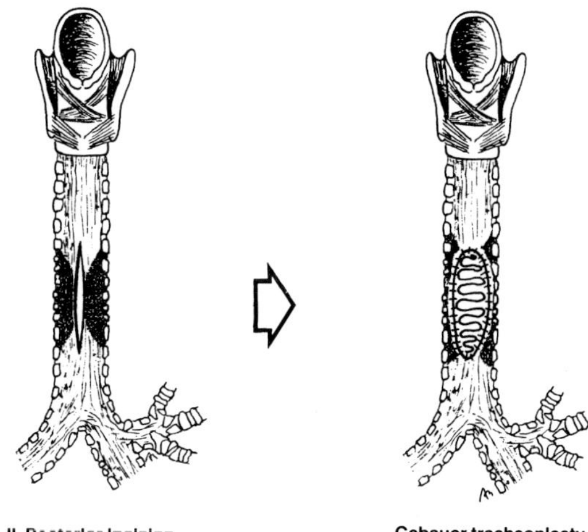
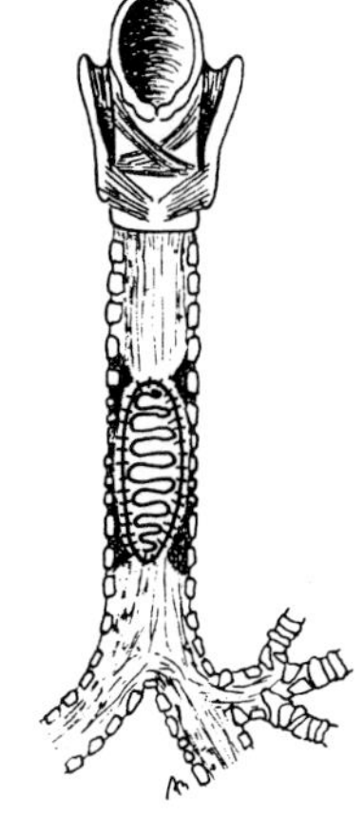

II. Posterior incision | **Gebauer tracheoplasty**

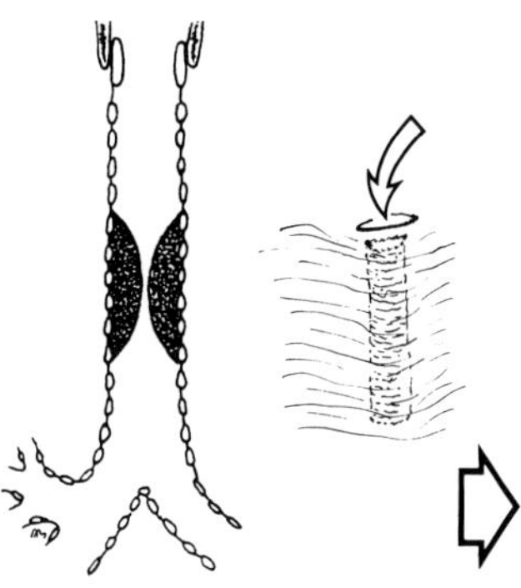

III. Tracheoplasty, step one: a bone fragment is implanted into the skin near the affected portion of the trachea

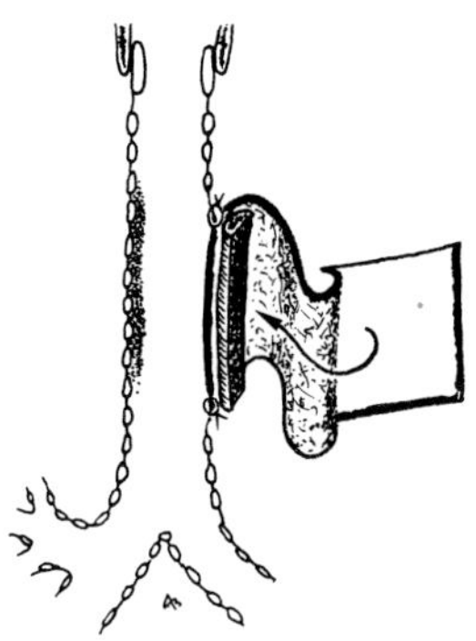

Tracheoplasty, step two: the flap of bone and skin is folded on to the trachea and sutured.
N.B. *This technique is only suitable for non-annular stenosis*

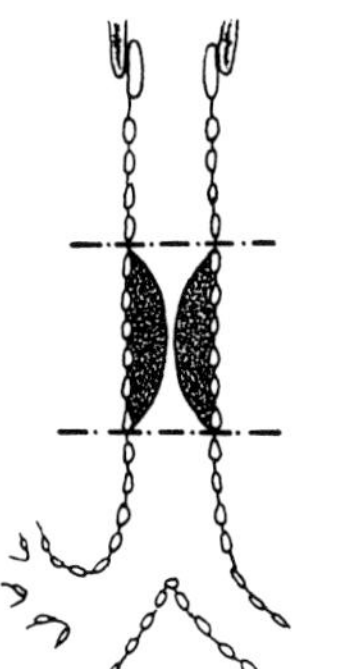

IV. Resection of unlimited length

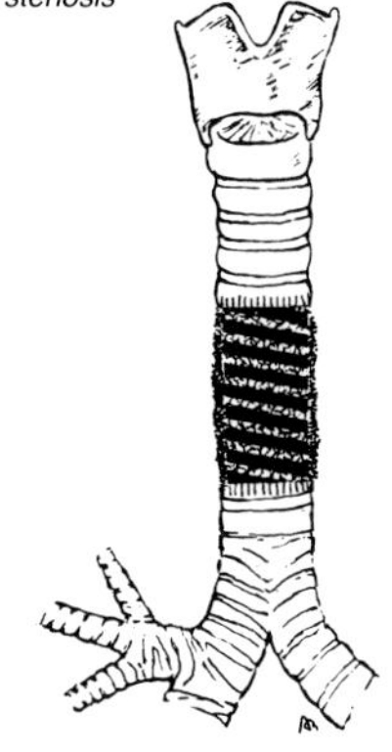

Interposition of a **reinforced prosthesis** (this technique is still experimental)

Bronchial rupture

Like many other types of chest trauma, bronchial rupture has become more common over the last thirty years. It now occurs in 1.5% of serious chest traumas.

Our figures show that 82% of bronchial ruptures occur in males; the injury has also been reported in infants. In one case, a three-week-old rupture with stenosis was successfully repaired in a baby of 13 months.

Between 1848 and 1926, some twenty bronchial ruptures were found at **autopsy:** the injury, therefore, was assumed to be uniformly fatal. However, when Krinitski happened on a complete cicatricial stenosis of the right main-stem bronchus during the autopsy of a 31-year-old woman who had been crushed under a cart during childhood, the idea of survival through spontaneous cicatrisation began to be accepted.

Throughout the next twenty years, bronchial rupture was diagnosed in **living** patients. As surgical techniques developed, it gradually became clear that late excision of infected pulmonary tissue below the stenosis could be abandoned in favour of an earlier approach to the rupture itself.

811

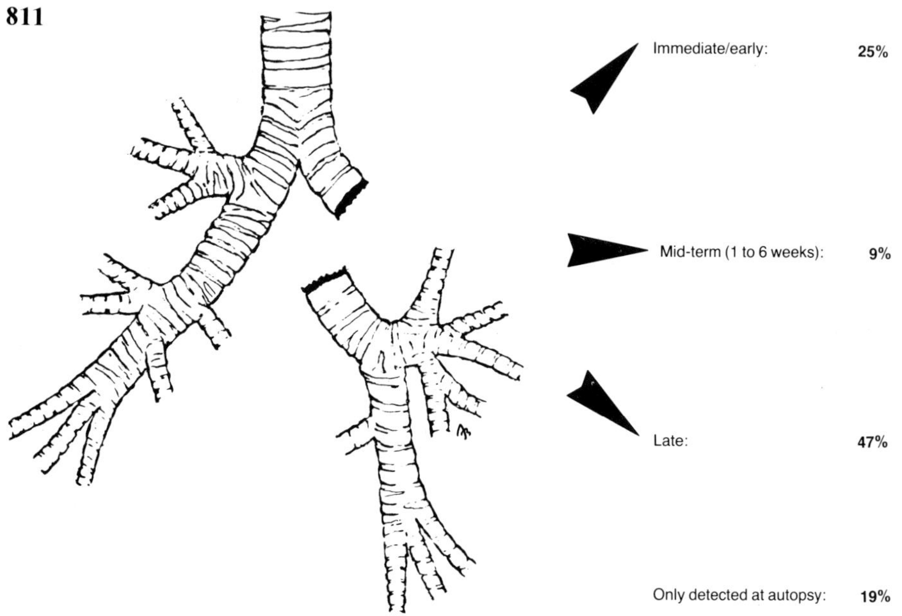

811 Early mid-term and late diagnosis of bronchial rupture. (According to Dor's historical survey, 1964, $n = 210$)

Successful **early repair** of a ruptured bronchus was first reported in 1951. Since then, great advances have been made in the management of all types of tracheal and bronchial injuries. The principles of surgical management are now clearly defined.

It must be emphasised, however, that the prognosis of these injuries is probably poorer than the literature suggests: contributors are often those who have been successful, and many cases do not have long-term follow-up.

Types of accident

Bronchial rupture implies an extremely violent accident. For example:

		of all cases
a car accident		33%
– car driver	22%	
– car passenger	11%	
a crush-injury		28%
a motorcycle accident		22%
a fall from several floors		17%

About 15% of patients with bronchial rupture also have a fracture of the first rib; therefore, any patient presenting a fractured first rib – an unusual injury – should be examined for tracheo-bronchial injury (as well as for aortic rupture and injuries to the brachial plexus and cervical column).

Biomechanics

Tracheobronchial rupture is sometimes the result of a *sudden change in pressure within the airways.* Explosions – especially of anaesthetic gas – and over-inflation of intubation tube cuffs are common causes. The damage – be it a fissure, a tear or an avulsion – often occurs at the junction of the membranous and cartilaginous walls.

Animal experiments show that the principal cause of bronchial rupture in closed chest traumas is the sudden *transverse widening of the thorax* during a frontal **crush-injury.** The immediate cause of rupture is the **lateral displacement of the lungs** which severs one or other of the main-stem bronchi.

Rupture can be prevented either by lateral retention of the chest walls, or by liberation of the lungs from the chest wall before the impact (by the creation of a bilateral pneumothorax, for example).

Bronchial rupture is both more frequent and more severe when the *glottis is closed*: if a weight of approximately 25 kg is dropped on to the anterior chest wall of an anaesthetised and intubated dog, bronchial rupture occurs in 15% of cases; when the endotracheal tube is clamped, the incidence of rupture rises to more than 70%.

812

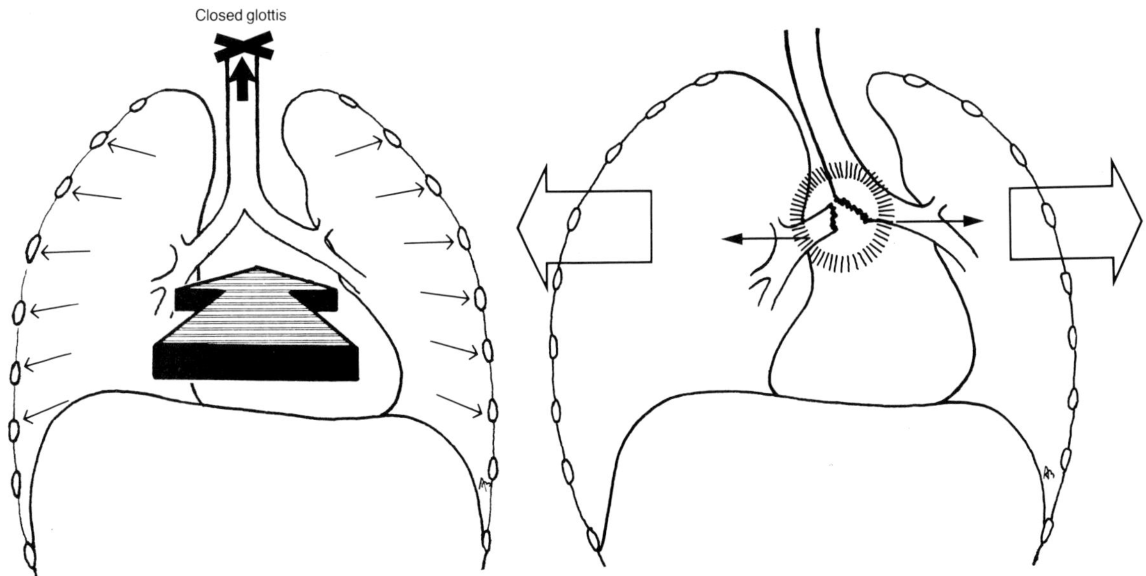

Anteroposterior compression causes transverse widening of the thorax; traction on the lungs opens the angle of the carina and tears one of the main-stem bronchi.

Animal experiments show that this type of rupture can often be prevented by:

– creating a *bilateral pneumothorax* before compression is applied
– *opening the glottis* at the moment of impact
– *lateral retention* of the chest walls

812 Biomechanism of rupture of main-stem bronchi during frontal crush-injury.

The biomechanism of bronchial rupture explains 1) why it is the proximal portion of the main-stem bronchus that ruptures, 2) why the stumps are usually neither contused nor gashed, 3) why this type of rupture so often occurs in young and supple people, especially children, usually without any parietal damage and 4) why bronchial rupture and tracheal rupture so rarely co-exist.

Rupture of a main-stem bronchus is nearly always accompanied by rupture of the bronchial arteries, but the pulmonary artery is rarely damaged; this detracts substantially from the theory that bronchial rupture results from the direct crushing of the bronchi between the sternum and the vertebral column.

Diagnosis

Contrary to what one might expect, only about 40% of bronchial ruptures are diagnosed in the first 48 hours. The figure would be higher if all likely cases were rigorously investigated at the outset.

One third of all bronchial ruptures occur in *children or adolescents* with supple thoracic cages; a further third occur in *young adults*.

X-rays are useful, but often unspecific. The points to look for are a gaseous syndrome and/or atelectasis (see page 11).

Bronchial rupture has a variety of clinical forms. For example:

- a *spectacular* form with a severe gaseous syndrome, suffocation, haemoptysis . . .
- a *typical* form with a complete, but not life-threatening gaseous syndrome,
- a *discreet* form where the gaseous syndrome is slight and haemoptysis intermittent or absent,
- a *deceptive* form where most of the signs are absent,
- a *late* form consisting mainly of bronchiectasis or atelectasis due to stenosis.

Pneumothorax is the most frequent sign. It is usually ipsilateral but occasionally can be contralateral – especially when it is the left main-stem bronchus that ruptures. This eventuality is not so rare as might be thought.

The pneumothorax produced by a major bronchial rupture is unlikely to cause suffocation so long as the patient is in spontaneous respiration; air moves freely through the rupture, so the pneumothorax remains 'open'.

However, if the patient is intubated and especially if he is ventilated with positive pressure, the pneumothorax quickly becomes *compressive*. Resuscitation of patients with bronchial rupture is, therefore, both difficult and dangerous.

Atelectasis is usually a late sign; it is always ipsilateral.

Stenosis often occurs early and usually leads to *bronchiectasis* and distal parenchymal infection. Bronchiectasis seems to occur more quickly when stenosis is incomplete (see **830e, 830f**).

813

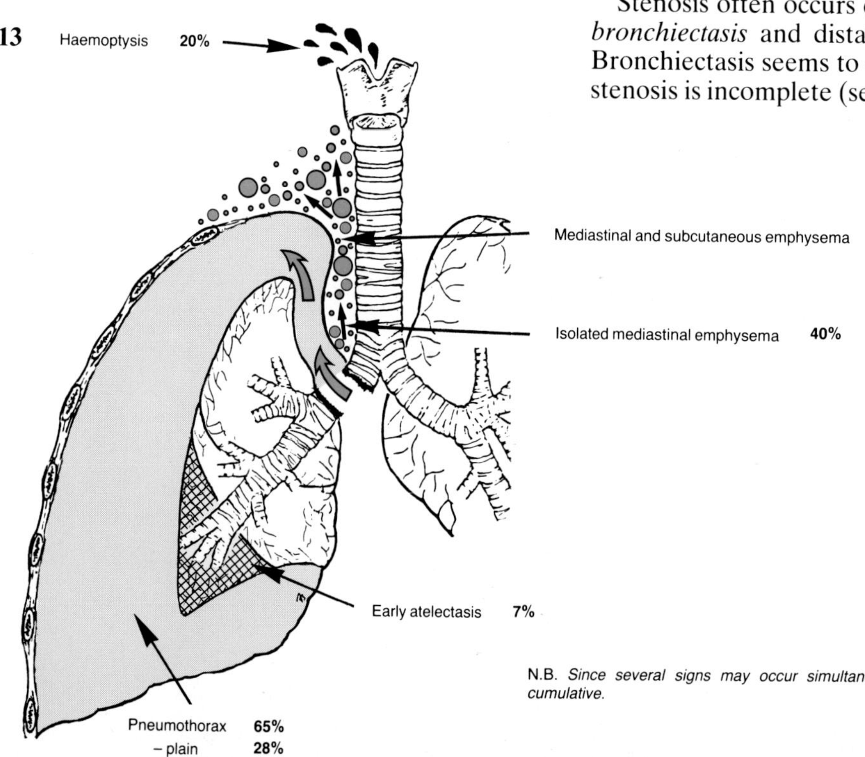

N.B. *Since several signs may occur simultaneously, the percentages given are not cumulative.*

813 Initial signs of bronchial rupture (Literature review, $n = 309$)

814a

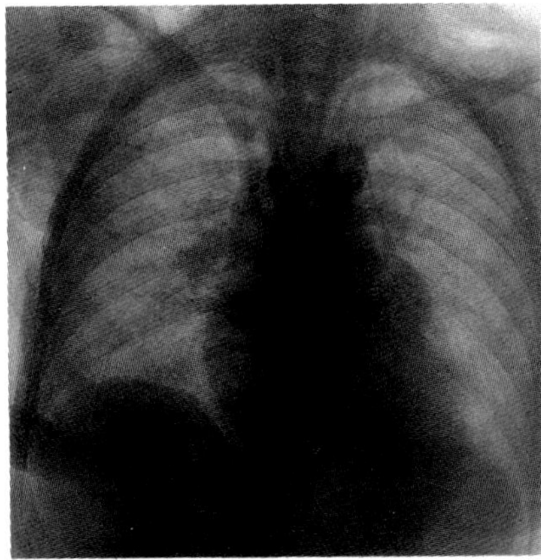

C.N. ♀ 29 yrs. 3 Oct. 1970

814b

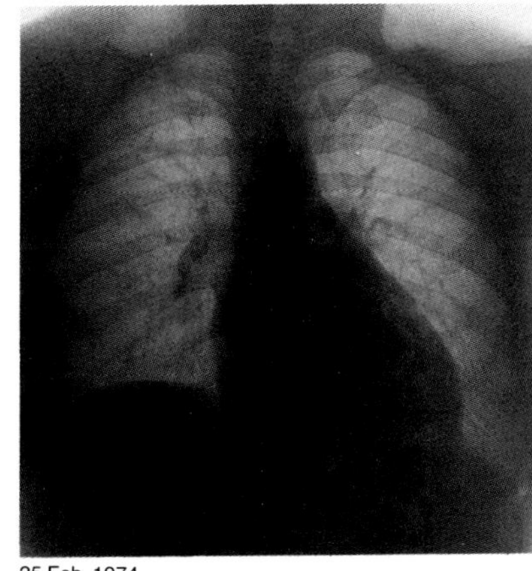

25 Feb. 1974

814a Rupture-dislocation of the intermediate right bronchus, following a suicide attempt from the fourth floor. On admission, the patient presents moderate mediastinal and subcutaneous emphysema, but **no pneumothorax.** Emergency right thoracotomy for direct bronchial repair. Recovery.

814b Follow-up X-ray, four years later.

815a

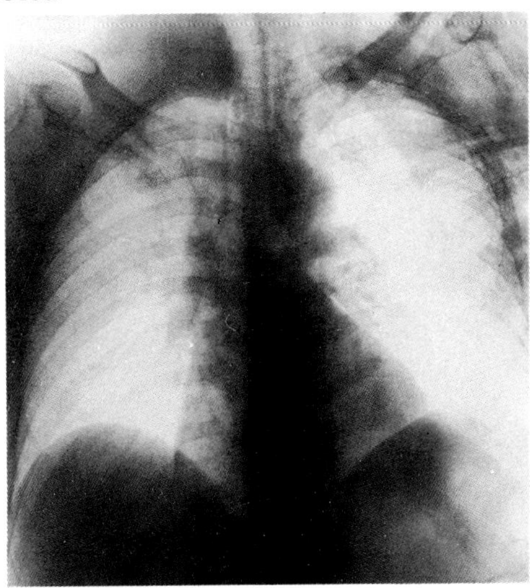

B.A. ♂ 47 yrs. 1 May 1974

815b

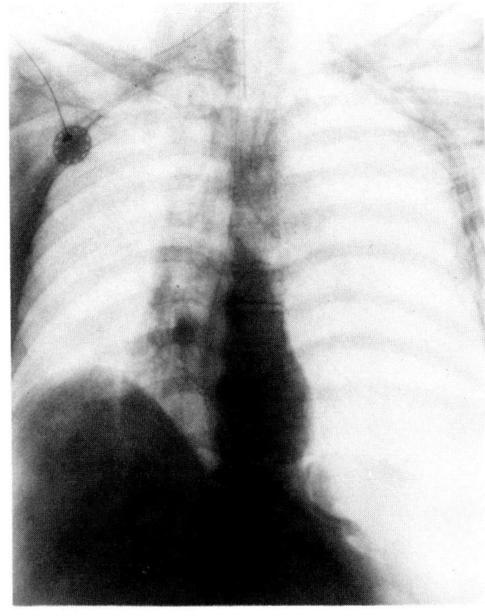

1 May 1974

815c

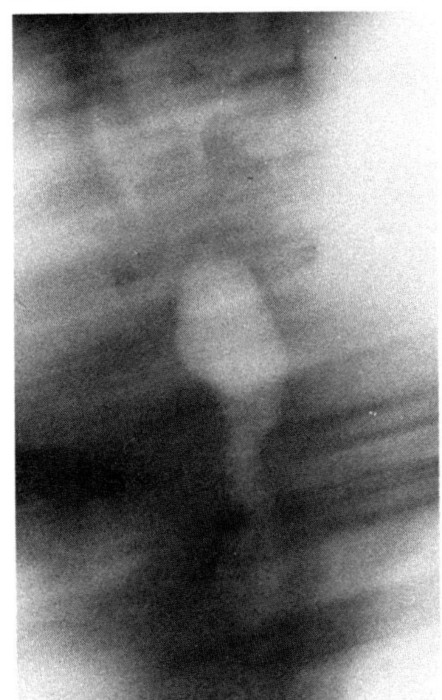

9 July 1974

815d

13 May 1975

815d The healed trachea.

815a Partial rupture of the left upper lobe bronchus giving rise to a **tension pneumothorax** during resuscitation. On admission, the patient (a motorcyclist knocked over by a lorry) displays moderate subcutaneous emphysema (see Volume 1, **478, 536**), and a flail chest with paradoxical motion.

815b Thirty minutes later – after resuscitation and *intubation with positive pressure ventilation* – a tension pneumothorax displaces the mediastinum to the right, inverts the left hemidiaphragm and causes a pleural hernia and massive subcutaneous emphysema. Pleural drainage proves insufficient. Tracheostomy and emergency thoracotomy.

815c The repaired bronchus heals but early tracheal stenosis – 74% in diameter and 93% in cross-section – has to be excised through a combined cervical and trans-sternal approach.

816a F.R. ♂ 21 yrs. 3 Dec. 1973

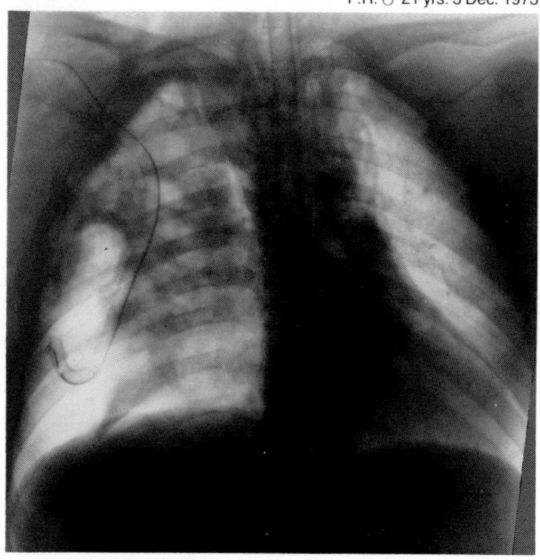

816b 14 Dec. 1973

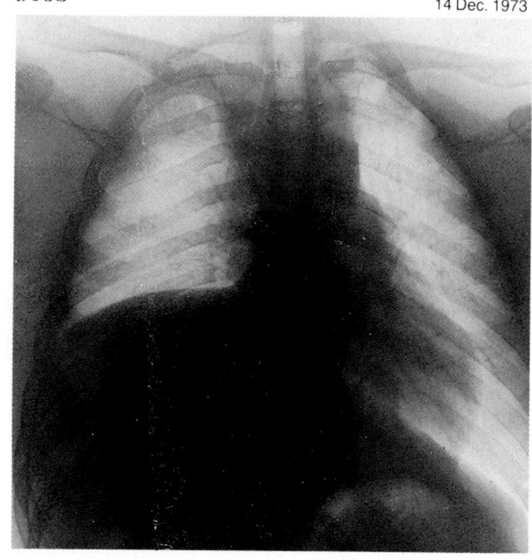

816a Rupture of the right upper lobe bronchus with a **massive air leak through the pleural drain.** The right upper lobe has been transfixed and lacerated by a chest tube (intended to drain a pneumothorax). The bronchial rupture and pulmonary laceration combine to leak massive volumes of air.

816b Recovery without sequelae after an emergency upper lobectomy.

817a

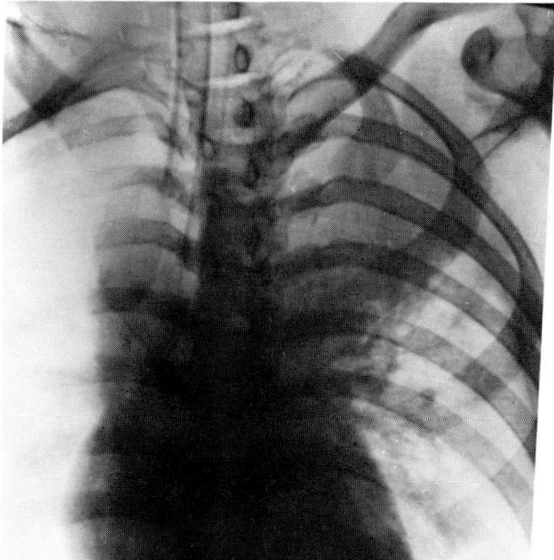

B.D. ♀ 21 yrs. 7 Feb. 1971

817b

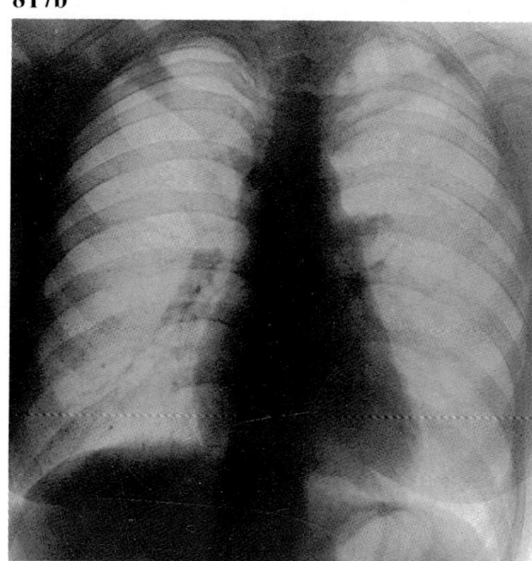

23 Feb. 1972

817a Bronchial rupture with **early atelectasis** in a car driver involved in a head-on collision. The patient was admitted with an incomplete rupture of the mucosa of both the trachea and the left main-stem bronchus (3 cm from the carina). Atelectasis quickly develops in the left upper lobe, presumably as a result of a haemorrhage within the bronchi. A left thoracotomy is performed on the unconfirmed suspicion of damage to a major vessel. The bronchial rupture is treated conservatively.

817b Complete recovery one year later.

Localisation

Rupture usually occurs within 2.5 cm of the carina. It is slightly more common on the right than on the left.

A number of pathological types of bronchial injury can be distinguished:

- complete *rupture* (whether total or partial) is usually transverse and is sometimes accompanied by dislocation of the distal portion of the bronchial tree,
- mucosal (and sometimes muscular) *laceration* without damage to the bronchial cartilages (incomplete rupture),
- *fracture* of the external cartilages not affecting the internal layers (incomplete rupture).

818

Pathology of bronchial rupture

COMMON TYPES

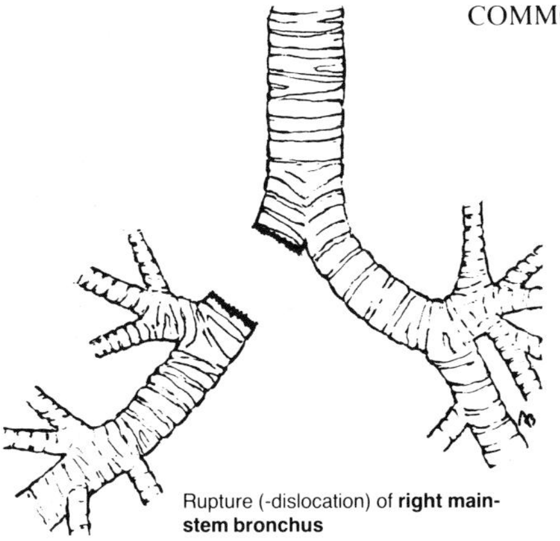

Rupture (-dislocation) of **right main-stem bronchus**

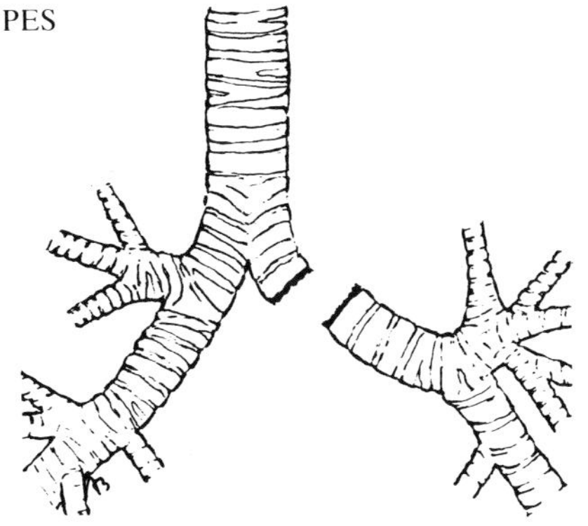

Rupture (-dislocation) of **left main-stem bronchus**

LESS COMMON TYPES

More complex variant

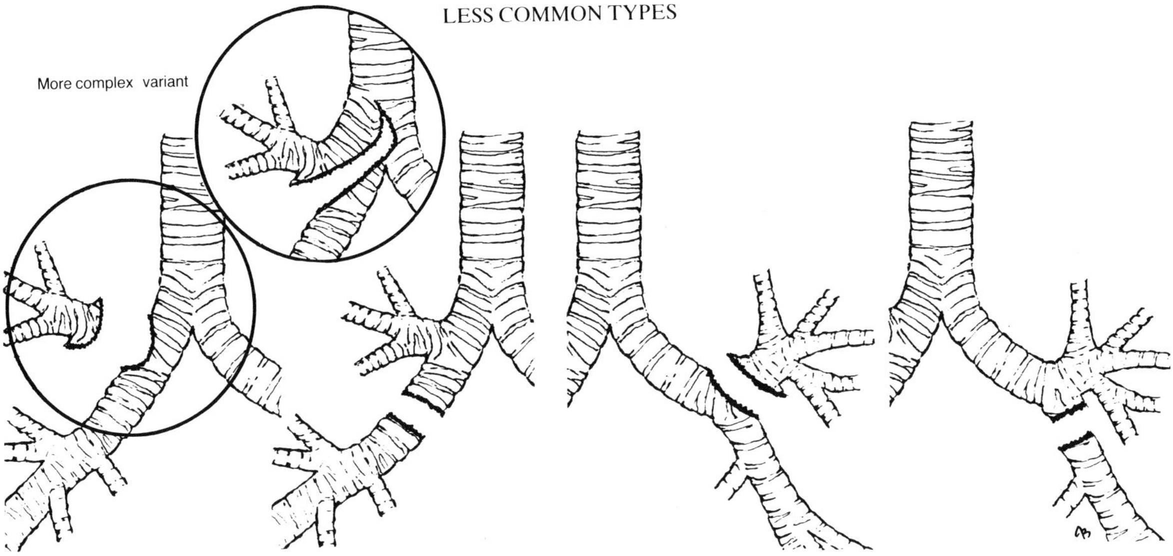

Rupture of **right upper lobe bronchus**

Rupture of **intermediate bronchus** (or below)

Rupture of **left upper lobe bronchus**

Rupture of **left lower lobe bronchus**

RARE TYPES

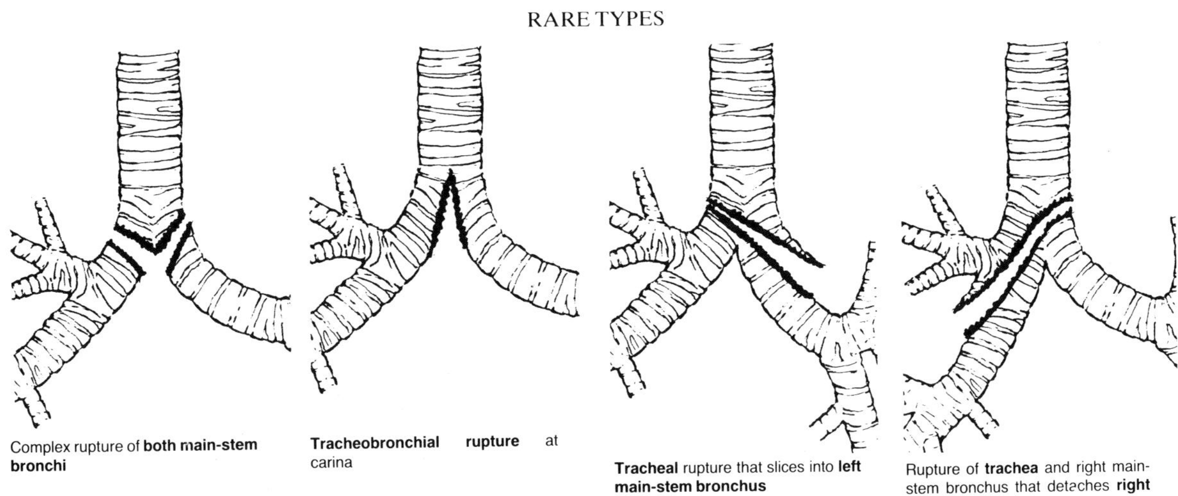

Complex rupture of **both main-stem bronchi**

Tracheobronchial rupture at carina

Tracheal rupture that slices into **left main-stem bronchus**

Rupture of **trachea** and right main-stem bronchus that detaches **right upper lobe bronchus**

819

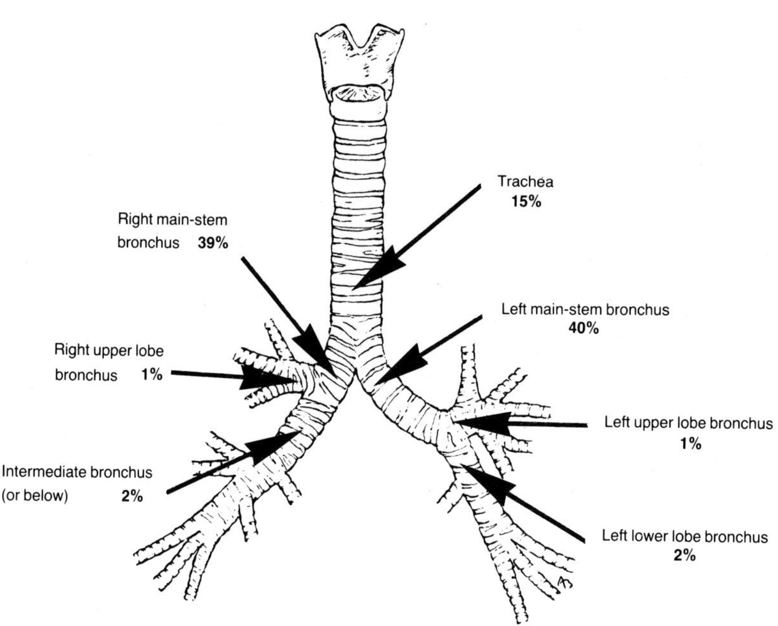

819 Tracheobronchial ruptures: General localisations (literature review)

820

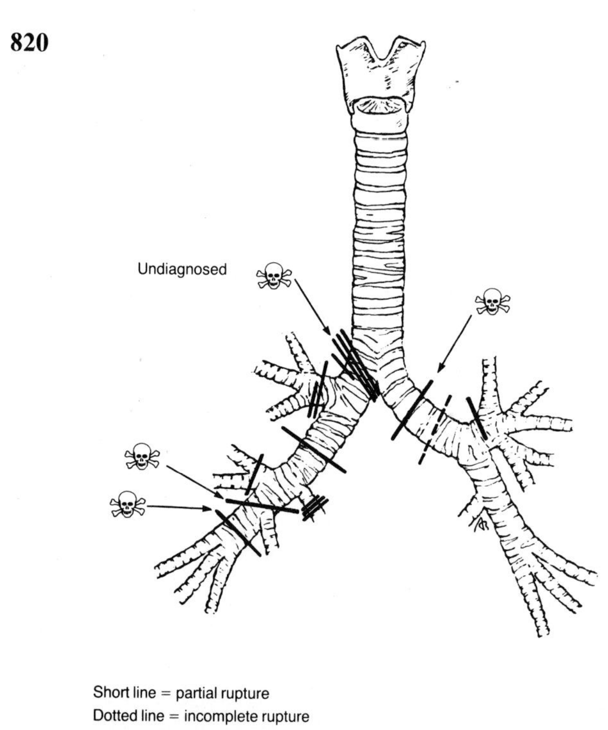

820 Rupture of major bronchi: specific localisations (in our material, $n = 16$).

821

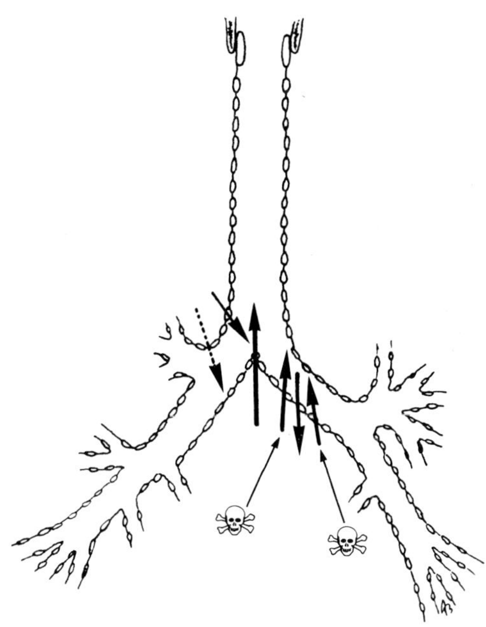

821 Perforation of major bronchi: localisation (in our material, $n = 6$).

Management

The following steps are recommended:

- immediate *resuscitation* with transfusion, oxygen administration, pleural drainage and, when necessary, mediastinal decompression.
- detailed *endoscopic examination* before tracheal intubation,
- early, direct *surgical repair*.

If a suspected or known bronchial rupture is accompanied by a pneumothorax, the pleural cavity should be drained before bronchoscopy. Care is needed for pleural aspiration can be dangerous; instead of inducing the lung to re-expand, suction may aspirate the entire air-intake and cause fatal asphyxia. The larger the rupture, the greater the likelihood of asphyxia during pleural aspiration.

If the pleural drain gives issue to large volumes of air, suction should be discontinued and the drain left in a water-seal bottle (Bülau). In the event of a massive air leak through the pleural drain, immediate intubation with a White or Carlens tube occasionally can save the patient's life. It is worth noting, however, that these tubes are too large to be used in young patients or children.

Bronchial rupture should be dissected and then repaired by direct, end-to-end anastomosis. It is best approached from the side of the pneumothorax (whether the pneumothorax be ipsi- or contra-lateral).

In instances where direct repair is impossible, it can be necessary to resect pulmonary parenchyma and/or to perform a sleeve resection. Every effort should be made to reimplant the intact lobes.

822

Early surgical repair of bronchial rupture

I. DIRECT REPAIR

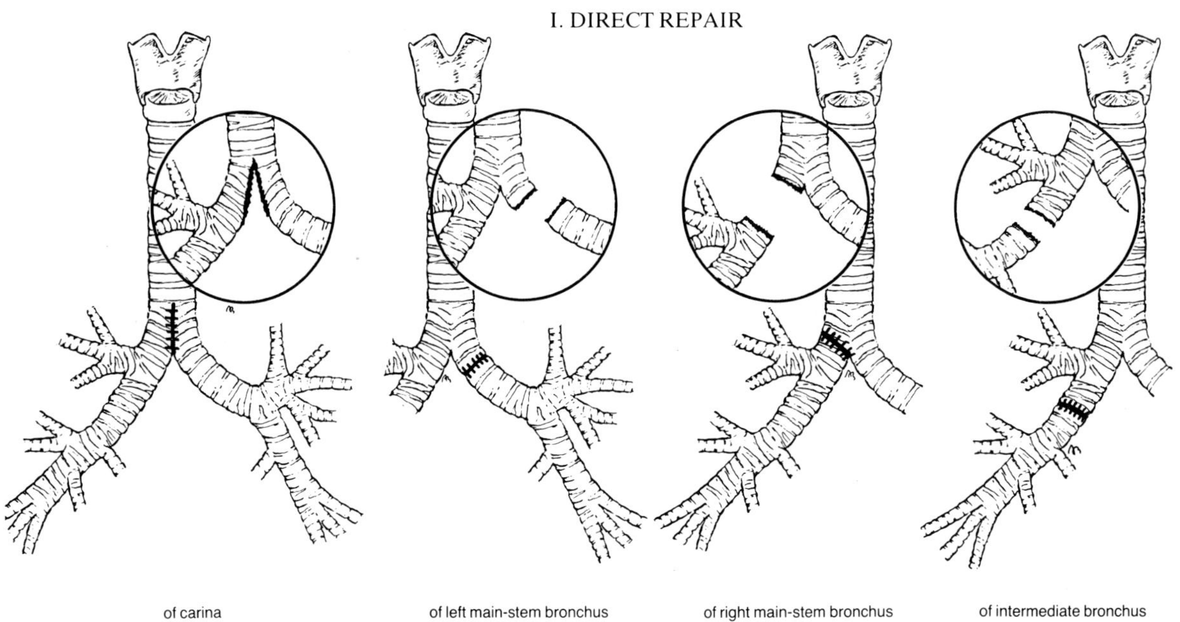

of carina | of left main-stem bronchus | of right main-stem bronchus | of intermediate bronchus

II. PULMONARY EXCISION (WITH POSSIBLE SLEEVE RESECTION OF BRONCHUS)

823

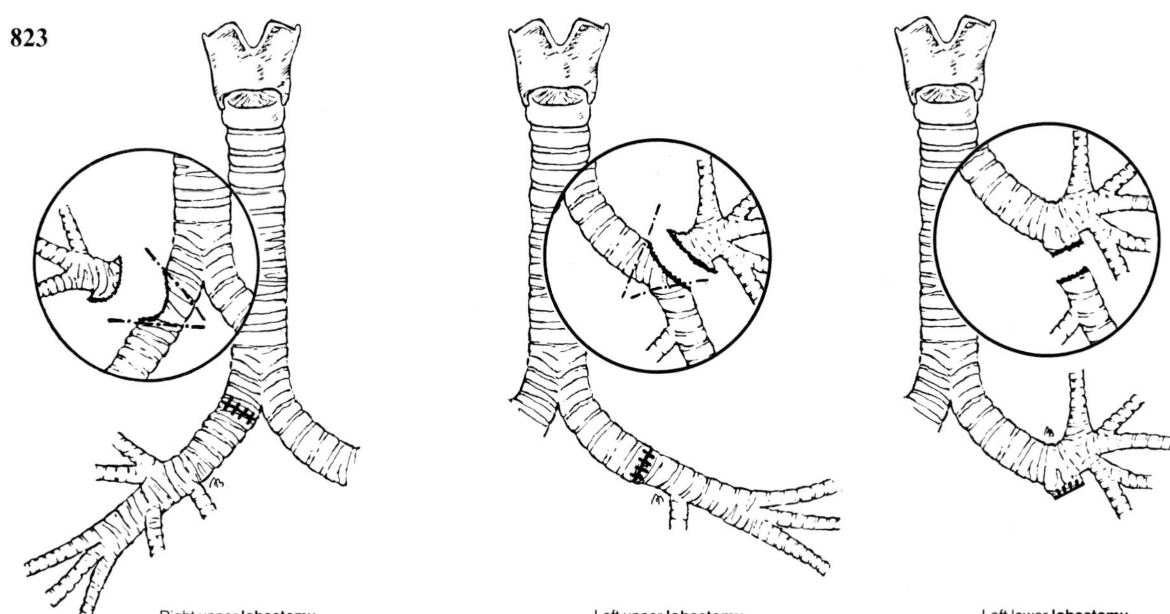

Right upper **lobectomy** | Left upper **lobectomy** | Left lower **lobectomy**

824

III. COMPLEX REIMPLANTATION

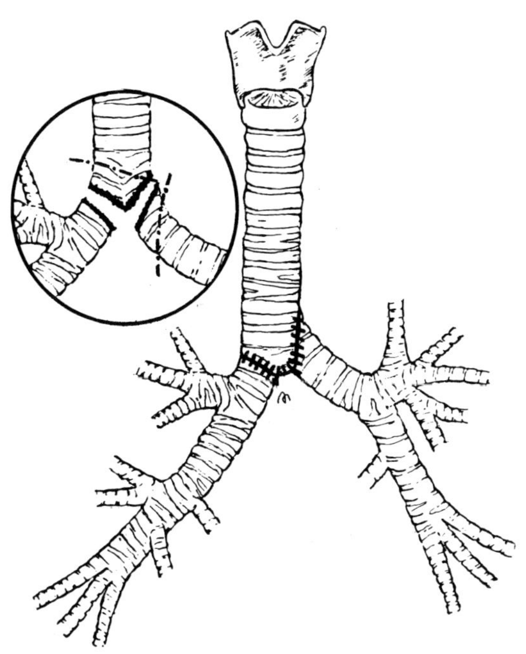

Direct repair of right main-stem and **reimplantation** of left main-stem into trachea

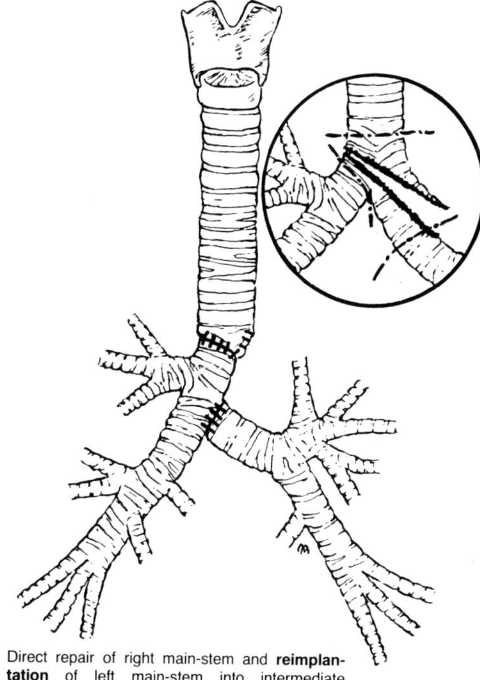

Direct repair of right main-stem and **reimplantation** of left main-stem into intermediate bronchus

IV. COMBINED EXCISION AND COMPLEX REIMPLANTATION

825

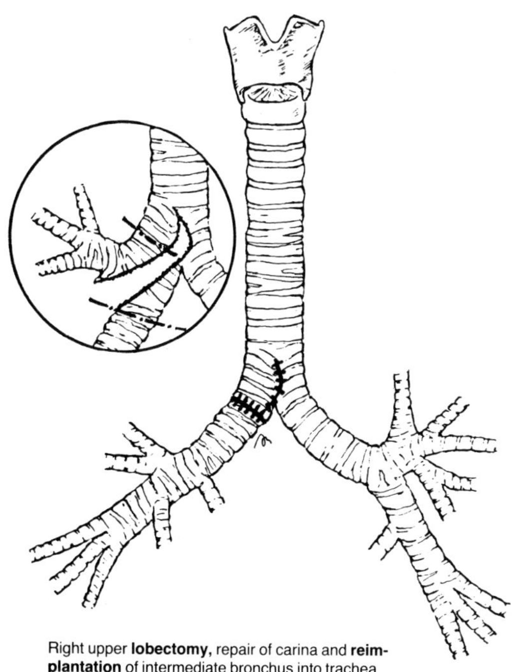

Right upper **lobectomy,** repair of carina and **reimplantation** of intermediate bronchus into trachea

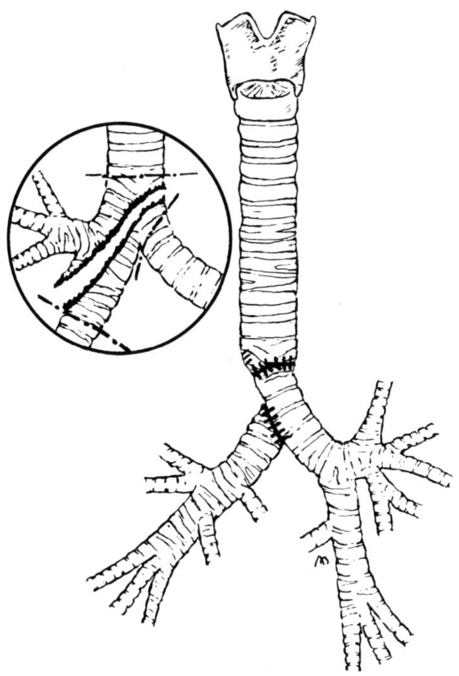

Right upper **lobectomy**, direct repair of left main-stem and **reimplantation** of intermediate bronchus into left main-stem

Evolution

Mortality is high. Even today, as many as 30 to 50% of patients alive on arrival are irretrievable. Death is usually early, and generally the result of asphyxia; the immediate cause can be either a highly compressive pneumothorax or a massive air-leak through the pleural drain.

On the other hand, patients who survive initially and are amenable to immediate surgery usually recover without complication. However, in view of the threat of late stenosis, no patient can be declared fully recovered until at least six months after surgery (see **828, 830**).

826a T.M. ♂ 27 yrs. 20 June 1975

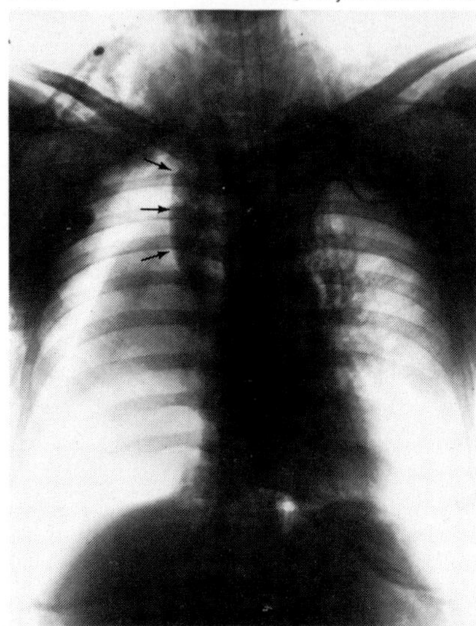

826a Rupture of right main-stem bronchus due to crush-injury. Immediate repair. Late stenosis. The patient was crushed between a fork-lift truck and a hydraulic press. Despite bilateral pleural drainage, there is a tension pneumothorax on either side. The anterior parts of both hemidiaphragms are inverted and there is massive subcutaneous emphysema.
(Fribourg Hospital)
N.B. A rupture of the subclavian artery and a mediastinal haematoma (→) will only be recognised five months later (see ***1003****).*

826b

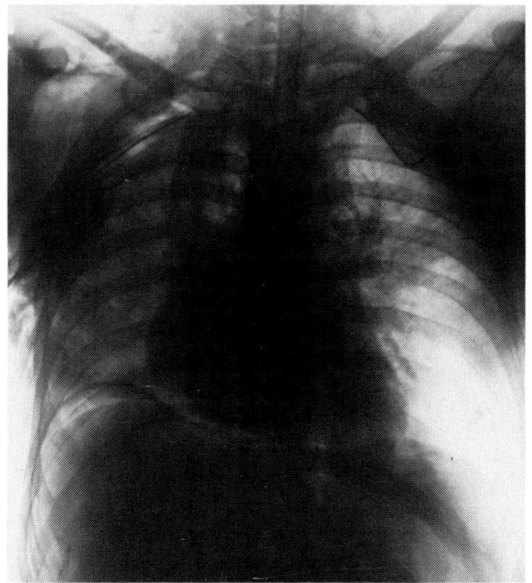

20 June 1975

826b The right lung re-expands after the introduction of a second pleural drain. The X-ray shows increasingly serious mediastinal emphysema (that has led to a pneumoperitoneum), and severe bilateral pulmonary contusion. A massive air-leak causes asphyxia. The patient has two cardiac arrests during a tracheobronchoscopy that reveals a longitudinal tear of the lower trachea and a dislocated rupture of the right main-stem bronchus.

826c

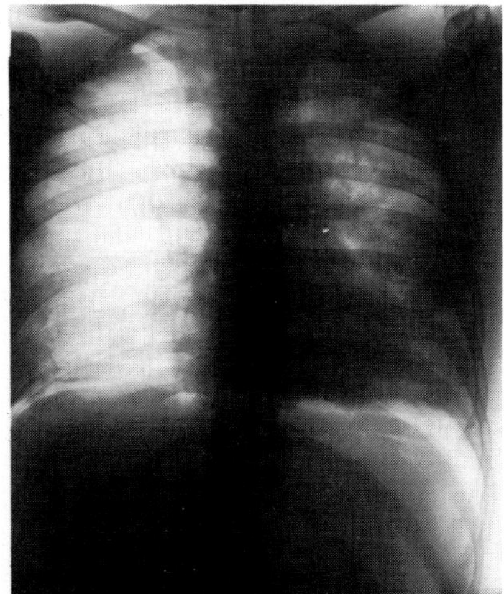

1 July 1975

826d

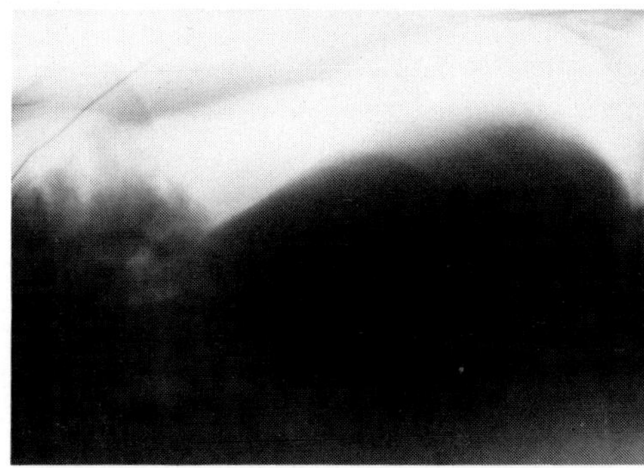

1 July 1975

826c The right lung is fully functional after direct repair of the bronchial rupture. The left lung remains radio-opaque despite positive pressure ventilation. The massive pneumoperitoneum persists.

826d The pneumoperitoneum seen with the patient lying on his left side. (Inselspital, Berne.)

826e

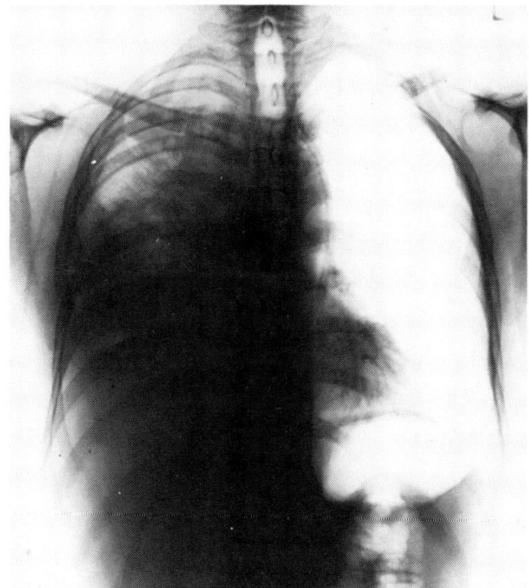

17 Nov. 1975

826f

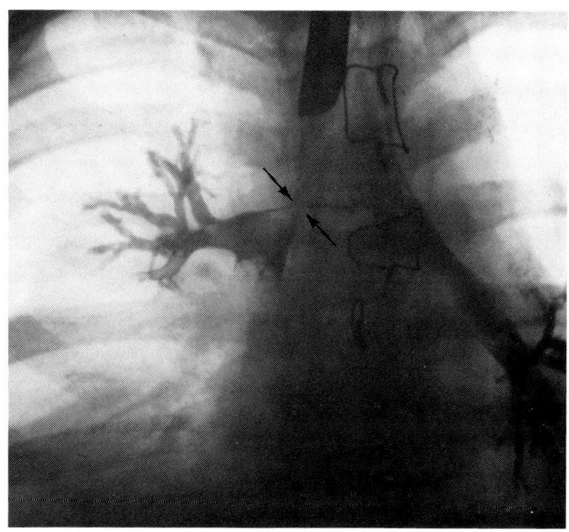

17 Nov. 1975

826g

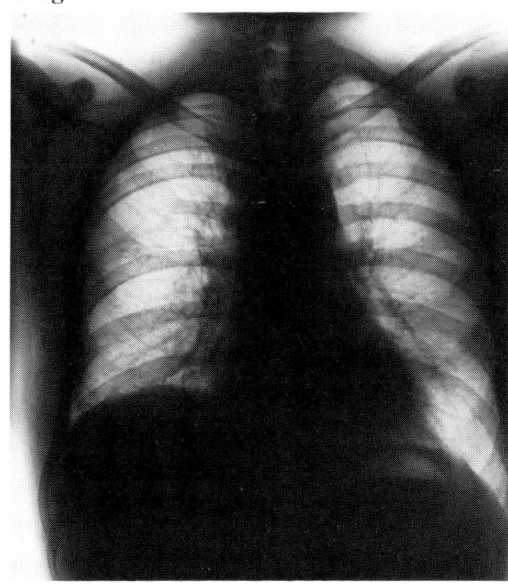

3 Dec. 1975

826e Five months after the accident, atelectasis of the right lung causes severe hypoxia.

826f Bronchography shows stenosis of the right main-stem bronchus at the suture line. Endoscopic cauterisation and excision of several granulomas from the sutures allow temporary re-expansion of the lung.

826g For three years, the right lung remains fully functional, but bronchial stenosis then recurs and right lung function is completely lost.

827

Spontaneous evolution of undetected bronchial rupture

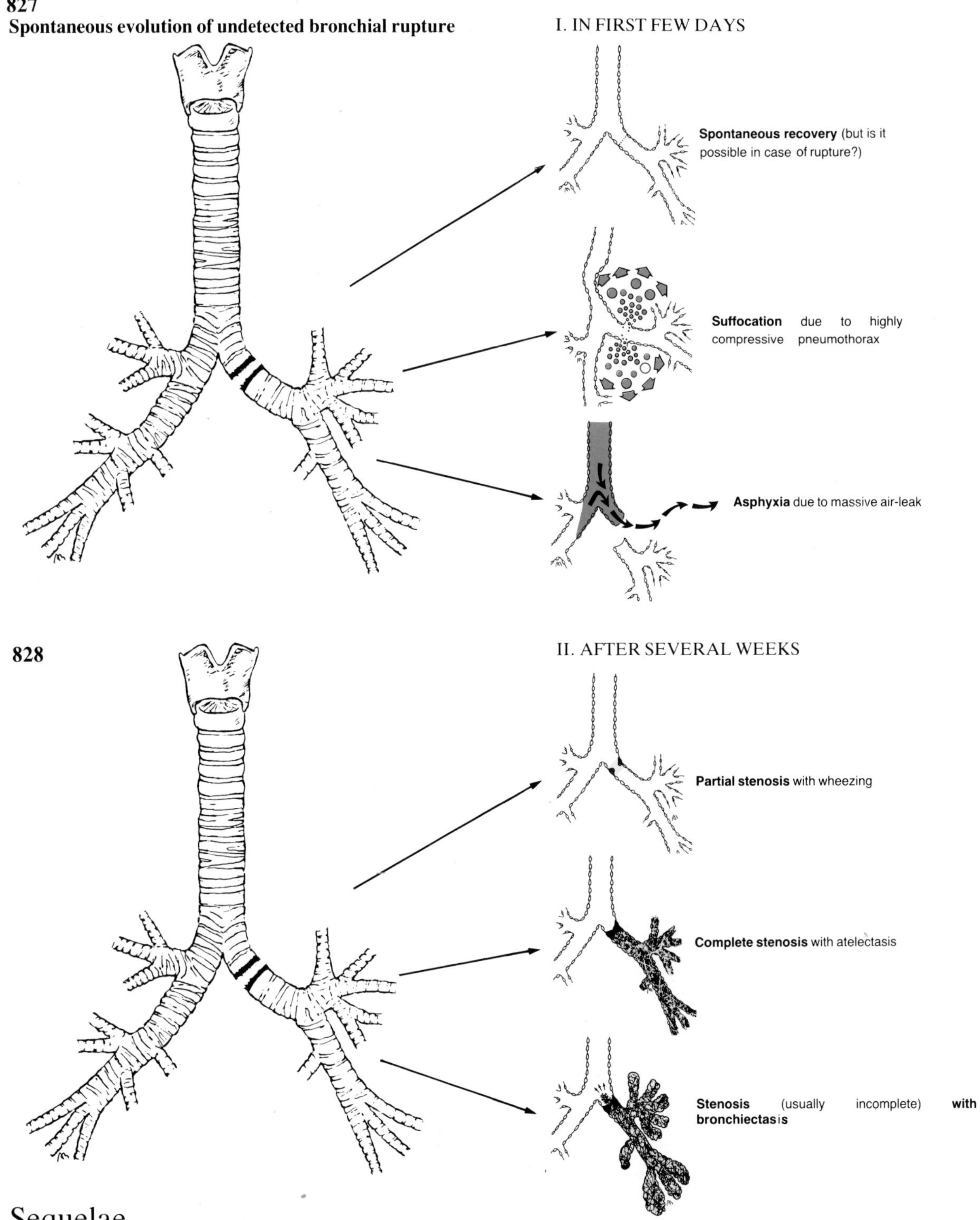

Sequelae

Some bronchial injuries, particularly tears, can heal without sequelae. Untreated ruptures, on the other hand, nearly always evolve through hypertrophic cicatrization to subtotal or total stenosis.

In cases where the distal portion of the bronchial tree has dislocated over several centimetres, stenosis is aggravated by the scarring of peribronchial tissues.

Partial bronchial stenosis can be relatively well tolerated (see **826g**). It is frequent, however, for the territory below the stenosis to become infected and to cause episodes of pulmonary suppuration. This, in turn, tends to aggravate the stenosis and induce gradual bronchiectasis with lung abscesses.

829
Treatment of post-traumatic bronchial stenosis

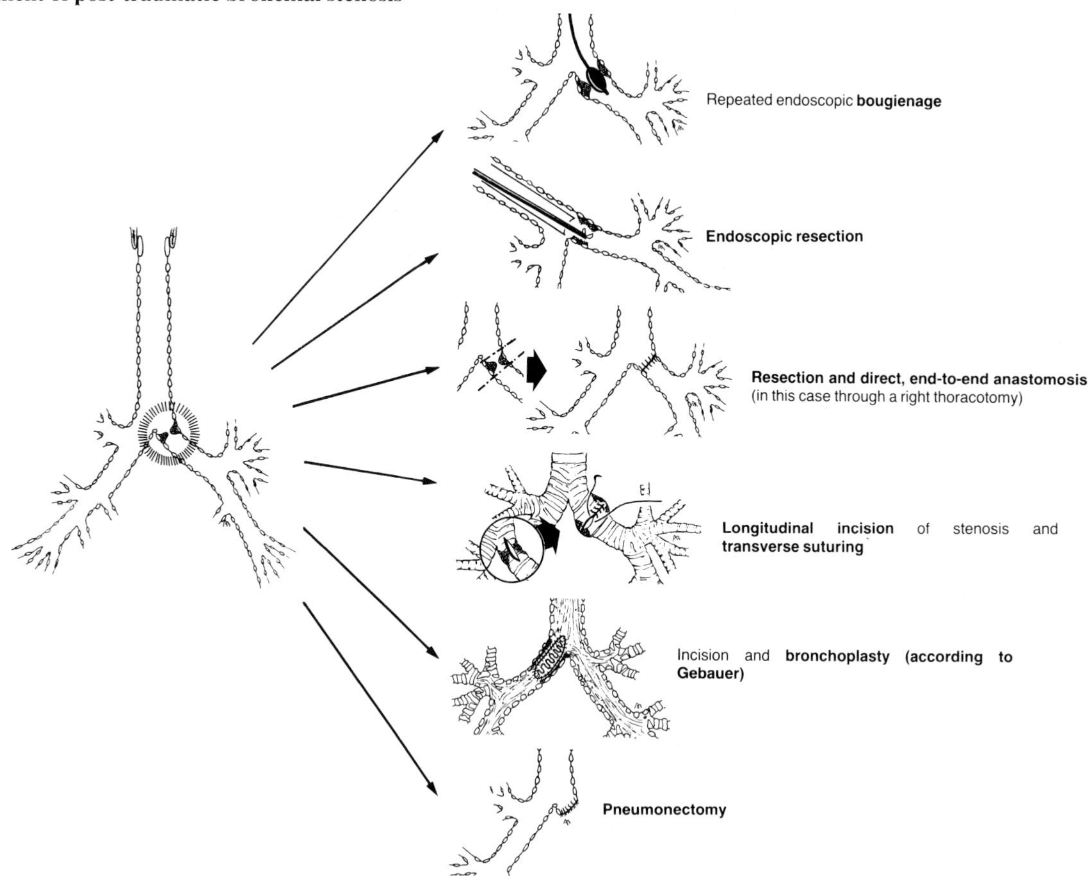

In cases of complete stenosis, bronchiectasis arise not from infection but from the fact that the sealed bronchi continue to secrete mucus until they are full to capacity (see **830h**).

Occasionally, when the pulmonary parenchyma has not been damaged too severely, it can be reventilated by excision of the stenosis and end-to-end anastomosis. However, reventilation is sometimes unavailing, for inactivity soon destroys the capacity of the alveolar walls to transfer oxygen.

Both during rupture and repair, the fine and sensitive nerves going to the distal portion of the bronchial tree are often torn. The resultant *decrease in bronchial sensitivity* entails the loss of the cough reflex, and the accumulation and possible infection of the mucus secretions. This is an aspect of bronchial rupture about which little is known.

The bronchial arteries, too, are nearly always either torn as the bronchus ruptures or ligated during repair. Experiments on dogs suggest that the pulmonary vessels can supply the necessary blood, but they also show that interruption of the bronchial arteries predisposes to late bronchiectasis.

Post-traumatic bronchial stenosis occurs in one or other main-stem in 75% of cases and very often results in the functional exclusion of one lung. The repercussions are three-fold:

- **respiratory** – 50% reduction in vital capacity or maximum ventilation.
- **cardiac** – such a large reduction in the vital capacity or in maximum ventilatory volume demands vigorous compensatory effort from the heart.
- **circulatory** – because of extensive vascular shunting.

The right-to-left shunt caused by pulmonary exclusion is aggravated by a left-to-right shunt from the dilated bronchial arteries to the pulmonary veins. Post-traumatic bronchial stenosis, therefore, is seriously incapacitating.

At present, bronchial rupture with stenosis is treated by:

– resection with end-to-end anastomosis in	73% of cases
– lobectomy in	8% of cases
– pneumonectomy in	18% of cases
– conservative treatment in	2% of cases

830a

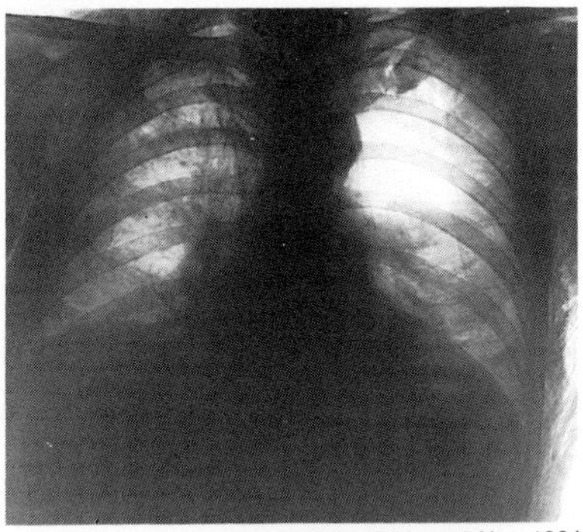

B.A. ♂ 54 yrs. 5 Nov. 1964

830b

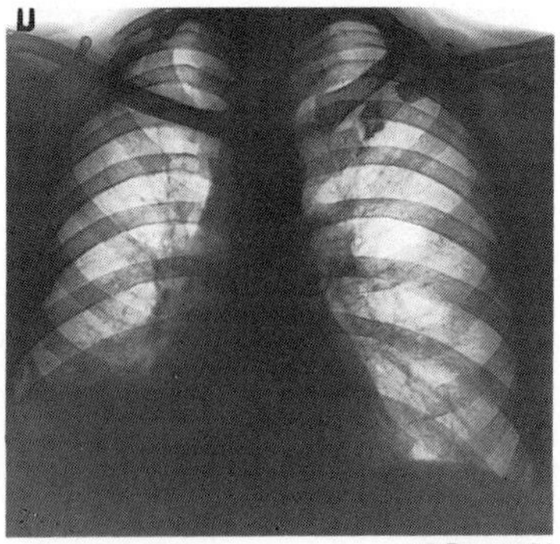

18 Dec. 1964

830c

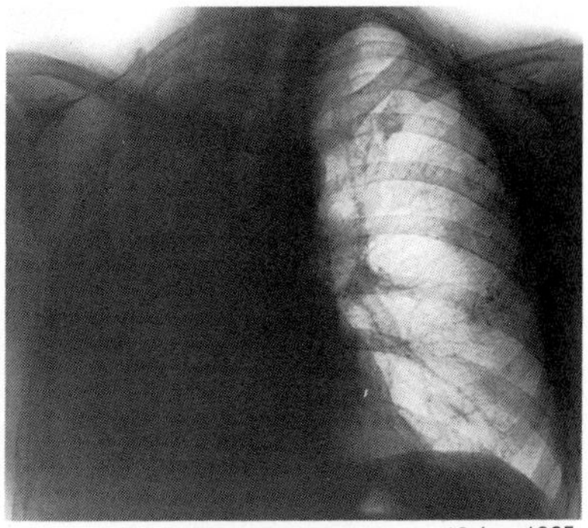

13 Jan. 1965

830d

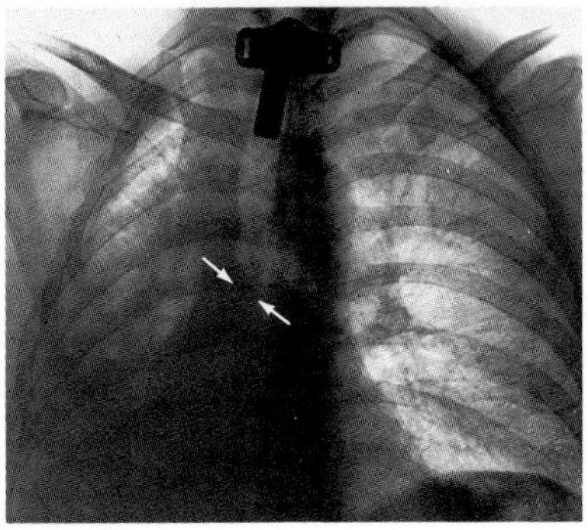

15 Jan. 1965

830e

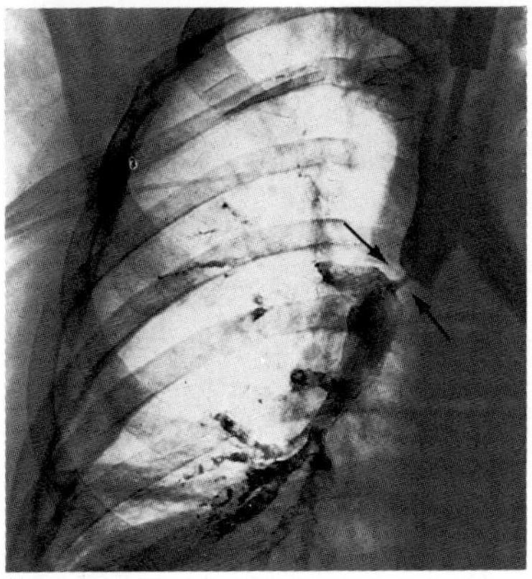

27 Jan. 1965

830f

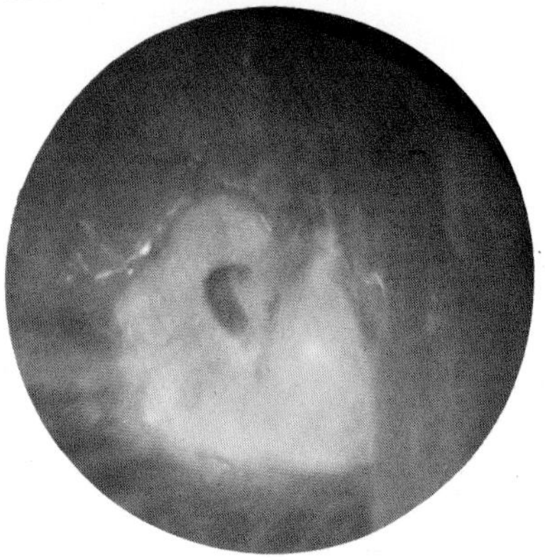

27 Jan. 1965

830g

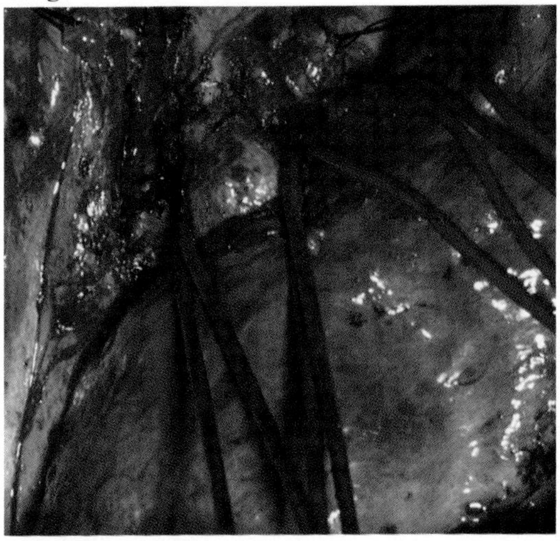

2 Feb. 1965

830h

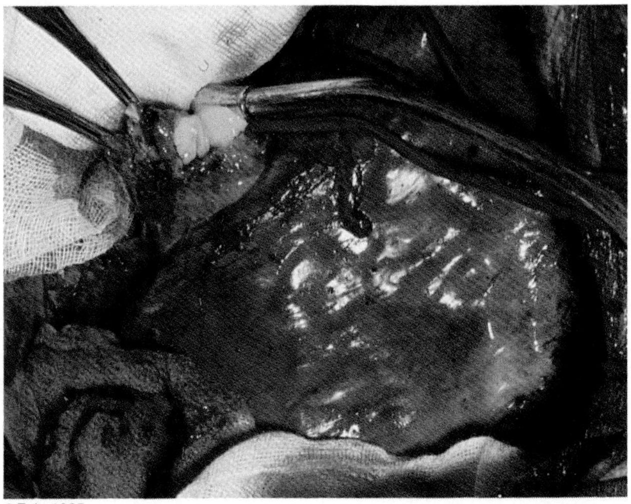

2 Feb. 1965

830a Spontaneous cicatricial stenosis 10 weeks after undetected rupture of right main-stem bronchus. The patient sustained a violent impact against the steering wheel of his car when he hit a tree without braking. On admission he presented subcutaneous emphysema, a flail chest with paradoxical motion, a left pneumothorax and fractures of the vertebral column and clavicle.

830b Six weeks later, the patient's X-ray is apparently satisfactory.

830c However, complete atelectasis of the right lung appears two months after the accident. The paradoxical motion persists.

830d The upper lobe re-expands to some extent after a tracheostomy for bronchial toilet. It is clear from the air bronchogram that the right main-stem bronchus is occluded (→), but this passed unnoticed at the time.

830i

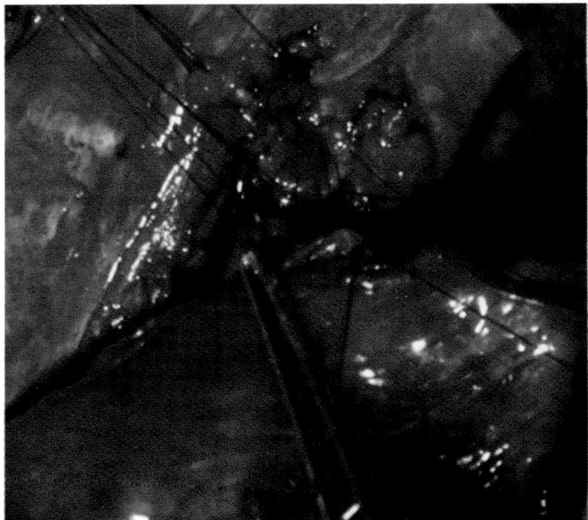

2 Feb. 1965

830 l

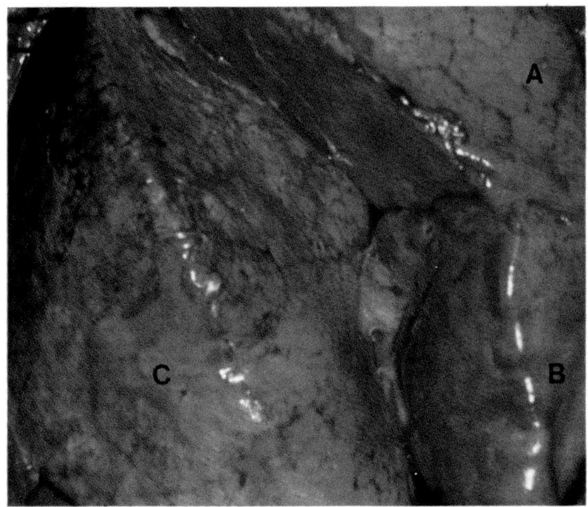

2 Feb. 1965

830k

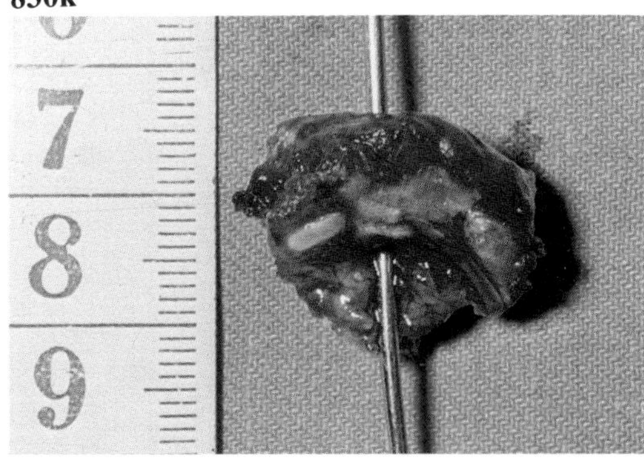

2 Feb. 1965

830e A full ten weeks elapse before bronchography is performed: total rupture of the right main-stem bronchus has resulted in almost complete stenosis (→). Below, the sealed bronchial tree is dilated by accumulated mucus.

830f Endoscopic view of the fibrous, cicatricial stenosis.

830g Right thoracotomy to prepare the main-stem bronchus and lower trachea.
N.B. Complete atelectasis of the right lung.

830h Mucus wells up when the bronchus is opened below the stenosis.

830i The stenosed area is excised, and end-to-end anastomosis achieved.

830k The bronchial lumen has a diameter of 1mm (Operative specimen).

830 l Repair leads to the immediate re-expansion of the upper (A), middle (B) and lower (C) lobes of the right lung.

830m

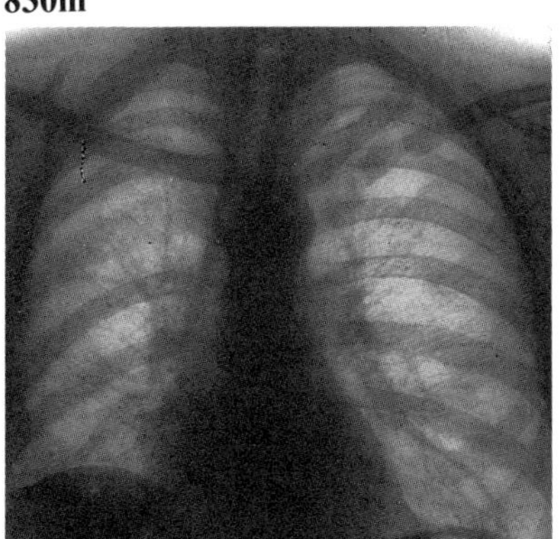

21 Apr. 1965

830n

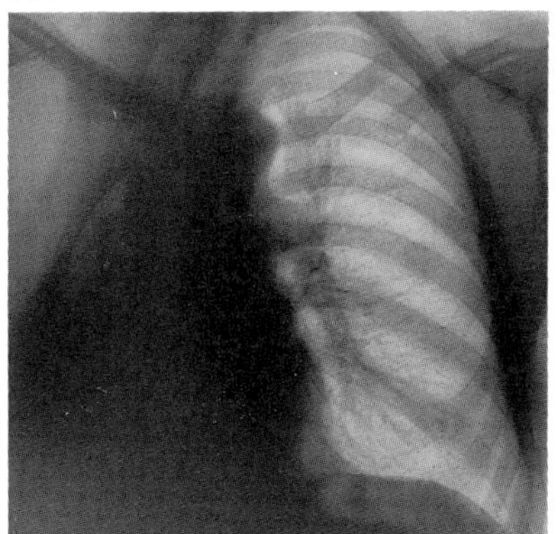

18 Oct. 1965

830m Subsequent partial dehiscence of the suture line does not affect ventilation initially but . . .
830n . . . residual empyema ultimately will necessitate a right pneumonectomy and an upper thoracoplasty. Recovery with major ventilatory sequelae.

Open wounds of the trachea and major bronchi

Open wounds of the trachea usually occur in the neck. The cause can be a bullet, a piece of shrapnel, a knife, a razor or any other sharp instrument. Peace-time injuries are often due to suicide or murder attempts but, even in areas with a high crime rate, this type of wound is rarely seen on the operating table. There are several reasons for this:

- the trachea is largely protected by the lower mandible and sternum;
- both the cervical and thoracic portions are highly mobile and are more easily displaced than injured;
- serious wounds tend either to be immediately fatal, or to be accompanied by fatal damage to vital adjacent organs.

If the tracheal wound is small, and if there is no accompanying injury to the great vessels, the risk of asphyxia is small. The likely signs are coughing and haemoptysis, rapidly followed by massive subcutaneous and mediastinal emphysema.

A large wound, on the other hand, takes the form of a tracheostome, or even of total section. The risk of asphyxia and massive haemorrhage is correspondingly high.

Most open tracheal wounds require emergency repair, though very small wounds occasionally can be left to cicatrize spontaneously. The damage is best evaluated endoscopically.

Depending upon the circumstances, it can be prudent to protect the tracheal sutures for about ten days with a tracheostomy or a nasotracheal tube. It is often necessary to drain subcutaneous emphysema.

Stab or gunshot wounds of the major bronchi are almost invariably accompanied by fatal mediastinal injuries. However, on the rare occasion when death is not immediate, the bronchial wound can be treated surgically as a rupture or perforation.

831

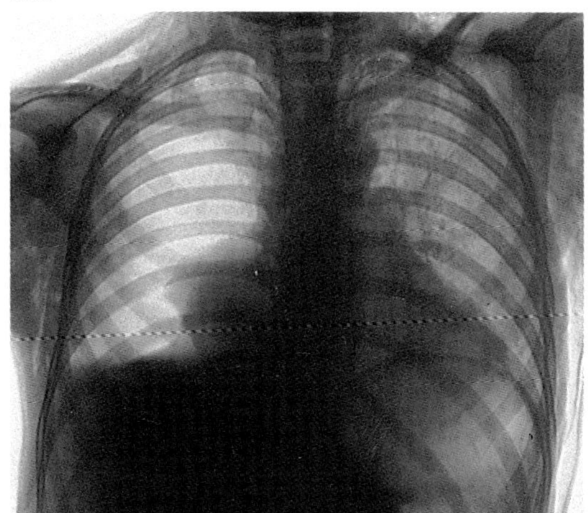

D.L. ♂ 9 yrs. 6 Feb. 1953

831 Tracheobronchial perforation by impalement. The child was lying on a sledge when it hurtled into a car. The starting-handle penetrated the neck low-down on the right, and perforated the junction between the trachea and the right main-stem bronchus. On admission, the child was in respiratory distress and had a complete right pneumothorax with massive subcutaneous emphysema.

Immediate right thoracotomy for tracheobronchial repair. Recovery. No sequelae on 26-year follow-up.

8 Trauma of the heart and pericardium

Incidence

Any chest trauma can result in injury to the heart and/or pericardium: seemingly slight contusion of the anterior chest wall, for example, can cause rhythm disturbances, ischaemia, myocardial infarction, rupture . . . with all their potentially fatal complications.

As the volume of traffic on the roads has increased, so injuries to the heart and pericardium have become more frequent. Today, 6% of all serious chest injuries include damage to the heart, and over 67% of all cardiac traumas are the result of road accidents (40% of which involve car occupants).

75% of the victims are males; their average age is 37 years.

Diagnosis

The admission of a patient with an injury to the heart or to its pedicles is often dramatic. Examination and emergency treatment are immediately the surgeon's responsibility.

Cardiac tamponade in particular demands swift and subtle diagnosis. In cardiac tamponade, shock is cardiogenic and should not be mistaken for hypovolaemic shock, for which the treatment is essentially different.

Tamponade

Symptoms:
- mid-thoracic constrictive **pain**
- severe **dyspnoea,** easing in the sitting position

Signs:
- head, neck and upper chest **cyanosis**
- **dilatation of the jugular veins,** sometimes increasing on inspiration
- **hypotension** and a decrease in the arterial pressure-differential
- **tachycardia**
- **paradoxical pulse** with a 10 to 20mm Hg drop in arterial pressure at the end of the inspiratory phase (Kussmaul's pulse). However, this sign is of little practical value: it is difficult to interpret in the general agitation that surrounds a severe chest case and, in fact, a reliable assessment can be achieved only on the rare occasion when arterial pressure can be monitored continuously by direct catheterisation
- **muffled heart sounds** with occasional pericardial rub. This sign again is often difficult to interpret, for the audibility of heart sounds depends fundamentally upon the physical constitution of the patient. Moreover, concomitant parietal and/or pleuropulmonary damage sometimes entirely precludes sensitive auscultation.

Paraclinical data:
- **central venous pressure** rises above 20cm H_2O (and sometimes as high as 40cm H_2O)
- **the electrocardiogram** shows a QRS wave of low voltage, especially in the precordial leads
- **standard chest X-ray** may usefully demonstrate other thoracic injuries, but usually offers little specific evidence in cases of *acute* heart trauma. The emergency X-ray is usually obtained from short distance, in difficult conditions and with the recumbent patient in incomplete inspiration: all these factors predispose to pseudo-widening of the mediastinum (see page 130). Nevertheless, in the case of *subacute* or *chronic* tamponade, the classic radiological signs of pericardial effusion are usually clear
- **ultrasonography or echography** can document pericardial effusion within minutes – provided, of course, that the necessary technicians are available
- **computerised tomography** can be used to investigate the possibility of an intrapericardial fluid collection
- **a pericardial tap** releasing pressurised blood or fluid provides confirmation of tamponade.

832

832 Post-traumatic cardiac tamponade is due to:
(in our material, n = 36)

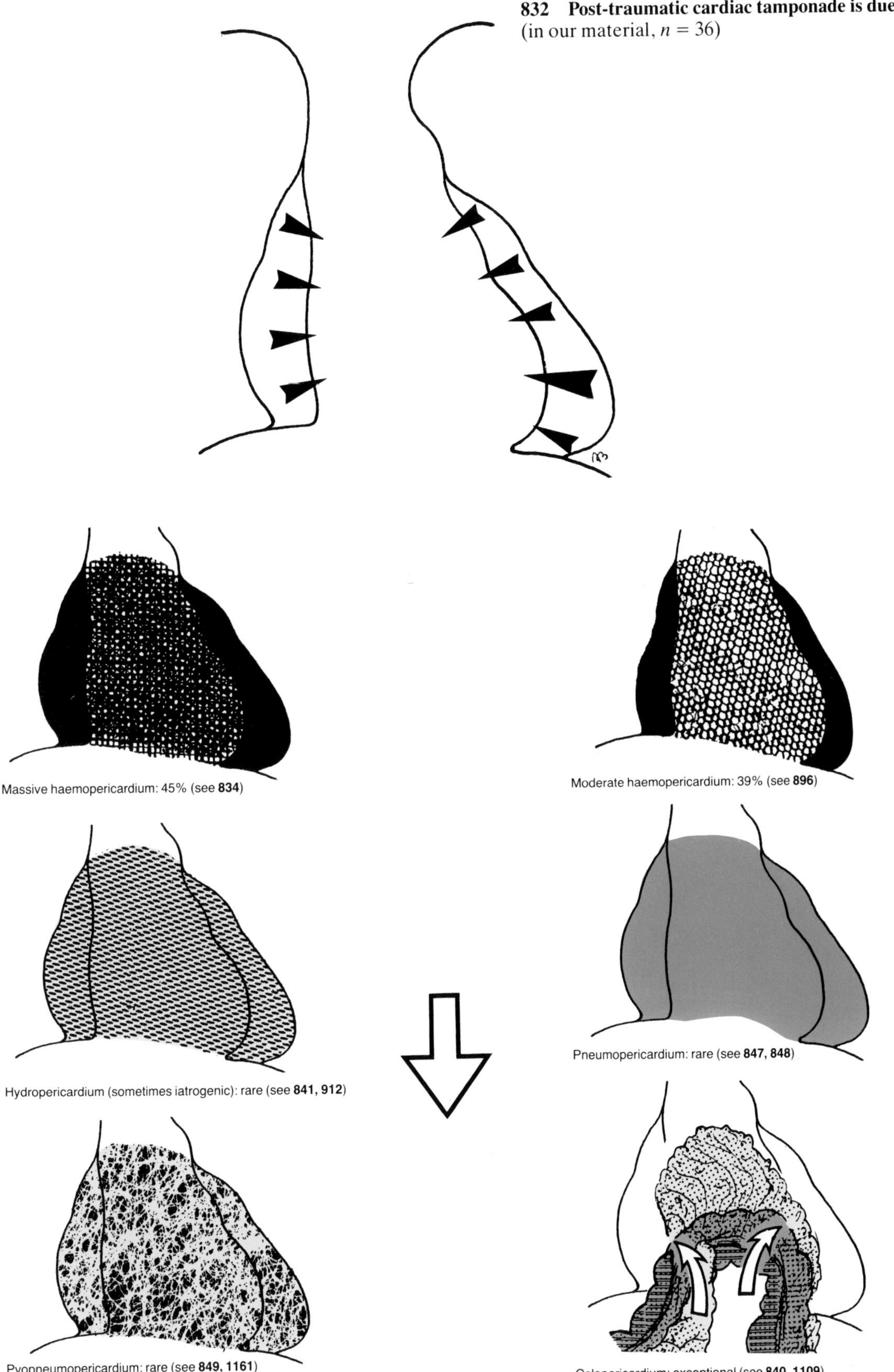

Physiopathology

833

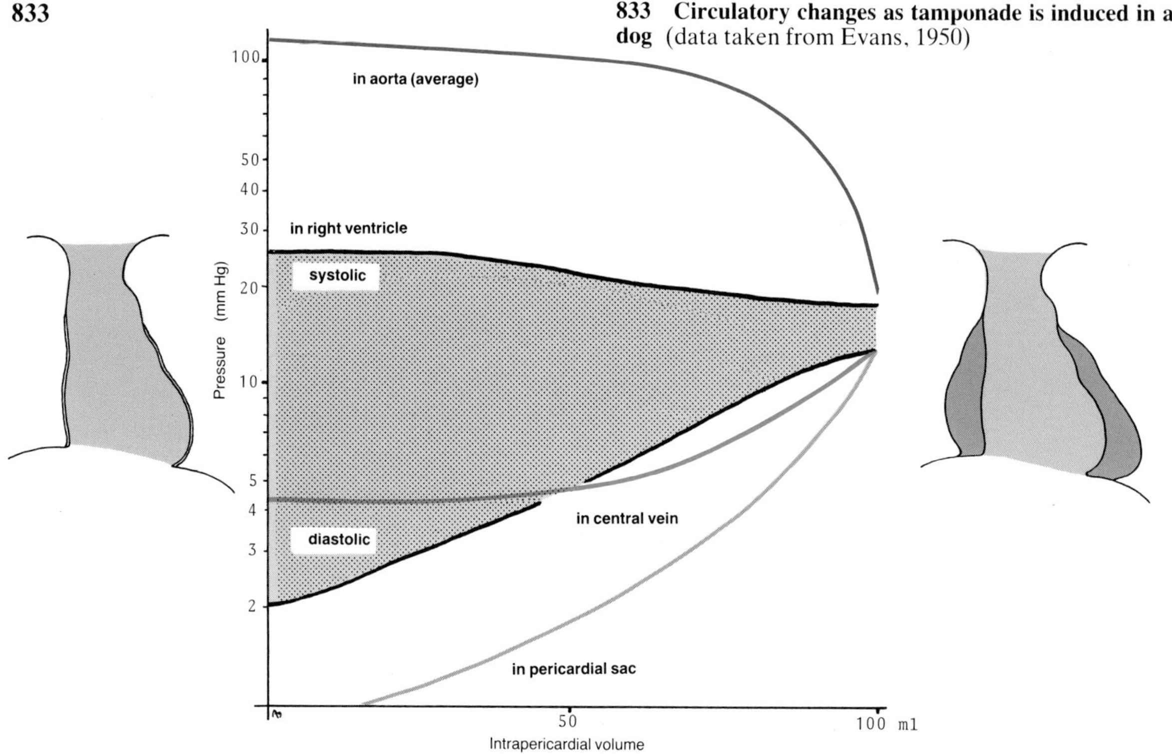

833 Circulatory changes as tamponade is induced in a dog (data taken from Evans, 1950)

Acute tamponade

The triad (1) cardiogenic shock, (2) high central venous pressure and (3) muffled heart sounds, suggests acute tamponade and calls for immediate pericardiocentesis. Aspiration of only a few ml of pericardial fluid usually results in a dramatic clinical improvement (see **837**).

834 Cardiac tamponade due to 600 ml clotted haemopericardium. The outline of the heart is only slightly enlarged. Death from accompanying brain injuries a few minutes after admission.

834

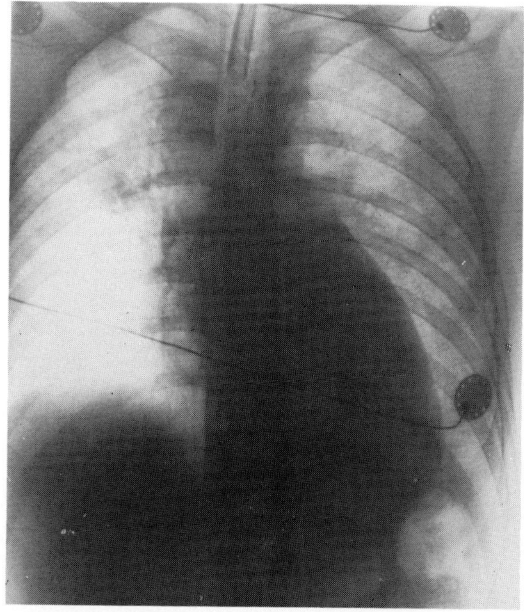

Subacute and chronic tamponade

Diagnosis of subacute or chronic tamponade is less pressing and, as a rule, relatively straightforward; the clinical signs are less marked than in the case of acute tamponade, but the radiological and ultrasonographic signs are usually clear.

Only rarely is haemopericardium the cause of subacute or chronic tamponade. There are a number of other more common causes (see **832, 841**).

Management

Resuscitation

As for initial resuscitative manoeuvres, a compromise is to be found between rapid transfusion (or perfusion) in the case of haemorrhagic shock, and restriction of intravenous fluids in the case of cardiogenic shock (tamponade, cardiac contusion). Pre-operative resuscitation should be as brief as possible.

Pericardiocentesis

Pericardiocentesis on suspicion of haemopericardium is *falsely negative* in *25% – 40% of cases*; this is often because the haemopericardium has clotted, or because the needle becomes obstructed during puncture. On the other hand, the tap is *falsely positive* in about *15% of cases*. In any event, pericardiocentesis is *rarely competely effective*; pericardiotomy shows that blood (be it liquid or clotted) persists in large quantity in most cases where the pericardial sac was thought to have been evacuated completely.

Emergency surgery is indicated, therefore, regardless of the origin of the tamponade, regardless of whether the initial trauma was open or blunt and regardless of whether the blood in the pericardium is dark or bright red.

At the beginning of the century, when surgery was still little developed, conservative treatment prevailed and few operations were performed: 60% of patients died.

It has since become evident that a favourable prognosis depends upon early intervention. Surgery alone makes it possible to identify and treat the source of the bleeding. The delay should be as short as possible – the time to prepare a theatre and to undertake the necessary resuscitative manoeuvres.

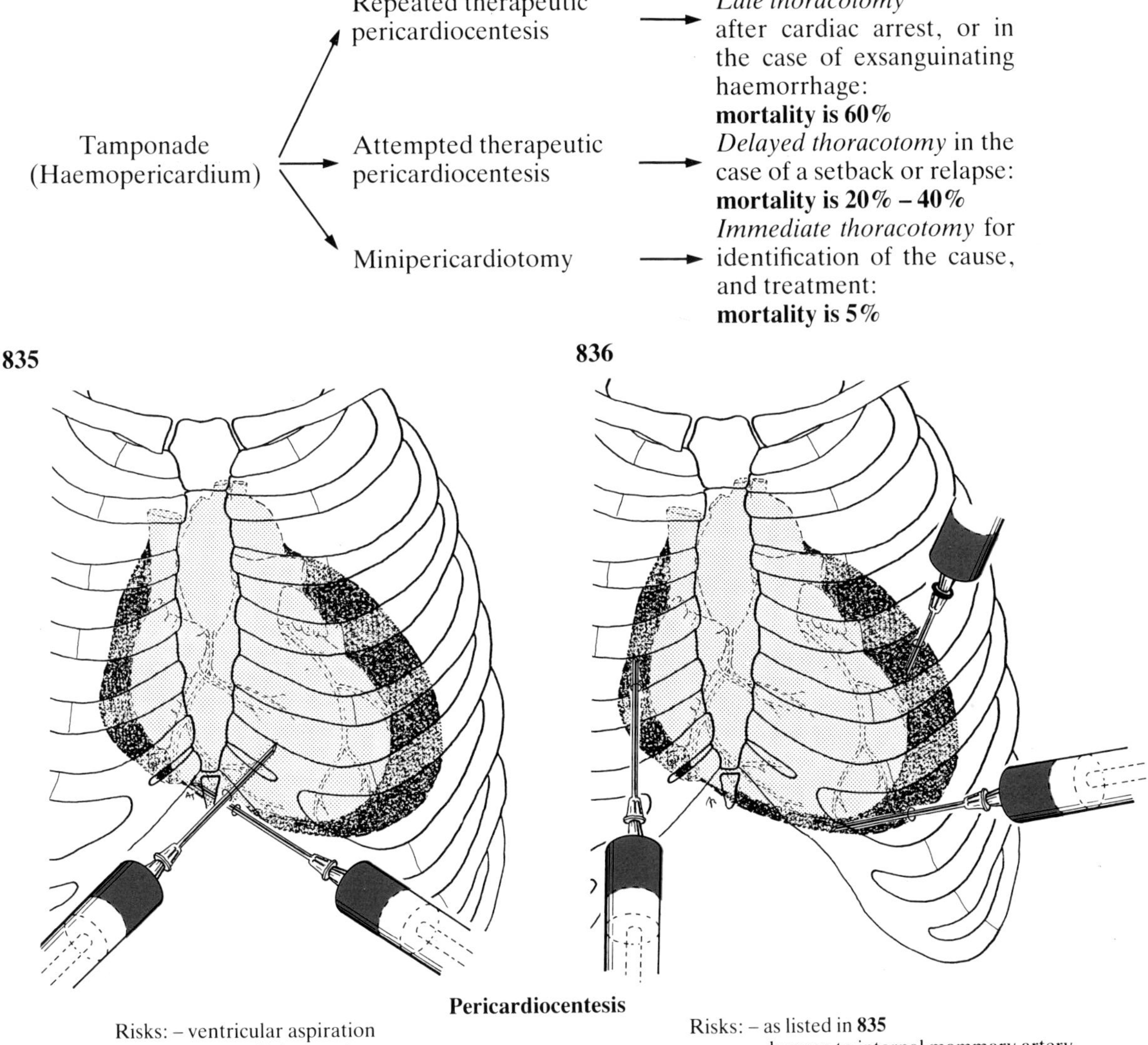

Pericardiocentesis

Risks: – ventricular aspiration
– myocardial wound
– coronary artery section

835 Classic subxiphoid approach

Risks: – as listed in **835**
– damage to internal mammary artery

836 Left intercostal approach – high (4th space) or low (6th space), or high right intercostal approach.

837

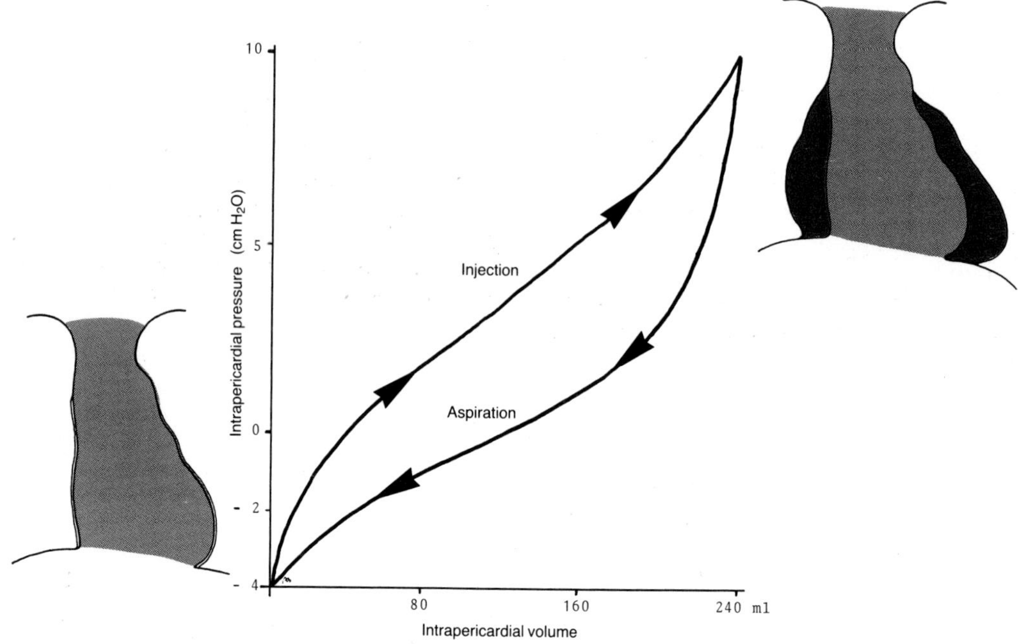

837 During pericardiocentesis, intrapericardial pressure falls faster than it rose (drawn on Morgan's data, 1965).

838

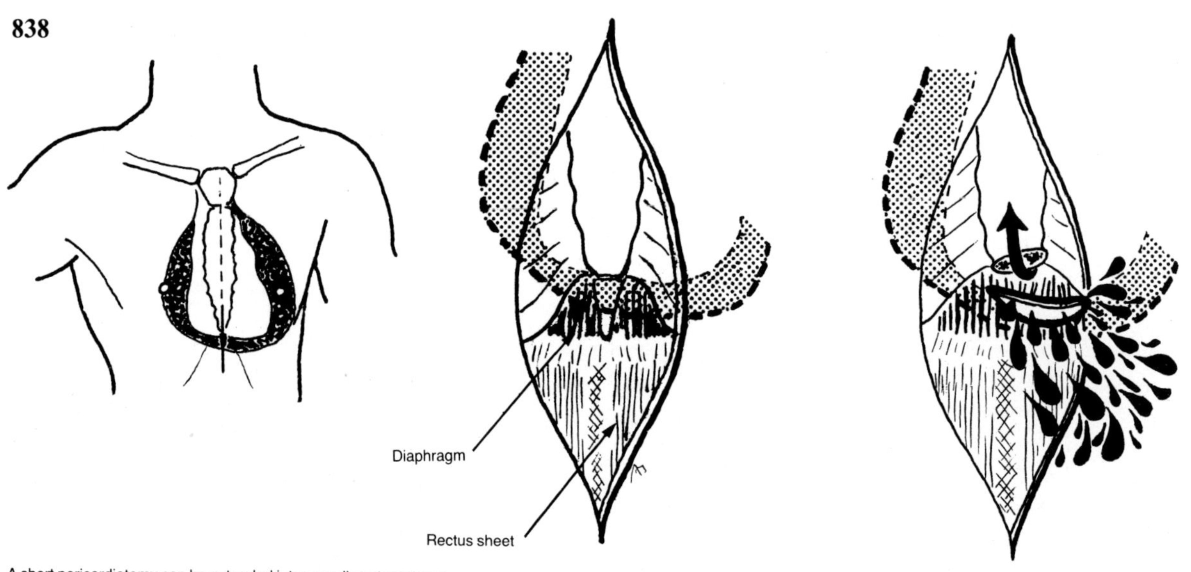

838 Exploratory minipericardiotomy for cardiac tamponade

Continuous drainage of the pericardium for non-bloody effusion

This can be effected by means of a fine drain, but the procedure is not recommended because of the attendant risks and nursing difficulties.

Indeed, if one or more pericardiocentesis can completely suppress the subacute or chronic tamponade, continuous drainage is superfluous.

Direct surgical approach

According to the location of suspected injuries – taking account of X-ray findings and, in cases of perforation, of the position of the entry (and exit) wound – an anterolateral thoracotomy (in the 4th or 5th intercostal space) on the side of the lesion is to be recommended. If the injury is known to be within the pericardial sac, a median sternotomy may be preferred.

As far as possible, aggravation of previous damage to the thoracic walls should be avoided during pericardial exposure. However, at the same time, scope should be left for exploring and treating injuries to adjacent structures. The possible necessity of subdiaphragmatic exploration should be kept in mind.

839

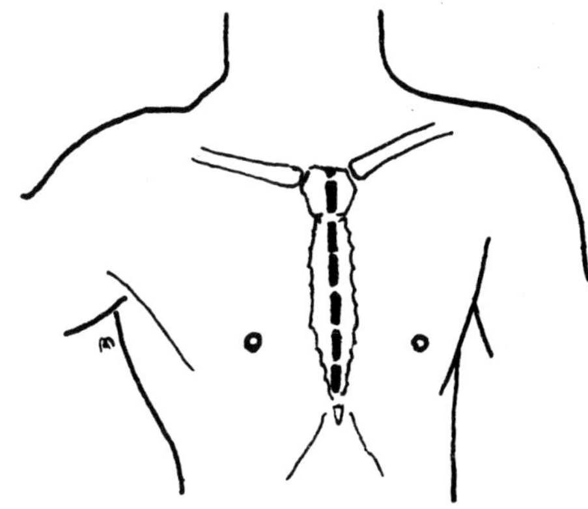

When the cause is known to be cardiac or pericardial

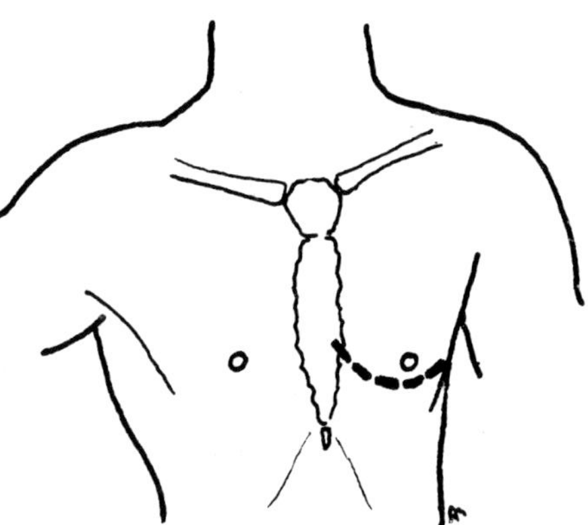

When the cause is unknown

839 Surgical approach for cardiac tamponade

840

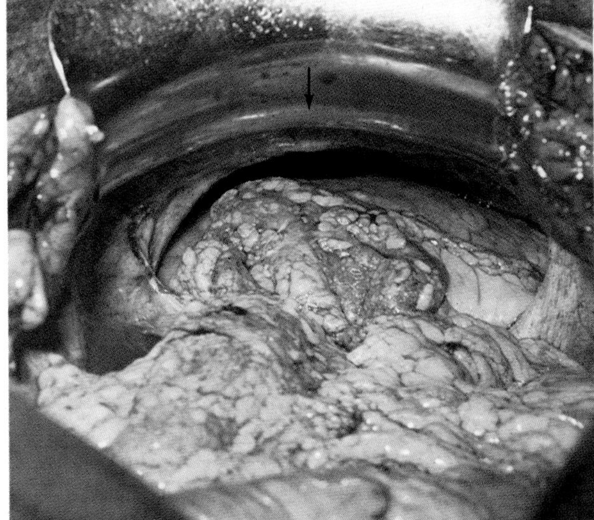

N.P. ♂ 69 yrs. 22 Oct. 1975

840 Subacute cardiac tamponade caused by omentum and transverse colon herniated through a ruptured diaphragm and pericardium: the photograph was taken through a median laparotomy after partial reduction of the hernia. The position of the xiphoid process below the retractor is arrowed. (See also **854, 1109**).

Pericardial injuries

In our experience, 4% of severe chest trauma patients present a pericardial injury.

Non-bloody pericardial effusion

Non-bloody pericardial effusions include:
- **hydropericardium,** generally after an ill-documented trauma (see **841**),
- **effusion** when a central venous catheter perforates a heart chamber (see **912**),
- traumatic **chylopericardium** after rupture of the thoracic duct (exceptional),
- **pyopneumopericardium** through broncho- or oesophagopericardial fistulisation (see **849, 1161**).

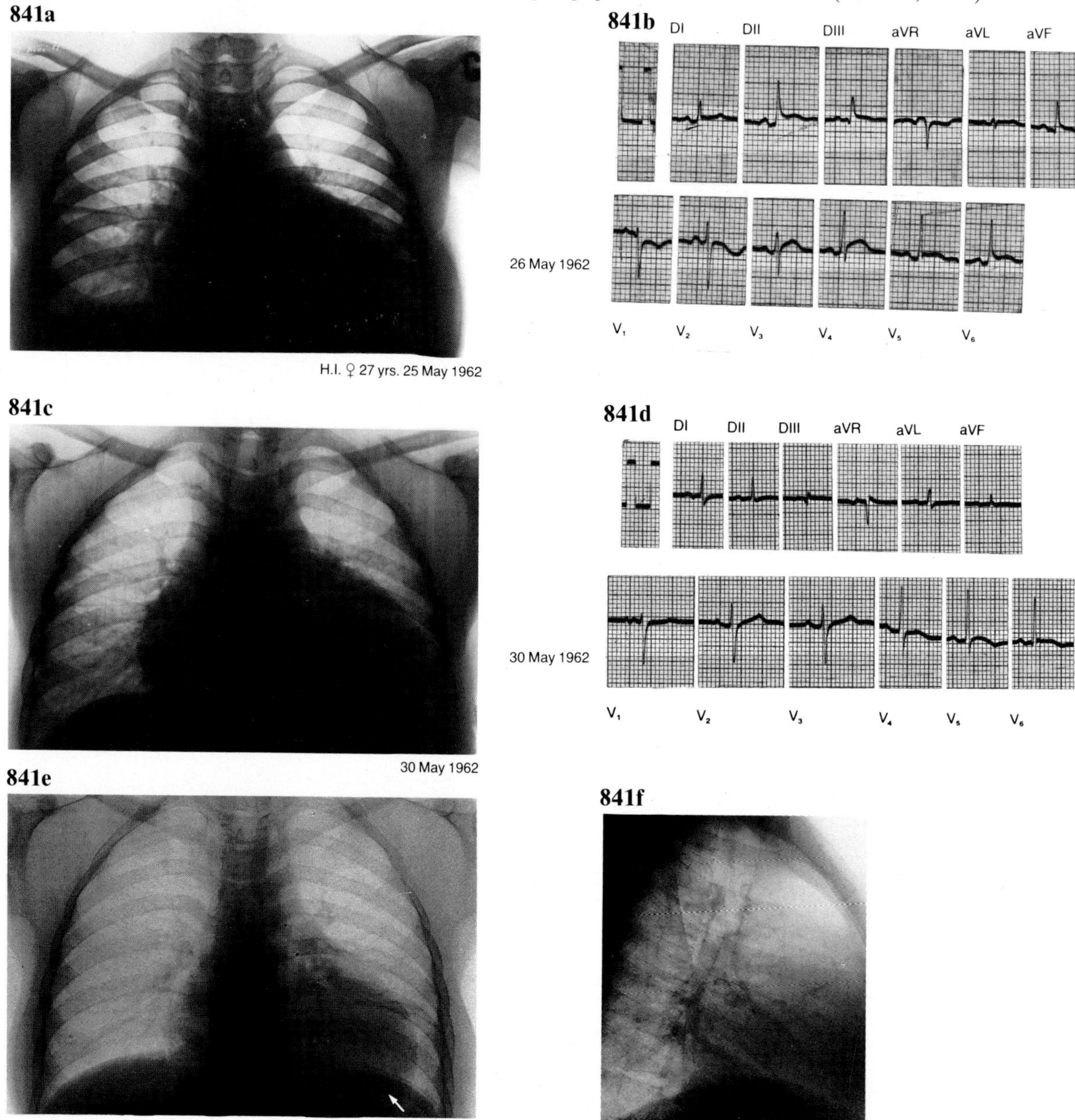

841a Subacute tamponade by intentional needle perforation of left ventricle in a schizophrenic woman. The injury passed undetected for 10 weeks. The initial X-ray shows a significant but cryptogenic pericardial effusion. Tamponade is moderate. **841b** Voltage is low. **841c** The effusion increases: there is no cardiac insufficiency but both the superior and inferior venae cavae are compressed. **841d** The potentials are still of diminished amplitude. **841e** Conservative treatment (diuretics, cortisone, digitalis) leads to clinical and radiological improvement. The cause of the low-grade tamponade is still unidentified; a viral disease is thought most likely. **841f** This lateral X-ray is considered normal.

841g

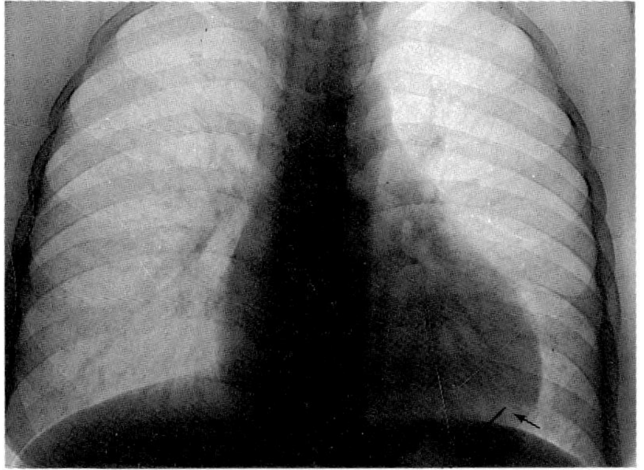

9 June 1962

841h

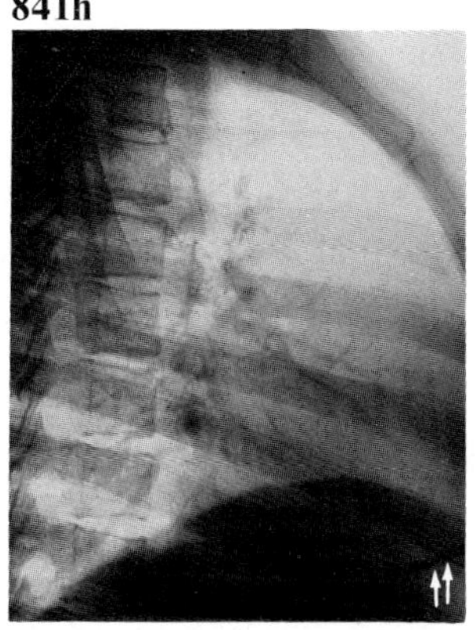

13 June 1962

841i

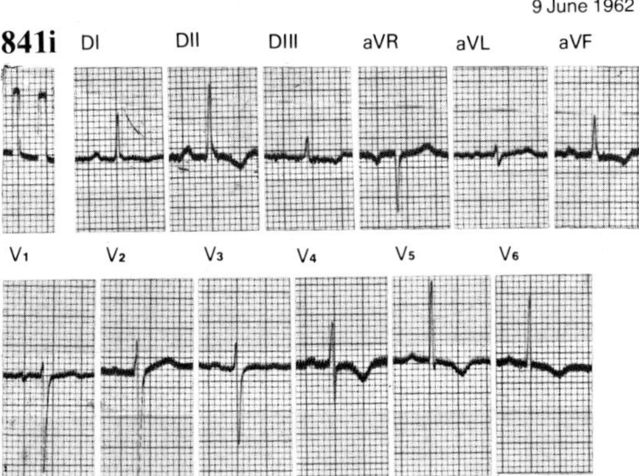

28 June 1962

841g The effusion gradually diminishes.

841h With this X-ray the foreign body (→) is finally identified; during suicidal delirium about ten weeks earlier, the young schizophrenic patient planted a needle deep into her chest, just below her left breast. The needle went through the pericardium and the apex of the left ventricle. Though this X-ray was exposed only once, the beating of the heart has resulted in a dual image of the needle. A left thoracotomy reveals inflammatory, constrictive pericarditis, but no haemopericardium. The foreign body is removed and the pericardium fenestrated.

841i The patient recovers clinically, but as with the pre-operative trace, the post-operative ECG shows abnormalities in the repolarisation phase. These are probably due to the pericarditis.

Haemopericardium

Haemopericardium without tamponade is a common injury – it is frequently seen during autopsies of car crash victims. In patients who survive, it is generally quickly reabsorbed with negligible repercussions. The typical haemopericardium observed at surgery is the result of a haemorrhagic injury of the heart or its intrapericardial pedicles; in most cases, it is compressive and results in acute tamponade. Exceptionally (3% – 10% of cases), compressive haemopericardium does not involve injury to the heart or to the intrapericardial vessels; in these cases, bleeding usually stops before the patient comes to surgery.

In cases of haemopericardium with tamponade, the pericardium can be punctured as soon as possible to decompress the heart. This procedure itself sometimes may suffice to prevent recurrence. When puncture gives rise to massive bleeding, emergency surgery is indicated – usually to repair a ruptured auricle, ventricle or coronary artery.

In general, if tamponade is documented, surgical haemostasis and treatment is indicated (see page 85).

842

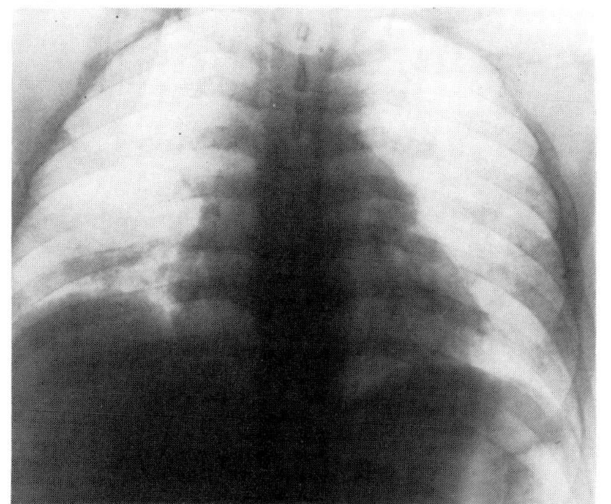

P.A. ♂ 32 yrs. 15 Sep. 1967

842 Traumatic haemopericardium with tamponade. The typical X-ray appearance. Death was due to an associated rupture of the carotid artery.

843a

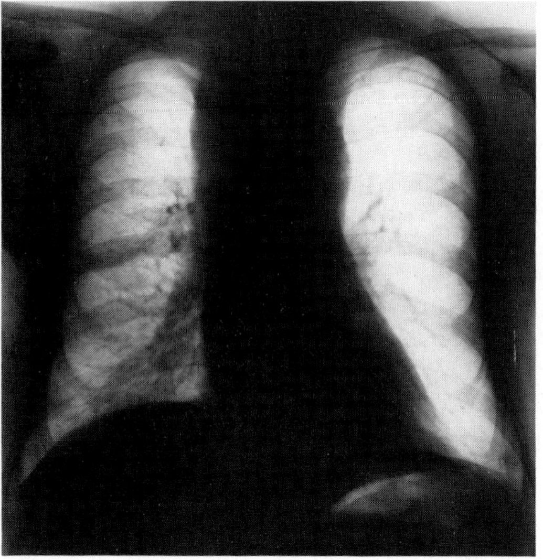

G.E. ♂ 43 yrs. 8 May 1970

843a Haemopericardium with tamponade and haemomediastinum (with superior vena cava syndrome and recurrent nerve paralysis) of cryptogenic, non-cardiac, non-traumatic origin. Initial X-ray.

843b

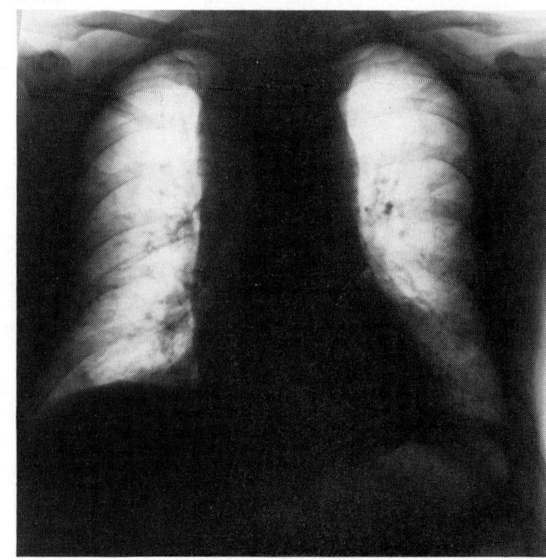

9 May 1970

843b The upper mediastinum has widened, and the outline of the pericardium has become triangular. A catheter is visible in the superior vena cava.

843c

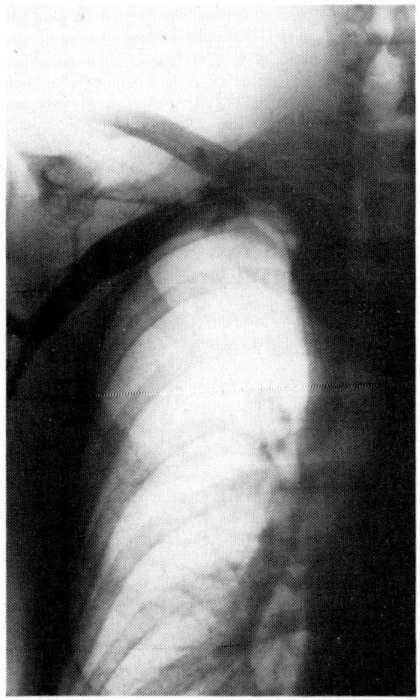

13 May 1970

843c The catheter enters the superior vena cava, but the contrast material is blocked at the right subclavian vein.

843d

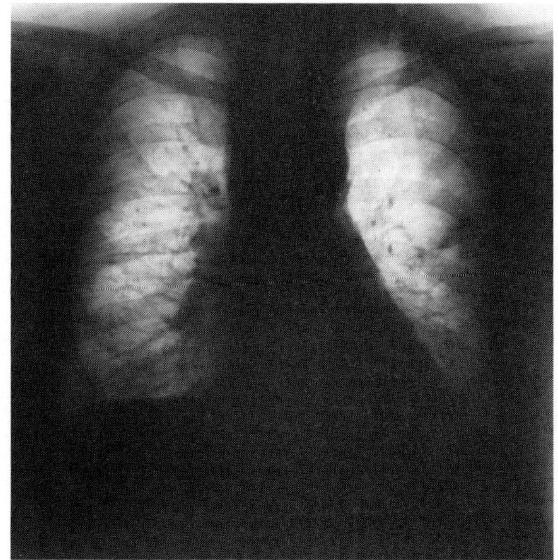

27 May 1970

843d Recovery follows evacuation of the haemopericardium and haemomediastinum through a combined cervical and right thoracic approach.

Pneumopericardium

A distinction must be made between pneumopericardium and pericardial emphysema.

Pericardial emphysema is a particular localisation of mediastinal emphysema (see Volume I, **479 – 497**) between the pericardium and the pleura.

Pneumopericardium is a condition where air is present in the pericardial sac. Pneumopericardium usually arises from tension pneumothorax, air escaping into the pericardial cavity through a small pleural rupture. It can usually be decompressed through pleural drainage. Tension pneumopericardium is exceptional; when it occurs, it can cause slight tamponade.

Pneumopericardium without lateral rupture of the pericardium is usually iatrogenic. It is a rare and sometimes fatal complication of the following procedures:

- pleural puncture,
- puncture of the sternal bone marrow,
- thoracotomy with pericardiotomy,
- mechanical ventilation (barotrauma).

Isolated cases of broncho- or oesophagopericardial fistulisation have been reported.

844

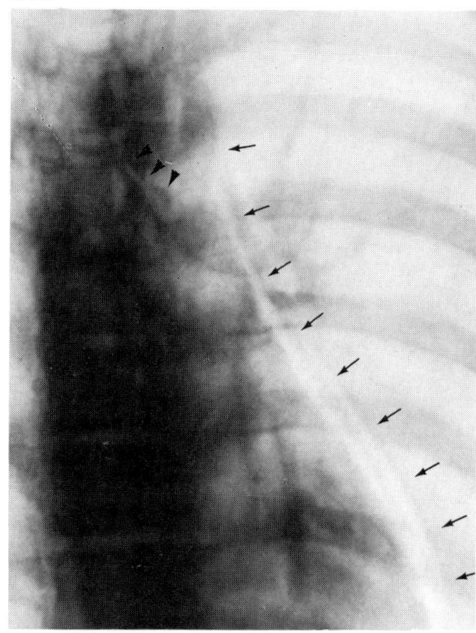

C.J. ♂ 20 yrs. 24 July 1966

845

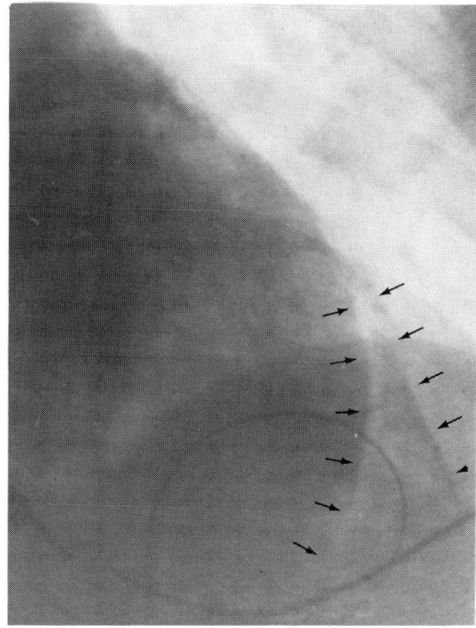

B.R. ♂ 55 yrs. 11 May 1973

846

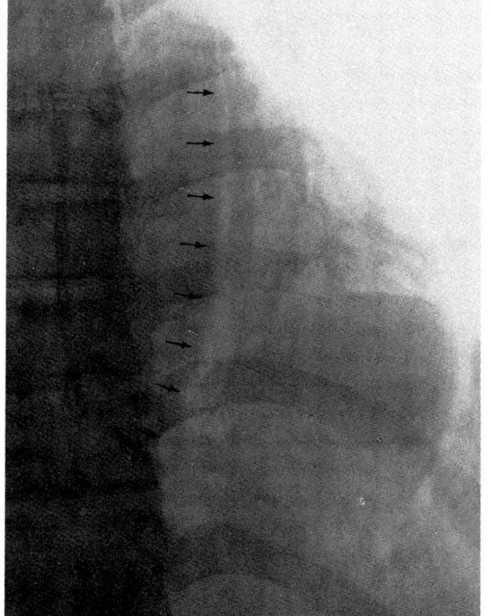

M.R. ♂ 1977

844 Moderate pericardial emphysema along the main pulmonary artery and left ventricle (→). Notice the double outline of the left main-stem bronchus (◀).

845 Emphysema dissecting the fatty **part of the pericardium.**

846 Periaortic emphysema at the hiatus.

847

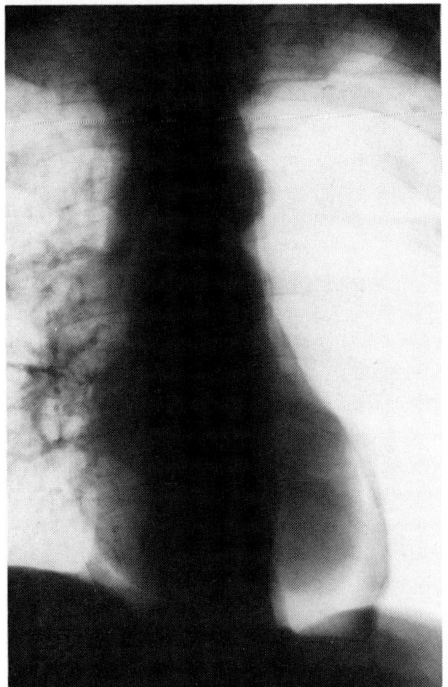

L.J. ♂ 59 yrs. 30 Mar. 1979

847 Pneumopericardium after intrapericardial left pneumonectomy. No clinical sign of tamponade.

848

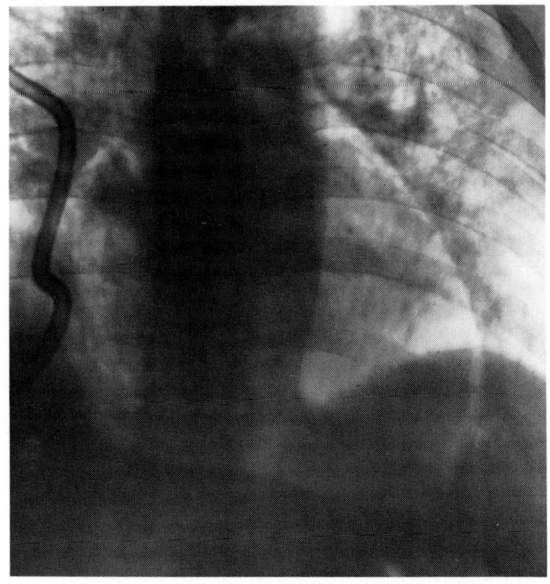

A.R. ♂ 53 yrs. 16 Dec. 1965

848 Tension pneumopericardium caused by a tension right pneumothorax (already drained) with a possible pericardial tear. Pleural drainage sufficed for a sound recovery (see Volume I, **543**).

849

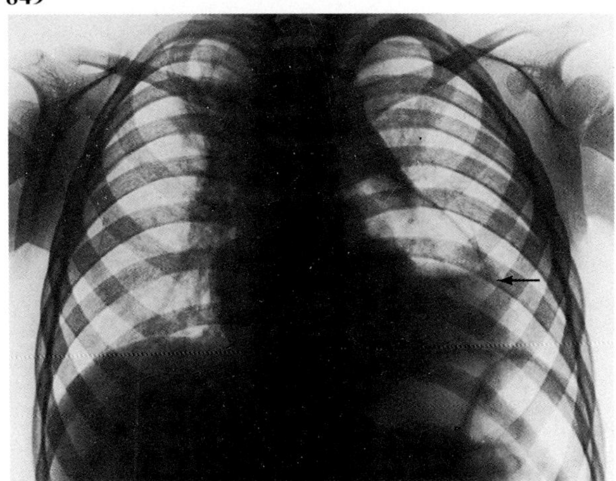

G.C. ♂ 2 yrs. 7 Nov. 1958

849 Pyopneumopericardium with oesophagopericardial fistula caused by alkaline corrosion of the oesophagus. This standing X-ray was obtained after repeated bougienage, and pericardial paracentesis: the hydro-aeric level is marked (→).

Post-traumatic and callous pericarditis

The commonest cause of callous, constrictive pericarditis is *inadequate drainage*. Emergency surgery for acute haemopericardium – with pericardial aspiration and toilet – usually obviates this complication.

It used to be thought that callous pericarditis was the result of *low-grade infection of haemopericardium* and, in particular, that post-traumatic calcification of the pericardium implied tuberculous infection. However, it has since been established in animal experiments that infected haemopericardium does not necessarily lead to constrictive pericarditis. Clotting – which is especially common after mesothelial injuries – is now generally considered the prime causal factor. Fluid haemopericardium, on the other hand, is quickly reabsorbed without complication.

Clinically, late constrictive pericarditis produces a classic Pick's syndrome.

In most cases, *pericardiotomy with decortication* has swift and lasting results.

850

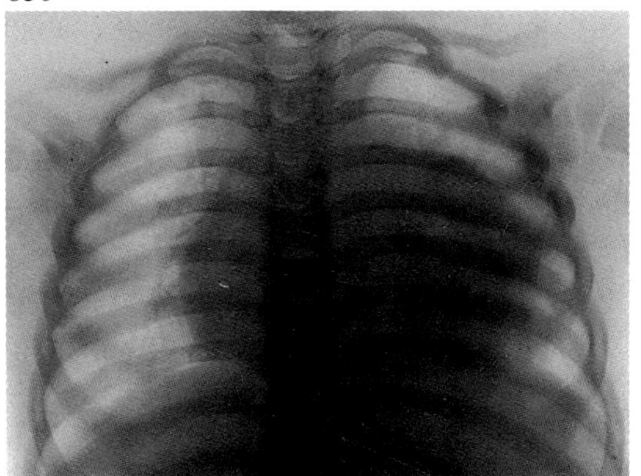

G.C. ♂ 2 yrs. 10 Nov. 1958

850 Pericardial tamponade due to purulent pericarditis (oesophagopericardial fistula after alkaline corrosion). Left thoracotomy for pericardial and pleural drainage. Multiple postoperative complications (see **849, 1161, 1162, 1215**). Death.

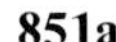

851a H.J. ♂ 38 yrs. 19 Aug. 1958

851a Late constrictive pericarditis. Major chest wall damage was inflicted 15 years previously by an exploding shell. A fragment pierced the thorax from behind, damaging the ribs, diaphragm and liver. Repeated pleural aspirations were followed one year later by a right thoracotomy, but the foreign body was not detected. Since then, the patient has suffered from serious respiratory difficulties, and developed chronic suppurative disorders with empyema necessitatis.

851b 19 Aug. 1958

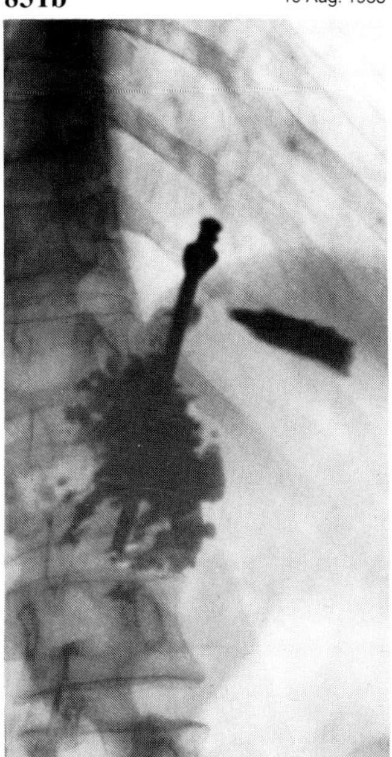

851b A sinogram shows the shrapnel lodged inside the pericardium. A second thoracotomy is performed for removal of the foreign body, rib sequestrectomy, pericardial and pleural toilet and Spühl-drainage. Recovery.

851c

851c The shell fragment.

Rupture

Lateral (pleural face)

Small lateral rupture of the pericardium doubtless frequently passes unnoticed, particularly when (as is usually the case) there is no phrenic nerve injury and no pleural or pericardial effusion. It is worth noting that when the pericardial wall has ruptured, pleural drainage can also clear the pericardium (see **848**).

On the other hand, **large lateral rupture** of the pericardium, with or without tear of the phrenic nerve, is rare. It occurs in violent deceleration accidents and is usually fatal, either because of accompanying severe multiple injuries, or because of haemodynamic disorders: opportunities for clinical observation are rare. There is a potential danger of intrapleural dislocation of the heart, and it is usually at this stage that diagnosis is made.

However, it must be added that dislocation of the heart is usually the consequence of **surgical incision** of the pericardium for pulmonary resection.

The principle of surgical treatment is to re-position the heart and then to suture the pericardium. Re-positioning can be difficult if the pedicles are twisted and the heart dilated (this often happens relatively early on); such cases require contra-incision of the pericardium. When the rupture is sutured, a window should be left to forestall secondary tamponade.

853a Dislocation of heart following pericardiotomy. A malignant teratoma of the superior, anterior mediastinum infiltrated the left lung. It is excised through a median sternotomy, and a left pneumonectomy is performed through a broad incision in the pericardium.

852

852 Dislocation of heart into left pleural space after lateral rupture of pericardium.

853a

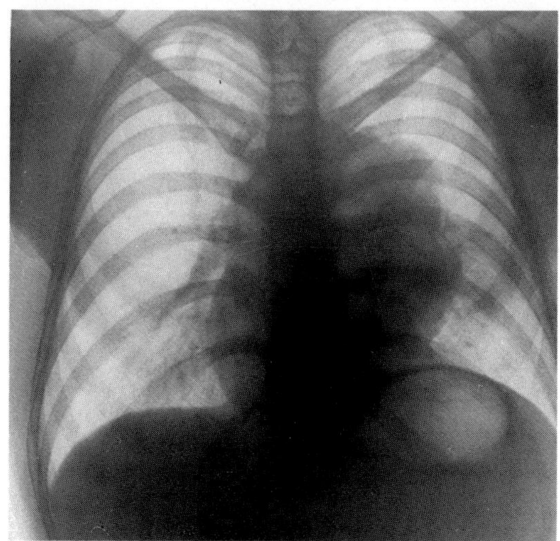

G.F. ♂ 25 yrs. 4 April 1970

853b

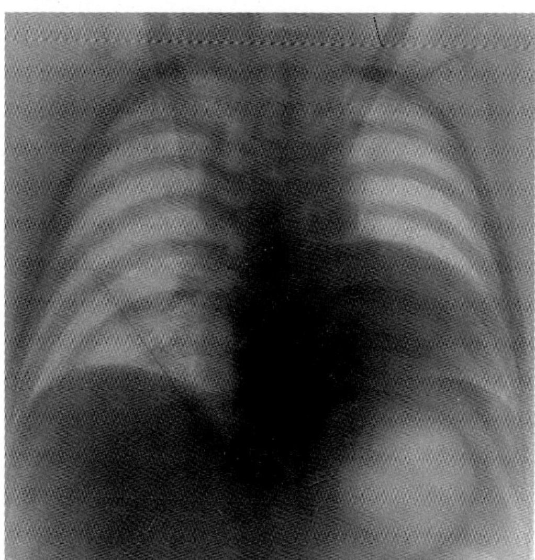

16 April 1970

853b The postoperative X-ray shows the heart dislocated through the pericardial window into the left pleural cavity. The chest is reopened and the pericardium is sutured afresh.

853c

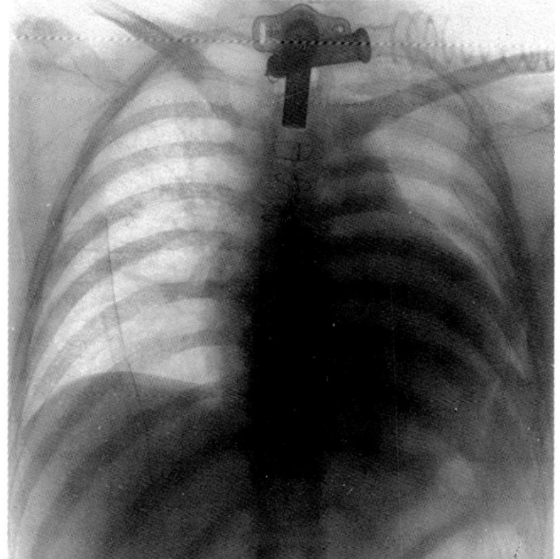

18 April 1970

853c Recovery with survival of five years (death due to recurrent malignancy).

Inferior (diaphragmatic face)

Rupture of the inferior pericardium is accompanied by a rupture of the central part of the diaphragm; the mechanism is that of transverse diaphragmatic rupture (see **1036**). The colon, omentum and sometimes, also, part of the stomach or of the left lobe of the liver migrate into the pericardial sac.

Rupture of the inferior pericardium usually causes subacute tamponade with slight and elusive symptoms and signs. It is well tolerated in most cases; indeed, there have been reports of its remaining undetected for more than 20 years. Radiological diagnosis is difficult.

The rupture can be sutured easily through an upper abdominal approach. Attempts through a left, right or even bilateral thoracic approach have met with major difficulties.

854a

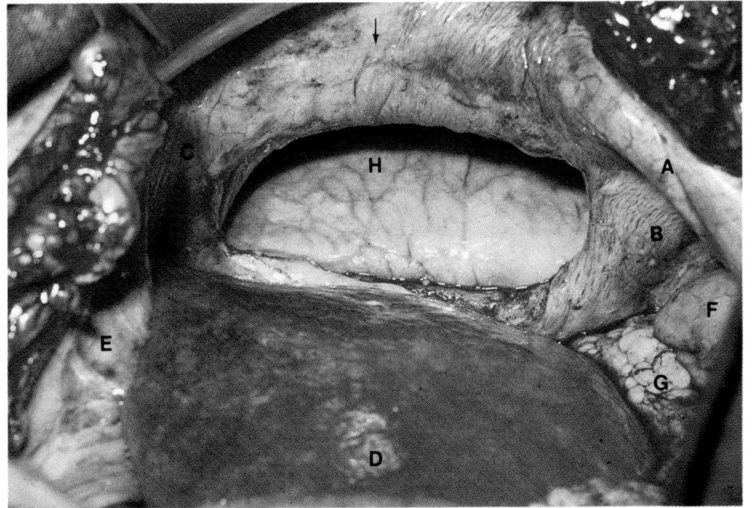

N.P. ♂ 69 yrs. 22 Oct. 1975

854a Transverse rupture of inferior face of pericardium and diaphragm after a violent lateral impact. The left costal margin (A), both hemidiaphragms (B and C), the left lobe of the liver (D), the triangular ligament of the liver (E), the stomach (F), the greater omentum (G) and the right ventricle (H) are seen through a laparotomy.
The arrow marks the position of the xiphoid appendix. The photograph was taken after reduction of the omentum and colon out of the pericardial sac (see **840**).

854b

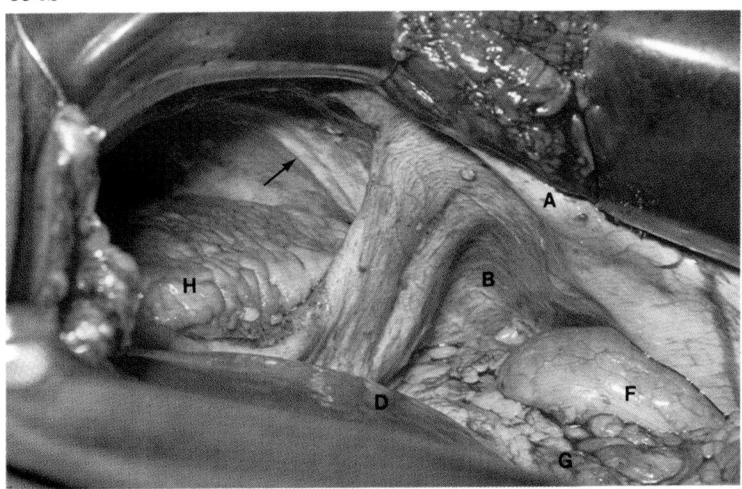

22 Oct. 1975

854b Both lateral faces of the pericardium are intact: the left phrenic nerve is arrowed. (For X-rays, see **1109**.) Repair, drainage. Recovery.

Blunt heart injuries

In Switzerland (particularly in the Lausanne region), blunt trauma of the heart is six times more frequent than open trauma.

Modern examination techniques have shown that serious injury to the heart after a blunt trauma is less frequent than slight or transitory damage; also, certain forms of permanent damage are not incompatible with survival.

A violent **impact** to the lower anterior chest wall can injure the heart either at the point of impact, or on the opposite side. In each case, the thoracic cage is often undamaged.

Under certain circumstances, anteroposterior **crush-injury of the thorax** can also seriously damage the heart or its valves when, trapped between the sternum and the vertebral column, the heart is distorted beyond the limits of its elasticity.

The following table shows the types of heart injury presented by patients admitted alive after a direct impact or violent deceleration:

Type of heart injury	Incidence (in our material, $n = 65$)
Concussion and simple contusion, as diagnosed by ECG or at autopsy	51.5%
Contusion complicated by:	
– arrhythmia	14%
– traumatic infarction or coronary wound	8%
– injury to the septum (ASD, VSD)	8%
Transmural laceration	14%
Valvular damage	3%
Dislocation of the heart	1.5%

855

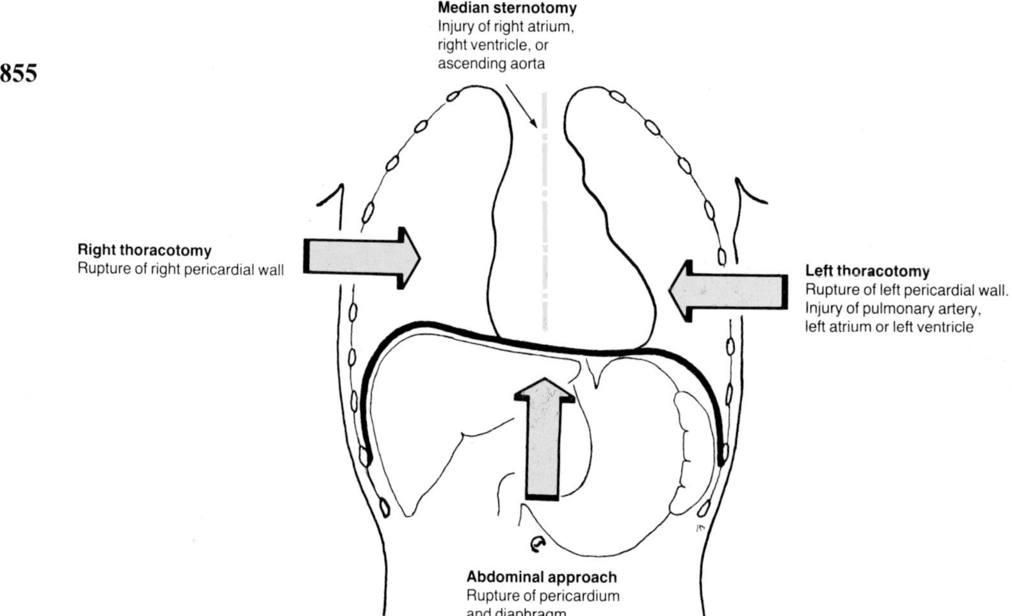

855 Surgical approaches to cardiac and/or pericardial injuries

Aetiology

There are various possible mechanisms:
- **direct blow** to the precordial region: a bucking horse, punch or kick, fiercely struck football or tennis ball, external cardiac massage . . .
- **deceleration**: compression of the heart against the sternum during an impact – against the steering wheel or dashboard, or during a climbing accident, for example . . .
- **crush-injury**: between the buffers of two railway carriages, under the wheel of a lorry, under a tractor, accidental burial, landslide . . .
- **extrathoracic compression**: compression of the abdomen or lower limbs, blast-injury.

Associated injuries

856

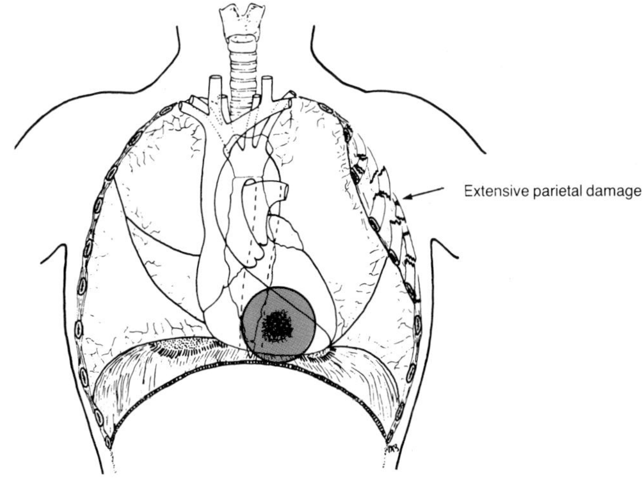

856 Injury **almost always** accompanying heart trauma (in over half of our cases)

857

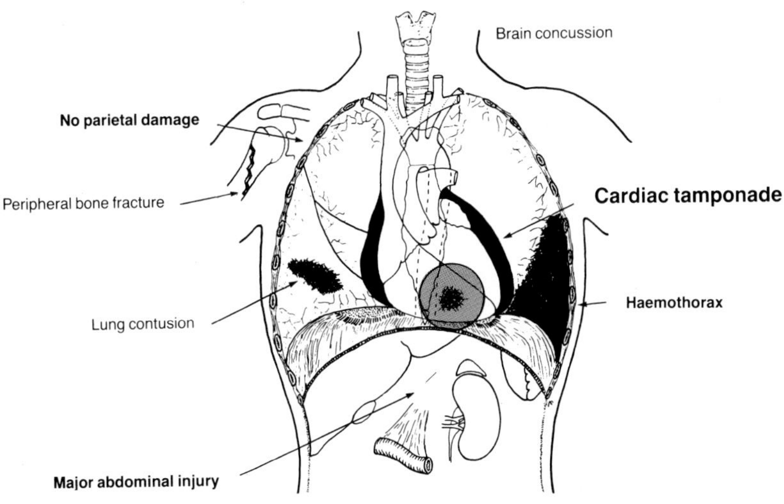

857 Injuries **often** accompanying heart trauma (in a quarter to a half of our cases)

858

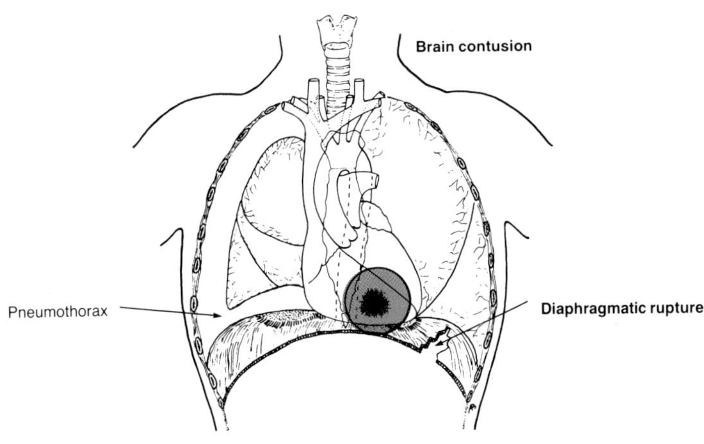

858 Injuries **sometimes** accompanying heart trauma (in a tenth to a quarter of our cases)

859

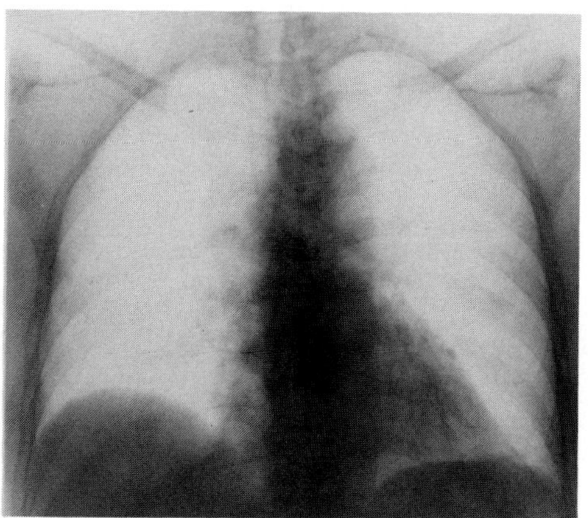

H.C. ♀ 53 yrs. 26 Mar. 1964

859 Cardiac contusion without injury to thoracic cage. Car accident. The X-ray is normal. Recovery in 10 days.

860a

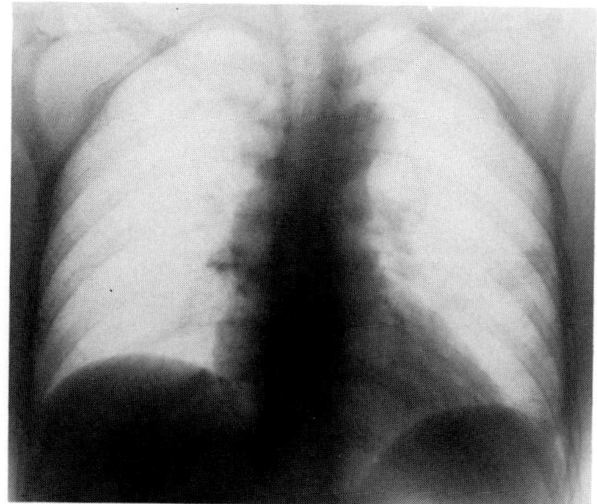

J.O. ♀ 47 yrs. 16 July 1970

860a Myorcardial contusion with two fractured ribs in a car passenger. The pelvis and femur are also fractured.

860b

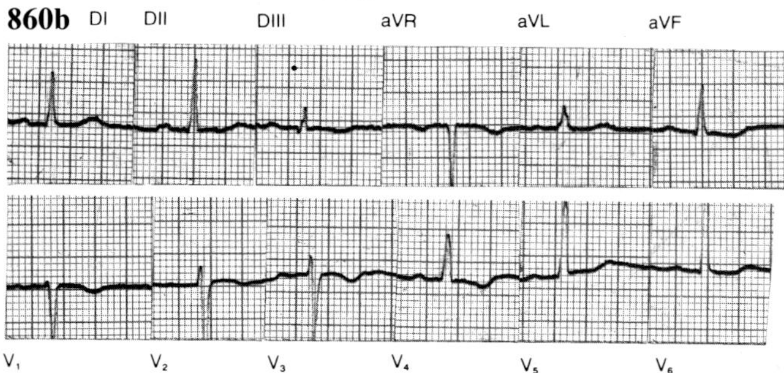

860b The trace shows disturbances in the repolarisation phase with negative T waves in DIII, aVF and in the precordial derivations, from V1 to V4.

861

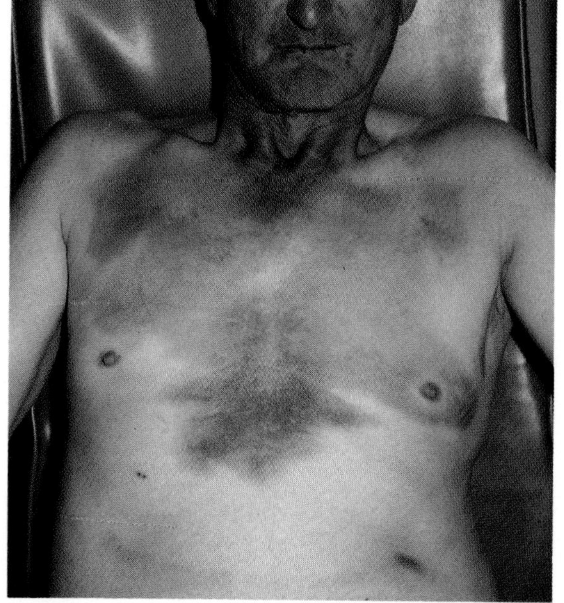

B.V. ♂ 67 yrs. 1970

861 Steering wheel syndrome: fracture of sternum and cardiac contusion. The patient was catapulted against the steering wheel of his car when, driving at 45 km/h, he collided head-on with a car of similar size travelling at 120 km/h. The boss of the wheel fractured the sternum (ecchymosis), and the rim has left a clear imprint on the abdomen. ECG indicates cardiac contusion. Recovery.

Mortality

In our material, mortality among heart trauma patients is 49%.

Death is directly attributable to the heart trauma in 17% of cases.

Concussion

The concept of cardiac concussion is empirical but nonetheless controversial. A violent impact to the precordial or cardiac region of an animal has been shown to cause fatal cardiac arrest without any histologically discernible injury (Goltz' experiment).

The term cardiac concussion should be reserved to describe acute post-traumatic cardiac failure without histological evidence of injury. Cardiac insufficiency manifests itself as fleeting electrical disturbances: arrhythmia, ventricular overload, signs of ischaemia, momentary heart block, etc.

Since patients with cardiac concussion usually survive, the diagnosis cannot always be proven. Unless there is an early and repeated ECG record, slight contusion should be assumed.

Ultimately, the distinction between the two is very fine and, indeed, the point is academic so long as the patient survives.

Contusion

Cardiac contusion resulting from blunt trauma can take the form of:

- *subendocardial or subepicardial haemorrhage* that is usually asymptomatic except for possible secondary thrombosis,
- *partial laceration* of the endocardium with subsequent clotting. Late and potentially fatal embolism sometimes occurs (usually in the third week),
- *intramyocardial haemorrhage* whose consequences depend on its localisation; arrhythmia is the most common result,
- *injury* (thrombosis or rupture) to a branch of *coronary artery* causing a localised infarct or, later, a cardiac aneurysm, (see page 106),
- a particularly violent impact causes complete, *transmural rupture* (see page 107).

Electrocardiographic evaluation of cardiac contusion is often difficult. The typical trace consisting of unspecific disturbances of variable duration could be attributable equally to hypovolaemic shock or to tachycardia. Both conditions are frequent in multiple injury patients.

The most reliable means of assessment is to compare successive ECGs.

However, according to circumstances, a degree of uncertainty may remain as to the relationship between the trauma and the cardiac injury monitored by the ECG. Indeed, although standard X-rays, clinical observation and specialised examination may all produce useful additional data, there is often insufficient evidence for a firm diagnosis.

Treatment of cardiac contusion, even if slight and clinically unimpressive, is the same as for an infarct: rest, close clinical and paraclinical observation, frequent auscultation and restriction of intravenous fluids. Anticoagulants are also sometimes required.

Certain anamnestic or clinical indications **should immediately suggest** cardiac contusion. They are:

- head-on car crash (front seat occupant),
- violent deceleration of a belted driver or passenger, even when the patient appears injury-free,
- sudden, post-traumatic angina, typical or atypical,
- precordial ecchymosis, however slight,
- sternal fracture, with or without compression fracture of a thoracic vertebra,
- arrhythmia, however fleeting,
- rupture of the aorta or diaphragm.

As an incidental finding

In some multiple injury cases, cardiac contusion is only diagnosed at autopsy. According to some pathologists, the incidence of cardiac contusion in deceleration fatalities can reach 50%.

Cardiac contusion in itself, however, is rarely fatal.

Except when there is no other traumatic injury, the causal relationship between contusion and death is difficult to establish.

862a

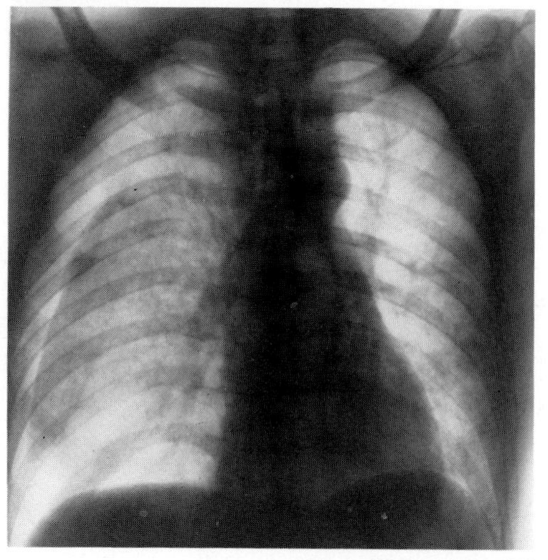

C. P.–A. ♂ 35 yrs. 14 Mar. 1970

862a Cardiac contusion in a driver involved in a head-on collision. Bilateral lung contusion and a right pneumothorax are associated with severe damage to the head and skeleton.

862b

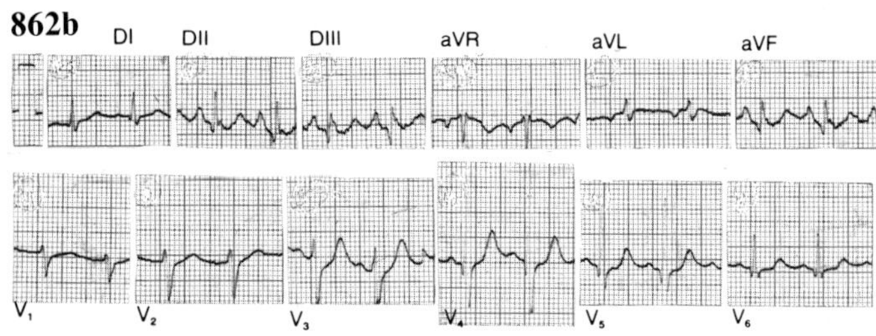

14 Mar. 1970

862b The admission ECG is almost normal. Autopsy three days later reveals a subendocardial haemorrhage in the right atrium and severe contusion of the left ventricle.

863

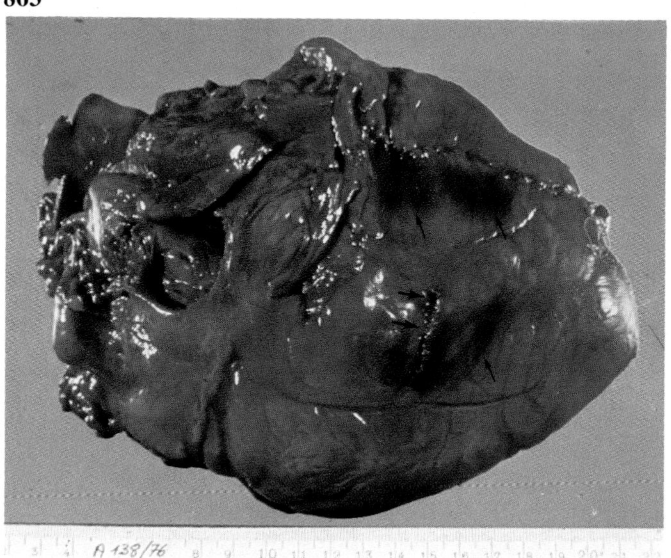

N.A. ♂ 62 yrs. 25 Feb. 1976

863 Contusions (→) and incomplete rupture of right ventricle (→) after blunt trauma. (Death on arrival.) (Institute of Pathology, Lausanne.)

With conduction disturbances and arrhythmia

Cardiac contusion very often entails conduction disturbances or arrhythmia. These conditions are usually short-lived, if not fleeting. They can take various forms.

A non-fatal *impact* or deceleration inflicted on a young rabbit causes:

- ventricular tachycardia in 65% of cases
- nodal rhythm in 14% of cases
- first-degree AV block in 16% of cases
- complete AV block in 10% of cases
- momentary asystole in 2% of cases
- elevation of the ST segment in 31% of cases

Most of these disturbances in the animal's ECG are temporary.

864a

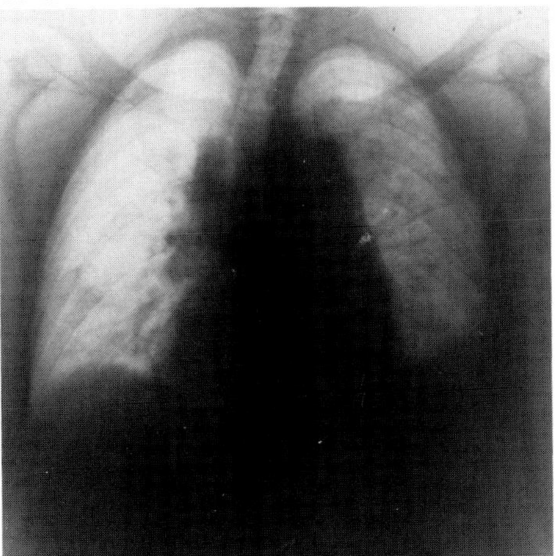

864b

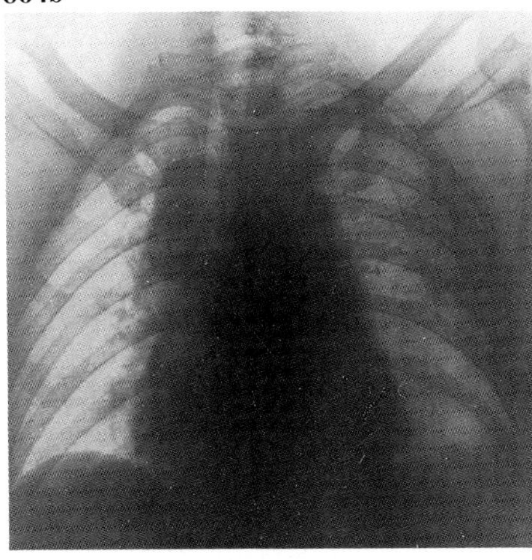

864a Cardiac contusion with tachycardia. When transferred to the University Hospital, this patient had a left haemothorax, shock and tachycardia (heart beat of 160 per minute).

864b Shortly after admission, the outline of the heart appears triangular, and a haemopericardium is suspected. A thoracotomy reveals no mediastinal injury and no haemopericardium. However, there is a 500ml haemothorax and tachycardia persists after the operation. A second thoracotomy three days later is followed by cardiac arrest; resuscitation is unsuccessful. Autopsy reveals extensive myocardial contusion with a haematoma 3cm in diameter in the right atrium, close to the sinus node.

865a

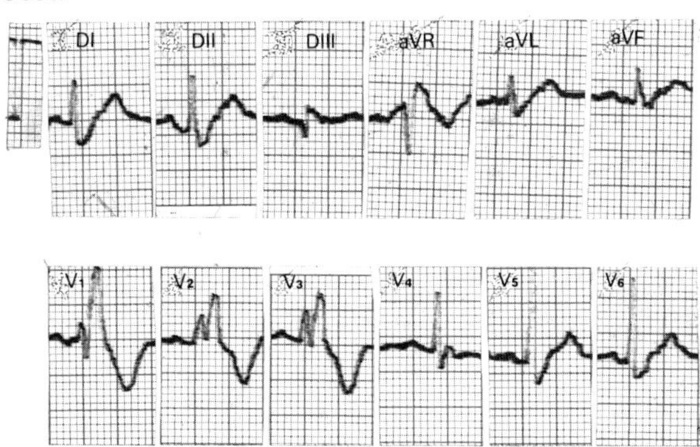

865b

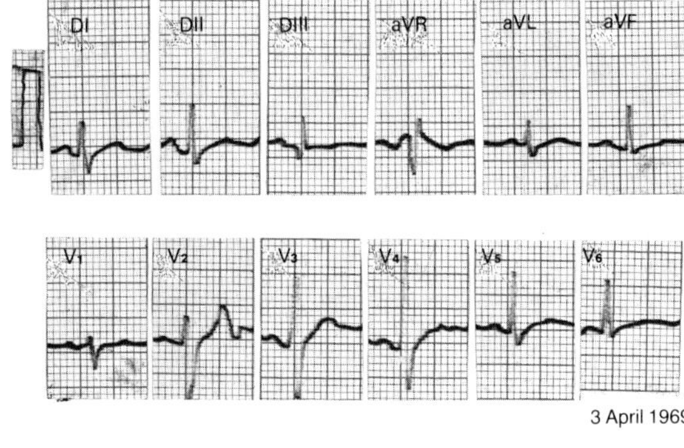

865c

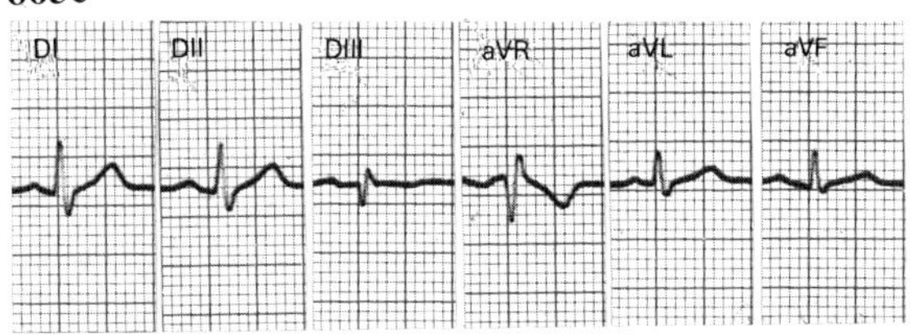

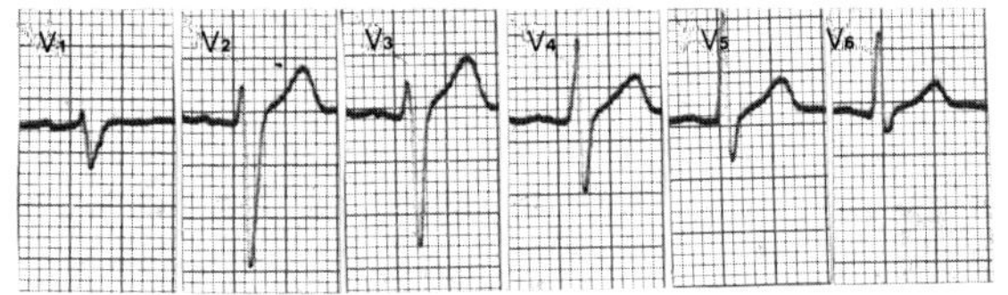

865a Momentary complete right bundle branch block (RBBB) due to myocardial contusion (steering wheel and dashboard syndrome).

865b The following day, there is clinical evidence of fat embolism and severe hypoxia. X-ray shows the outline of the heart to be enlarged, but the ECG indicates that the RBBB has disappeared.

865c Return to normal one month later.

866

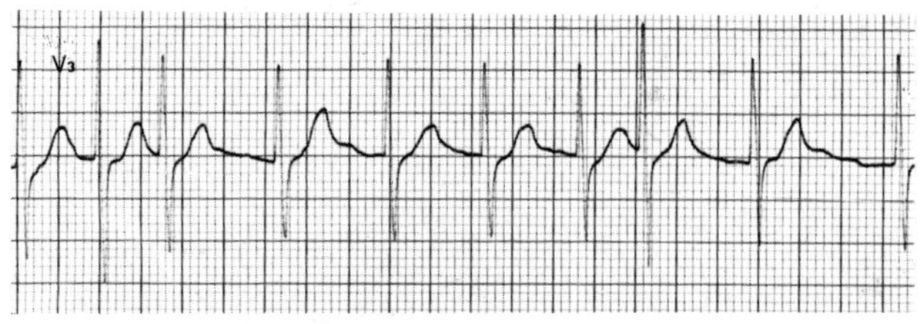

B.M. ♂ 49 yrs. 21 April 1976

866 Post-traumatic atrial fibrillation persisting for several days in a multiple injury patient under controlled ventilation for a flail chest with paradoxical motion (for chest X-ray, see Volume I, **528**). Sinus rhythm returns a few days later. Recovery.

867a

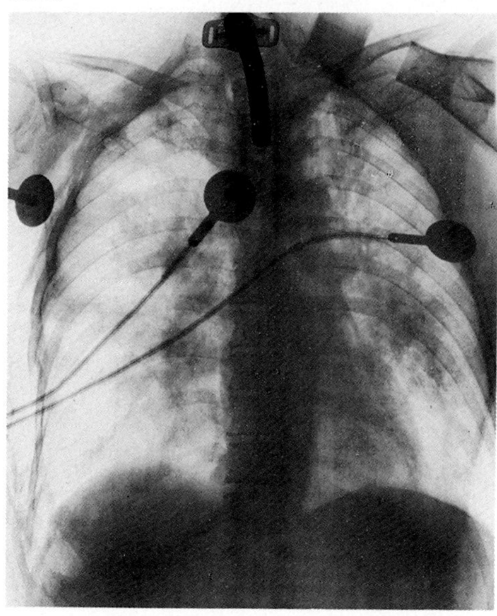

J.R. ♂ 66 yrs. 26 Jan. 1967

867a Post-traumatic RBBB, AV block and bigeminy. Cardiac contusion, pulmonary contusion and a flail chest with paradoxical motion were sustained in an impact against the steering wheel.

867b The trace shows the RBBB with depression of the ST segment, particularly in the left precordial leads, a first degree AV block and numerous ventricular extrasystoles. Other sections of the trace show episodes of bigeminy.

867c The RBBB block disappears. The trace shows high amplitude P waves in DII, DIII, and aVF. The ST segment has returned to normal.

867d Bigeminy persists despite a further improvement in the trace. Death three weeks later (bronchopneumonia, tracheo-oesophageal fistula, perforated stress ulcer). Apart from the myocardial contusion, autopsy also reveals an ulcerated atheromatous plate on the right coronary artery.

867b

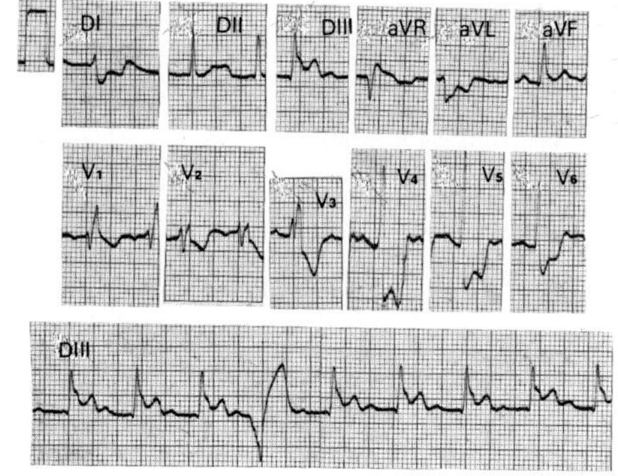

26 Jan. 1967, 10hrs.

867c

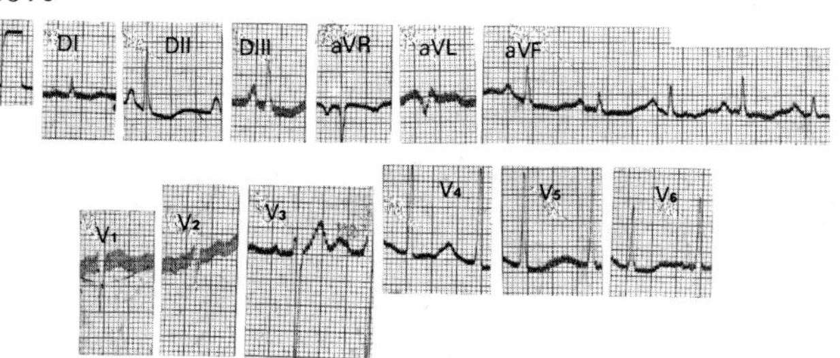

26 Jan. 1967, 14.30hrs.

867d

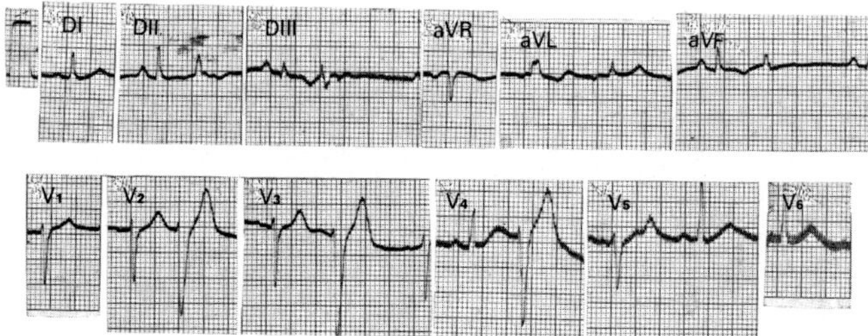

27 Jan. 1967

868a

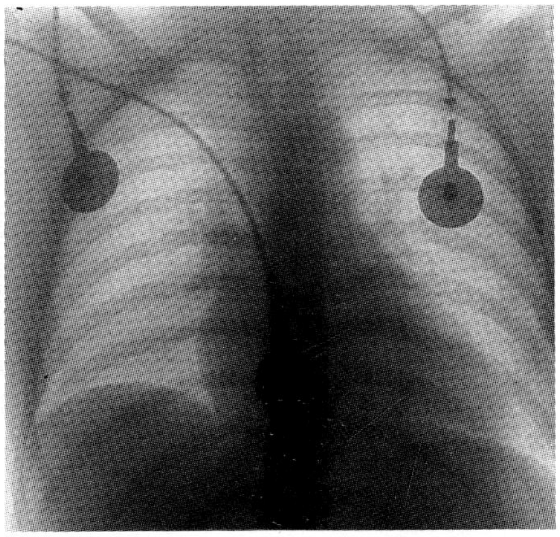

Z.E. ♀ 33 yrs. 22 Oct. 1967

868b

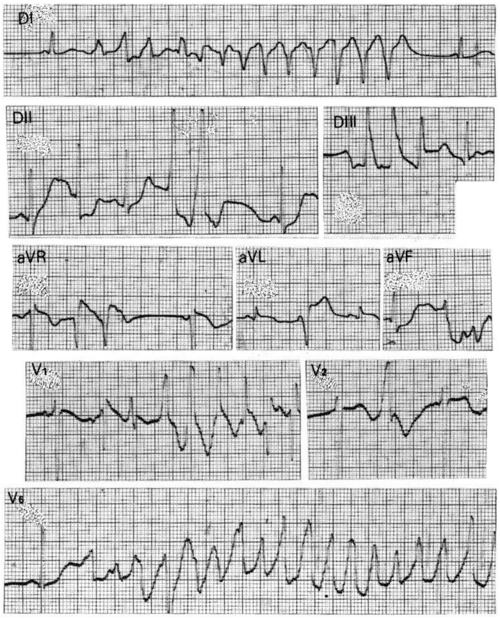

DI

DII DIII

aVR aVL aVF

V1 V2

V6

22 Oct. 1967

868c DII DIII aVR aVL aVF

V1 V2 V3 V4 V5 V6

aVR

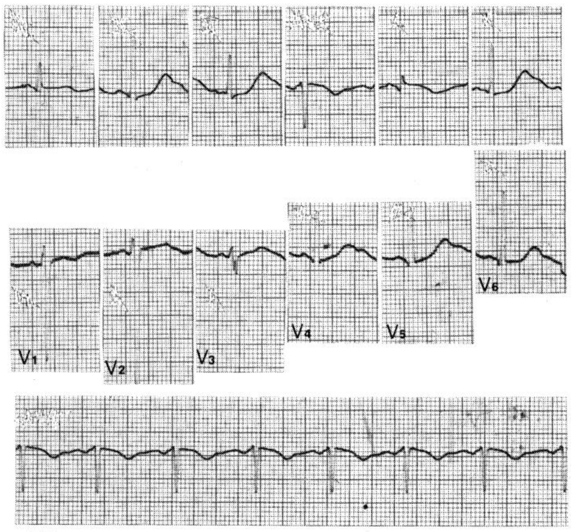

23 Oct. 1967

868d DI DII DIII

aVR aVL

aVF

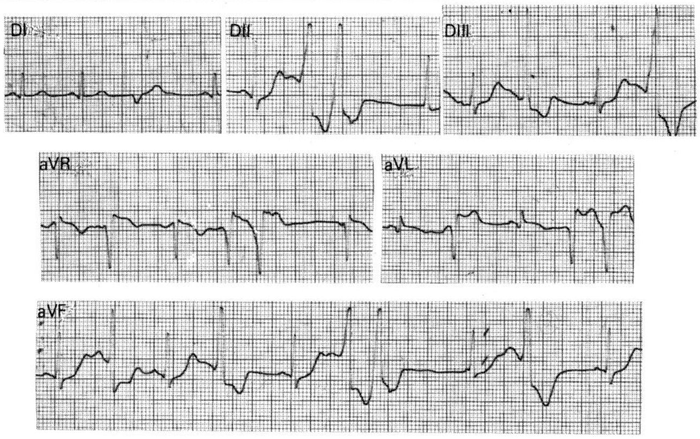

23 Oct. 1967

868e

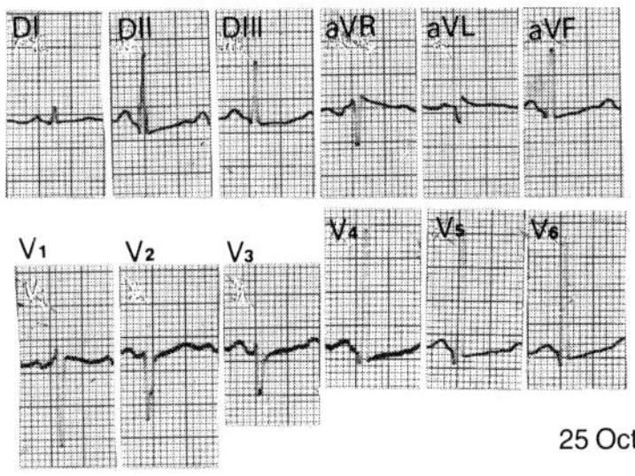

DI DII DIII aVR aVL aVF

V1 V2 V3 V4 V5 V6

25 Oct. 1967

868f DI DII DIII aVR aVL aVF

V1 V2 V3 V4 V5 V6

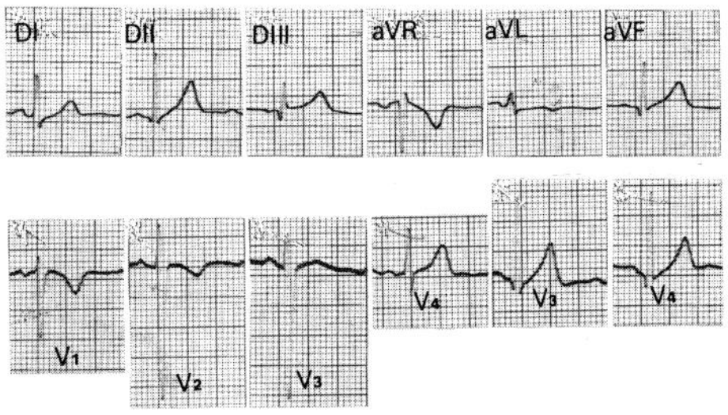

8 Nov. 1967

14 Oct. 1968

868g

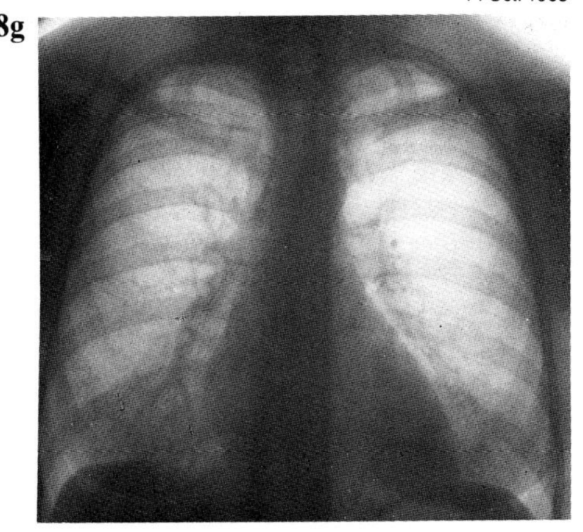

868a Salvoes of ventricular extrasystoles with ventricular fibrillation. Recovery. Cardiac contusion, with temporary cardiomegalia, was sustained in a fall from a jeep.

868b One hour after admission, ECG documents episodes of ventricular tachycardia.

868c Twelve hours after admission, sinus rhythm is restored but disturbances in the repolarisation phase persist . . .

868d . . . and are followed after a further twelve hours by salvoes of ventricular extrasystoles.

868e Disturbances in the repolarisation phase persist two days later.

868f Clinical recovery is accompanied by the appearance of Q waves in DIII and aVF.

868g Eleven months later, the outline of the heart has returned to normal.

With ischaemia

Ischaemia is the main electrocardiographic finding in cases of major cardiac contusion. Changes in the ECG are often permanent.

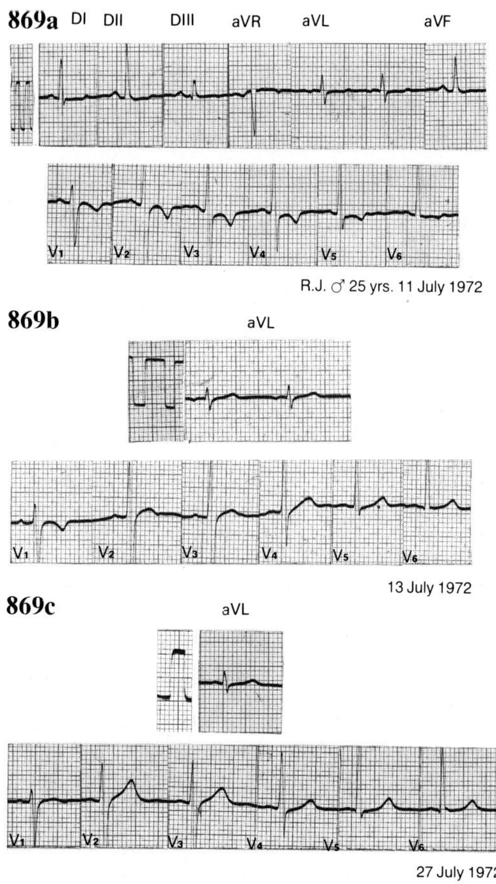

869a Cardiac contusion with acute ischaemia of the anterior myocardium in the passenger of a car which rolled over several times. On the 3rd day, the ECG shows negative T waves.

869b Positive T waves reappear in the precordial leads two days later.

869c Three weeks later the trace returns to normal.

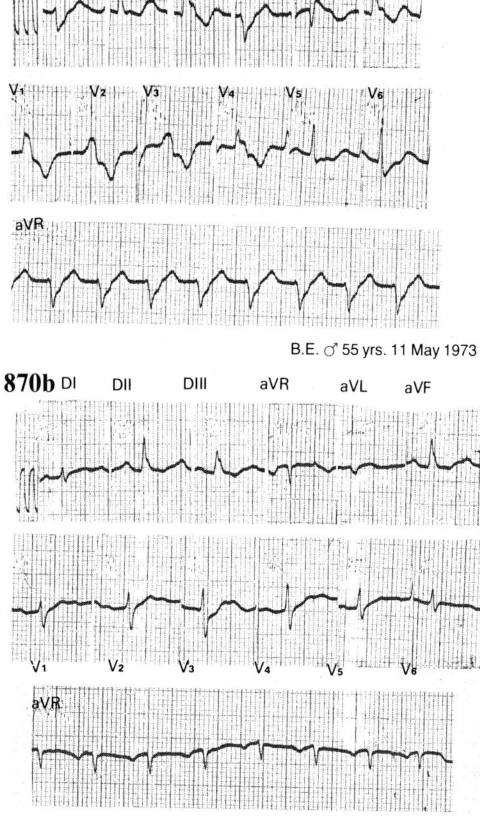

870a Cardiac contusion with RBBB and signs of ischaemia. (Steering wheel syndrome.)

870b The ECG returns almost to normal within 24 hours. The patient died the next day from numerous other injuries.

With infarction

Traumatic injury to a coronary artery (or one of its branches) can cause *acute obstruction* either through incomplete rupture, rupture with intimal flap, or subepicardial rupture-dislocation.

Post-traumatic coronary obstruction is most frequently seen in people with a previous history of arteriosclerotic disease, but acute thrombosis of a healthy coronary artery is also known to occur (see page 111).

The result of post-traumatic coronary obstruction is infarction. The clinical and electrical signs are usually the same as for any other type of infarction. However, the prognosis of this type of infarction is often aggravated by other associated cardiac injuries.

871a

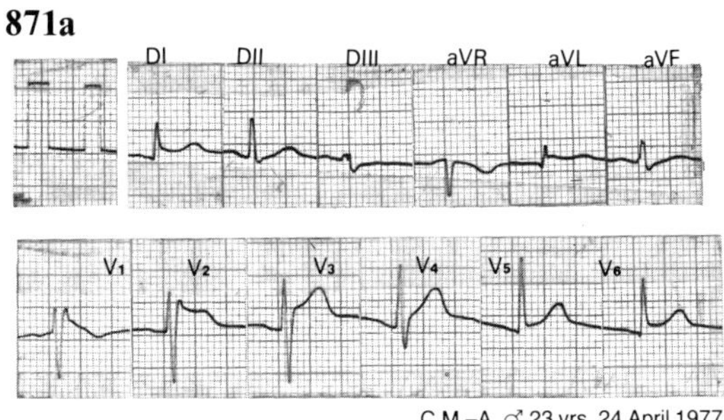

871a Traumatic anteroseptal infarct accompanied by an isthmic rupture of the aorta (see **955**): ECG on admission. Reversible cardiac arrest occurred nine hours after the accident, shortly before the aorta was repaired.

871b

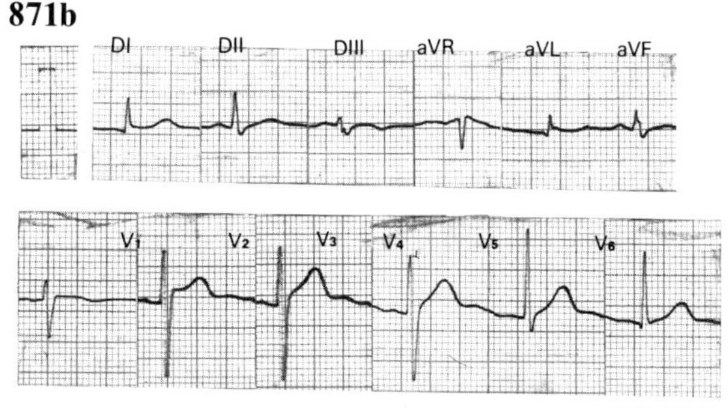

871b Four days later, the RBBB and the ST segment elevation have disappeared. Full recovery.

872

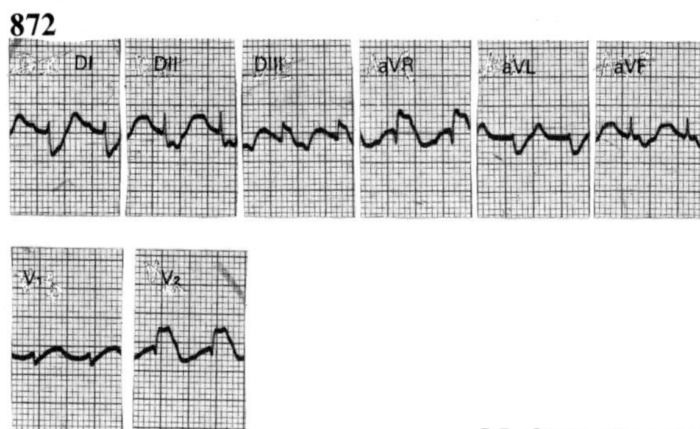

872 Post-traumatic myocardial necrosis with a Pardee wave in V2. Motorcyclist knocked over by a car. Extensive injuries to the chest, abdomen and extremities. Death from pulmonary oedema three days after the accident. Haemorrhagic necrosis of the septum confirmed at autopsy.

873

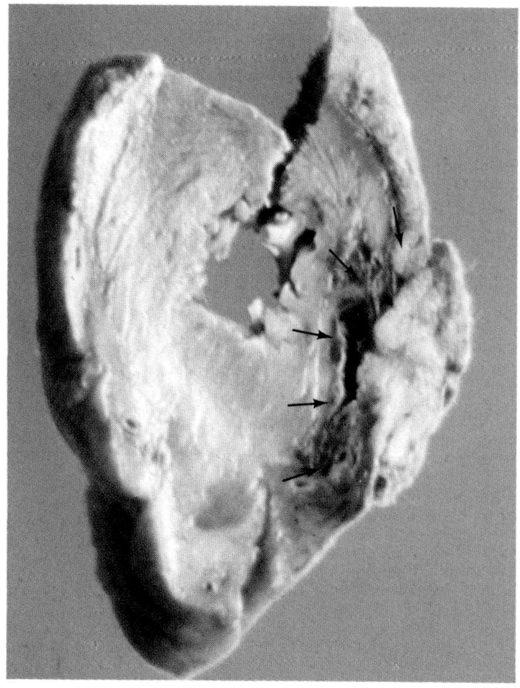

V.J. ♂ 19 yrs. 19 April 1968

873 Post-traumatic infarct (→) at apex of left ventricle, with secondary (3rd week) transmural necrosis and sudden acute tamponade due to rupture. Immediate sternotomy to repair the left ventricle. Death 14 days later from pneumonia. (See **883**.)
(Institute of Pathology, Lausanne.)

With cardiac aneurysm

Cardiac aneurysm is a late complication of post-traumatic infarction. The damaged portion of the ventricle thins, dilates and then evolves into an inert pouch which expands passively when the heart contracts. Blood accumulates in the pouch during systole, seriously reducing cardiac output. Moreover, the accumulated blood tends to clot.

It is advisable to excise large cardiac aneurysms if they have resulted in cardiac failure. Surgery also obviates the danger of peripheral systemic embolism. In some instances, however, the pouch is of such dimension that there is insufficient healthy myocardium to permit excision. Post-operative recurrence is not uncommon.

874a C.P. ♂ 39 yrs. 23 June 1971

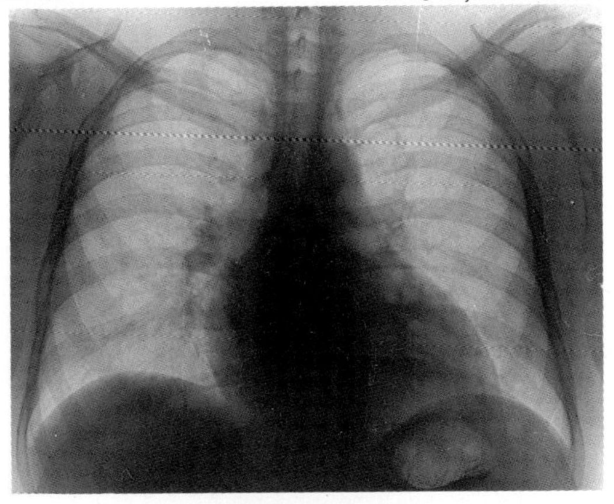

874b 31 July 1971

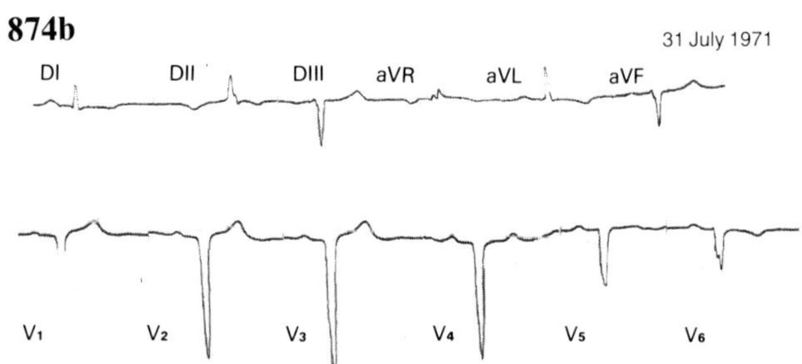

874a Post-traumatic aneurysm of left ventricle. Injury was caused by a blow from an opponent's knee during a soccer match. Pain was initially attributed to a sternal fracture . . .

874b . . . but an ECG reveals a large anterior infarct. An anterior cardiac aneurysm soon develops, principally involving the left ventricle.

874c

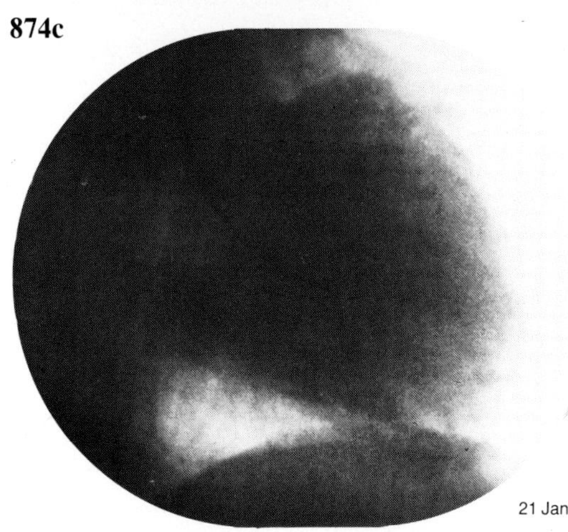

21 Jan. 1972

Left ventriculogram; diastolic phase.

874d

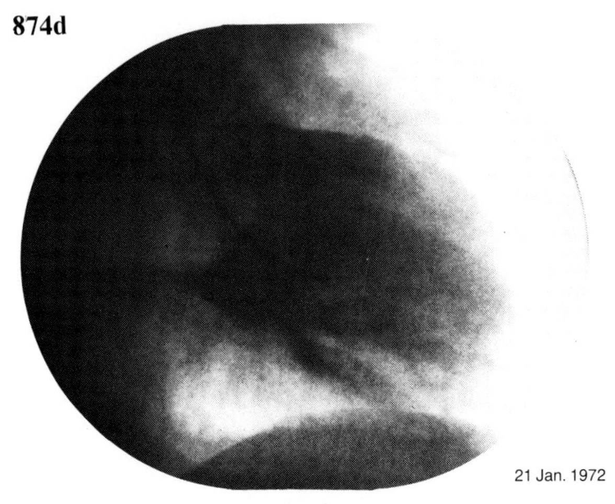

21 Jan. 1972

Systolic phase.

874e

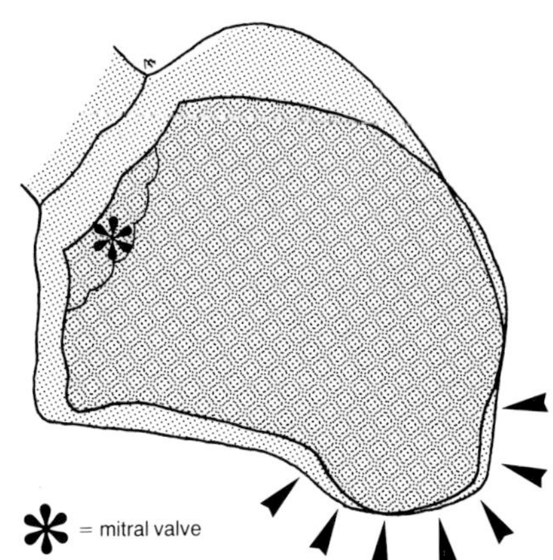

21 Jan. 1972

874e The drawing shows the two phases superimposed. The aneurysm is large and located at the apex of the left ventricle. Catheterisation shows cardiac function to be excellent, and the patient displays no symptoms.

874f

DI DII DIII aVR aVL aVF

V1 V2 V3 V4 V5 V6

24 Mar. 1975

874f Ventriculographic examination four years later shows no change in the size of the aneurysm. Cardiac function is still excellent and the ECG unchanged. The condition is still asymptomatic.

Rupture

Traumatic rupture of the heart can involve any of the chambers and/or valves. The various ruptures and avulsions can occur singly or in combination and involve:
- an **arterial valve,**
- an **atrioventricular valve,**
- the **papillary muscles or chordae tendineae,**
- an **atrial wall,**
- a **ventricular wall,**
- the **septa,** causing a sudden left-to-right shunt; the gravity of such a rupture depends upon its size and localisation; rupture of the ventricular septum is generally more serious than rupture of the atrial septum.

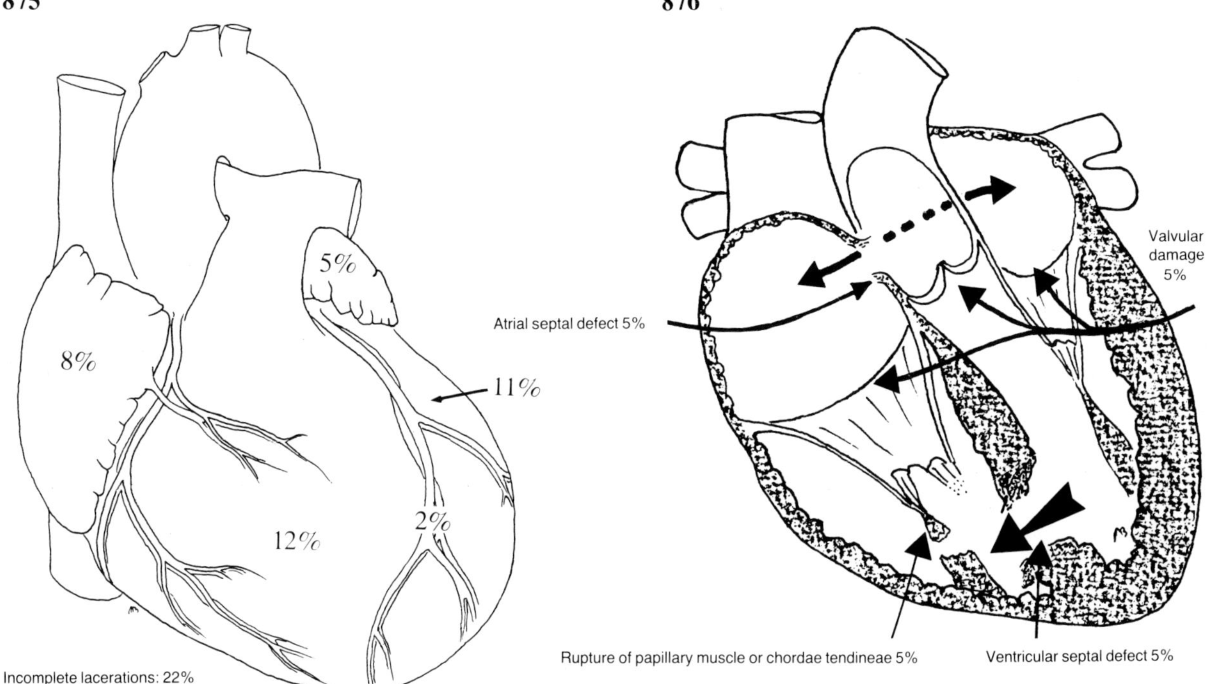

875 Rupture of external heart walls in autopsy material (Literature review)

876 Intracardiac ruptures in autopsy material (Literature review)

The mechanism of cardiac rupture is the same as that of cardiac contusion; the decisive factor is the degree of violence. On rare occasions rupture can result from a relatively non-violent trauma: for example, from over-vigorous external massage of a weak heart, or from puncture-laceration of the heart on a vertebral osteophyte. Older people in particular are prone to this type of injury.

Rupture of an atrial or ventricular wall is seen frequently on the autopsy table: the victims are often young and healthy. Only exceptionally is the thoracic cage damaged.

Overall, transmural rupture is fatal in 94% of cases:
- atrial rupture is immediately fatal in 81% of cases
- right ventricular rupture in 98.5% of cases
- left ventricular rupture in almost all cases
- rupture of more than one chamber in almost all cases.

Moreover, it has been established in autopsy studies that rupture of a cardiac chamber is accompanied by rupture of the aorta in 25% of cases. Animal experiments have shown that a fatal blow (or deceleration):

(1) to the *mid-sternum very rarely* produces a cardiac injury but causes a total rupture of the aorta in *88% of cases*;
(2) to the *lower sternum* produces a cardiac rupture in *35% of cases* and a *serious* pulmonary laceration in *84% of cases*.

877

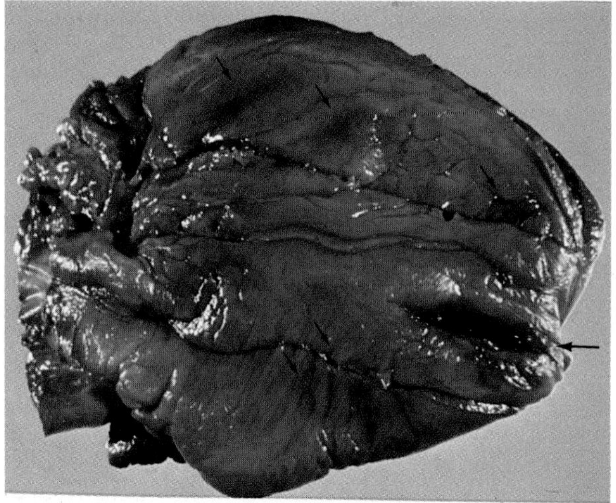

877 Transmural rupture of right ventricle by blunt trauma. Contusions (←) are accompanied by a 4cm transmural rupture (←) close to the right coronary artery.
The patient died 10 minutes after a motorcycle fall. (Institute of Pathology, Lausanne.)

N.A. ♂ 62 yrs. 25 Feb. 1976

Auricles

It has been shown that about 20% of patients with atrial rupture survive long enough for repair to be effected. Every case of apparently uncomplicated cardiac contusion, therefore, should be further investigated for the possibility of atrial rupture.

878

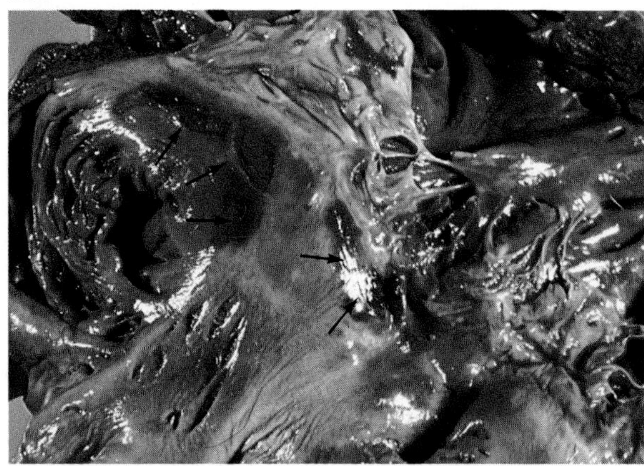

878 Incomplete ruptures of right atrium in an old man who died from a ruptured aorta shortly after admission (see **975**). (Institute of Pathology, Lausanne.)

J.G. ♂ 77 yrs. 10 Feb. 1978

879

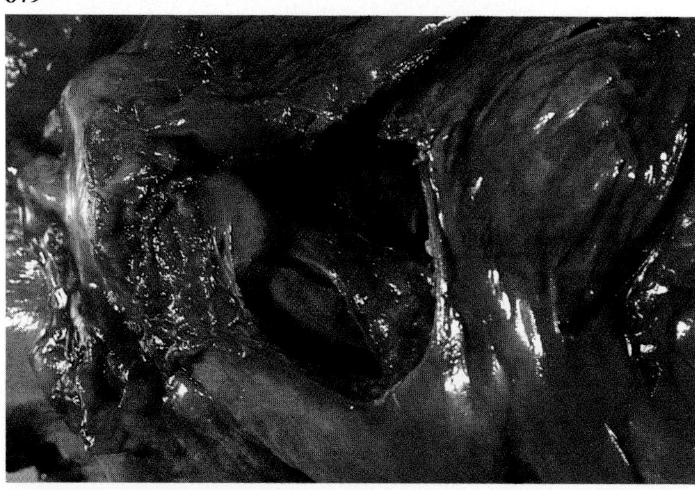

879 Large, complete rupture of right atrium found at autopsy in the victim of a motorcycle accident, who survived for 10 minutes. (Institute of Pathology, Lausanne.)

N.A. ♂ 62 yrs. 25 Feb. 1976

880

Haemostasis by means of:

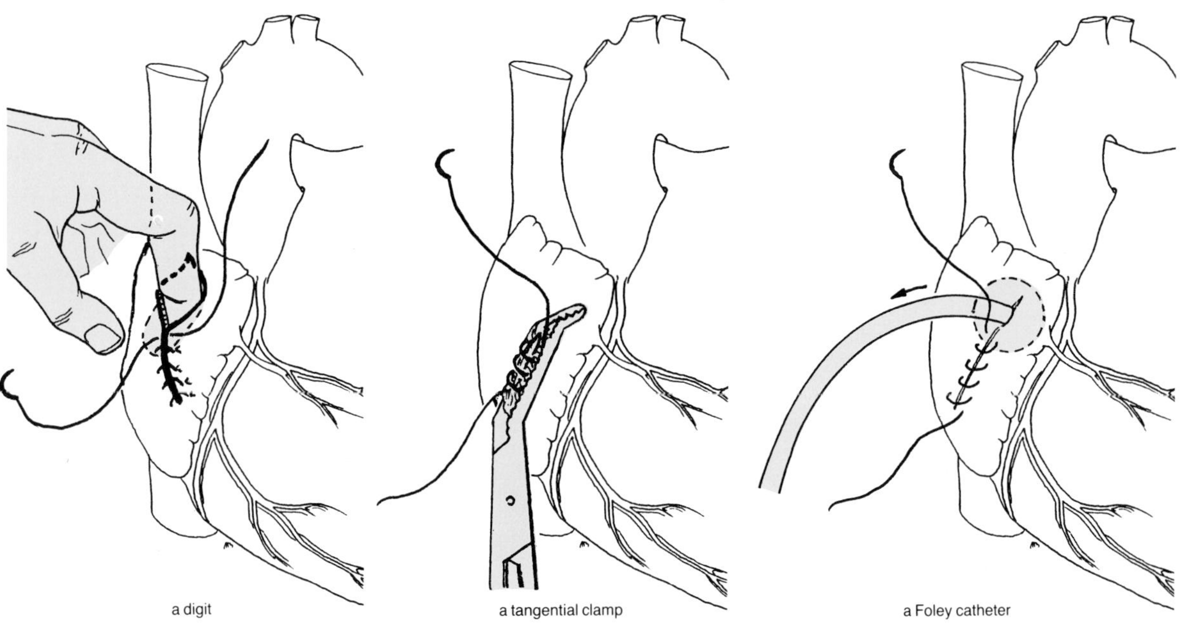

880 Repair of atrial rupture (or wound)

Ventricles

All but the smallest ventricular ruptures by blunt trauma are *immediately* fatal. Survival is so rare that to our knowledge only about ten cases of traumatic right ventricular rupture and a single case of left ventricular rupture have been repaired successfully. In the latter case, a lateral rupture of the pericardium allowed 4000 ml of blood to drain into the left pleural cavity, so forestalling fatal tamponade.

Depending upon its localisation, a traumatic infarct can cause *delayed* rupture with acute tamponade two to three weeks after the initial trauma.

881

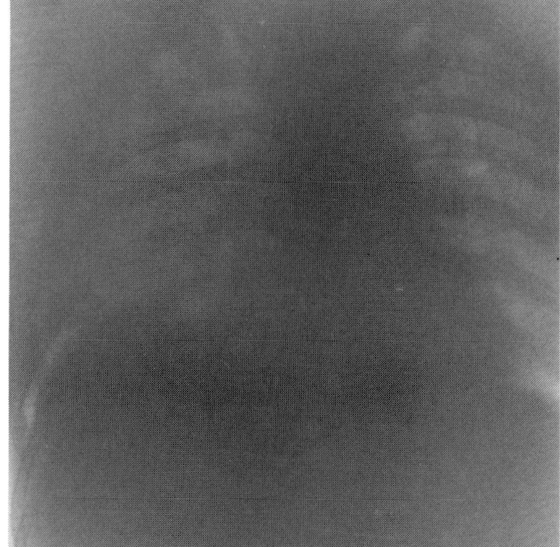

881 Transmural rupture of right ventricle with tension haemopericardium in a car driver involved in a collision with a lorry; he died during resuscitation. Despite indubitable tamponade, the poor quality X-ray shows no significant enlargement of the heart.

M.A. ♂ 44 yrs. 23 Feb. 1968

882

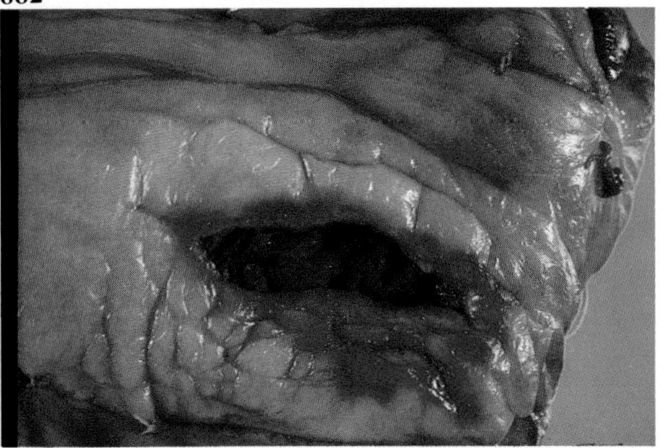

N.A. ♂ 62 yrs. 25 Feb: 1976

882 Anterior transmural rupture of right ventricle with tears of parietal pericardium following a blunt trauma. No cardiac tamponade. Death due to haemorrhage. (Institute of Pathology, Lausanne.)

883

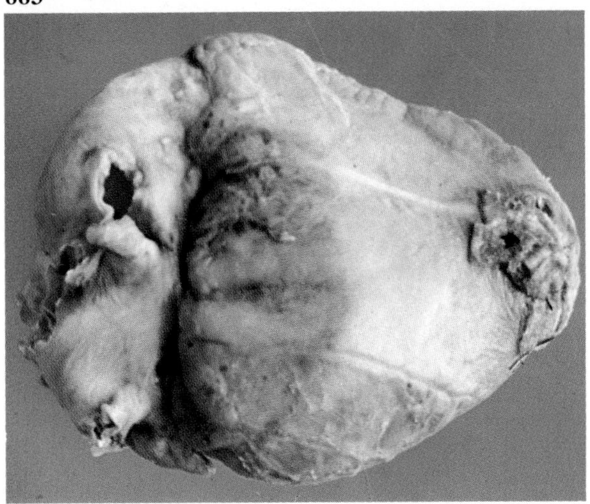

V.J. ♂ 19 yrs. 19 April 1968

883 Secondary rupture of left ventricle. Three weeks after a blunt thoracic trauma, an infarct of the apex of the ventricle ruptured causing cardiac tamponade. Median sternotomy; repair. Death 14 days later due to associated cerebral injuries and bronchopneumonia. (See **873, 903**.) (Institute of Pathology, Lausanne.)

884

Haemostasis by means of:

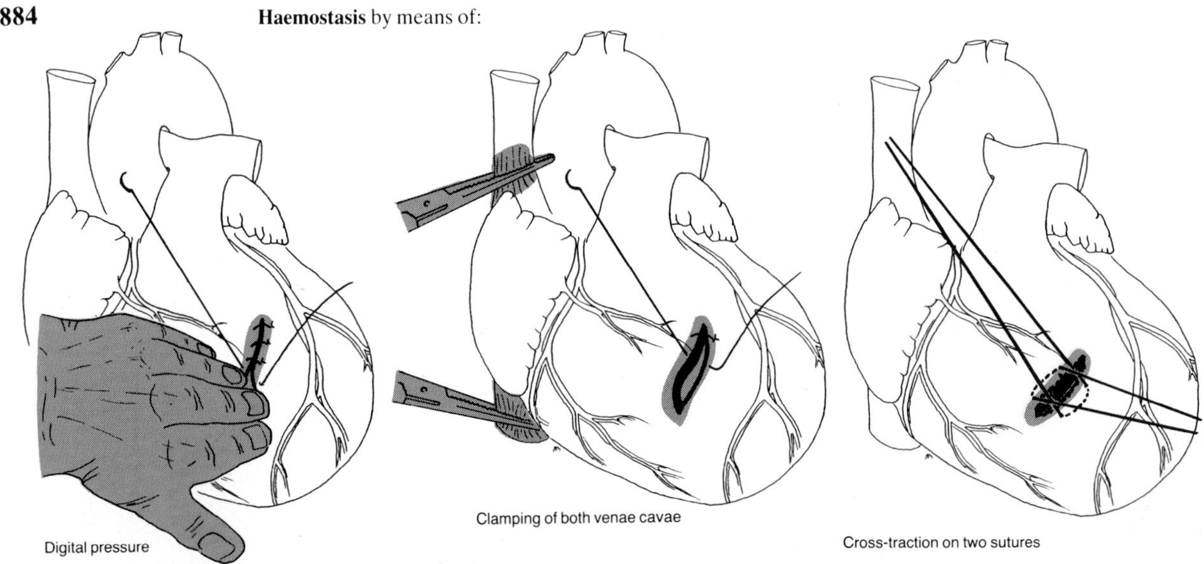

884 Repair of ventricular rupture (or wound)

Septa, with shunts

Rupture of the cardiac septum by blunt trauma can become manifest immediately, or after a delay.

Traumatic atrial septal defect (ASD) usually occurs when the chest is crushed sufficiently to compress the heart between the sternum and the vertebral column. The prognosis is determined by the extent of the damage to the thoracic cage and viscera.

The symptoms and signs of traumatic ASD are the same as those of congenital ASD. Surgical treatment is also the same but it should be remembered that traumatic ASD is accompanied, almost invariably, by other life-threatening injuries. Indeed, traumatic ASD is often only discovered at autopsy.

Traumatic ventricular septal defect (VSD) results either from violent compression of the heart (in which case it appears immediately) or from secondary necrosis of a septal infarct caused by heavy contusion (in which case its appearance is delayed). It is seen most commonly in young males involved in car accidents.

Symptoms arise at the moment shunting begins. This can be weeks after the accident. The clinical repercussions and the evolution of traumatic VSD depend upon its localisation and, above all, upon its dimensions.

The surgical indication and technique of repair are the same as for congenital VSD. Suturing – when necessary – is often easier as traumatic VSD is usually situated in the muscular part of the septum, near the apex of the heart.

About 20% of traumatic VSDs are sufficiently small to be well tolerated for years; indeed, in some cases, repeated catheterisation has documented spontaneous closure. About two thirds of cases have to be operated on because of the severity of the shunt. As for the rest, cardiac failure is rapidly fatal.

885

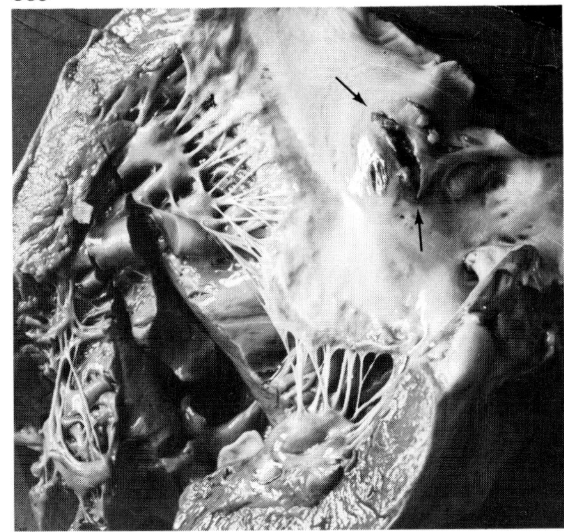
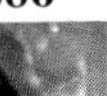

D.R. ♂ 20 yrs. 17 Aug. 1956

885 Post-traumatic atrial septal defect first seen on the autopsy table seven days after the patient was involved in a motorcycle accident. Death was due to a number of other haemorrhagic injuries and to a crush syndrome. (Institute of Pathology, Lausanne.)

Coronary arteries

Post-traumatic **thrombosis** of a healthy coronary artery is exceptional. Previous coronary disease is a significant predisposing factor. Although the chronology of the two causal factors is clear, their relative importance is often difficult to establish. The result is infarction (see page 104).

On the other hand, **traumatic rupture** of a healthy coronary artery is not infrequent. The result is high pressure tamponade with myocardial ischaemia below the rupture. Unless the rupture is very distal, immediate death is inevitable.

886

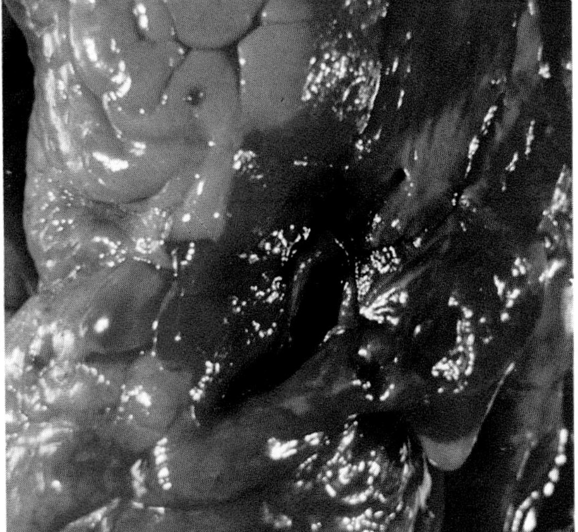

C.J. ♂ 40 yrs. 23 May 1974

886 Rupture of right coronary artery by blunt trauma. Haemopericardium and haemomediastinum. Death shortly after admission. Autopsy specimen. (Institute of Pathology, Lausanne.)

Valvular damage

Valve rupture is most frequent in males between the ages of 50 and 70 years. Healthy valves are no less susceptible than valves weakened by endocarditis.

Rupture of the aortic valves has been known for a long time; it is the most commonly documented valvular injury.

In cases of severe multiple injury, it is often the sole cardiac injury. The most likely cause is a 'water-hammer effect' created by a wave of high pressure within the aorta or the left ventricle. This mechanism is not of the same intensity in the low pressure vessels and chambers; these valves, therefore, rupture only exceptionally.

Rupture of the aortic valve causes rapidly worsening cardiac insufficiency. Early surgery is indicated – within a few weeks of the injury at the latest. Operative procedure is the same as for a non-traumatic defect.

The atrioventricular valves can rupture or be avulsed during a crush-injury. Diagnosis is difficult. Provided the accompanying injuries permit, the damaged valve should be repaired as soon as diagnosis has been made.

Traumatic rupture of the *papillary muscles or chordae tendineae* results in immediate and severe valvular insufficiency; the mitral valve is the valve most often affected. Insufficiency is so acute that it often proves fatal within a matter of hours. Many ruptures are only detected on the autopsy table.

887

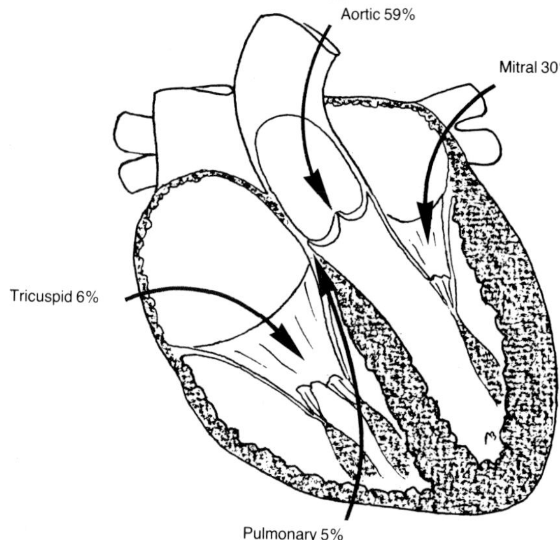

887 **Valve rupture** by blunt cardiac trauma (Literature review).

888

The resultant aortic insufficiency is usually critical.

888 A healthy **aortic valvule** can rupture at its free edge or be avulsed at its base.

889 Post-traumatic insufficiency of a **mitral or tricuspid valve** can be caused by:

889

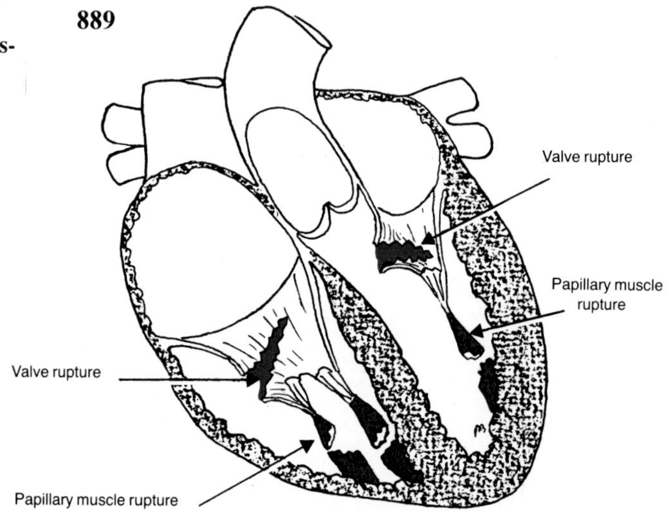

890

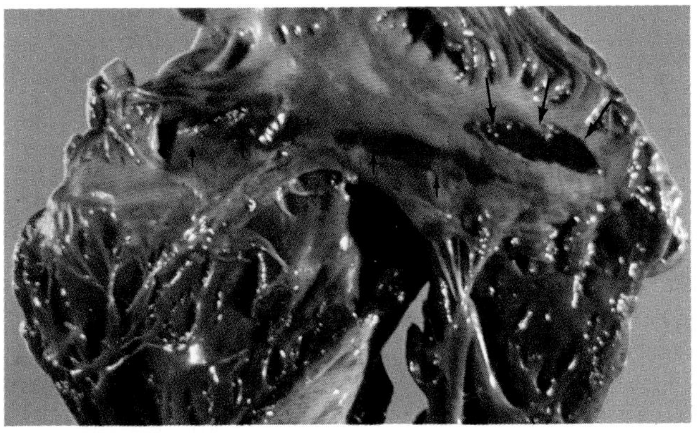

C.J. ♂ 40 yrs. 23 May 1974

890 Partial rupture of tricuspid valve (→) with subendocardial ecchymosis (→) after a blunt trauma. The patient, a car-passenger, died shortly after admission. (Institute of Pathology, Lausanne.)

Open wounds of the heart

(see also Volume I, chapter 3)

Until the end of the 19th century, wounds of the heart were considered fatal. Today, even large wounds can be overcome.

According to our figures, 90% of stab and gunshot wounds occur in males with an average age of about 30 years.

Aetiology

Most heart wounds result from suicide and murder attempts. The proportion of each varies in different countries and regions.

Mortality rates

At least 80% of heart wounds are fatal on the scene of injury.

891

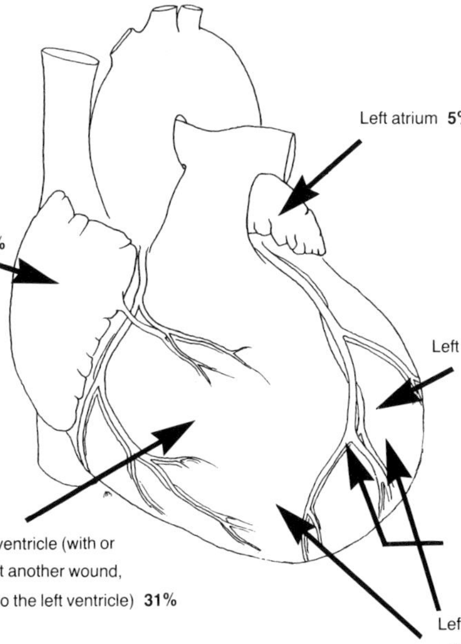

Left atrium **5%**

Right atrium **9%**

Left ventricle (at least) **32%**

Right ventricle (with or without another wound, except to the left ventricle) **31%**

Coronary artery **2%**

Left and right ventricle with a septal injury **21%**

891 Localisation of **heart wounds** in victims **dead** on arrival at hospital (Figures taken from Sugg, $n = 366$).

892 Victims of heart wounds **dying after admission** die from:

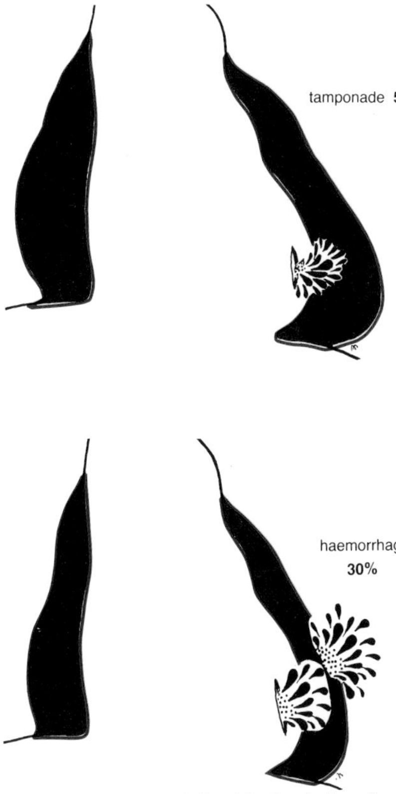

tamponade **57%**

haemorrhage **30%**

some other cause (pulmonary oedema, air embolism, infarction due to section of a coronary artery . . .) **13%**

893a

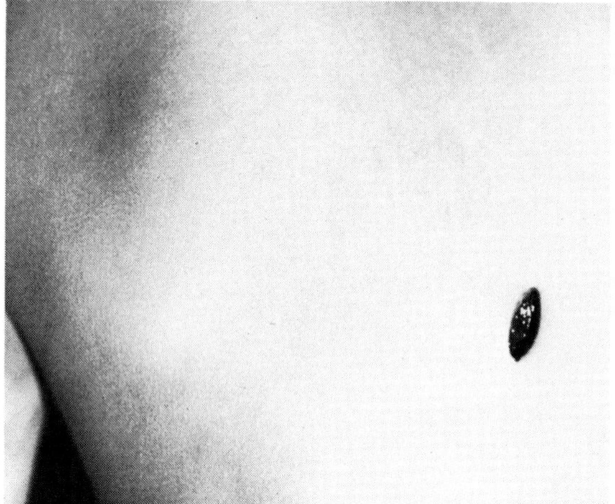

F. A.–S. ♀ 9 yrs. 18 April 1972

893b

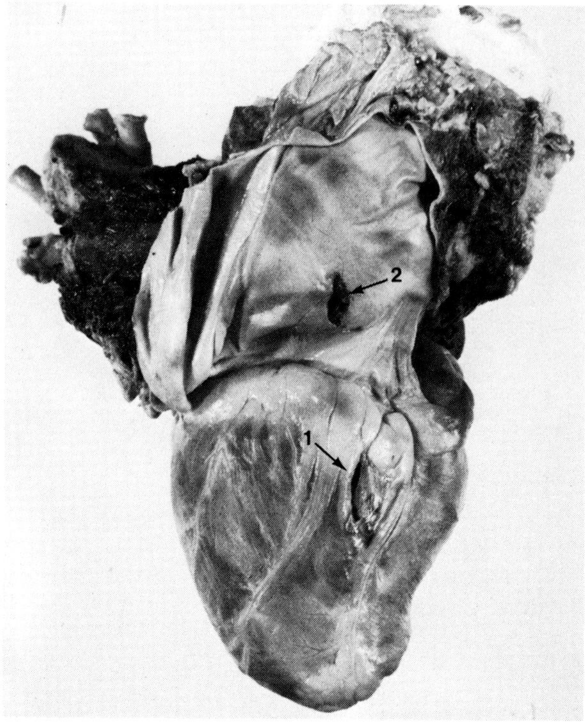

18 April 1972

893a Left ventricular wound with tamponade. Death. The murderer's knife entered to the left of the vertebral column.

893b The autopsy specimen shows a large wound of the left ventricle (→ 1). The posterior pericardial wound (→ 2) was too short to allow the haemopericardium to drain into the pleura (see also **1014**).

893c

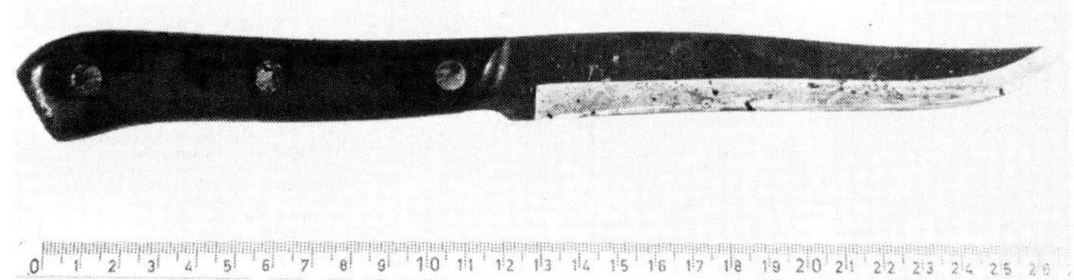

Mortality varies according to the instrument used. A review of the literature ($n = 459$) shows that 89% of gunshot wounds, and 61% of stab wounds are fatal before the victim reaches hospital.

Localisation

If heart wounds are categorised according to the damaged chamber (and given that when two chambers are damaged, only the more serious injury is considered) their relative gravity may be shown thus (figures taken from Sugg, $n = 428$):

Injury to:	dead on arrival	die later	survive
left ventricle	93%	6%	1%
right ventricle	84%	3%	13%
valve/ coronary artery	88%	7%	5%
atrium/ pericardium	52%	12%	36%

894 Localisation of **heart wounds** in victims **alive** on admission (Literature review, $n = 52$).

894

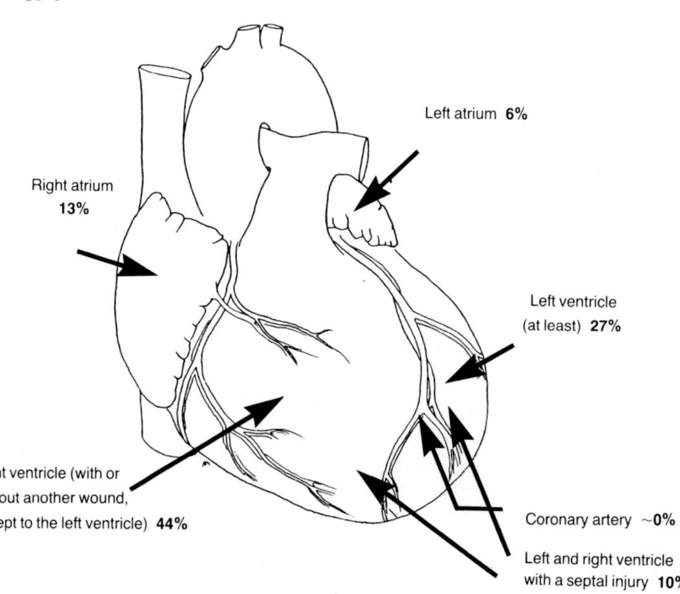

895a

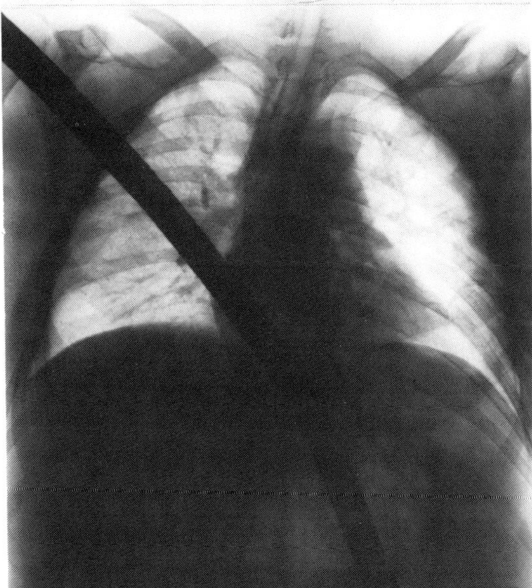

C.P. ♂ 30 yrs. 16 May 1978

895a Thoraco-abdominal impalement with pericardial perforation. The patient fell on a vine-rod which penetrated the chest, fracturing the 3rd right rib and tearing the right internal thoracic (mammary) artery.

895b

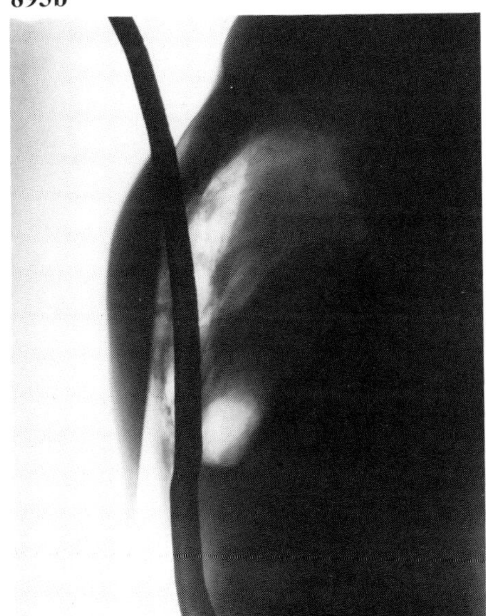

16 May 1978

895b After traversing the pericardium behind the sternum and displacing the heart . . .

895c

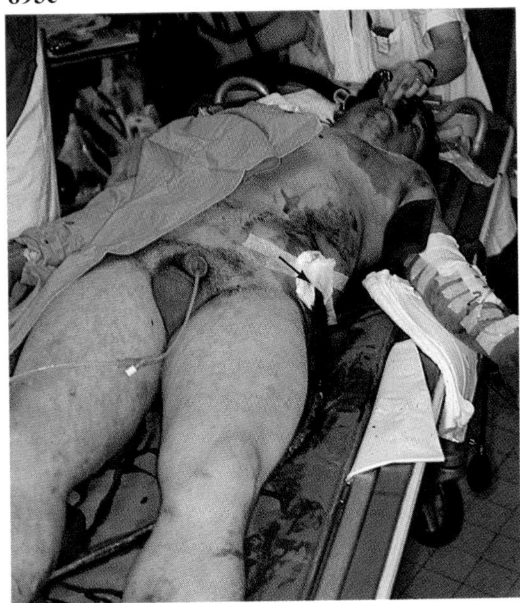

16 May 1978

895c . . . it emerged by the left lateral abdomen, without causing any intra-abdominal injury. Immediate partial median sternotomy for haemostasis of the internal thoracic (mammary) artery and evaluation of the damage. The heart is intact. Drainage, antibiotics.

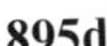

895d

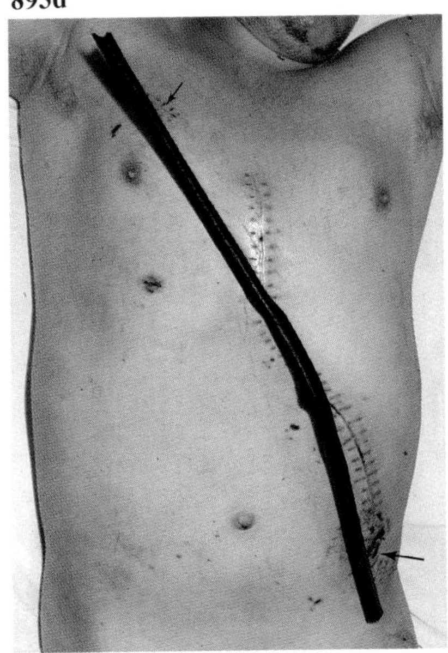

25 May 1978

895d The path of the stake reconstructed to show the points of entry (→) and exit (→). Anterior view, with the stake. Recovery.

895e

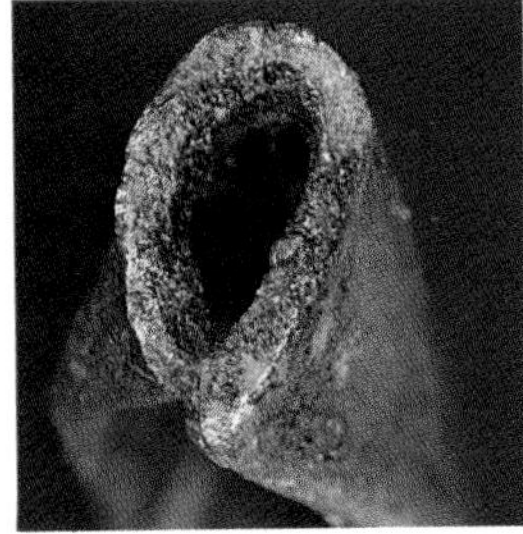

895e If the stake (shown actual size) had been sharp, damage would have been fatal.

896a

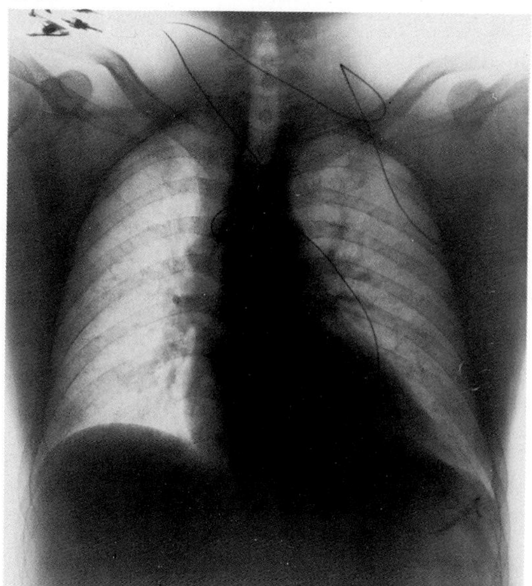

896a Stab wound of right ventricle with massive tamponade. The patient reported to a casualty department where the skin wound was considered superficial and sutured (!). Transferred to hospital, he displayed a slightly enlarged heart shadow.

896b

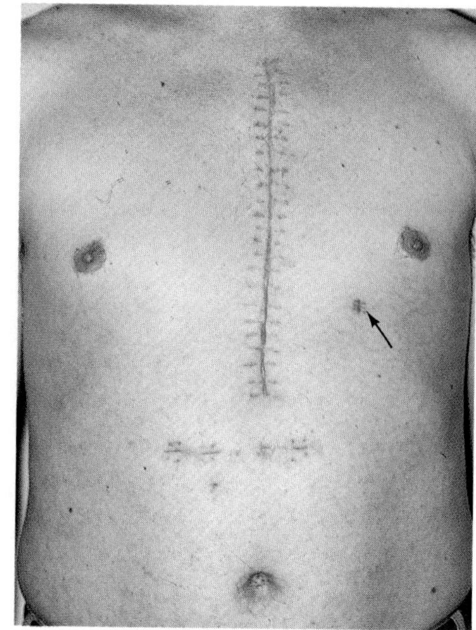

896b Cardiac arrest shortly after admission. An emergency median sternotomy leads to the discovery of a 500 ml semi-clotted haemopericardium and a wound of the right ventricle. Repair and internal cardiac massage. Recovery without sequelae.
N.B. The knife entered (→) 4 cm below and to the right of the left nipple.

897a

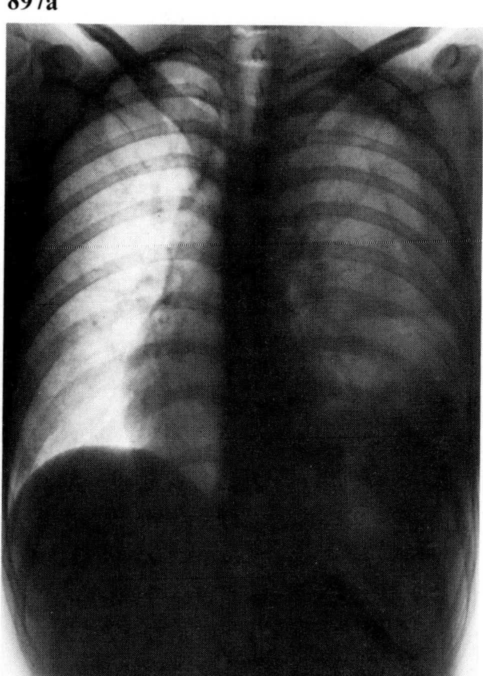

897b

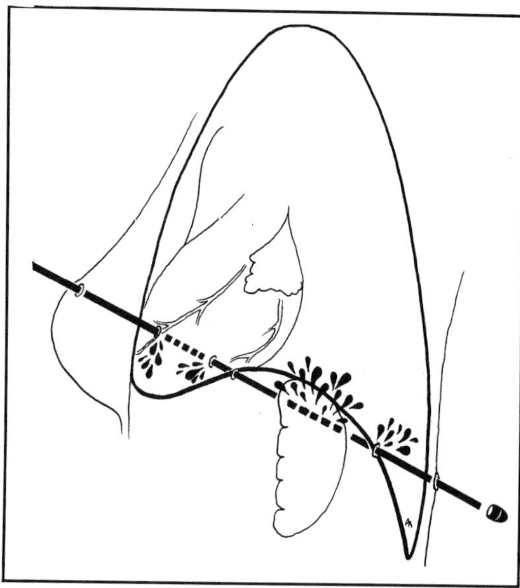

897b Path of the bullet.

897a Perforating wound of left ventricle by 7.65 mm middle velocity bullet, **with section of branch of left coronary artery**. The admission X-ray shows a compressive left haemopneumothorax with an inverted hemidiaphragm and mediastinal shift. Immediate left thoracotomy. After evacuating the 3000 ml haemothorax, the surgeon finds blood coming from the abdomen through two diaphragmatic wounds. Incision of the diaphragm reveals a haemorrhagic tear of the spleen: splenectomy and diaphragmatic repair. Subsequent incision of the pericardium discloses 100 ml of clotted blood. Having ceased to bleed, the transfixed left ventricle is sutured on dacron felt pledgets; the left diagonal artery responsible for the haemopericardium is ligated.

897c

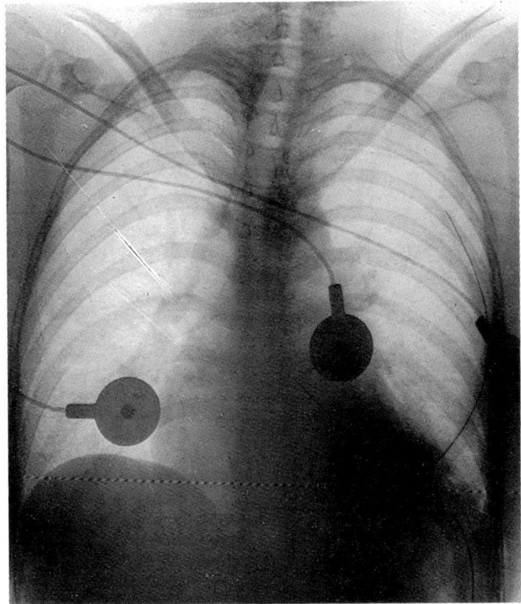

24 Dec. 1967

897c Postoperative X-ray.

897d

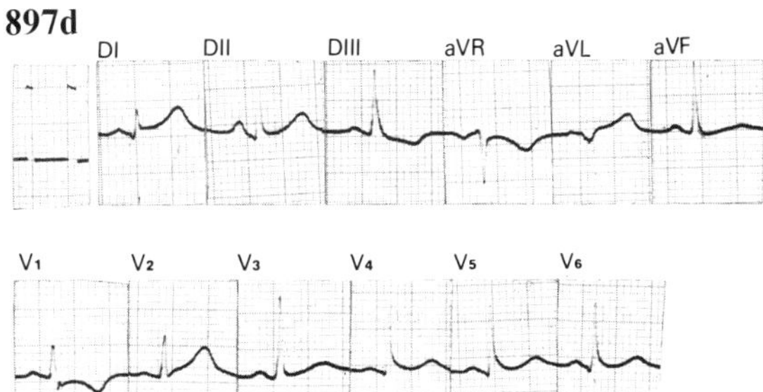

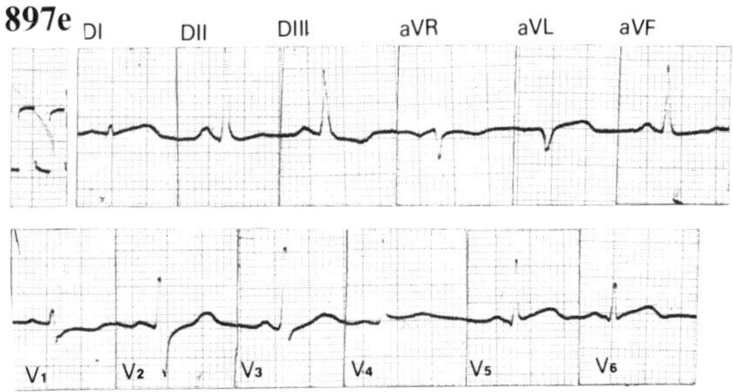

30 Dec. 1967

897d A subsequent ECG shows signs of anterolateral infarction (section of the left diagonal artery).

897e

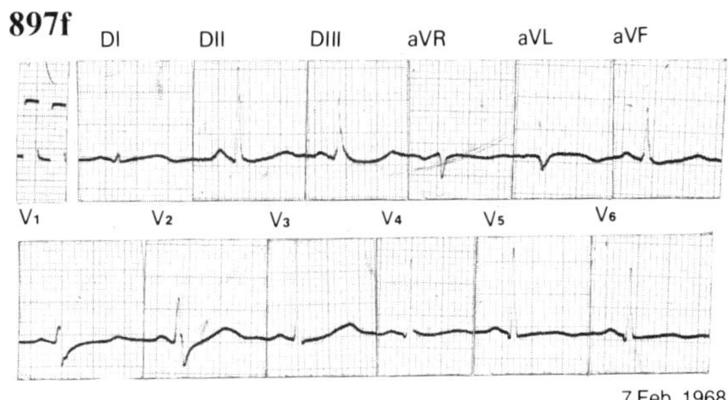

897e The ECG returns to normal with the exception of a QS complex in aVL. 6 Jan. 1968

897f DI DII DIII aVR aVL aVF

V1 V2 V3 V4 V5 V6

7 Feb. 1968

897f ECG six weeks after the accident.

897g

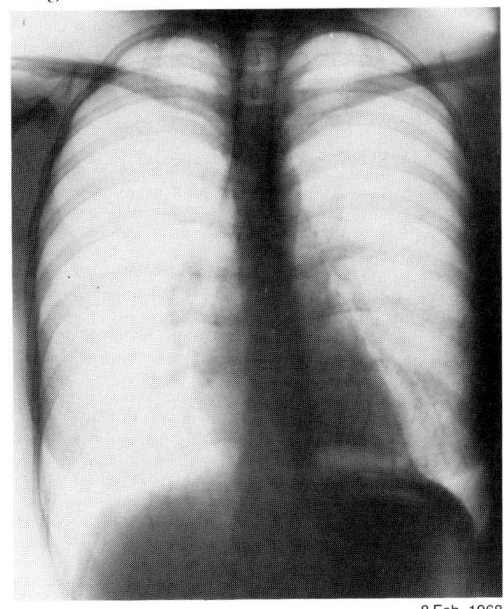

8 Feb. 1968

897g Recovery.

898 W.O. ♂ 60 yrs. 22 Mar. 1979

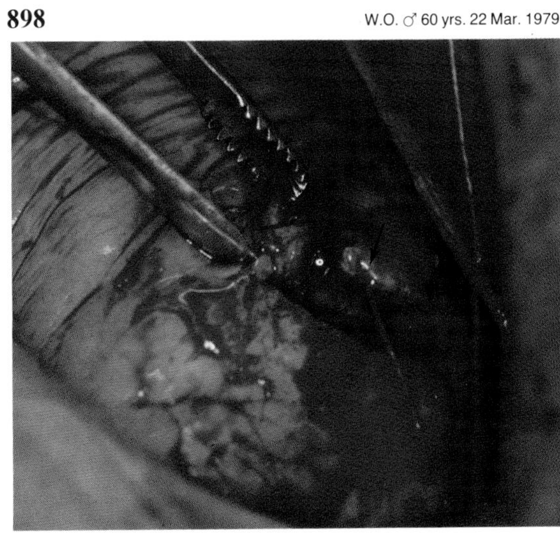

898 **Stab wound of left ventricle with section of branch (→) of interventricular anterior artery** and a 200 ml haemopericardium after a suicidal attempt. The blade did not enter the left ventricle. Ligation of coronary artery, repair of the myocardium. Recovery without noticeable sequelae.

Diagnosis

Immediately after a wound to the heart, a patient may:
- be almost completely free of symptoms,
- be in haemorrhagic shock,
- suffer acute cardiac insufficiency as a result of tamponade or valve injury,
- experience arrhythmia through a conduction tissue injury,
- suffer infarction due to section of a coronary artery,
- experience acute left-to-right shunting because of a perforated septum,
- be dead or dying with few external signs of injury.

The possibility of a heart wound should be investigated systematically whenever the precordial region has been injured. Methods of investigation include (1) questioning of the patient, (2) examination of the offending instrument, (3) reconstruction of the probable path of the bullet or knife, (4) estimation of the position of the patient at the moment of impact and (5) taking a standard X-ray and (6) a sinogram.

When a wound of the heart is accompanied by a lateral perforation of the pericardium, blood usually runs into the pleural cavity. Instead of tamponade, the result is a potentially massive haemothorax. Provided the blood loss is not life-threatening, the haemothorax should be drained by pleural aspiration.

899

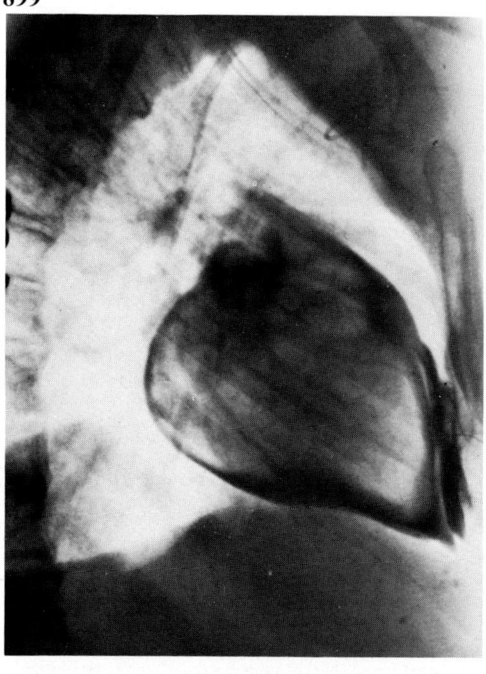

S. 1967

899 Stab wound of pericardium. Catheter sinogram. (Prof. F. Steichen, New York.)

900

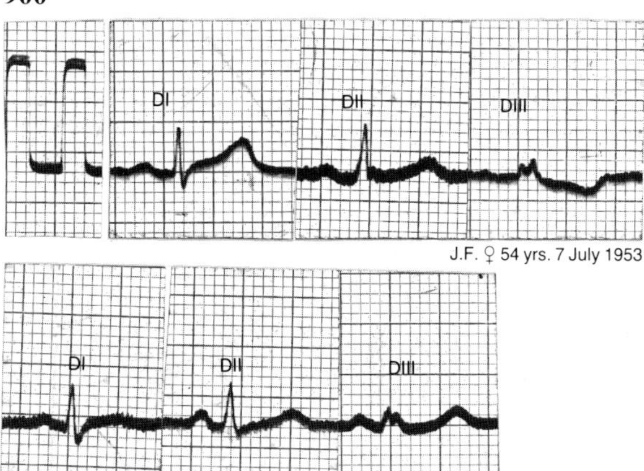

900 Perforation of left ventricle by a revolver bullet. Thoracotomy, repair. Recovery. Disturbances of the ECG are transient.

Management

A patient with a known or suspected **stab wound** to the heart should be operated upon immediately, either through a *left thoracotomy* or a *median sternotomy*. In cases of tamponade, *pericardiocentesis* can be helpful provided, of course, that the blood-loss from the pericardial drain does not endanger the patient's life.

Gunshot wounds, also, should be treated immediately. In almost every case, a direct approach is to be recommended – possibly after preliminary pericardiocentesis. The choice between *a left or right anterolateral thoracotomy* and a *median sternotomy* depends upon the location of the entrance (and exit) wound and upon X-ray evidence.

901

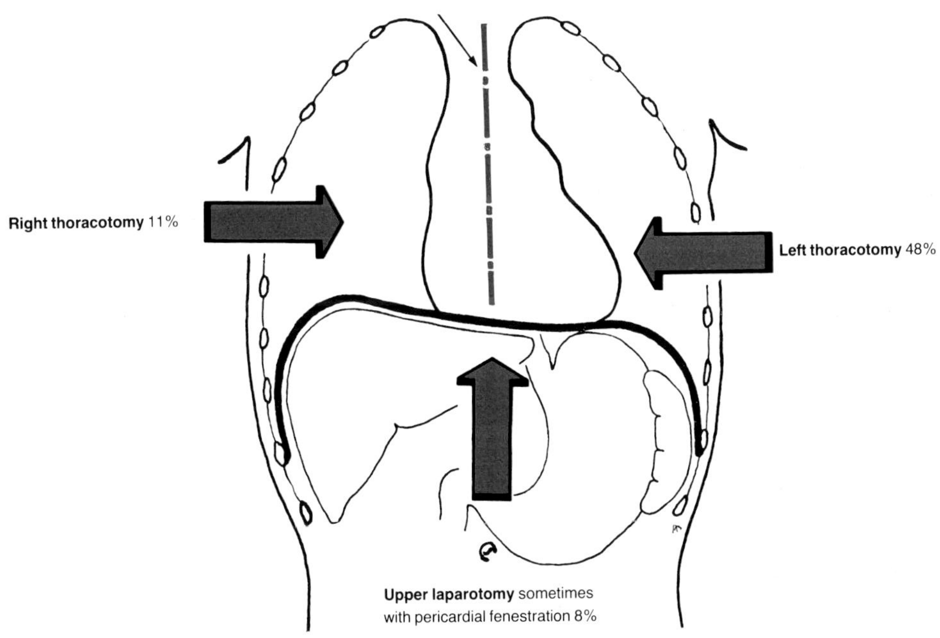

901 Surgical approaches to wounds of heart or intra-pericardial vessels (Literature review)

902

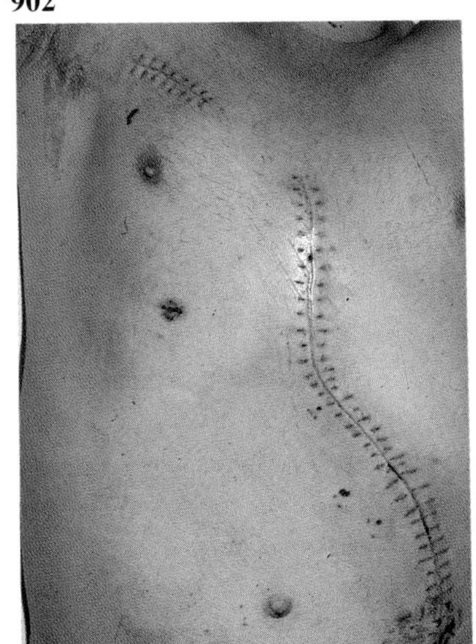

C.P. ♂ 30 yrs. 16 May 1978

902 The surgical approach can be complex. This impalement wound was explored initially through a partial median sternotomy. Incisions were then made along the line of the offending instrument and at the entrance and exit wounds (see **895**).

903

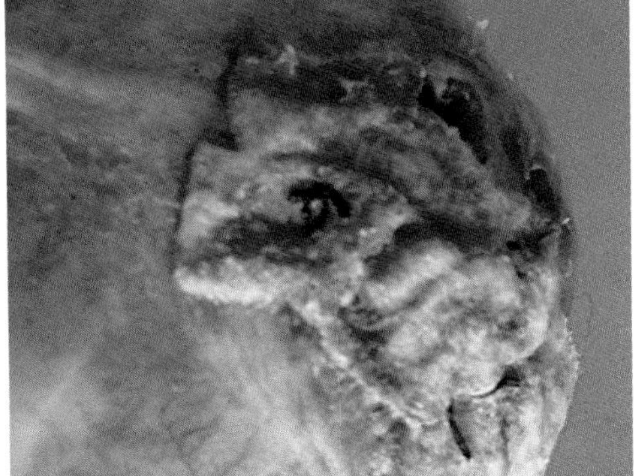

V.J. ♂ 19 yrs. 19 April 1968

903 It is useful to support ventricular sutures on dacron felt pledgets. (Institute of Pathology, Lausanne.)

Sequelae

Successful surgical repair of a heart wound by no means precludes the possibility of subsequent complications or sequelae. Long-term follow-up is vital in every case. In order of prevalence, the sequelae amenable to surgery are:

- initially undetected septal injuries which subsequently cause a left-to-right shunt,
- late vascular or cardiac aneurysm,
- unrecognised valvular injuries,
- intracardiac presence of a foreign body, with subsequent peripheral embolism (systemic or pulmonary),
- serofibrinous, purulent pericarditis – constrictive or, occasionally, callous,
- fistulisation between a coronary artery and vein or, between an artery and a cardiac chamber.

All of these conditions are dealt with separately elsewhere in this chapter, except the two covered below.

Perforation of the atrial or ventricular septum in a stab or gunshot wound of the heart is usually small and clinically well tolerated. Since it generally arises in otherwise healthy young men, the prognosis is usually better than for an equivalent congenital defect.

In some cases, an apparently slight precordial wound can have serious repercussions. The initial wound may heal after conservative treatment but subsequently lead to an **arteriovenous fistula**. Fistulas have been reported also between the aorta and the vena cava, the aorta and either right chamber, the aorta and the pulmonary artery, and between a coronary artery and vein.

These sequelae are, however, rare. Once diagnosed and investigated haemodynamically, they should be repaired without delay. The procedure required varies from case to case.

Electric injury of the heart

An electric shock of several seconds from an alternating current (of between 110 and 380 volts and 50 to 60 Herz) can cause fatal myocardial fibrillation. (Myocardial fibrillation occurring inside a hospital can be reversed by a second electric shock administered with a defibrillator.) Survivors usually suffer supraventricular tachycardia with repolarisation phase disorders for several weeks afterwards.

Occasional cases of myocardial infarction have been reported after electric burns in the precordial region. It is possible that infarction is sometimes the result of a direct, deep burn of the heart muscle itself. Late rupture of the right ventricle has been observed.

A high voltage electric shock generally has a more marked arc-effect. Burns are the most common result, but polymorphic ischaemic heart disorders also have been reported.

904

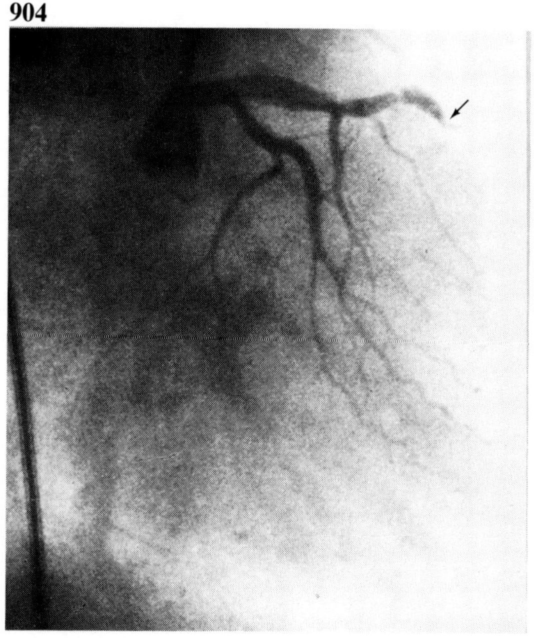

F.F. ♂ 49 yrs. 9 May 1975

904 Anterior septal infarct with complete thrombosis of anterior descending artery (→) caused by 220 volts electric shock. Symptomatic injury leading to stage III angina. Selective coronary angiogram.

Foreign body injury to the heart

There are numerous well-documented cases of foreign bodies that have migrated far from their initial point of entry into the vascular bed.

A bullet trapped between the papillary muscles or chordae tendineae can be well tolerated. It may remain silent for many years, producing nothing more than psychological side-effects. As a general rule, however, any foreign body (especially if it is greater than one centimetre in any of its dimensions) trapped in the heart or pericardium for more than a few days should be removed. In this way, many potential complications are avoided: serofibrinous pericarditis, pericardial emphysema, myocardial abscess, late haemorrhage and secondary pulmonary or systemic embolism.

Pulmonary or systemic embolus

A foreign body or bullet *directly* entering *one of the chambers of the heart* can pass either into the greater or into the lesser circulation.

The foreign body that is most frequently responsible for **pulmonary embolism** is an intra-cath fragment inadvertently sectioned during withdrawal through the needle. Pulmonary embolism of revolver bullets is also known. Low velocity gunshot wounds to the *abdomen or lower limbs* can imply non-transfixing venous wounds. The intravascular bullet readily migrates towards the heart, coming to rest either in the right ventricle or in a pulmonary artery.

The technique required to extract a foreign body from the right ventricle or atrium varies from case to case. Some fragments can be removed through the jugular vein under local anaesthesia and with the help of an image intensifier. Other cases demand thoracotomy (see **906**) or even extracorporeal circulation. If the patient is operated upon in the lateral decubitus position, a Swan-Ganz balloon catheter should be inserted to hold the foreign body in position, since it has been known for a bullet to switch sides, or even return to the right ventricle as the patient is prepared for surgery.

905a D.M.–L. ♀ 3 yrs. 20 Mar. 1972

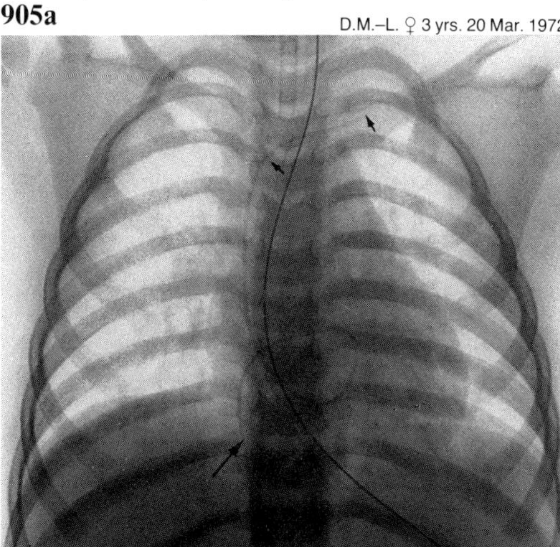

905a Transjugular extraction of catheter from pulmonary artery in a child. A piece of catheter sectioned in the leg has risen into the superior vena cava and the left innominate vein (→). The other end (**→**) is still in the inferior vena cava. The intervening coiled portion has traversed the tricuspid valve.

905b 20 Mar. 1972

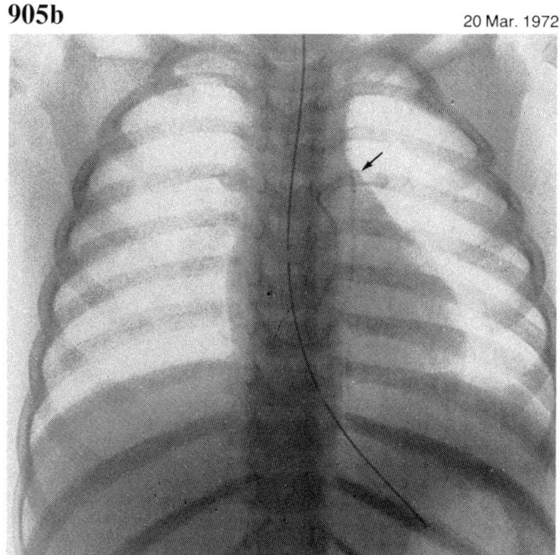

905b The flow of blood through the right ventricle drags on the loop and before long, the loop reaches the trunk of the pulmonary artery . . .

905c 20 Mar. 1972

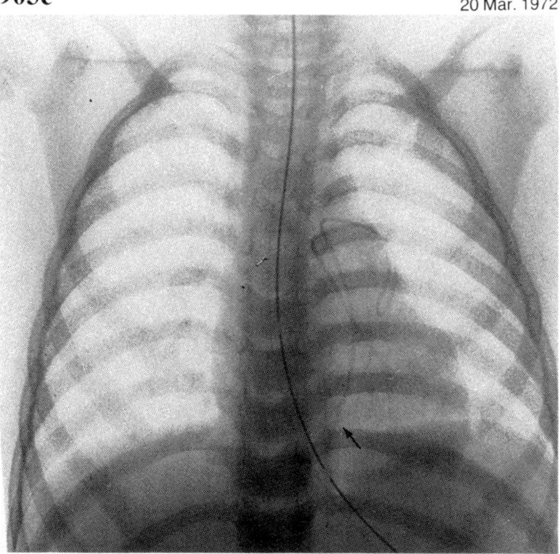

905c . . . and then enters the left pulmonary artery; the proximal part of the catheter remains in the right ventricle. The child shows no symptoms.

905d 30 Mar. 1972

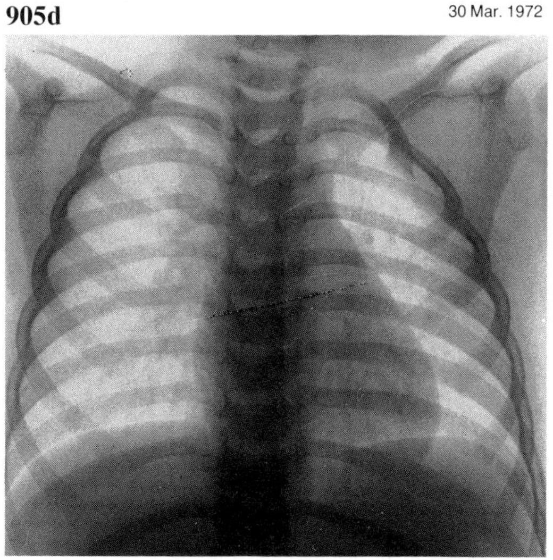

905d Recovery after transjugular extraction.

906a

G.S. ♀ 19 yrs. 26 April 1973

906b

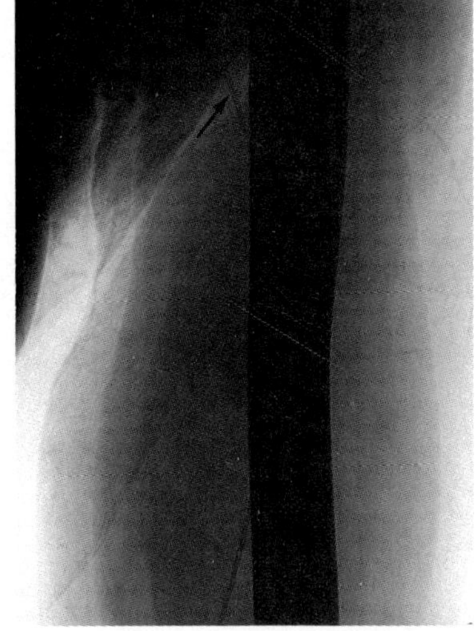

26 April 1973

906c

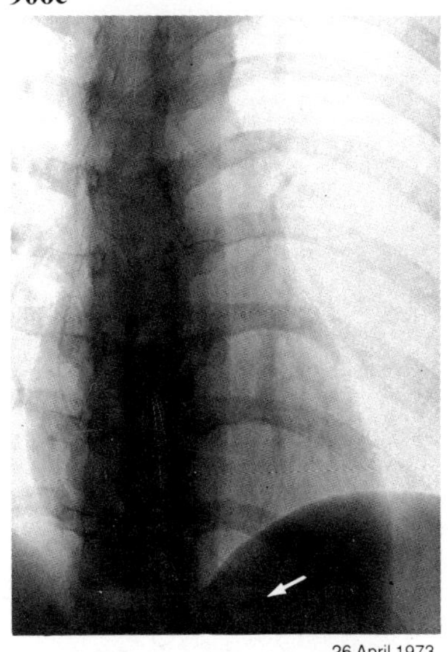

26 April 1973

906d

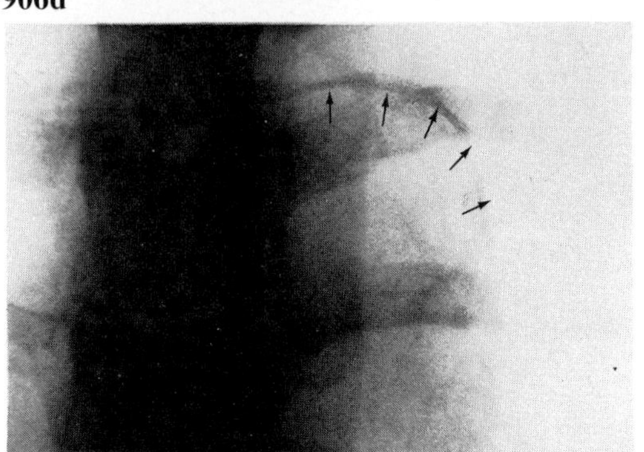

27 April 1973

906a Embolism of intra-cath fragment in pulmonary artery. Extraction by left thoracotomy. After a basilic vein puncture, the catheter was sectioned as it was withdrawn through its needle. A tourniquet (→) was applied immediately, but did not prevent the catheter from advancing towards the heart.

906b The catheter enters the brachial vein . . .

906c . . . and is then drawn into the left innominate vein, the superior vena cava, the right atrium and right ventricle (→).

906d Twenty-four hours later, it finally lodges at the bifurcation of pulmonary artery.

906e *N.B. On a standard chest X-ray, it is often very difficult to detect catheter embolism.*

906f The catheter has been removed through a left thoracotomy. Recovery.

906e

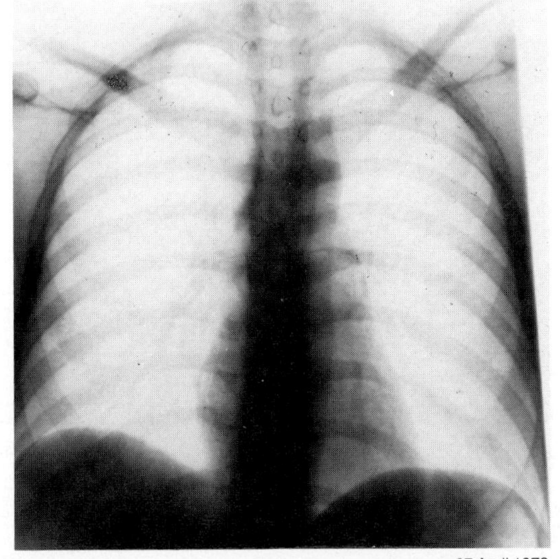

27 April 1973

906f

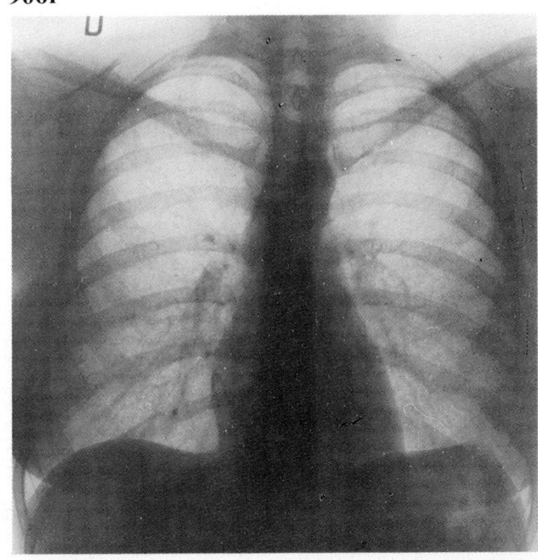

27 April 1974

Systemic embolism of a foreign body is less frequent. The embolus is usually a low velocity bullet or small fragment of shell that has arrived in the left heart, either directly through the atrial or ventricular wall, or via the pulmonary veins.

The clinical developments are the same as for any other type of systemic embolism. Once recognised and located, the foreign body should be extracted and a distal arterial thrombectomy performed.

The symptoms and signs arising from the heart wound vary from case to case. Repair is not always necessary.

907

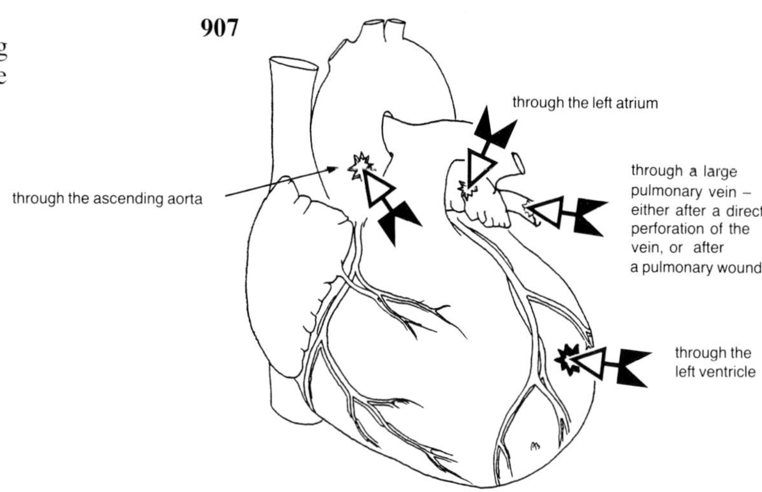

907 Potential emboli can enter the left heart in several ways

908

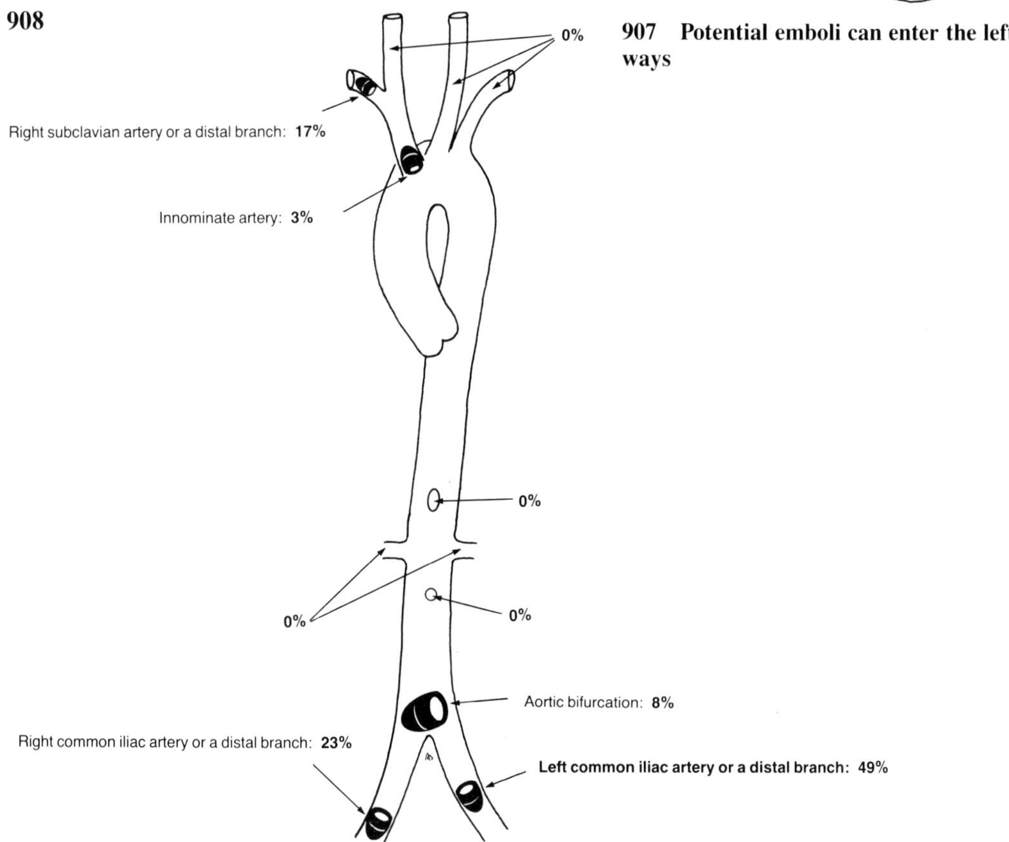

908 Final systemic localisation of bullet emboli (Literature review)

Perforation from within

The chambers of the right heart can be perforated from within during certain diagnostic or therapeutic manoeuvres. For example:

1. during cardiac catheterisation (a rare and benign injury),
2. during angiography (rare and benign),
3. from the displacement of a pacemaker electrode (a frequent injury, but relatively harmless),
4. when a central venous catheter perforates the heart wall and passes into the pericardial sac (infrequent, but extremely dangerous).

Perforation of the right atrium or ventricle is among the risks of **catheterisation** or **angiography**; it is usually detected immediately. Surgical repair is rarely necessary.

By pacemaker electrode

The endovenous introduction of a **pacemaker electrode** into the right ventricle can lead to slow perforation. Wherever the electrode is positioned, the ceaseless action of the myocardium is likely to drive it slowly through the wall into the pericardial sac.

Perforation can be diagnosed either from X-ray evidence or from the reduced efficiency of the pacemaker stimuli; hiccoughing (usually the consequence of direct stimulation of the diaphragm) is a frequent attendant sign.

The perforation is generally small and bordered by cicatricial tissue.

As long as the electrode remains occlusive, there is no effusion of blood into the pericardium and effusion remains moderate (50 to 100ml). Even when the electrode is withdrawn during surgery for epicardial implantation of new electrodes, bleeding is usually only minimal. Consequently, whenever pacemaker stimulation is ineffective, the electrodes can be re-positioned with little danger, even when perforation is suspected. For safety, this manoeuvre should be followed, nevertheless, by one or two days' hospital observation.

When perforation is indubitable and stimulation persistently ineffective, or when hiccoughing is exhausting the patient, a median sternotomy should be performed to suture new electrodes directly on to the epicardium.

909a

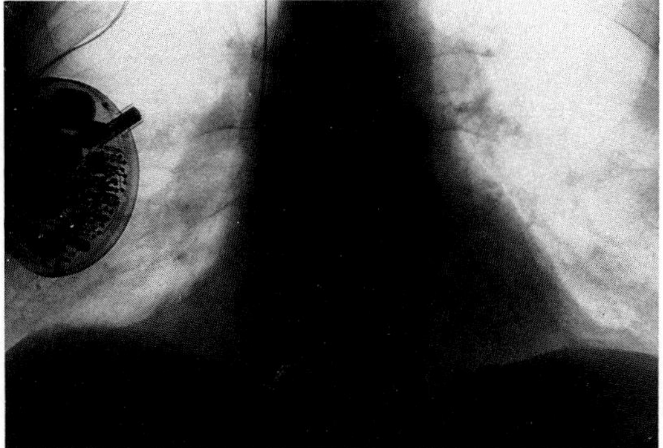

M. J.–P. ♂ 71 yrs. 18 Nov. 1974

909a Perforation of right ventricle by a pacemaker electrode. On this postoperative X-ray, the tip of the electrode is hidden by the shadow of the vertebral column.

909b

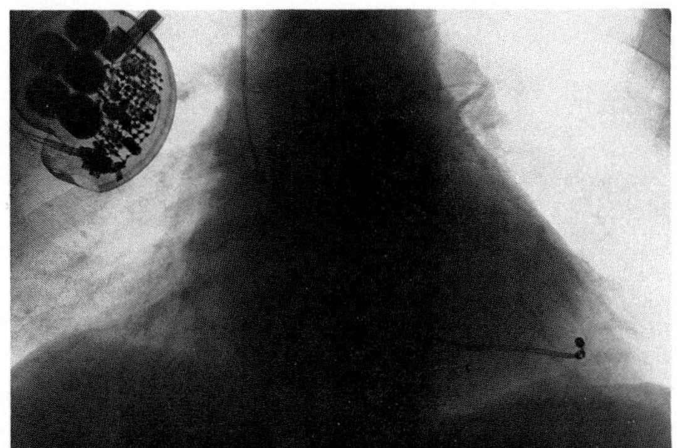

16 Dec. 1974

909b One month later, it has come into view. Ineffective pacing and the enlarged outline of the heart suggest perforation of the right ventricle.

909c

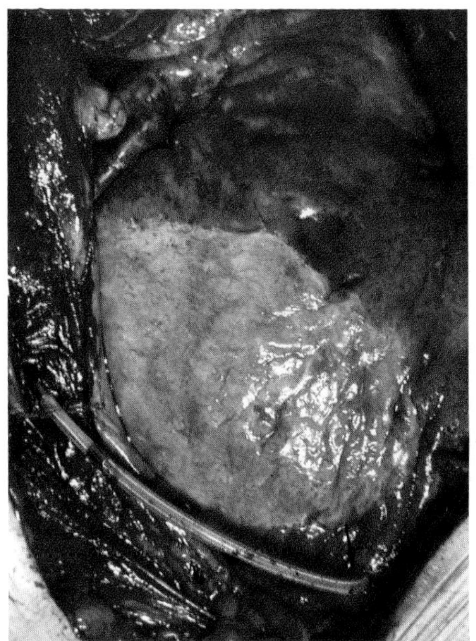

18 Dec. 1974

909c Median sternotomy: the electrode has perforated the apex of the ventricle (→), and penetrated 10cm into the pericardium. There is a slight fluid reaction, but no haemopericardium. After the electrode has been extracted and the ventricle sutured, fresh electrodes are applied to the epicardium. Recovery. (Prof. H. Sadeghi, Lausanne.)

By central venous catheter

Perforation by a central perfusion catheter can be extremely dangerous. It occurs when the catheter is inadvertently left inside the right ventricle or atrium instead of the vena cava. Central venous catheters are currently in widespread use; correct placement (see Volume I, page 53) always should be verified by X-ray.

Peforation of the heart by a catheter is in itself relatively harmless. The danger is that continued perfusion through the catheter rapidly leads to acute tamponade and death. The danger of tamponade is particularly high if the perfusion is administered by an automatic pump.

Moreover, this type of tamponade is often inadvertently rendered fatal by the administration of injections through the catheter itself (thought to be correctly placed).

There are only two reported cases of survival after this type of perforation and tamponade. The therapeutic steps are:

1. to **diagnose** the tamponade and the perforation with an over-exposed chest X-ray,
2. to stop the perfusion **without moving the catheter**,
3. to connect the catheter to a suction device to clear the tamponade,
4. to **withdraw** the catheter from the pericardial sac,
5. to **observe** the patient carefully to detect renewed tamponade (by secondary haemorrhage).

910 C.Y. ♂ 17 yrs. 9 Dec. 1973

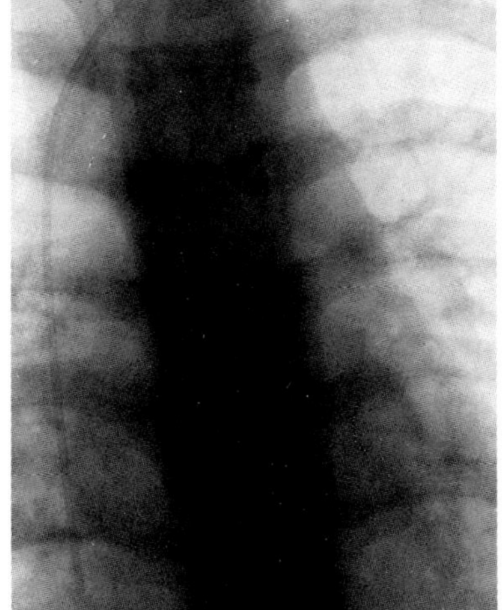

910 Central venous catheter in right atrium. There is a risk of perforation.

911 B.V. ♀ 65 yrs. 19 Mar. 1975

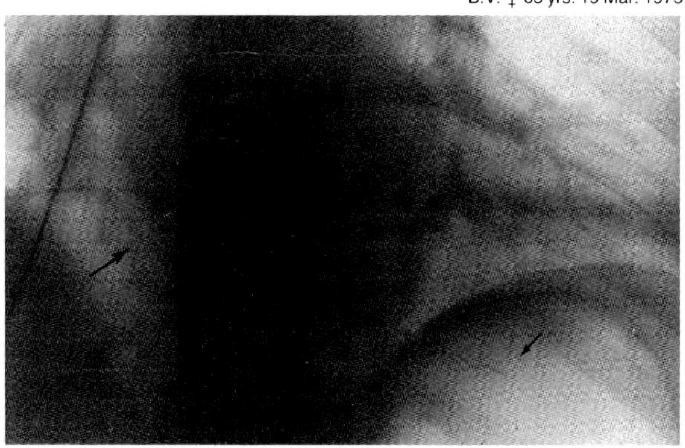

911 Intraventricular catheter. Superficial examination of this X-ray might suggest that the tip is close to the tricuspid valve (→); in fact, the tip of the catheter (→) can be seen to extend to the left of the vertebral column.

912a

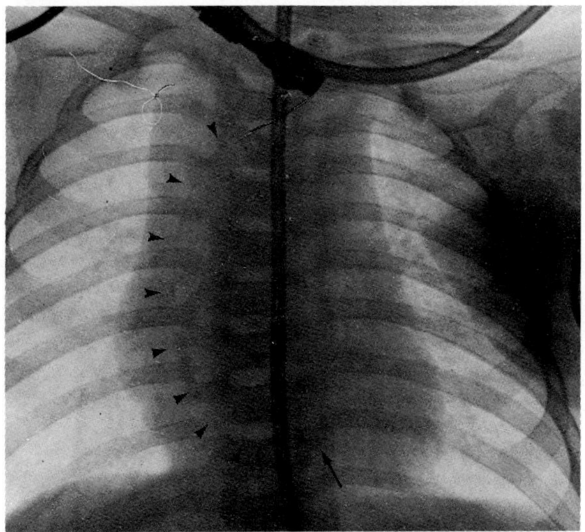

C.S. ♂ 5 mths. 16 Nov. 1970

912b

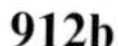

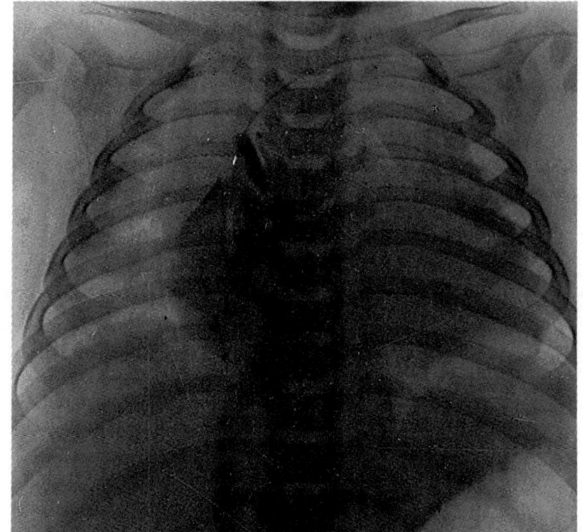

22 Nov. 1970

912a Fatal cardiac tamponade resulting from atrial perforation by central venous catheter and from infusion of fluid into pericardium in an infant with abdominal difficulties. A catheter has been inserted through a cut-down of the left cephalic vein. Opacified by contrast material, it appears to lie in the right ventricle (→).

It is withdrawn 4cm, sutured to the skin and then connected to an automatic perfusion pump.

912b Six days later, the child dies suddenly. The post-mortem X-rays shows massive enlargement of the heart and pericardium and a right pleural effusion. Contrast material introduced through the catheter has flooded the pericardium, indicating that the catheter was still 6cm too deep.

912c

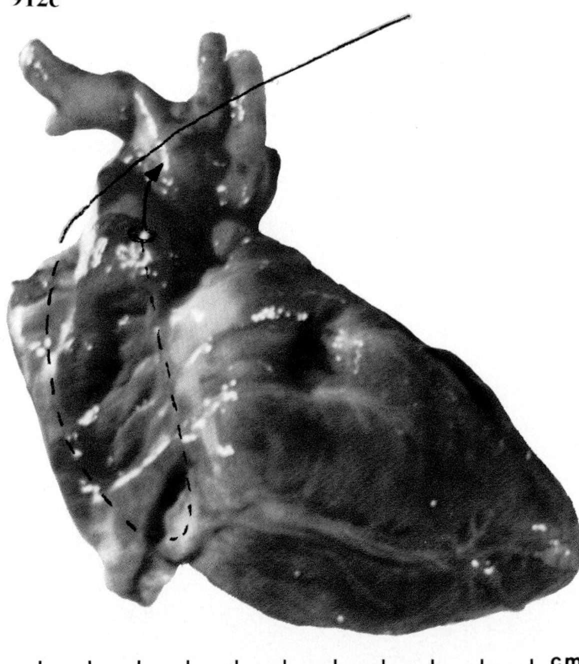

cm

22 Nov. 1970

912c Autopsy reveals pericardial tamponade caused by 40ml of perfusion fluid. Having circled within the right atrium, the catheter (cath) perforated the atrial appendage. (Dr. Z. Bozič, Lausanne.)

912d

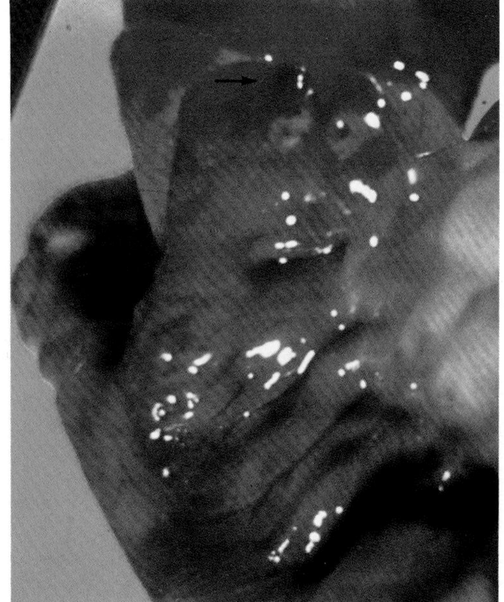

22 Nov. 1970

912d Close-up of the right atrium and its appendage: the wound is a neat puncture.

9 Trauma of the thoracic aorta and great vessels

Incidences

About a third of casualties dying on the scene of a road accident present an injury to the heart or thoracic aorta. Of those who reach hospital alive, 2% present a severe injury to the aorta and 1.8% an injury to the supra-aortic vessels.

In view of the high early mortality of aortic laceration, the importance of swift diagnosis and treatment for the small number of patients who survive initially cannot be over-stressed.

Major vascular surgery has advanced considerably since an aortic wound was first successfully repaired in 1948, and a rupture of the aortic isthmus in 1960. However, even today, the prime criterion for successful surgery is early diagnosis. The key to early diagnosis is always to suspect the injury even when it is only a faint possibility; acquaintance with methods of confirmation and confutation is, therefore, crucial.

Mediastinal widening

The standard, anterior view chest X-ray provides the basic evidence for the diagnosis of ruptures of the great thoracic vessels; the most important single sign is **widening of the upper mediastinum** due to a haemomediastinum. If this sign is present, an angiogram should be taken immediately to locate the vascular rupture.

However, caution is required. (1) **Pseudo-widening of the mediastinum** can be caused by certain technical factors – incorrect positioning of the patient on the X-ray table, for instance. (2) Widening of the mediastinum is not necessarily a sign of major vascular damage. It can also result, for example, from stasis in the superior vena cava (cardiac failure), or from atelectasis of an azygos lobe. (3) Genuine traumatic haemomediastinum can objectively diminish in size, giving a false sense of security.

913

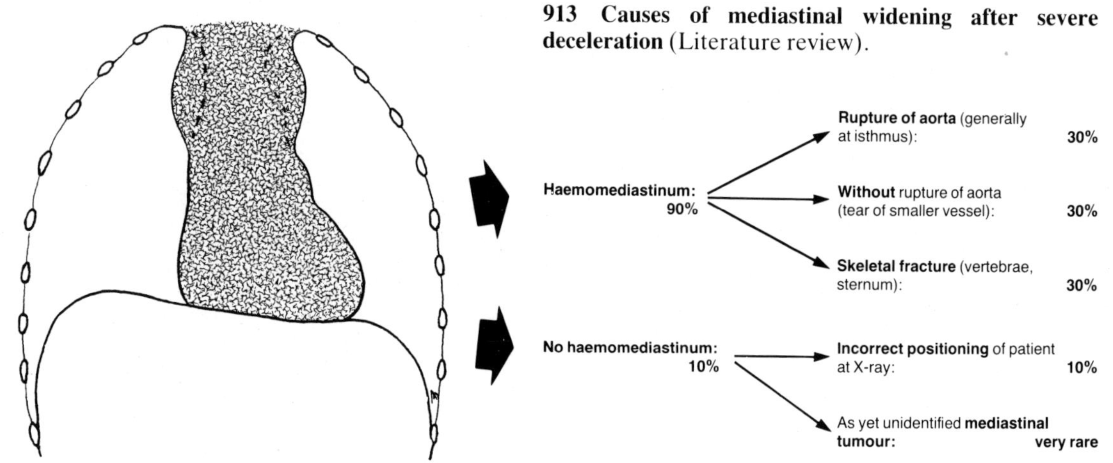

913 Causes of mediastinal widening after severe deceleration (Literature review).

Haemomediastinum: 90%
- **Rupture of aorta** (generally at isthmus): **30%**
- **Without** rupture of aorta (tear of smaller vessel): **30%**
- **Skeletal fracture** (vertebrae, sternum): **30%**

No haemomediastinum: 10%
- **Incorrect positioning** of patient at X-ray: **10%**
- As yet unidentified **mediastinal tumour: very rare**

914 Pseudo-widening of mediastinum due to **positioning** of patient

914

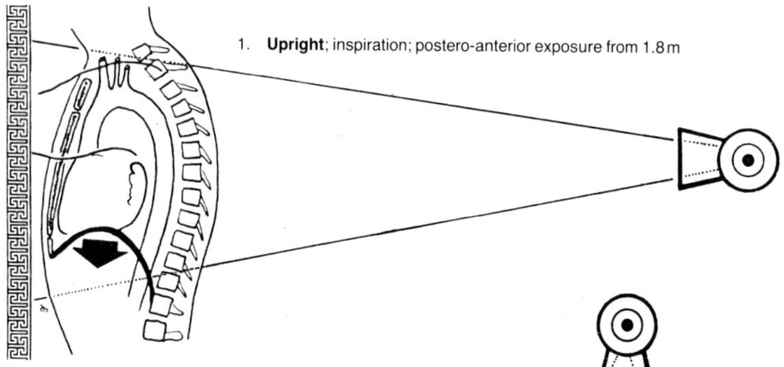

1. **Upright**; inspiration; postero-anterior exposure from 1.8 m

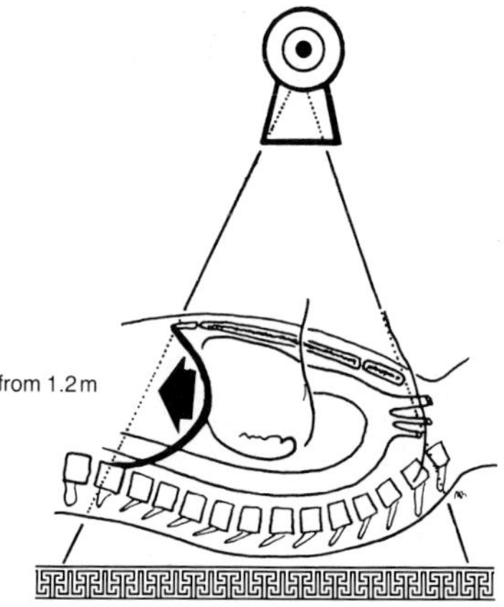

2. **Supine**; inspiration; anteroposterior exposure from 1.2 m

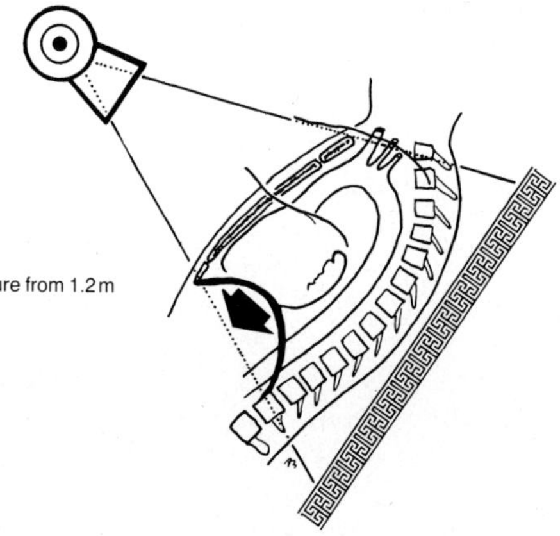

3. **Half-sitting**; inspiration; anteroposterior exposure from 1.2 m

N.B. All of the films opposite are of the same person.

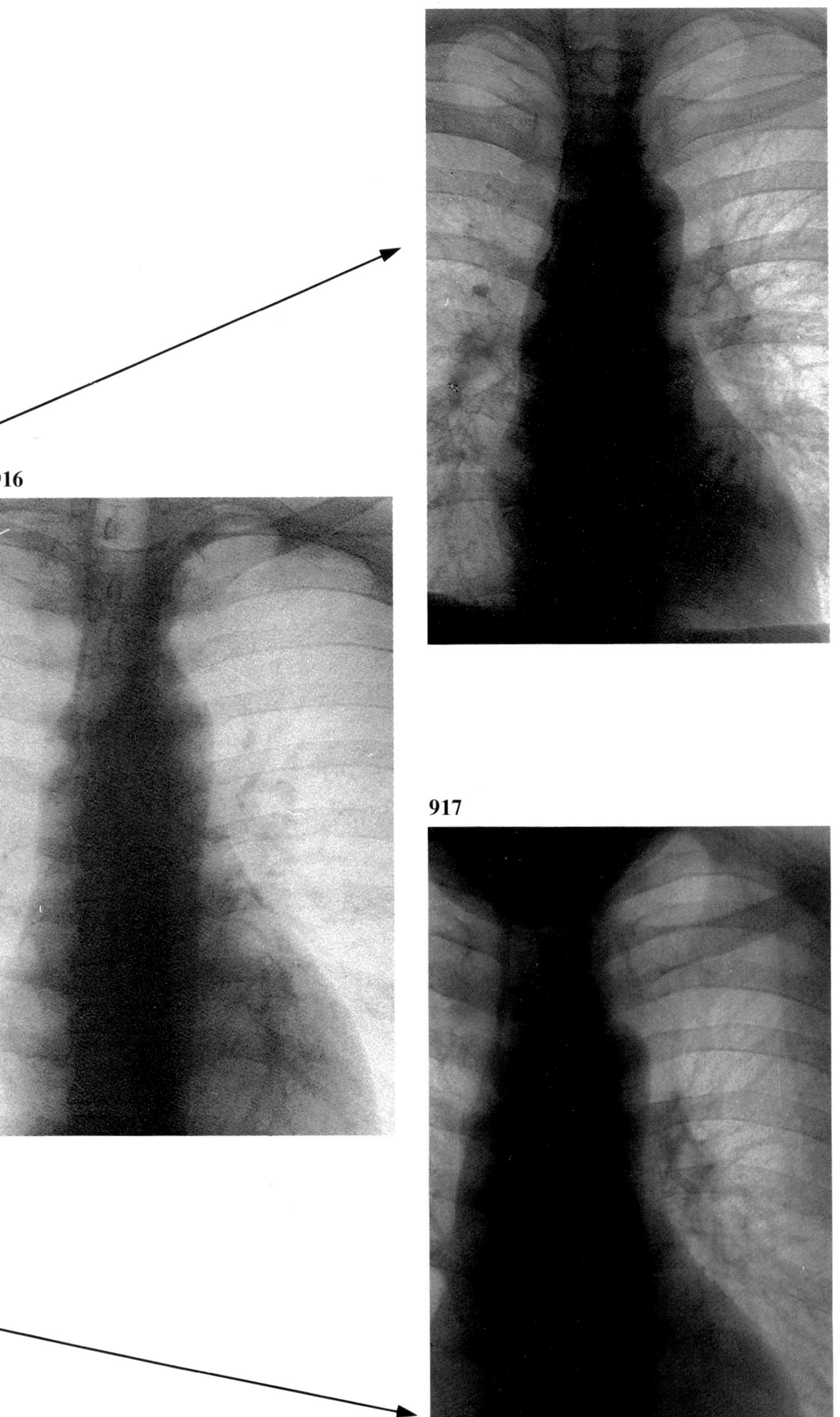
915
916
917

918 Pseudo-widening of mediastinum due to **respiratory phase**

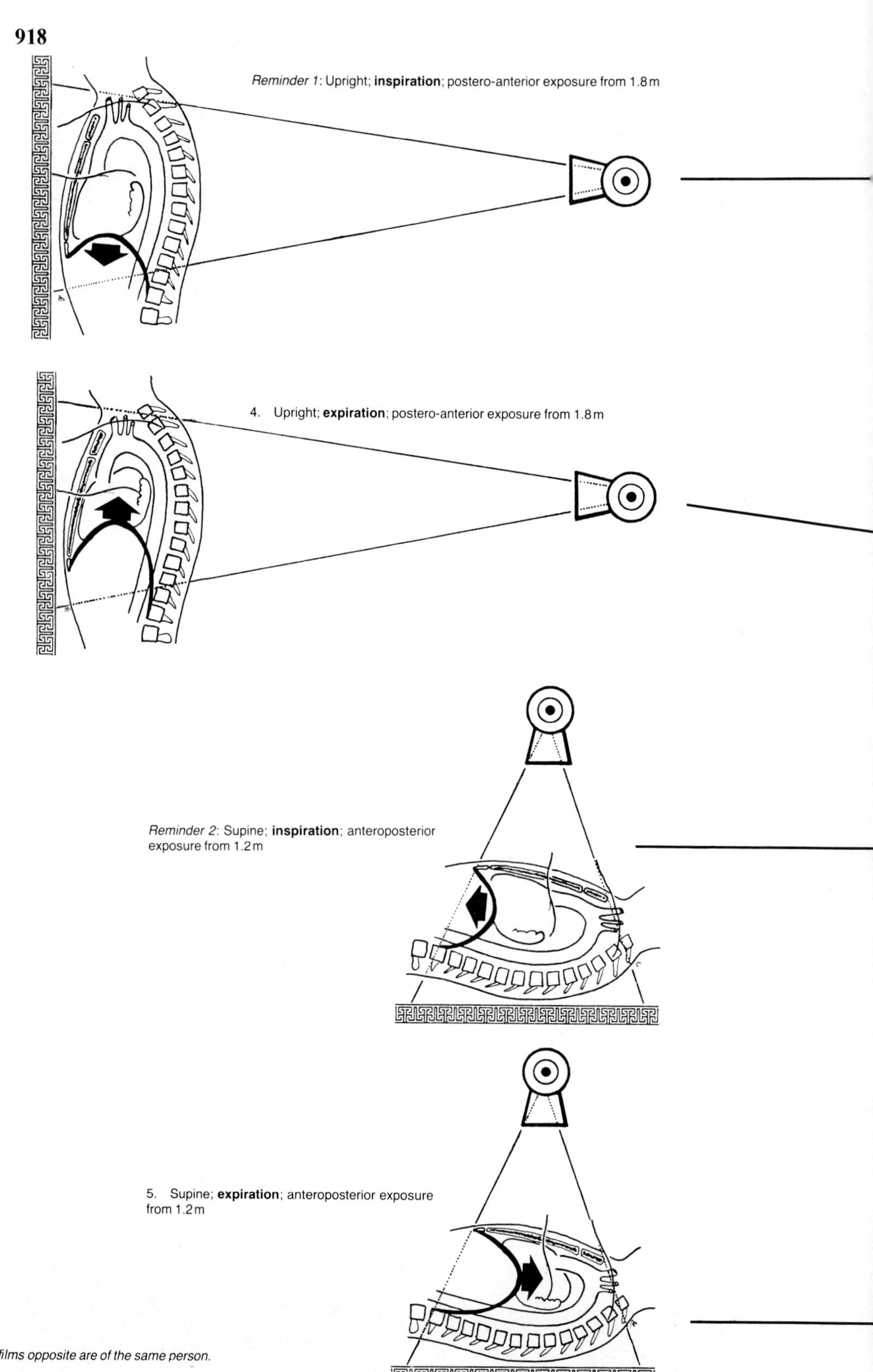

N.B. All of the films opposite are of the same person.

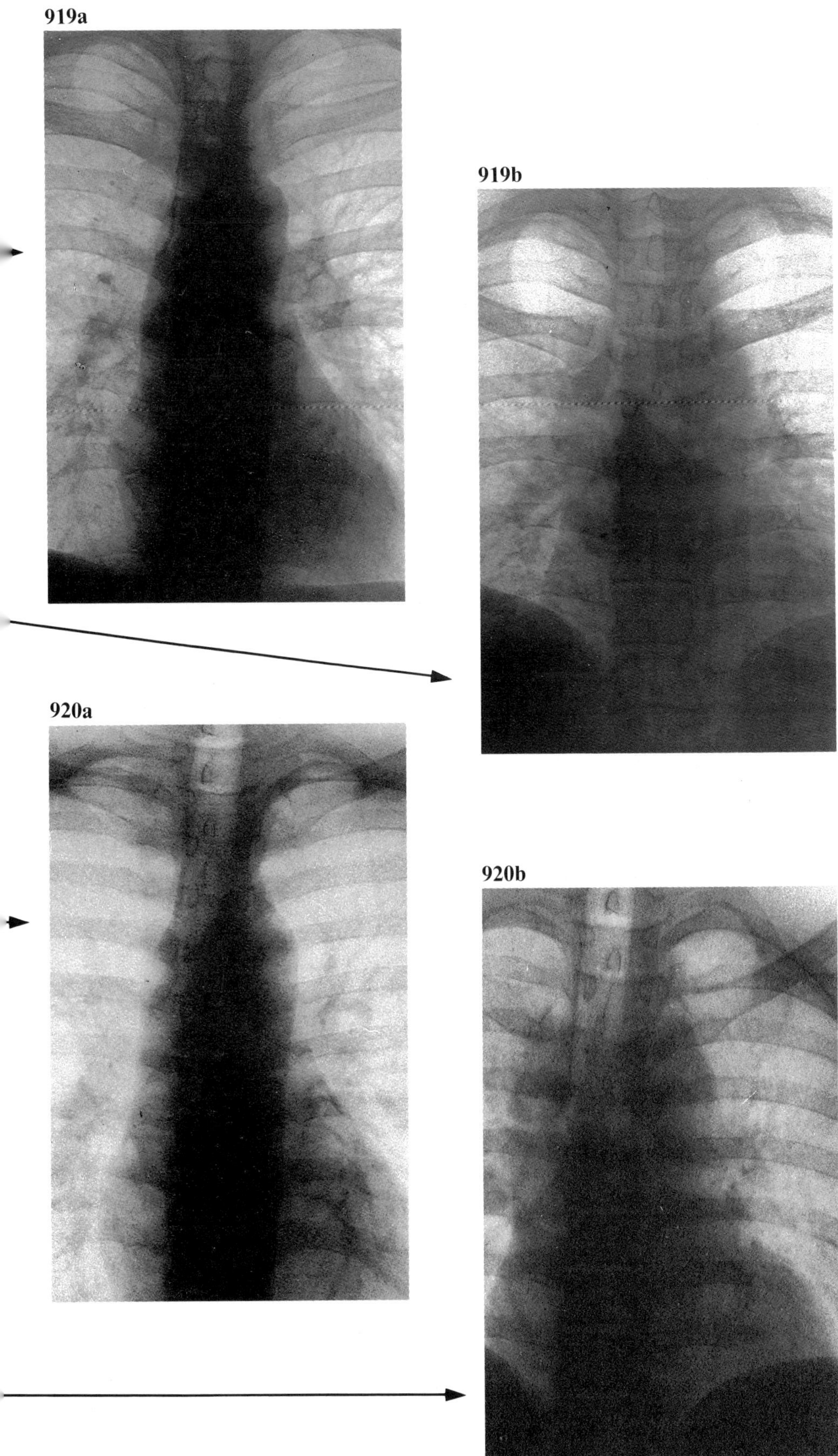
919a
919b
920a
920b

Mediastinal widening is the principal sign of aortic rupture. Corroborative signs are discussed on page 141.

921a

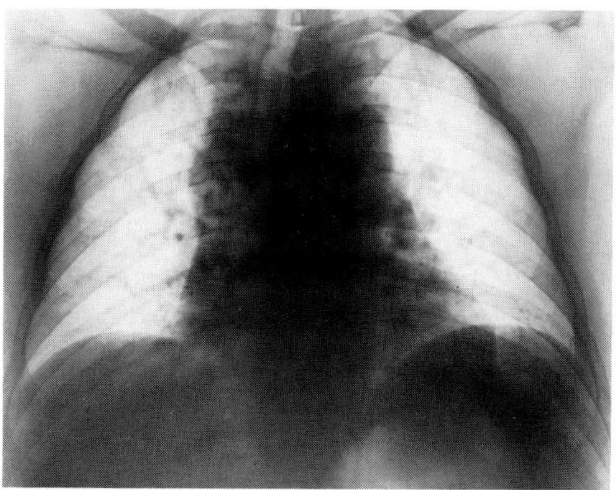

B.R. ♂ 47 yrs. 22 Jan. 1972

921a Pseudo-widening of mediastinum. Anteroposterior X-ray of a supine patient in semi-inspiration. The upper mediastinum is widened to the left of the trachea, but the aortic knob is clear and there is no pleural cap sign.

921b

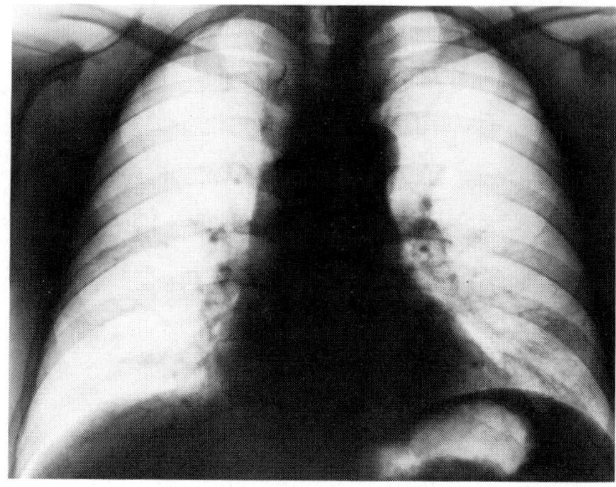

22 Jan. 1972

921b Upright, postero-anterior X-ray of the same patient in deep inspiration. The outline of the upper mediastinum is now normal.

922a

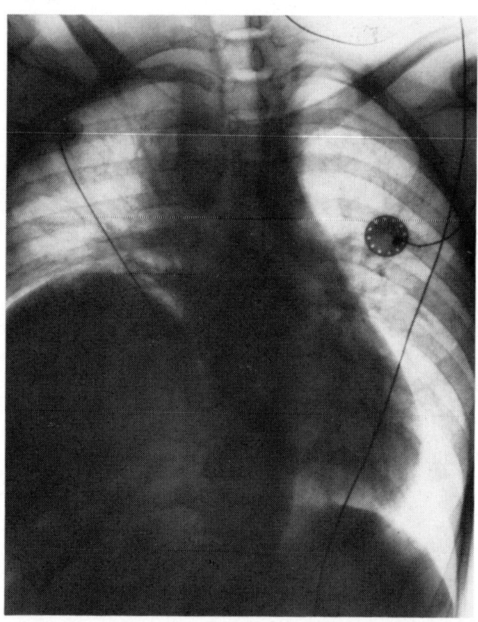

C.P. ♂ 19 yrs. 8 Dec. 1978

922a Pseudo-widening of the mediastinum produced by **azygos lobe atelectasis**. The atelectasis is due to compression of the lung from beneath by a complete hepatothorax.

922b

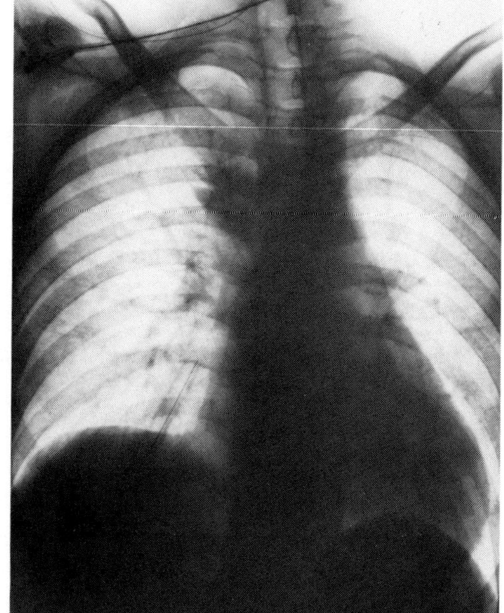

9 Dec. 1978

922b The atelectatic lung re-expands once the liver has been replaced and diaphragm repaired. The scissura and the azygos vein are both clearly visible. Recovery.

923

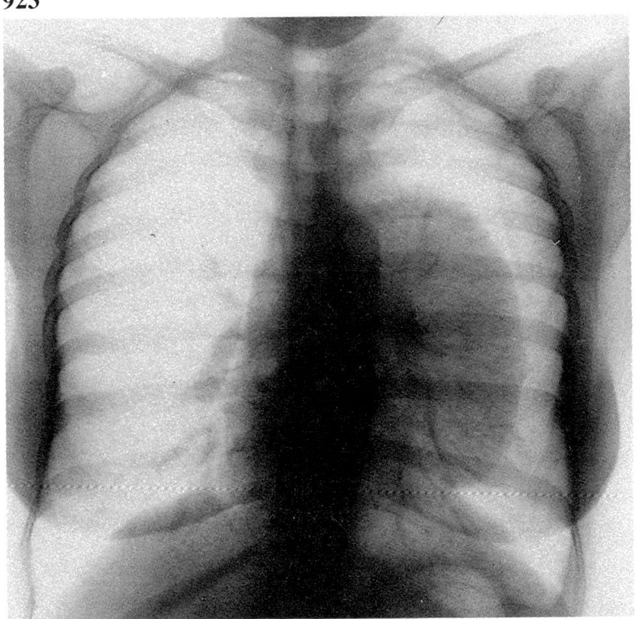

G.A. ♂ 45 yrs. 13 Sep. 1977

923 Pseudo-widening of the mediastinum produced by a **thymic tumour**. A car accident victim initially was thought to have a ruptured aorta. This diagnosis was later confuted when a Hodgkin's thymoma was discovered by serendipity.

924a

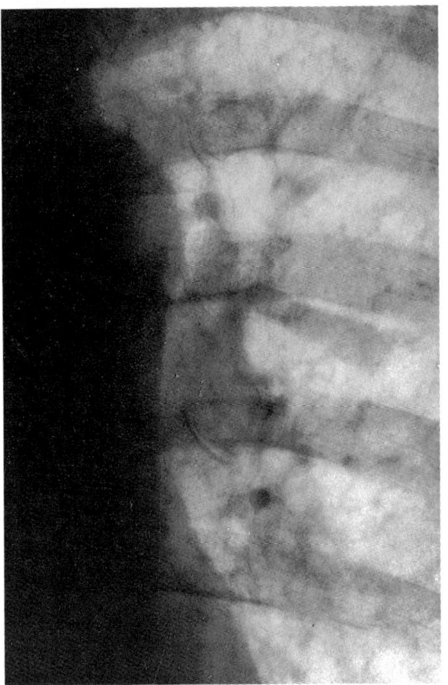

F.A. ♂ 54 yrs. 19 Aug. 1976

924a **Unexplained pseudo-widening** of the aortic knob. Admission X-ray of a car driver who had been thrown violently against the steering wheel in a high-speed collision with a lorry.

924b

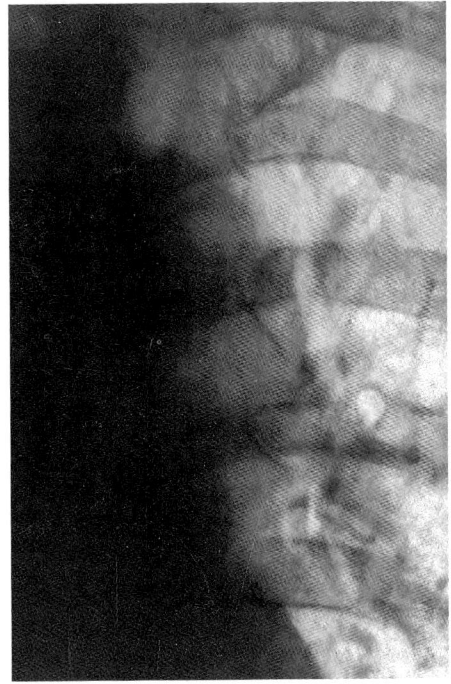

1 hr. later

924b The pseudo-widening seen here is due probably to the fact that this film was taken from a different angle. Exploratory thoracotomy: the aorta is intact.

925a

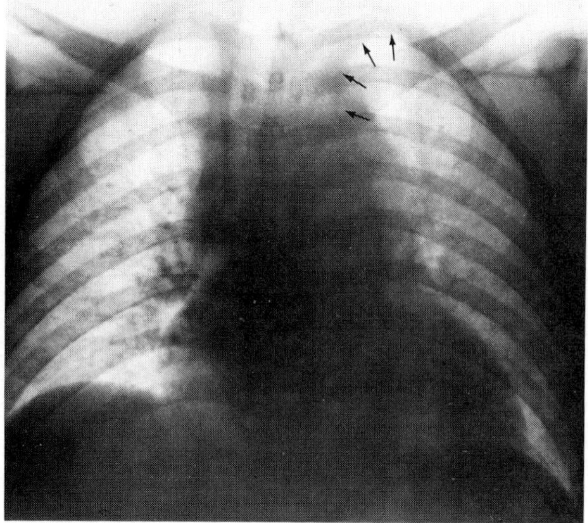

F.J. ♂ 19 yrs. 16 Oct. 1965

925b

20 Oct. 1965

925a Genuine leftward widening of mediastinum due to the haemomediastinum caused by a rupture of the aortic isthmus. The anteroposterior supine X-ray taken in semi-inspiration shows rightward displacement of the trachea, depression of the left main-stem bronchus, blurring of the aortic knob and the apical cap sign (→). **925b** Four days after the rupture was repaired, the outline of the mediastinum is back to normal.

926a

M.D. ♂ 22 yrs. 17 Sep. 1978

926b

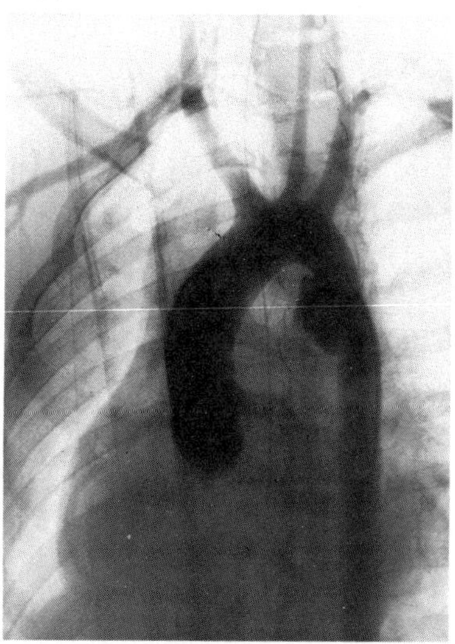

17 Sep. 1978

926a Genuine bilateral widening of mediastinum . . .

926b . . . due to an isthmic rupture of the aorta sustained in a 300 m hang-gliding fall. Remarkably, the young man survived initially. The rupture was sutured directly without difficulty, but brain death was pronounced the following day.

927

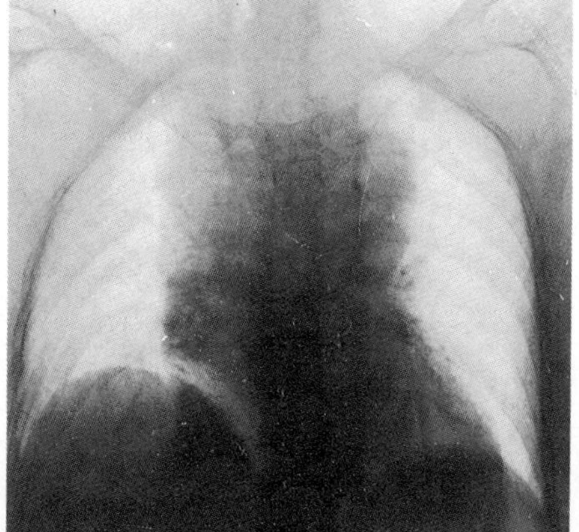

P.M. ♀ 66 yrs. 21 April 1965

927 Significant enlargement of upper mediastinum due to a rupture of the aortic isthmus diagnosed both clinically and radiologically. The patient is cerebrally dead and surgery is not undertaken. Death 12 hours later.

928a

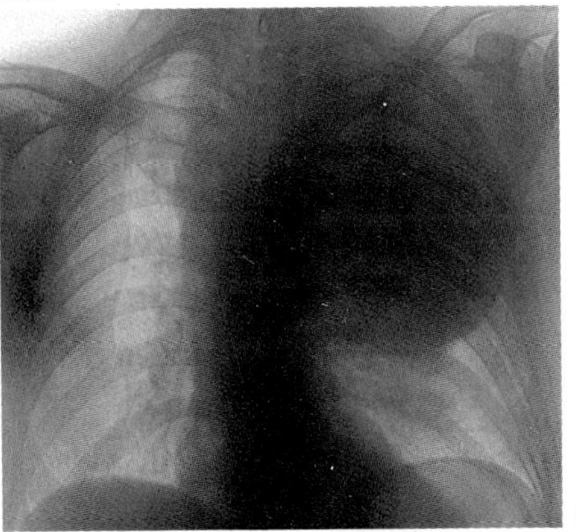

F.R. ♂ 44 yrs. 8 Feb. 1963

928a Massive leftward enlargement of upper mediastinum due to a rupture of the aorta sustained in a 40 km/h car crash. This X-ray was taken 6 hours after the accident. Thoracotomy, direct clamping, end-to-end anastomosis.

928b

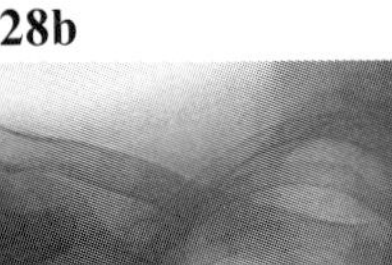

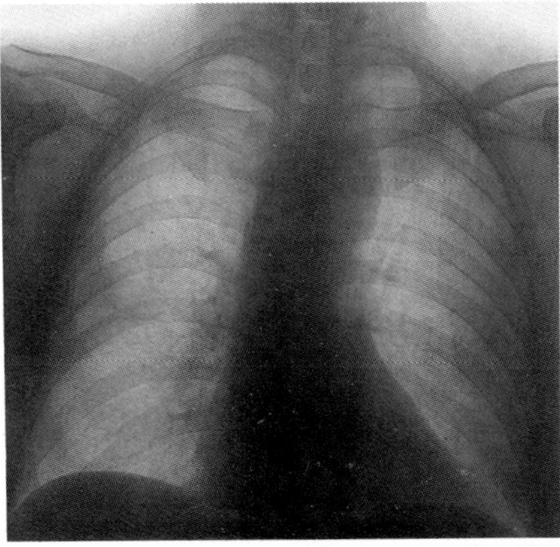

27 Feb. 1963

928b Recovery.

929a

M.J.–C. ♂ 27 yrs. 18 June 1966

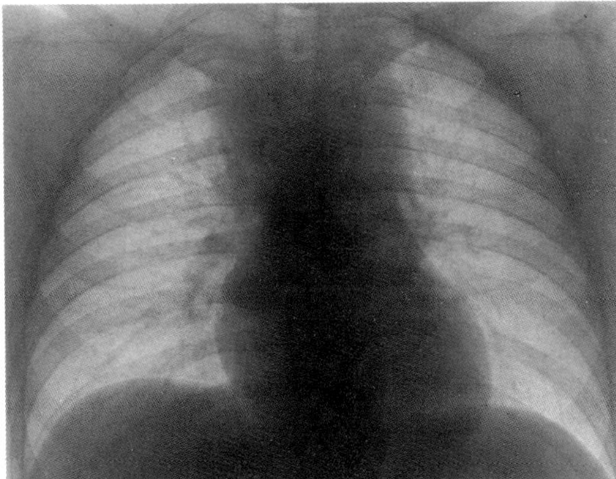

929a Haemomediastinum without vascular rupture. This haemomediastinum stems from haematomas due to fractures of the first 3 ribs and both clavicles. This is an unusual case, for skeletal damage to the upper thorax often implies an injury to the aorta (see **939**). The admission X-ray . . .

929b

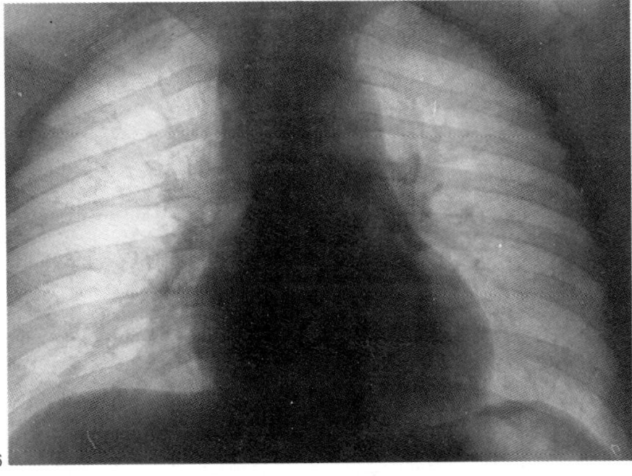

20 June 1966

929b . . . is followed by an angiogram that confutes suspicion of aortic or supra-aortic rupture. The widening diminishes . . .

929c

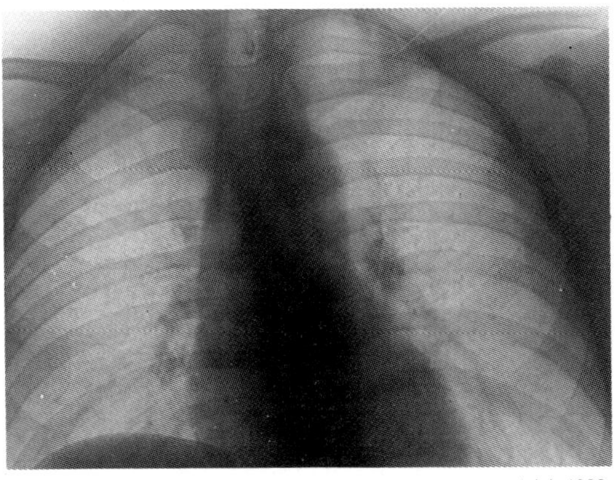

4 July 1966

929c . . . to disappear finally 2 weeks later.

930

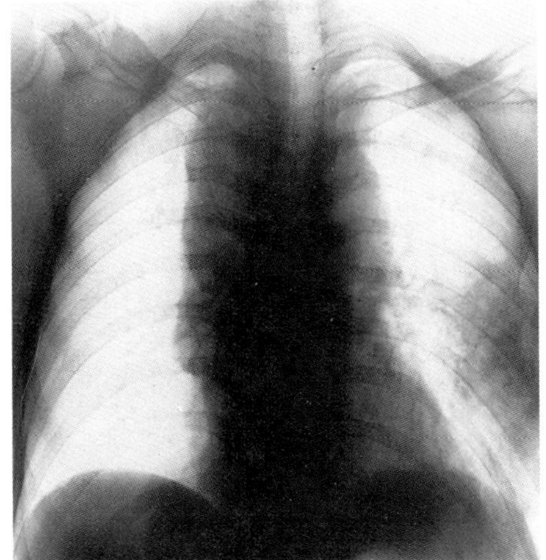

C.J. ♂ 30 yrs. 23 May 1974

930 Rightward widening of mediastinum caused by tears of the superior vena cava and a coronary artery.

Rupture of the aorta

In 1947, only 1% of the autopsies on car accident victims revealed a rupture of the aortic isthmus. Today the figure is above 15%. The number of reported operations is small (about 500) but increasing.

Indirect rupture of the aorta from deceleration can be variously localised (see **938**). Ruptures in certain localisations are immediately fatal; the incidence of any given localisation of rupture on the autopsy table is therefore markedly different from its incidence in surgical units.

931

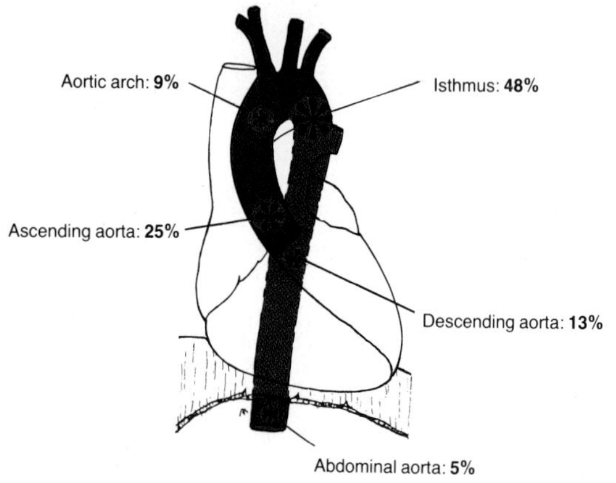

931 Localisation of indirect aortic rupture in victims **dead on arrival** at hospital (Parmley, $n = 258$).

932

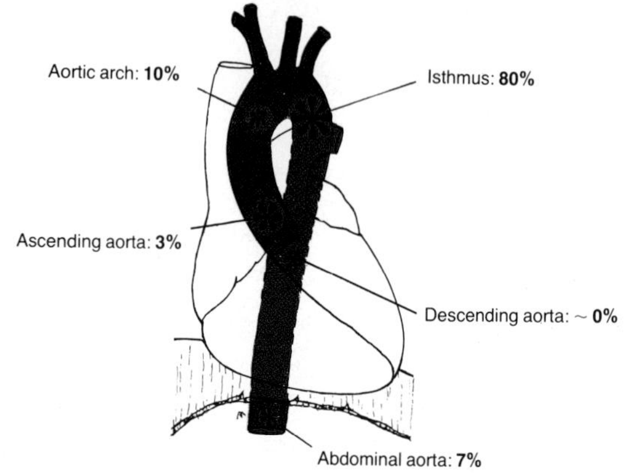

932 Localisation of indirect aortic rupture in victims **alive on admission to hospital** (in our material, $n = 32$)

Of those alive on admission, three-quarters are young men. Their average age is 38 years; by comparison, the average age for all chest trauma patients is 46. Two out of three are car accident victims, and the remaining third, usually, either have fallen from a considerable height or suffered a major crush-injury.

Two thirds are in shock when admitted.

In recent years, new restraint systems (air bags, for instance) have been developed to protect the occupants of motor vehicles during crashes. If these systems were to become obligatory, the survival rate in violent accidents would improve. As it is, conventional safety belts certainly have reduced the number of fatal cerebral injuries, but only at the cost of an increase in the number of pure deceleration injuries. Consequently, a significant decrease in the overall number of aortic, supra-aortic and cardiac ruptures is not yet foreseeable.

Types of accident

Ruptures of the aortic isthmus are usually the result of road accidents; 66% of victims are car drivers or passengers and about 30% are motorcyclists.

Although road accidents account for the vast majority of aortic ruptures, there are numerous other possible causes: for example, climbing accidents, runaway lifts, industrial crush-injuries.

Biomechanics

Indirect rupture of the aorta occurs in young men (60% are between 20 and 30 years of age) but, curiously, it is hardly ever seen in adolescents or children (2%).

Rupture usually requires an antero-posterior or vertical deceleration of around 80g. The exact force required is determined by: (1) the jerk of deceleration, (2) the nature of the surface coming into contact with the chest (the padding inside a car, for example) and (3) the phase of the heart's contraction at the moment of impact.

When a car travelling at about 100 km/h hits a rigid barrier and buckles over 50 cm (braking distance), the deceleration registered on the chassis of the vehicle is equivalent to 80 g (the critical threshold for aortic rupture).

933

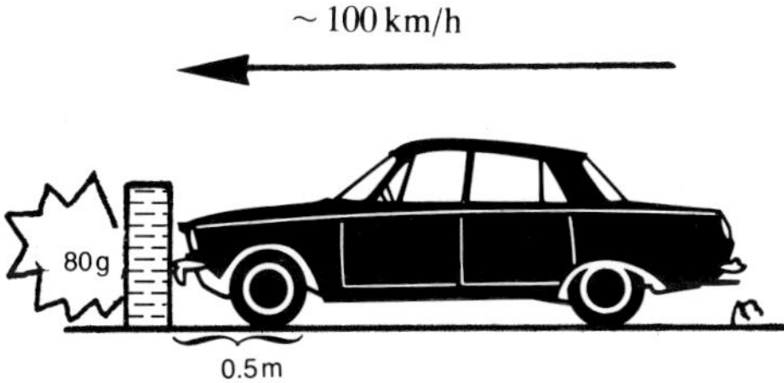

However, the deceleration of the occupant is significantly higher than the deceleration of the car. Consequently, when deceleration is measured on a **dummy** rather than on the chassis of the car, the critical threshold of 80 g is reached:

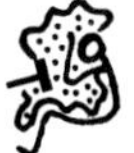

in an impact at ~ 90 km/h if the dummy is restrained by an **air bag,**

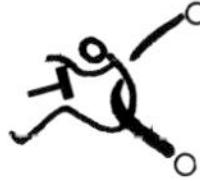

in an impact at ~ 70 km/h if it is restrained by a correctly worn **safety belt,**

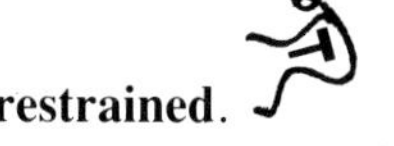

in an impact at ~ 40 km/h (or slower) if the dummy is **unrestrained**.

The histologists' observation that there is a weak point at the junction of the ligamentum arteriosum and the aortic isthmus has been corroborated by recent deceleration experiments on cadavers.

The same experiments have shown also that a healthy aorta is capable of withstanding pressures of up to 2000 mm Hg (2.6 atm), and that its resistance to lateral traction is greater than its resistance to longitudinal traction. When the aorta does rupture, it is the intimal and medial layers that give first, the adventitial layer being the strongest of the three.

For years it was thought that isthmic rupture resulted from the combination of a shock-wave (what might be termed a 'water-hammer' effect) with traction on the isthmus caused by forward displacement of the mobile heart and aorta. However, this hypothesis was clearly inadequate with respect to the anterior localisation of most partial ruptures of the isthmus.

934

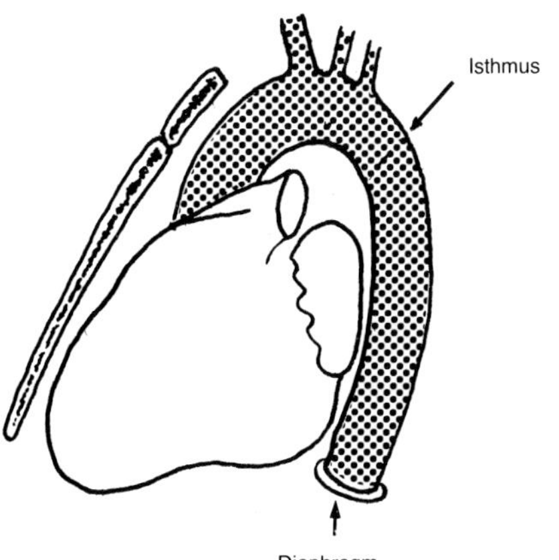

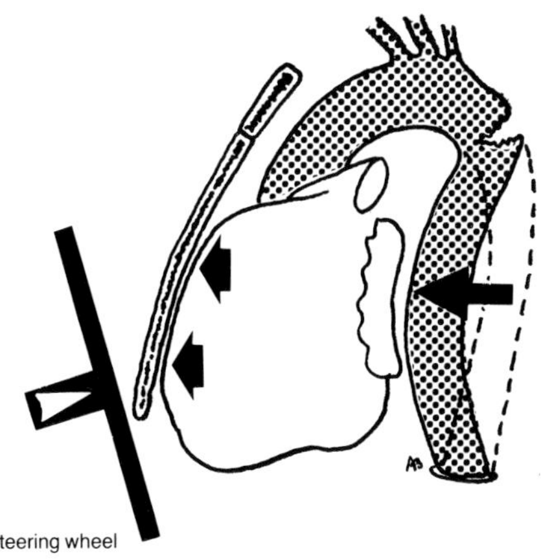

According to this theory, partial rupture ought to be posterior. The facts do not bear this out.

934 Obsolete biomechanical theory that indirect rupture of the isthmus results from 'water-hammer' effect.

On the basis of detailed cadaver experiments, Voigt has shown that most isthmic ruptures and/or ruptures of the ascending aorta are the result of a '*shovel mechanism*'. He also describes a '*shearing mechanism*' but regards this as very much less common.

The '**shovel mechanism**' can be described as follows. Because he is leaning backwards, the occupant of a car is thrown against the steering column (or dashboard) in such a way that the decelerating forces are applied to the base of his sternum along an upward and backward axis, and perhaps slightly to the right. The traction exerted on the descending aorta by the upward displacement of the heart ruptures the isthmus, either partially or totally. When deceleration is more violent or when the axis of the force is more vertical, the ascending portion of the aortic arch also ruptures (by flexion and compression against the upper thoracic cage).

Parietal damage is generally limited to fracture of the lower sternum and sometimes also of the false rib cartilages. Younger patients often present no parietal damage at all.

When the impact occurs along the same axes but slightly higher on the sternum, the result is different – fracture of the sternum and isolated rupture of the ascending aorta. This injury accounts for 10% of all immediately fatal ruptures.

935

935 Current '**shovel mechanism**' theory of **indirect** deceleration rupture of aortic isthmus:

Impact of driver against steering wheel

Impact of passenger against dashboard

936 **937** **938**

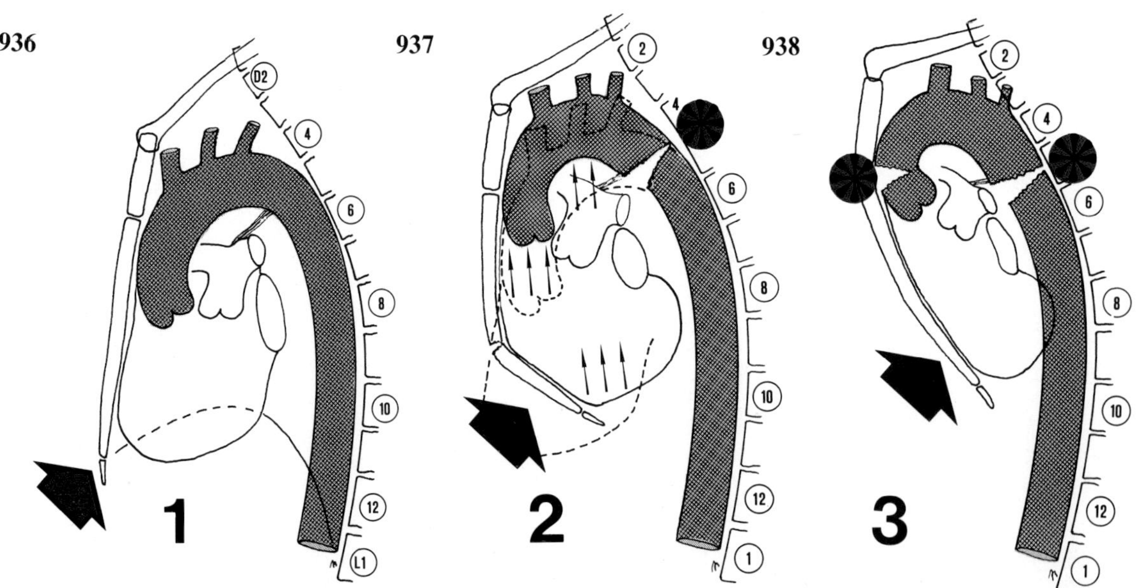

936 'Shovel mechanism' in action

937 Rupture of the aortic isthmus begins anteriorly and is caused by traction. In 45% of cases, it is accompanied by contusion and laceration of the heart.

938 If the impact is sufficiently violent, there is also the possibility of a subsequent anterior flexion-rupture of the ascending aorta.

The classic biomechanisms of aortic and diaphragmatic rupture differ only in the direction of the forces involved. This direction depends upon the position of the victim at the moment of impact: the victim of aortic rupture is leaning slightly *backwards*, while the victim of diaphragmatic rupture is leaning slightly *forwards*. Not surprisingly, the two injuries are sometimes associated (see **942**).

The less common '**shearing mechanism**' – whereby a shearing force applied to the uppermost portion of the rib-cage displaces the mediastinum and fractures both first ribs – results in rupture-dislocation of the aortic isthmus. Except for the direction of the forces, this mechanism is closely akin to the one whereby a tearing force to the neck or arms can avulse a major supra-aortic vessel (see **999**).

939

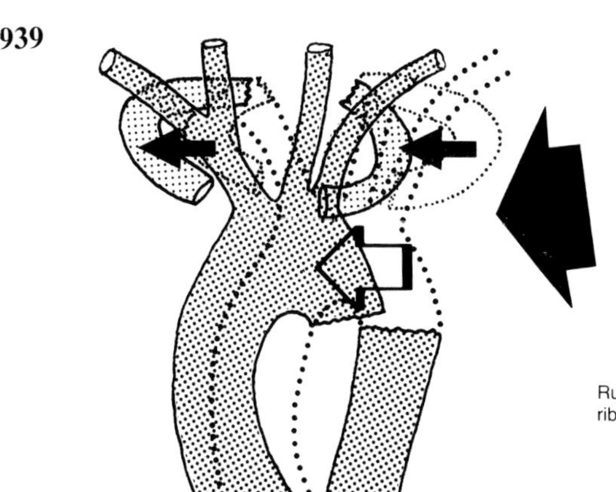

Rupture is caused by avulsion as the entire mediastinum is displaced. Both first ribs fracture.

939 Direct rupture-dislocation of aortic isthmus by **lateral impact** to upper thorax and shoulder.

Associated injuries

940

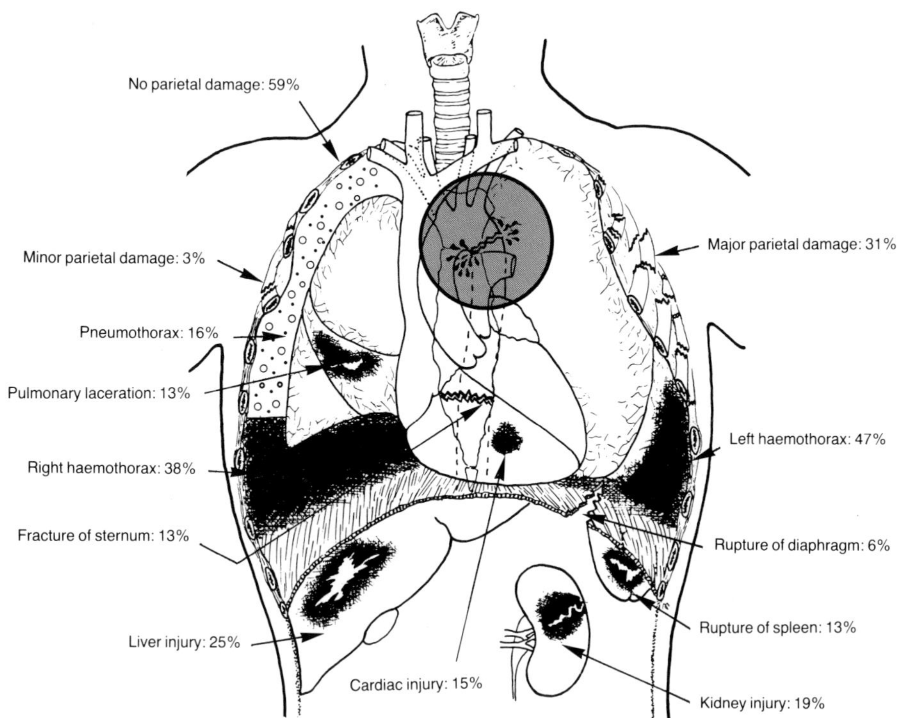

940 Injuries associated with aortic rupture and their incidence (in our material).

941a

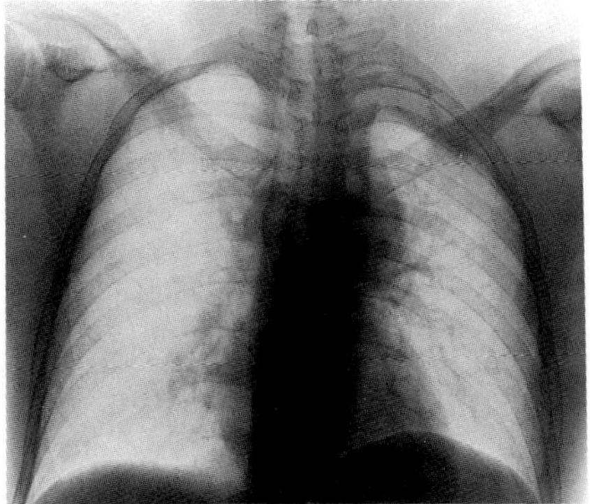

H.E. ♂ 32 yrs. 27 May 1967

941a Isthmic rupture of aorta with cardiac contusion. This admission X-ray clearly shows a widened mediastinum; rupture of the aortic isthmus is confirmed by an angiogram. Immediate repair.

941b

27 May 1967

941b In addition, the patient has a moderate traumatic myocardial infarct and extensive damage to his extremities.

941c

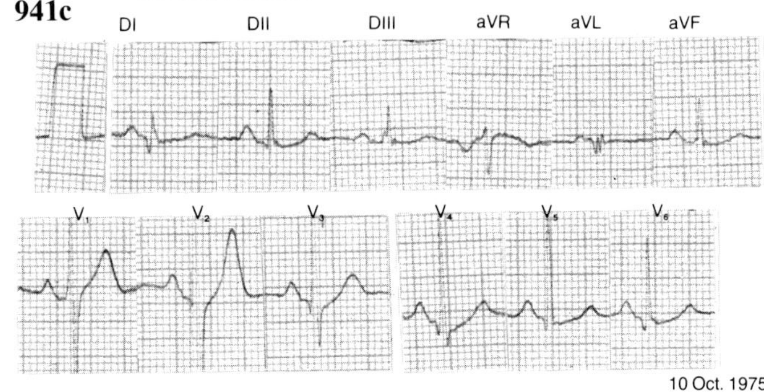

941c The ECG gradually improves, and the depressions in the S-T segment finally disappear (late control).

942

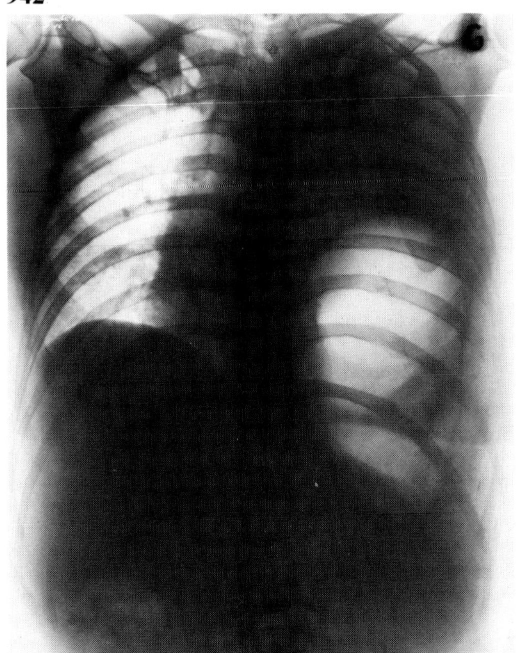

R.V. ♀ 42 yrs. 6 Nov. 1956

942 Rupture of diaphragm and aorta. The two injuries have similar mechanisms and are sometimes associated (see **1050**).

Symptoms and signs

A patient remaining conscious and lucid after a rupture of the aorta usually complains of **pain** high between the scapulae. The importance of this pain is often underplayed; even in the absence of radiological evidence, it is attributed frequently to parietal damage.

The expected clinical signs are not always found. In theory, they consist of a systolic murmur between the scapulae, a carotid sheath haematoma (see **954**) and a difference in pulse and arterial pressure between the two arms, or between the arms and legs. A rupture with an intimal or intimal and medial flap can give rise to pseudocoarctation or anuria and paraplegia.

Horner's syndrome and/or left recurrent nerve paralysis sometimes develop later.

943

943 Effect of isthmic rupture on **peripheral arterial pressure**.

Reduced pressure in **left arm**
(N.B. *reduced pressure in right arm usually signifies avulsion of innominate artery*).

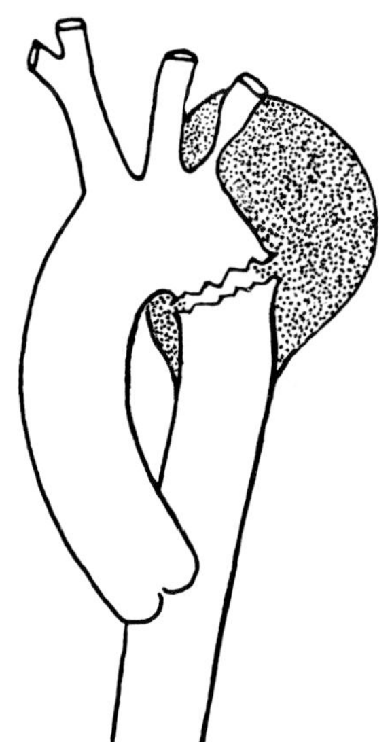

Reduced pressure in **lower limbs** (see **944**).

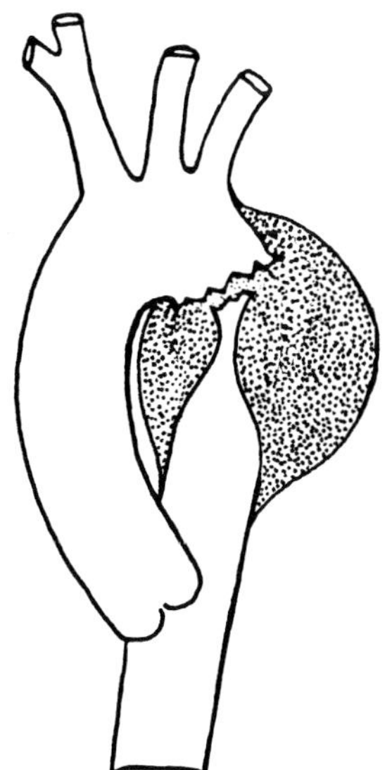

Pressure reduced virtually to nil in **distal aorta** (intimal flap, see **972, 975**).

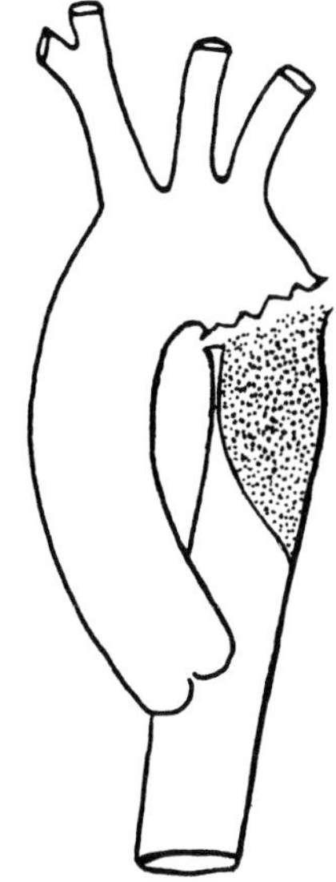

944

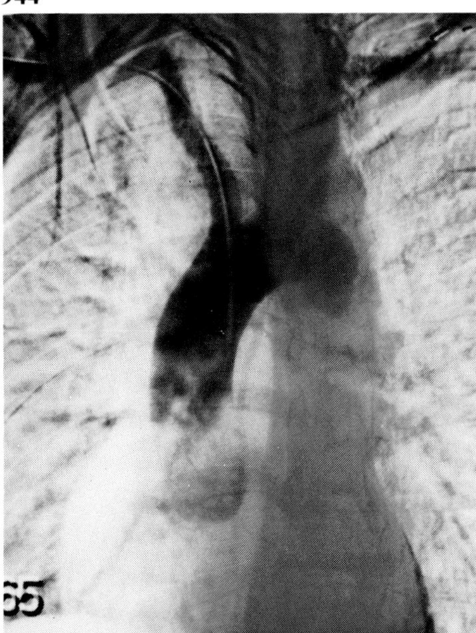

W.V. ♂ 26 yrs. 8 Feb. 1979

944 Distal aortic circulation can be interrupted if the haematoma surrounding a total rupture compresses and occludes the distal stump. In this patient, the absence of a femoral pulse was noticed when he became anuric and paraplegic 7 hours after injury. An angiogram taken after transfer to the University Hospital shows complete occlusion of the aorta at the isthmus. The aorta was repaired directly 15 hours after injury but the patient died from coagulation disorders shortly after the aorta was unclamped.

Arterial emboli generated in the aneurysmal pouch can become lodged in subdiaphragmatic arteries.

In practice, the clinical signs of aortic rupture are elusive, deceptive and inconstant, and their absence can be misleading. Accompanying parietal damage to the thorax is rarely obvious (a fact explained by the mechanism of the injury on the one hand, and by the bodily suppleness of its survivors on the other).

In many cases, victims of violent deceleration accidents present alarming extrathoracic injuries which distract attention from less apparent, but more life-threatening endothoracic damage. Aortic rupture, therefore, always should be presumed. The following signs should be looked for on the standard anterior X-ray:

- widening of the mediastinum [about 30% are due to a haemomediastinum resulting from total rupture of the isthmus (see **913**)],
- blurring of the aortic knob,
- the apical extrapleural cap sign,
- left haemothorax,
- rightward displacement of the trachea,
- depression of the left main-stem bronchus,
- rightward displacement of the oesophagus (or of a marked oesophageal tube),
- a double contour within the aortic knob signifying dissociation of the intimal and adventitial layers.

950a

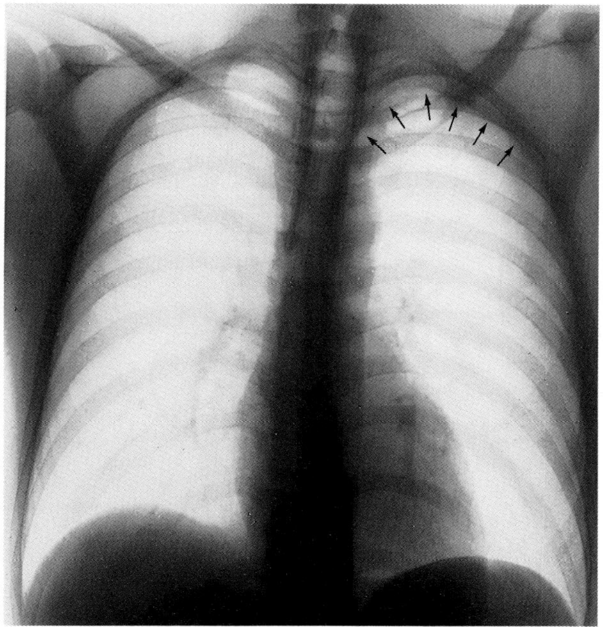

H.R. ♂ 24 yrs. 10 Sep. 1967

950a The apical cap sign is not pathognomic of isthmic rupture of the aorta. Here it is due to a fracture of the acromion.

950b

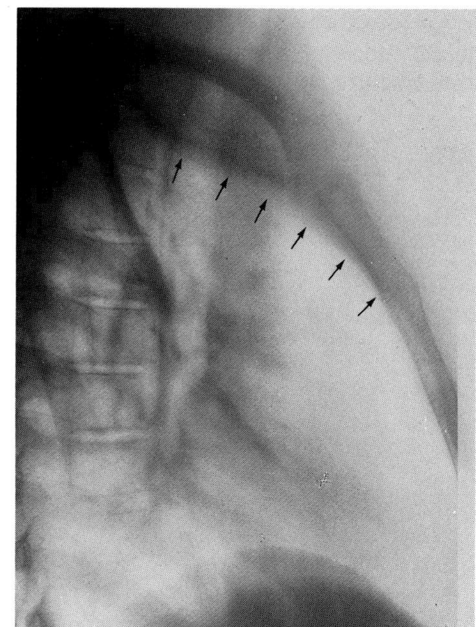

10 Sep. 1967

950b The haematoma extends anteriorly.

951

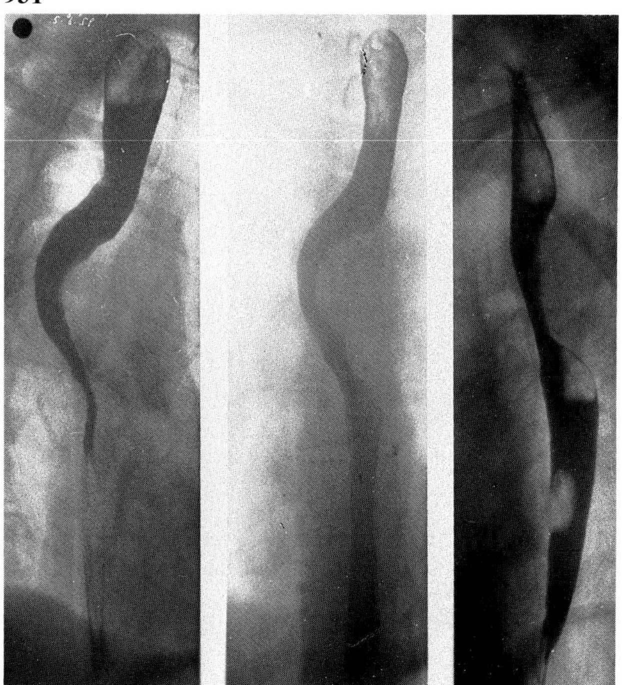

C.J. ♂ 38 yrs. 5 June 1959

951 Displacement of oesophagus by a post-traumatic pseudo-aneurysm of the aorta.

952

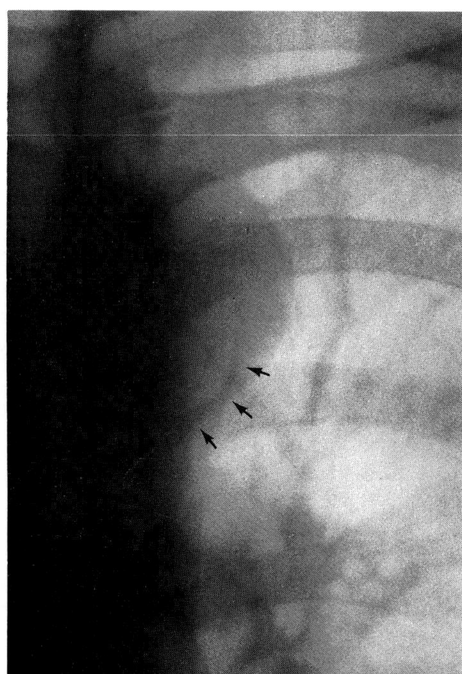

C.C. ♂ 49 yrs. 20 Feb. 1967

952 Separation of intimal and adventitial layers in a patient whose aortic arch has a calcified intima. On the standard X-ray, the curved line of the calcified intima (→) lies within the shadow of the haematoma or pseudo-aneurysm.

953

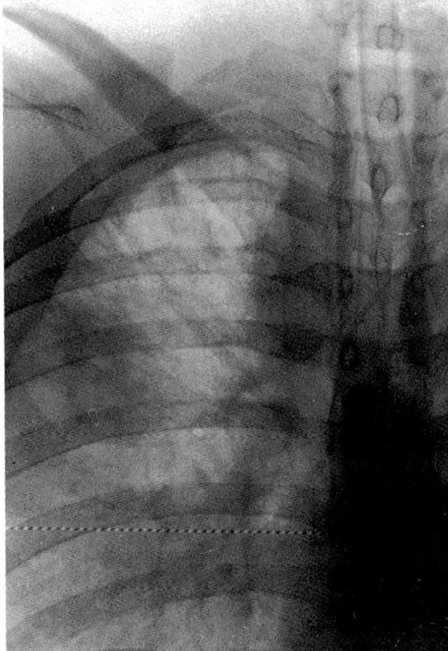

C.M.–A. ♂ 23 yrs. 24 April 1977

953 Right haemothorax accompanying an aortic rupture can mislead and distract attention.

954

1976

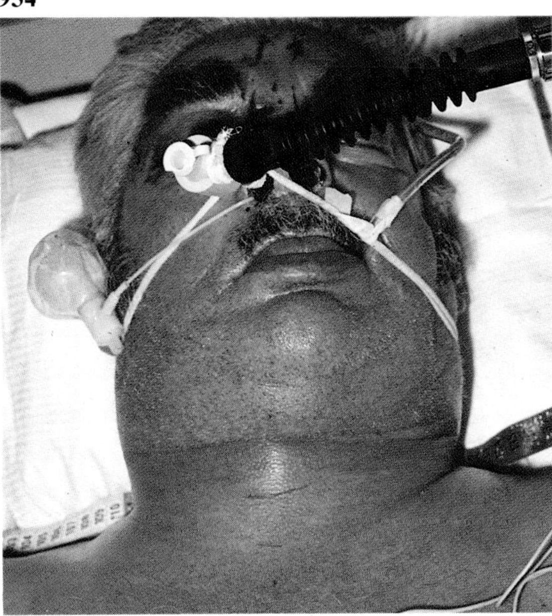

954 Haemomediastinum spreading to neck. This haemomediastinum is signalled clinically by a haematoma of both carotid sheaths. There is no damage either to the aorta or to any other great vessel. (Prof. J. Freeman, Lausanne.)

Final proof of aortic rupture is provided by **angiography**. There are, however, certain attendant risks:
(1) loss of time, (2) the risk of the catheter deviating through the rupture and (3) the possibility that the injection of dye suddenly may increase arterial pressure sufficiently to rupture the thus far intact adventitia and mediastinal pleura. Even if the widening of the mediastinum is relatively insignificant, early angiography is advisable. *Intravenous* injection of dye entails less risk than *retrograde arterial* injection: the impregnation of the aorta is less marked, but it is adequate in most instances, especially since the development of digital angiography.

Falsely positive angiography does occur, but only exceptionally (see **958**).

955a

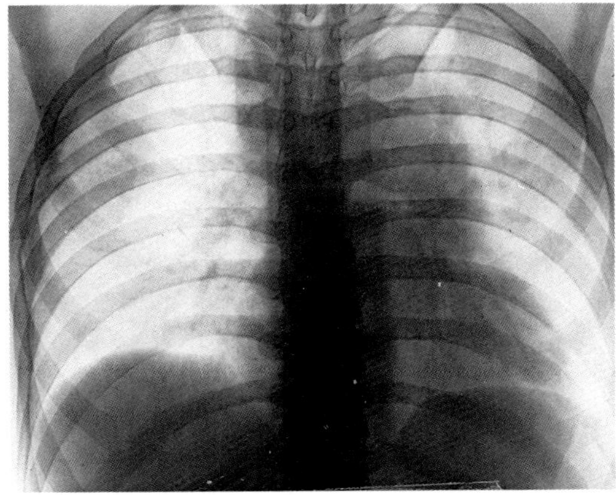

C.M.–A. ♂ 23 yrs. 23 April 1977

955a Widening of the mediastinum calls for angiography. The patient was thrown against the steering wheel of his car when he crashed at more than 100 km/h. The admission X-ray shows a significantly widened mediastinum. Sudden cardiac arrest due to cardiac contusion (see **871**). External massage proves effective after a few minutes. Transfer.

955b

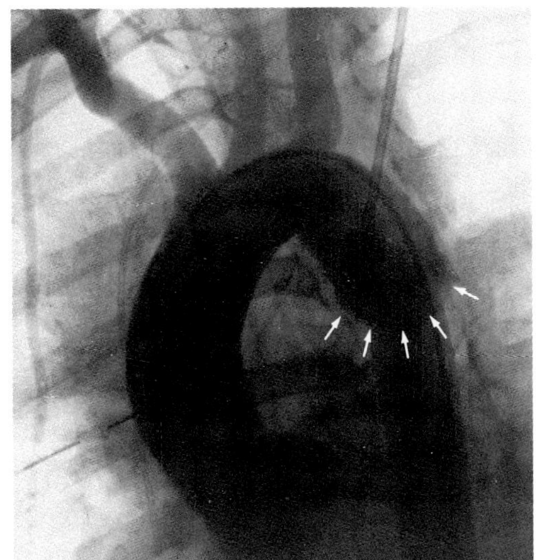

24 April 1977

955b An oblique angiogram clearly shows the rupture of the intimal and medial layers of the isthmus. The rupture is anterior. Extravasation is moderate.

956

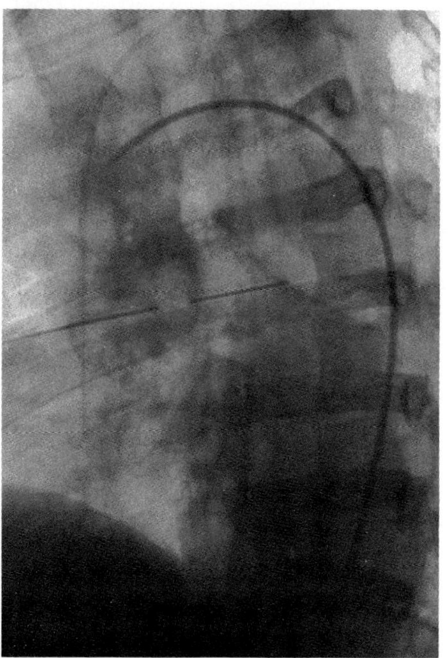

C.M.–A. ♂ 23 yrs. 24 April 1977

956 Danger of retrograde aortography. A Seldinger catheter has been threaded into the ascending aorta through the femoral artery. A total rupture of the aorta clearly would render this manoeuvre hazardous (see **957** and **967**). In this case of partial anterior rupture (see **955**), the risk is minimal since the catheter follows the broader curvature of the intact posterior wall.

957a

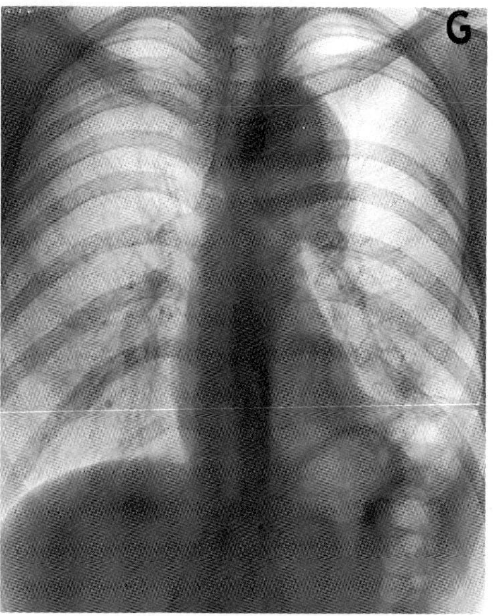

C.J. ♂ 38 yrs. 16 June 1959

957a Angiography catheter coiling within an 11-year-old post-traumatic pseudo-aneurysm of the aortic isthmus. The standard X-ray shows the shadow of the pseudo-aneurysm.

957b

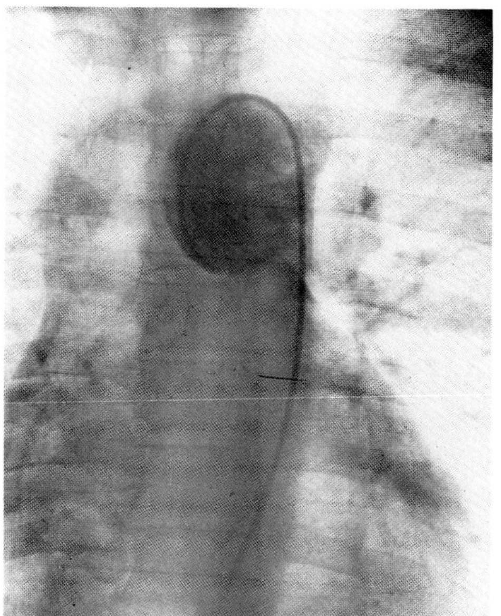

16 June 1959

957b The catheter (introduced through the femoral artery) spirals within the pseudo-aneurysm. Fortunately, no iatrogenic injury is sustained.

958a

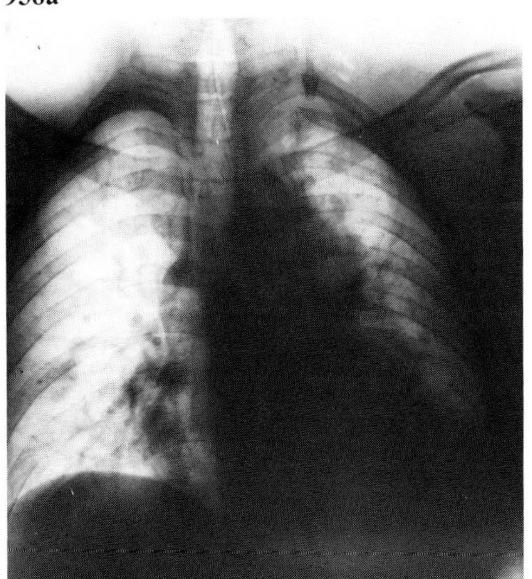

S.A. ♂ 35 yrs. 16 Oct. 1978

958a Arcography, on occasion, can be falsely positive. Three days after sustaining severe multiple injuries, this patient displays an enlarged upper mediastinum and a left haemothorax.

958b

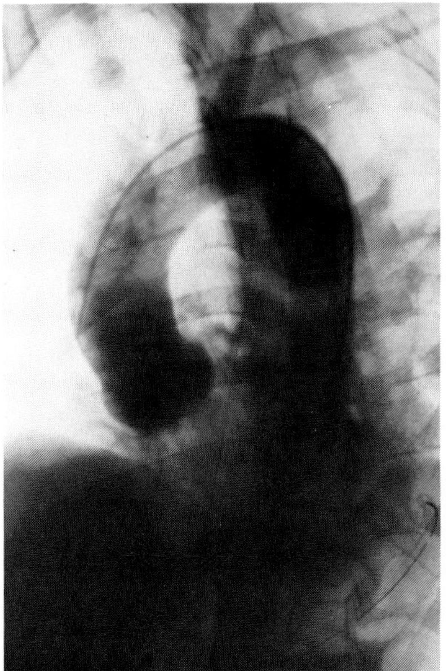

16 Oct. 1978

958b In the oblique projection, the isthmic region seems abnormal, so . . .

958c

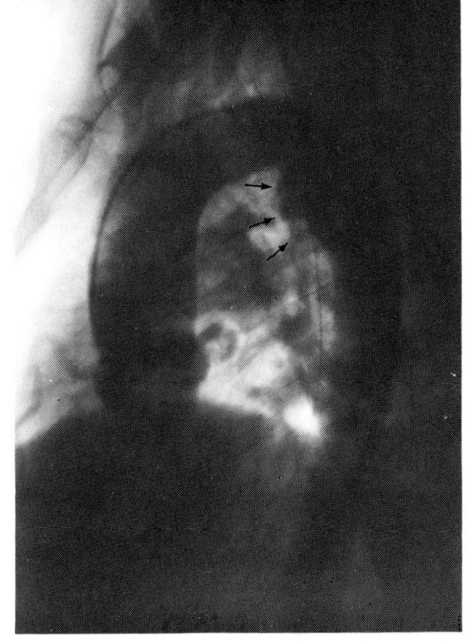

16 Oct. 1978

958c . . . a second, lateral film is taken. Extravasation seems to point to a classic isthmic rupture (→), but surgery shows the aorta to be intact.

Natural history and mortality

Most violent deceleration casualties with severe cardiac or vascular damage die on the scene of the accident. However, due to increasingly effective first-aid and transport, a growing proportion of casualties with life-threatening vascular damage survive long enough to be admitted to hospital: it is estimated that some 15% of aortic rupture victims are now admitted alive.

One result is that today's hospital mortality figures are artificially increased by the number of patients who are already hopeless on arrival and formerly would have died on the scene of the accident or in the ambulance.

A second, far more important result is the number who are now saved by a combination of proper in-transit care and early hospital treatment.

959

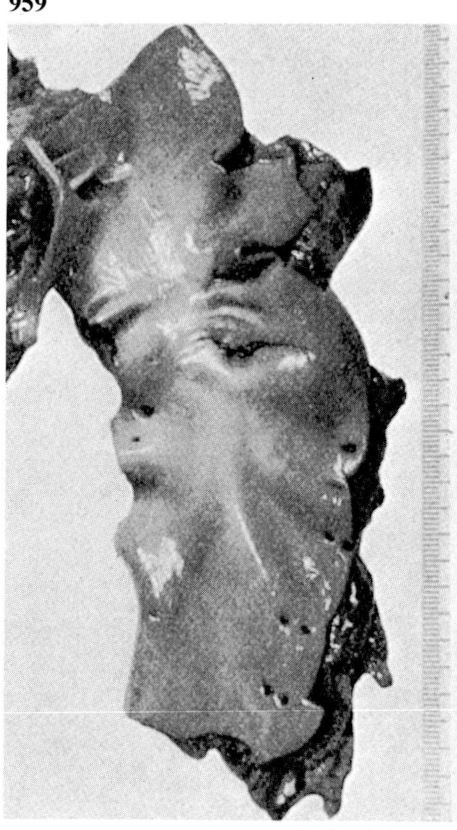

D.J. ♂ 30 yrs. 1958

959 Rupture of the aortic isthmus, however small, is usually fatal. This patient died five hours after a partial rupture (at a time when the injury was considered beyond the resources of surgery).

The natural history of aortic rupture is well-known. It is worth recalling, however, since an alarming number of patients are overtaken by sudden and fatal exsanguination even before aortic rupture has been suspected, let alone diagnosed. An untreated patient may well survive initially, but death is nonetheless inevitable after an unpredictable, often short delay. About 80% of aortic ruptures occur at the isthmus, and 55% are total.

At the beginning, the high pressure pulsating haematoma that surrounds the rupture is contained by the adventitia and the parietal pleura. Provided its walls are sufficiently resistant, the sealing haematoma then organises. This, the pseudo-aneurysm, usually provokes neither symptoms nor signs. Subsequently, the pseudo-aneurysm swells until it ruptures into the adjacent pleural cavity.

960

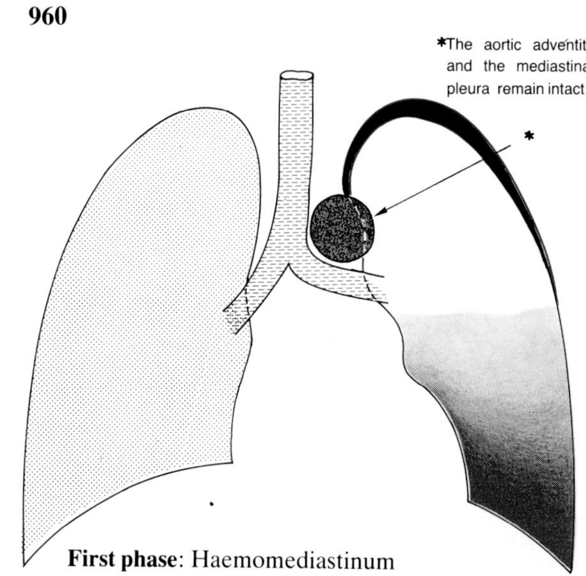

Natural history of isthmic rupture.

First phase: Haemomediastinum

961

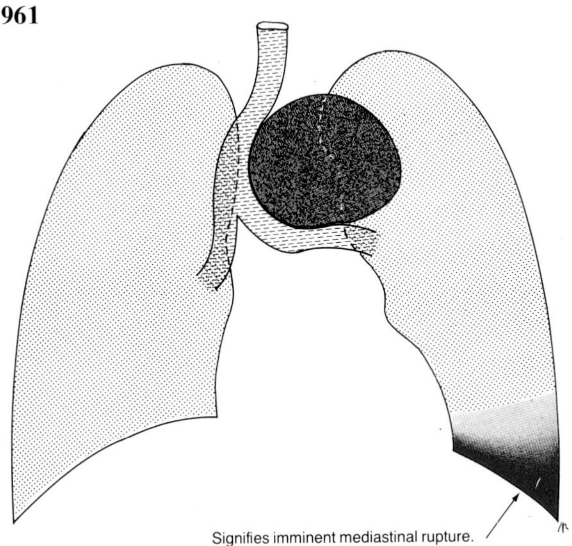

Free interval: Pseudo-aneurysm caused by organisation of haematoma.

962

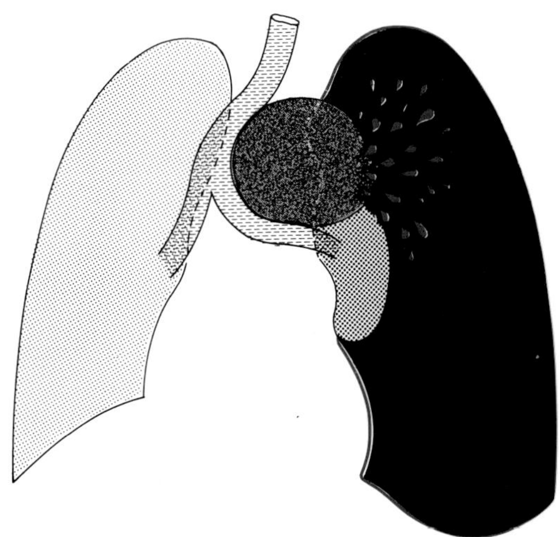

Second phase: Secondary rupture of mediastinum leading to exsanguination into pleural cavity.

Almost all aortic ruptures pass through two phases separated by a free interval: rupture of the intimal and medial layers (*first phase*), fast- or slow-growing pseudo-aneurysm (*free interval*), and rupture of the adventitial layer and mediastinum (*second phase*). The duration of the free interval is unpredictable; it can last for a few seconds or several years. In one case it lasted for 27 years.

Ruptures of the aorta can be classified conveniently according to the *timing of mediastinal rupture*. This, the second phase, can occur:

1. **immediately** (before admission to hospital).
2. **early** (within a few hours of admission): *acute pseudo-aneurysm*.
3. **after a delay** (between 24 hours and three weeks after admission): *fast-growing pseudo-aneurysm*.
4. **late** (after months or even years): *chronic, slow-growing pseudo-aneurysm*.

963

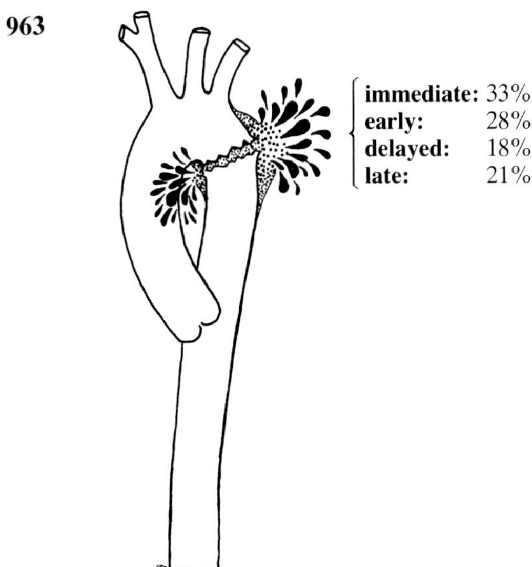

963 Timing of mediastinal rupture (second phase of aortic rupture).

964 Timing of exsanguination into pleural cavity (Parmley's study) (with percentages of survivors and non-survivors)

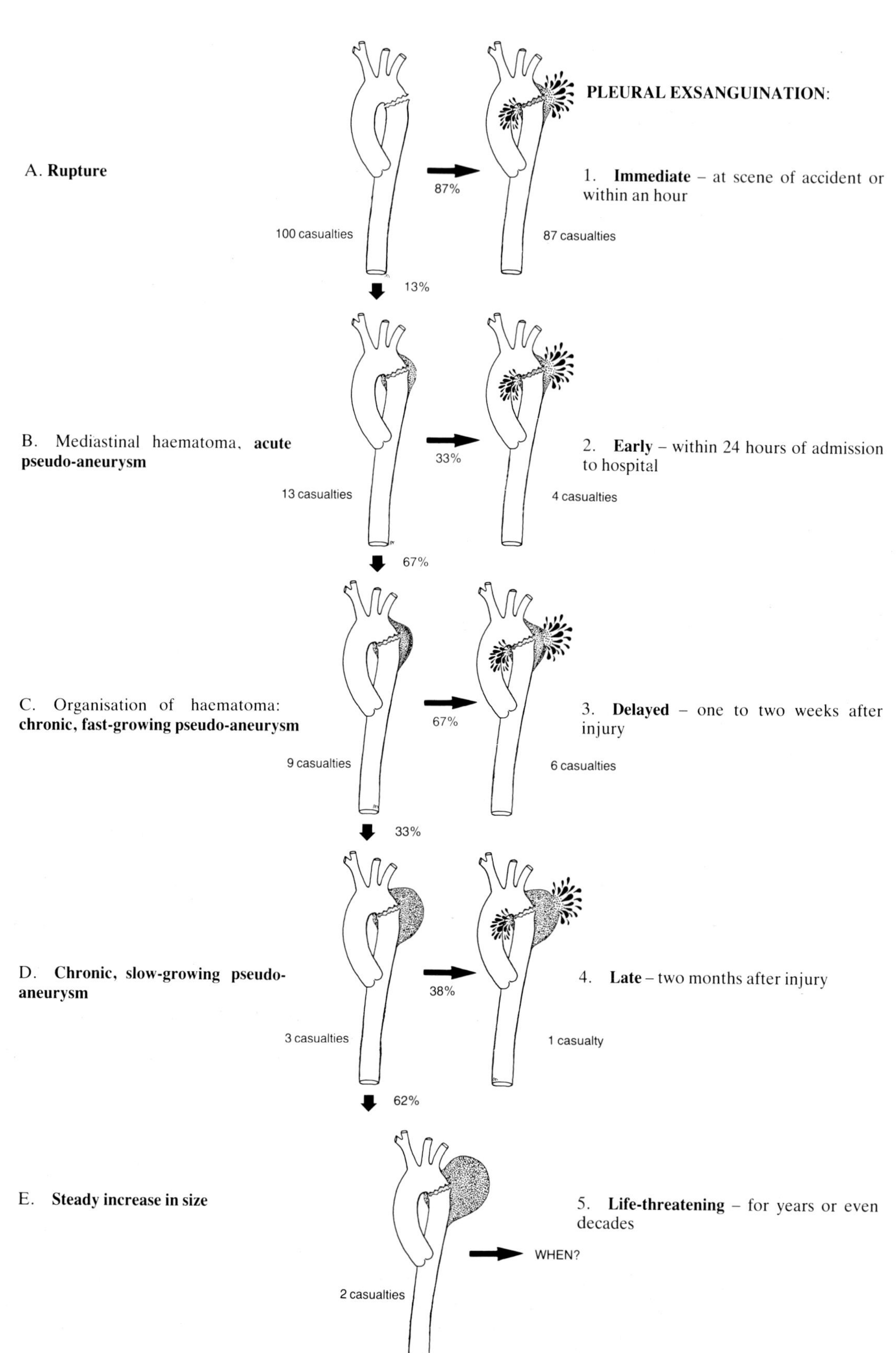

In the present state of knowledge, *immediate* or *early* exsanguination means certain death. In other words, aortic rupture is inevitably fatal in about 90% of cases.

Most patients with a *chronic, fast-growing pseudo-aneurysm*, on the other hand, can be cured provided the diagnosis is made: however, even in hospital a regrettable number of cases are **only diagnosed on the autopsy table**.

Patients with a *chronic, slow-growing pseudo-aneurysm* can undergo well-planned surgery.

Rupture into the pleural cavity

Sooner or later, the adventitia and parietal pleura containing the pseudo-aneurysm will rupture inevitably. This second phase of aortic rupture usually consists of a 10 to 15cm tear with massive pleural haemorrhage and rapidly irreversible shock.

In the vast majority of cases, death is immediate. On rare occasions, the haemothorax can clot and temporarily re-seal the ruptured aorta (see **969h** and Volume I, **574**), allowing a few hours' survival. Indeed, Inberg has reported the case of a patient with an exsanguinating haemothorax who was saved despite prolonged cardiac arrest; internal cardiac massage and massive transfusion were administered while emergency repair was performed without regard to asepsis.

965a

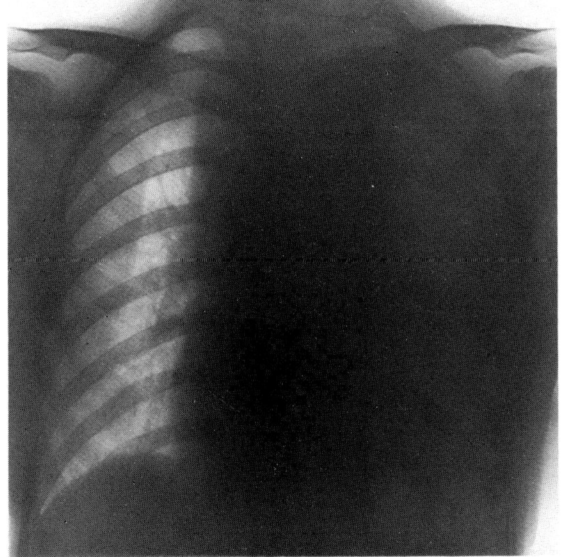

W.E. ♀ 19 yrs. 23 Aug. 1975

965a Total and complete rupture of the aortic isthmus can produce **immediate** bleeding into the left pleural cavity. This admission X-ray shows a massive left haemothorax (see Volume I, **66**).

965b

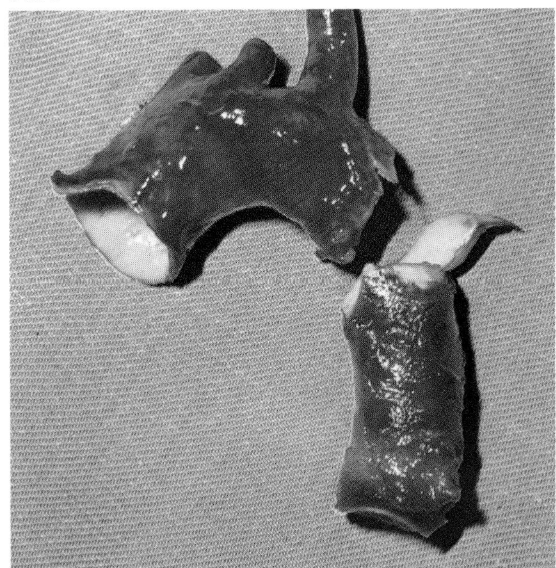

23 Aug. 1975

965b Repair of the aorta was attempted through a left thoracotomy but haemostasis proved impossible and the patient succumbed. Although this rupture is both total and complete, the patient survived longer than **959**, whose rupture was partial. (Dr M.Boumghar, Lausanne.)

966a

B.A. ♂ 59 yrs. 1 Jan. 1974, 04 hrs.

966b

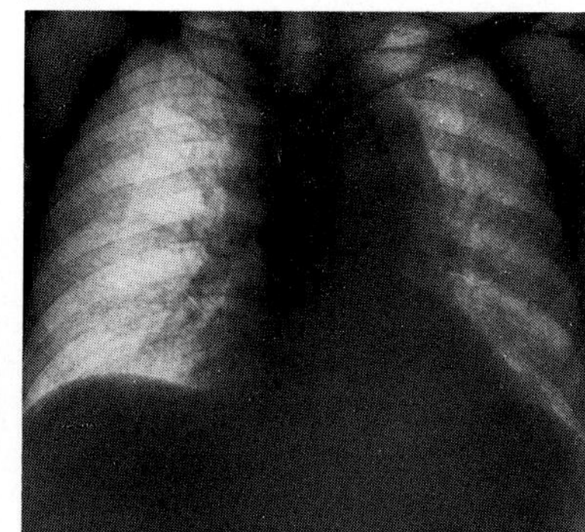

04.30 hrs.

966c

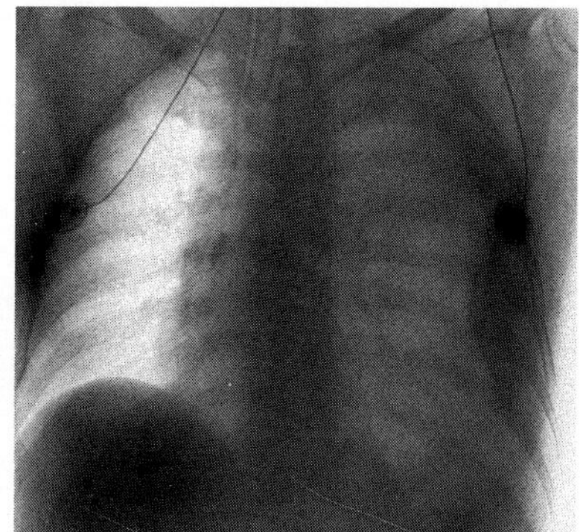

05 hrs.

966d

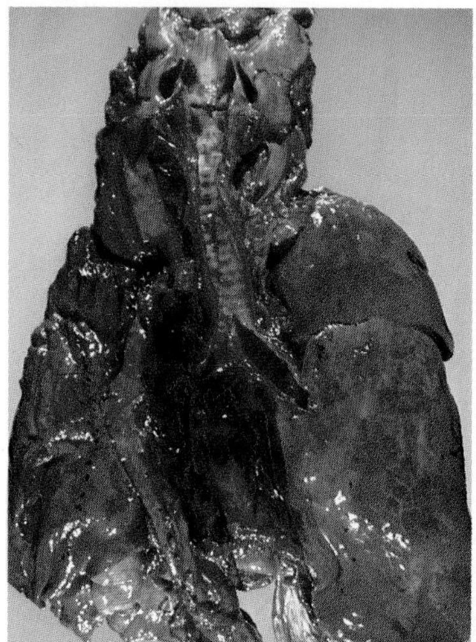

1 Jan. 1974

966e

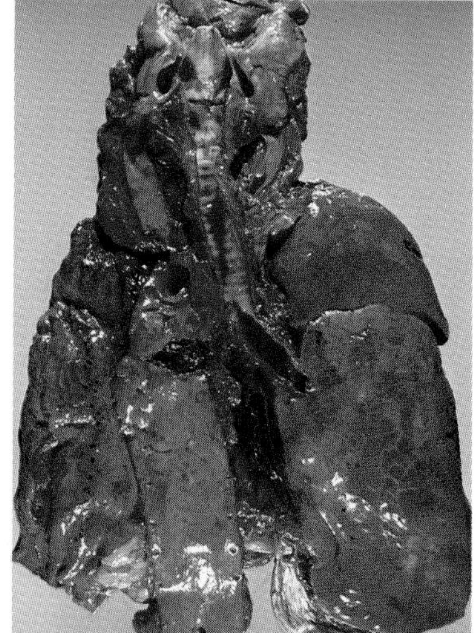

1 Jan. 1974

966f

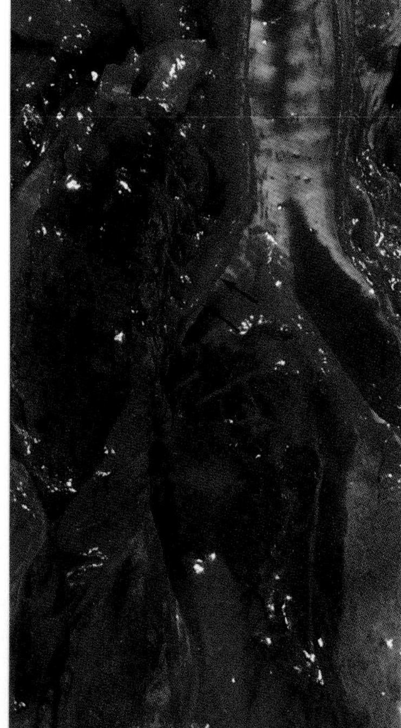

1 Jan. 1974

966g

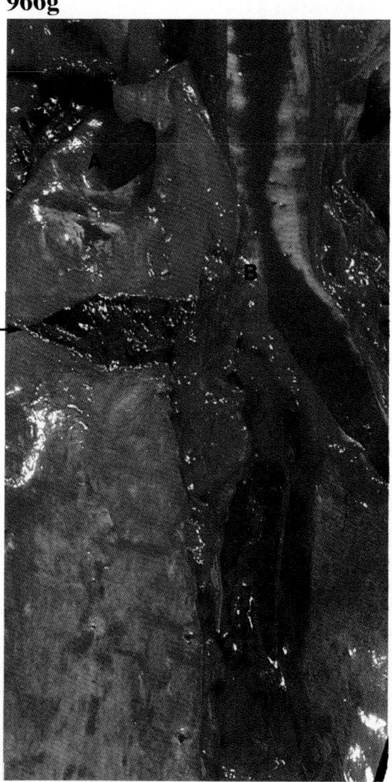

1 Jan. 1974

966a Rupture of the aortic isthmus followed by rupture of the mediastinum **shortly after admission**. This X-ray, obtained 15 minutes after the accident, shows a widened mediastinum.

966b In the next half hour, the mediastinum widens further and a left haemothorax develops.

966c The mediastinum ruptures (75 minutes after trauma) into the pleural cavity before an angiogram can be taken. Exsanguination. Death.

966d *Haemomediastinum*. The thoracic viscera are seen here from behind: the mediastinal haematoma has displaced the descending aorta to the left. (Institute of Pathology, Lausanne.)

966e The aorta has been opened to reveal an anterior rupture of the isthmus girdling three-quarters of the circumference.

966f The haemomediastinum has depressed and squashed the left main-stem bronchus (→).

966g Close-up of the rupture (→) situated just beyond the aortic arch (A), almost at the level of the carina (B). The aorta is seen here from behind.

967a

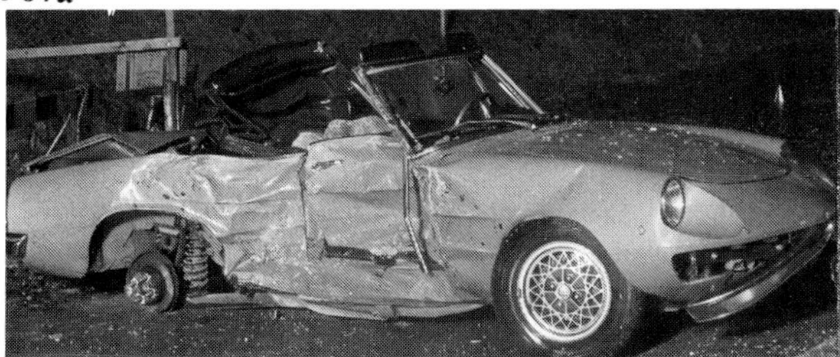

A.J.–R. ♂ 46 yrs 19 Nov. 1975

967b

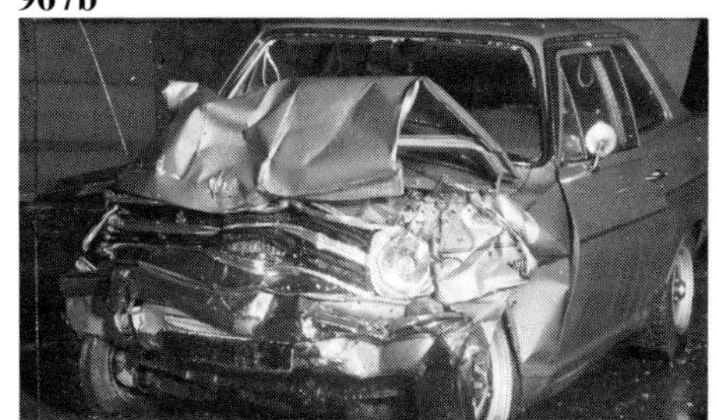

19 Nov. 1975

967c

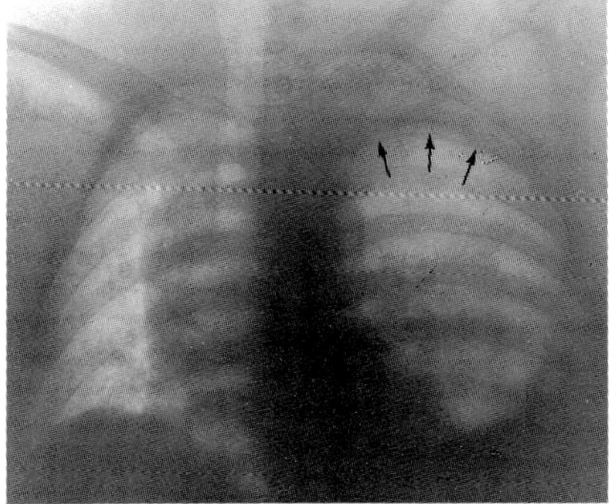

19 Nov. 1975, 21 hrs.

967d

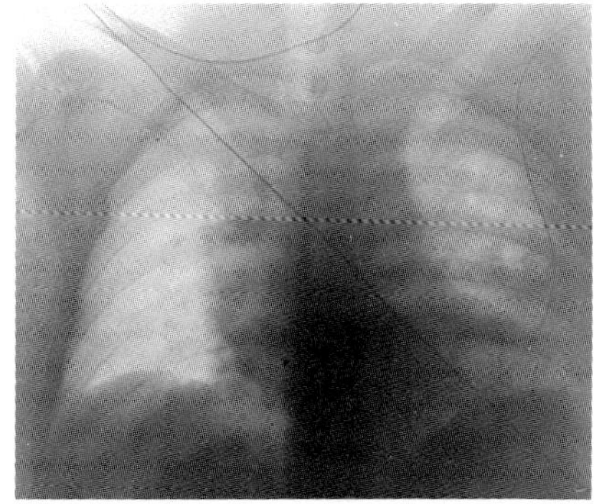

21.45 hrs.

967e

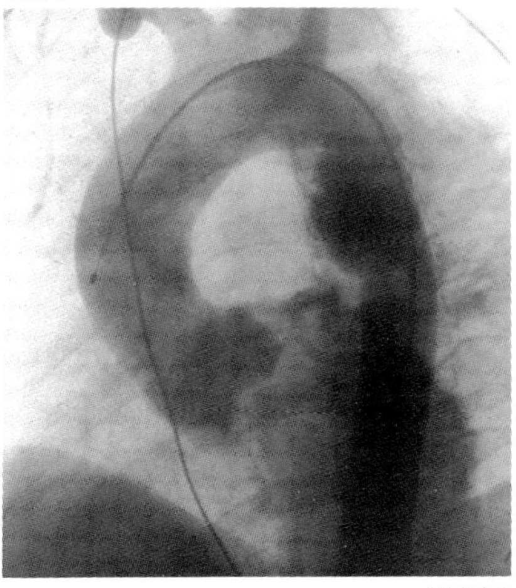

22.10 hrs.

967f

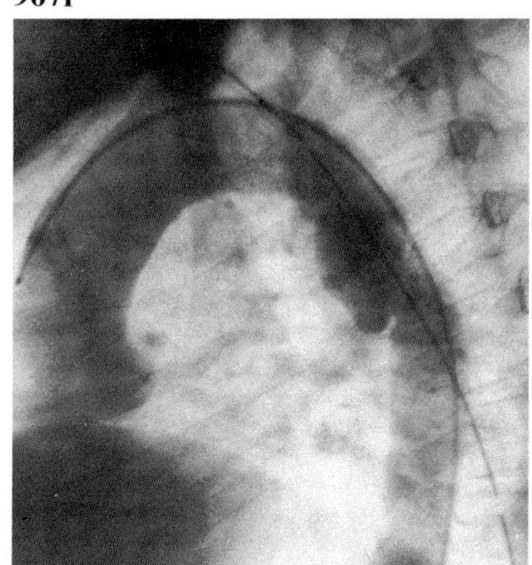

22.15 hrs.

967a Aortic rupture with secondary rupture of the mediastinum **during angiography**. This sports car skidded and was hit at about 100 km/h by the car in **967b**. The driver was found hanging over the right-hand door.

967c The admission X-ray shows mediastinal widening with the apical cap sign (→), a left haemothorax and rightward displacement of the trachea and mediastinum.

967d Mediastinal widening persists after pleural drainage.

967e The rupture is clearly evinced both on the oblique . . .

967f . . . and on the lateral angiogram.

The patient dies five minutes later from a massive haemorrhage into the left pleural cavity. It seems likely that the sudden pressure increase during angiography played a part in the fatal rupture of the pseudo-aneurysm.

About 10% of aortic ruptures give rise to a **right** haemothorax (with or without a left haemothorax) at some stage in their evolution. It is usually due to parietal damage, and sometimes can distract attention from the aorta.

An acute pseudo-aneurysm can exceptionally rupture into the right rather than into the left pleural cavity.

968a

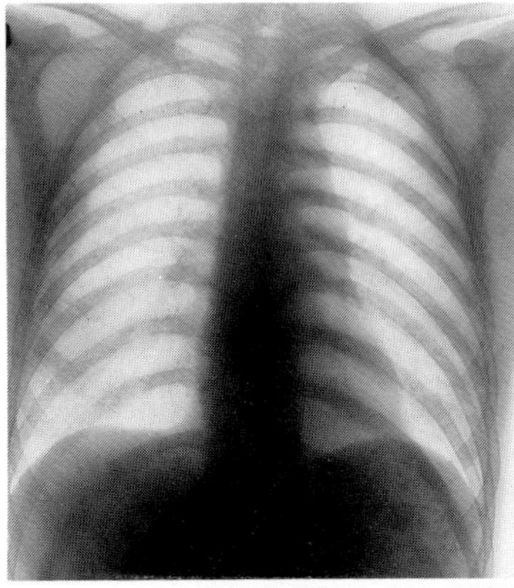

H.H.–P. ♂ 21 yrs. 16 April 1974

968b

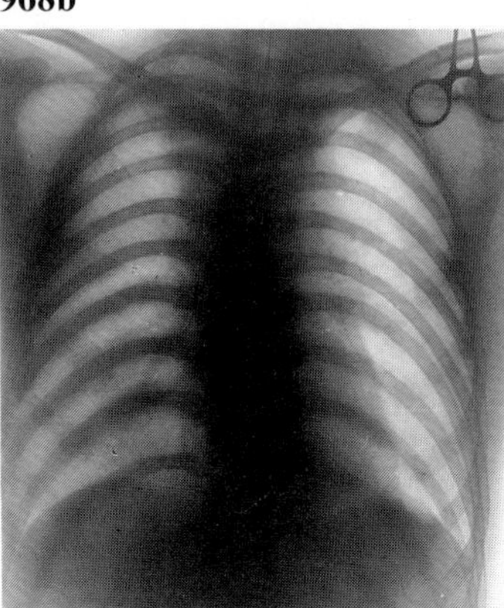

17 April 1974

968c

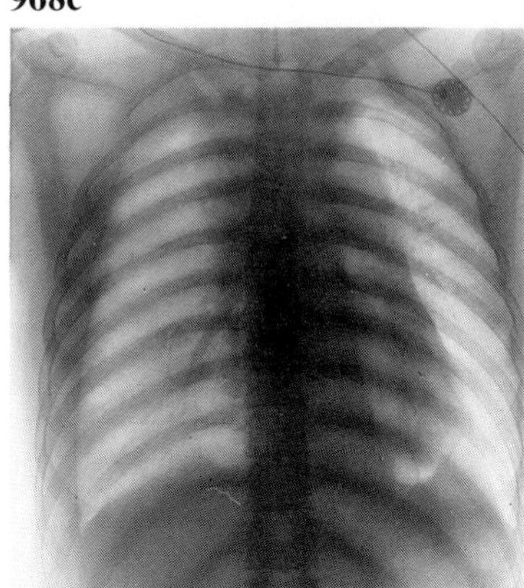

17 April 1974

968a Rupture of aorta into right pleural cavity. The admission X-ray of a decelerated lorry driver shows no mediastinal widening.

968b A right haemothorax appears the following day.

968c The haemothorax increases rapidly. A median sternotomy performed on suspicion of a disinserted supra-aortic vessel reveals an isthmic rupture of the aorta. The approach precludes repair. Death.

Post-traumatic pseudo-aneurysm

Post-traumatic aneurysms are called 'false aneurysms' because the aneurysmal pouch is formed by the conjunctive tissues surrounding the vessel. The adventitia often remains intact despite rupture of the internal arterial walls (the intima and media). So although the designation 'pseudo-aneurysm' has become current, the term 'organised haematoma' would be more correct.

An acute pseudo-aneurysm can either rupture into the pleural cavity or become chronic. The length of time a chronic pseudo-aneurysm will last before rupturing is highly unpredictable. Chronic pseudo-aneurysms can be classified according to whether they are fast- or slow-growing.

The radiological signs of a pseudo-aneurysm are usually evident (see **946**). Apart from the outline of the vascular mass itself, the important signs are rightward displacement of the trachea and possibly also of the oesophagus, and depression of the left main-stem bronchus. The larger the pseudo-aneurysm, the more obvious the signs. In older patients, the calcified intimal layer can be seen separate from the outline of the pseudo-aneurysm.

If an acute or chronic pseudo-aneurysm gives rise to even the slightest left haemothorax, danger is signalled: transudation of blood into the pleura implies an imminent risk of complete mediastinal rupture with exsanguination.

FAST-GROWING

969a

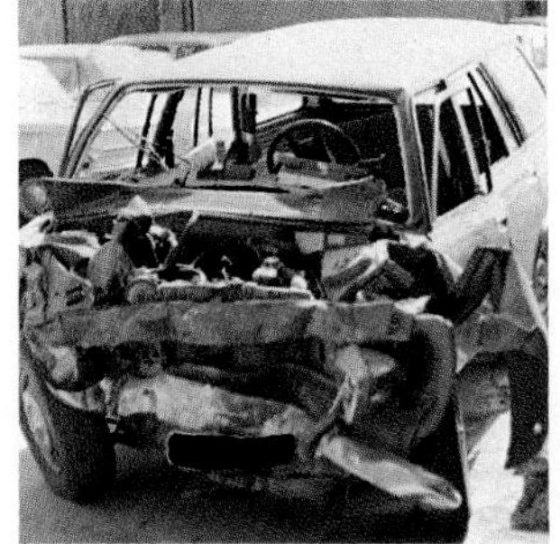

G.D. ♂ 36 yrs. 24 Jan. 1976

969b

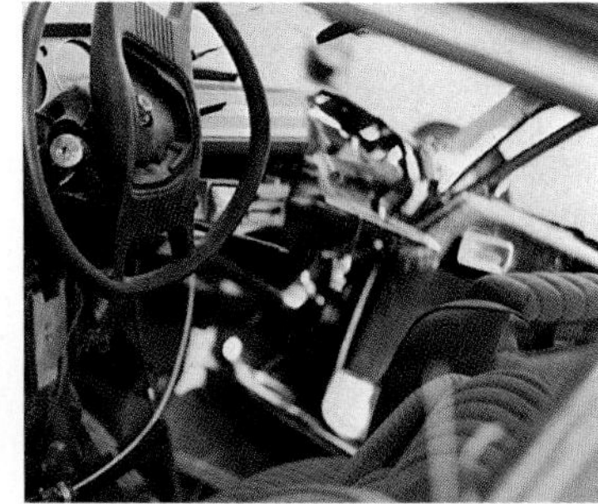

969a Total traumatic rupture of the aorta with a **fast-growing pseudo-aneurysm**. The patient was a passenger in this car when it crashed head-on at 100 km/h; he was wearing a safety belt.

969b The interior of the car after the ~ 80 g impact.

969c 25 Jan. 1976

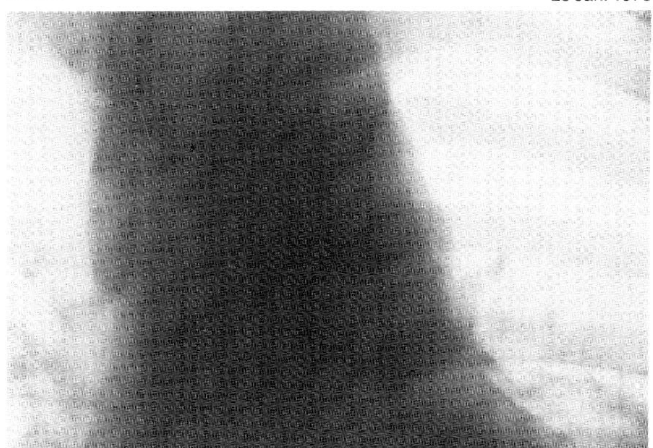

969c Development of fast-growing pseudo-aneurysm. The day after the patient was admitted to a district hospital, the outline of the mediastinum was considered normal.

969d 29 Jan. 1976

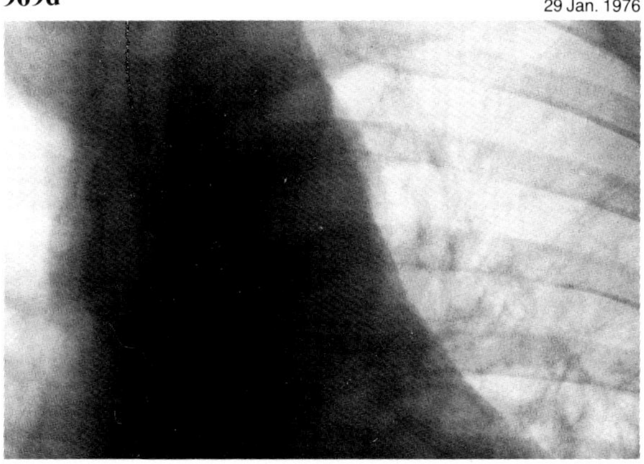

969d But by the sixth day, a slight protrusion can be seen in the wall of the aorta.

969e

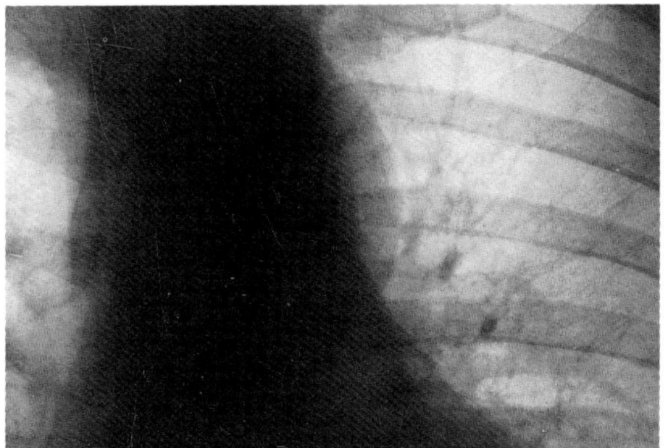

1 Feb. 1976

969e By the ninth day, the protrusion is sizeable.

969f

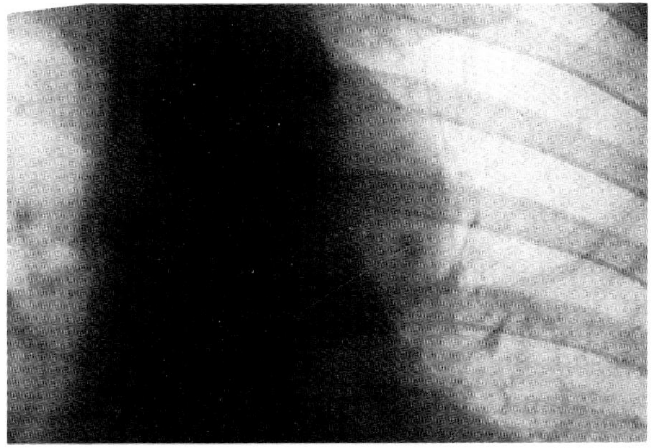

9 Feb. 1976

969f By the 16th day, the left main-stem bronchus is depressed . . .

969g

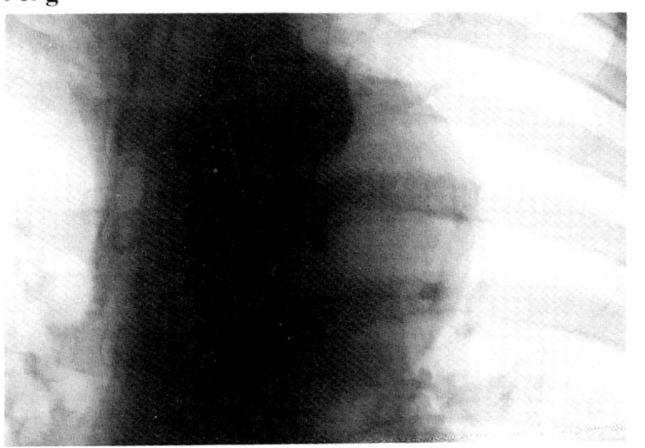

13 Feb. 1976

969g . . . and by the 20th day, the trachea is displaced to the right.

969h

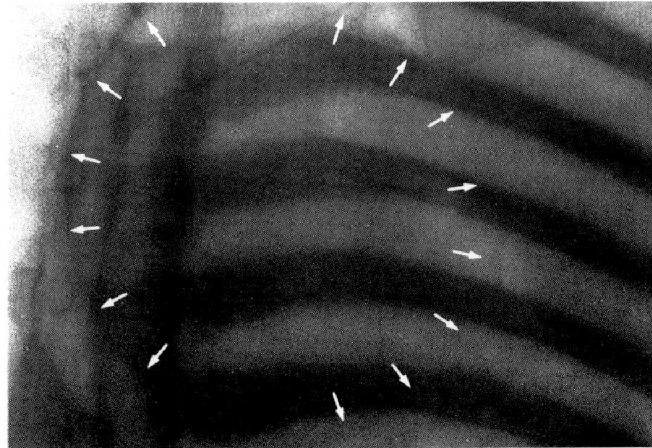

14 Feb. 1976

969h At the moment it ruptures into the left pleural cavity (on the 21st day), the pseudo-aneurysm measures 10cm in diameter (→). The patient is resuscitated on arrival at the University Hospital and surgical repair is attempted. Haemostasis proves impossible. Death. (See the complete X-ray picture Volume I, **574** and photograph of the rupture **978**.)

SLOW-GROWING

A slow-growing, chronic pseudo-aneurysm is potentially fatal at any stage (see **964**).

The slow growth of a pseudo-aneurysm does not necessarily imply a minor or partial rupture.

The walls of a chronic slow-growing pseudo-aneurysm are relatively stable; elective surgery usually can be performed under good conditions.

970a

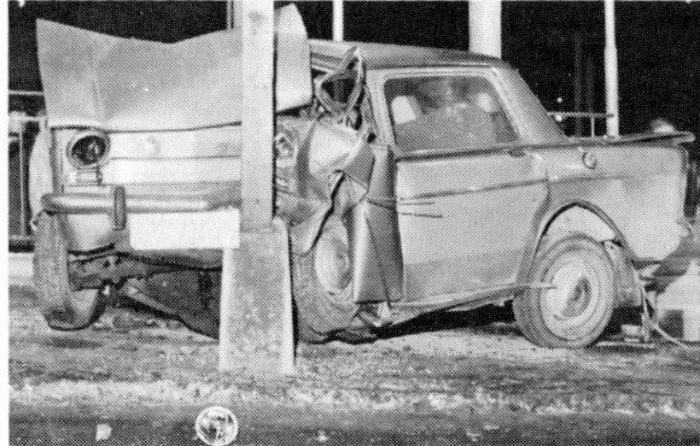

970b

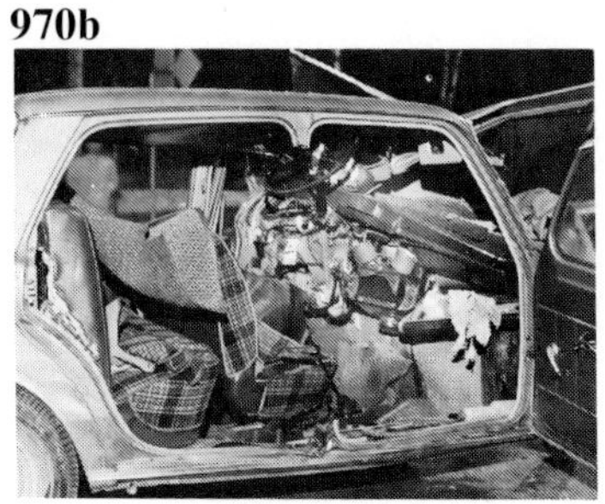

C.C. ♂ 49 yrs. 10 Jan. 1967

970c

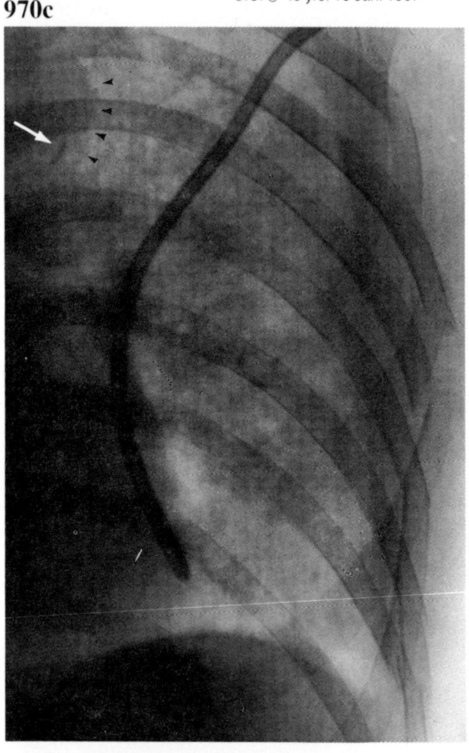

18 Jan. 1967

970a **Slow growth of pseudo-aneurysm** of the aortic isthmus over a period of nine years, without secondary rupture.

970b The patient drove into a pylon at 70 km/h.

970c An anterior flail chest with paradoxical motion, a left haemopneumothorax and left lung contusion are diagnosed. The calcified intima (→) of the aortic arch can be seen separate from the outline of the haematoma (←) produced by an as yet unrecognised partial rupture of the aortic isthmus.

970d The ensuing 9-year series of X-rays shows the gradual development of the pseudo-aneurysm. The distance between the intimal and adventitial layers increases progressively.

970d

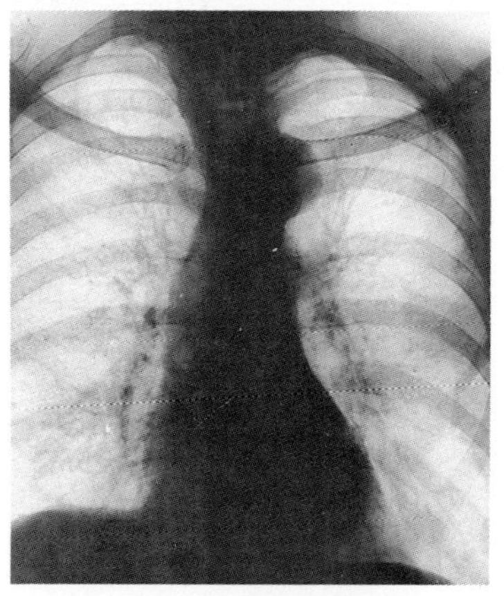

29 Aug. 1967

970e

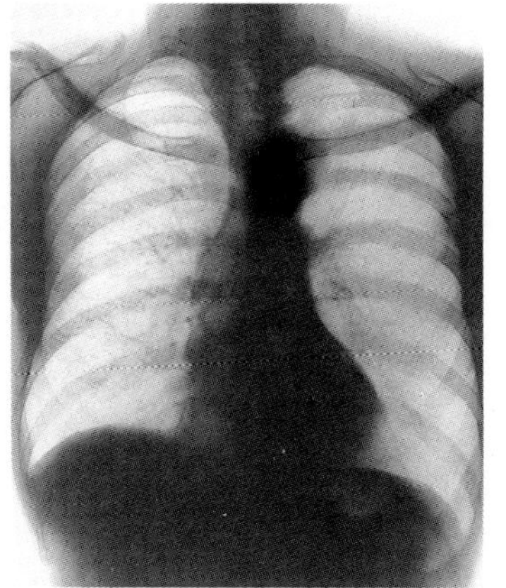

21 June 1974

970f

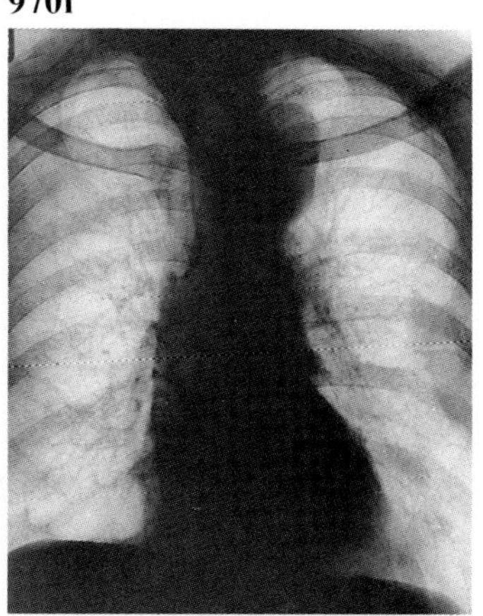

10 Feb. 1976

970g

29 Aug. 1969

970h

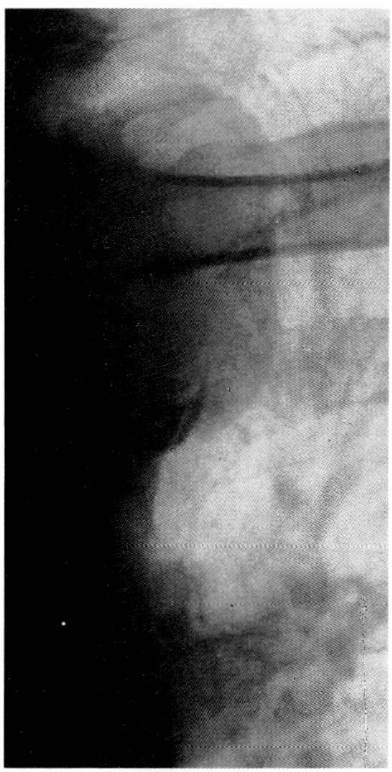

21 June 1974

970i

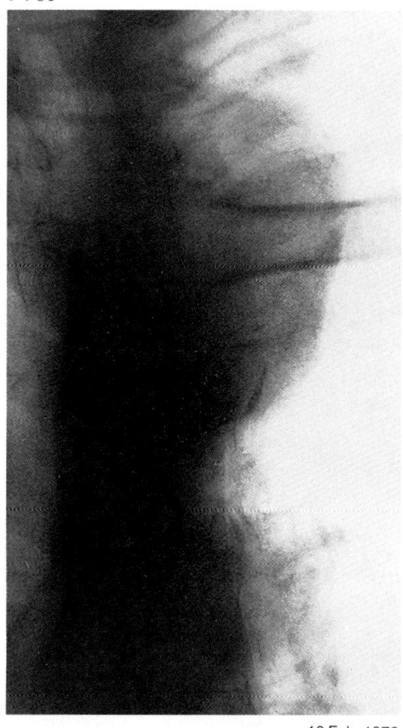

10 Feb. 1976

970j The pseudo-aneurysm is seen here through a left thoracotomy. The aortic arch (A), the left subclavian artery (B) and the descending aorta (C) have all been secured on small rubber drains. (Prof. H.Sadeghi, Lausanne.)

970k The resected aortic isthmus and pseudo-aneurysm are replaced by a dacron graft (see **982**).

970 l The pseudo-aneurysm contains organised clots. Recovery.

970j

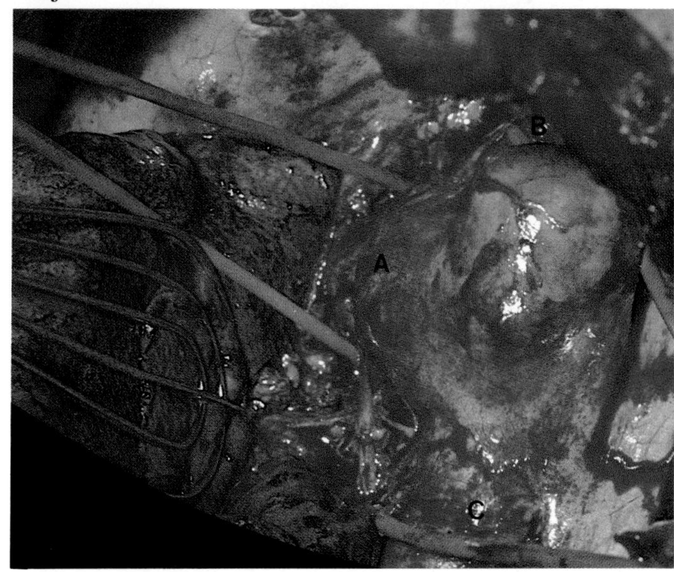

31 May 1976

970k

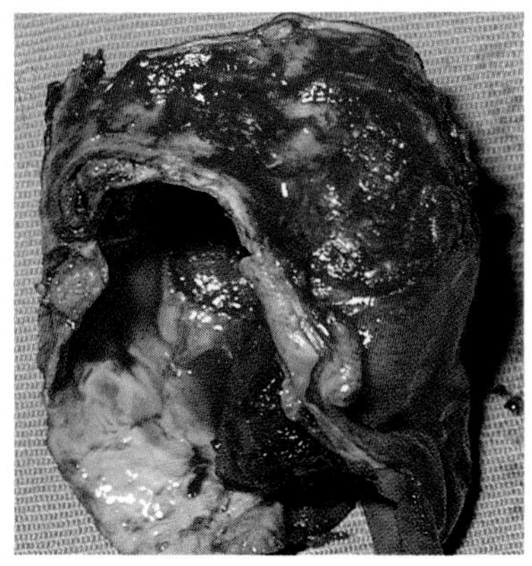

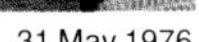

31 May 1976

970 l

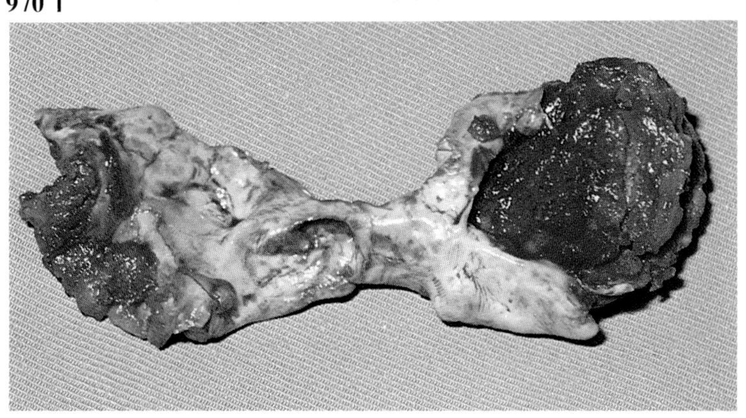

31 May 1976

971a

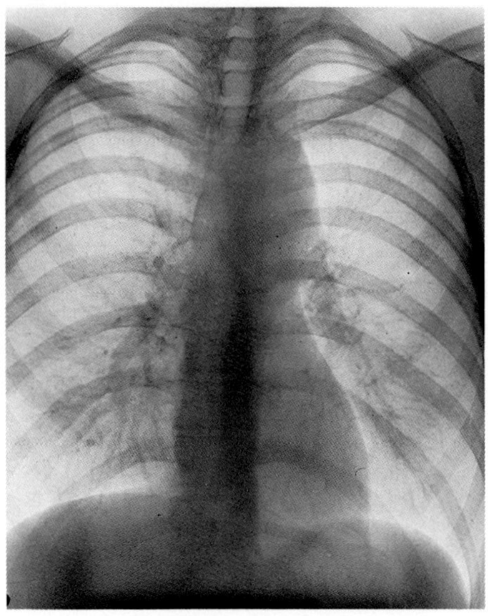

971b

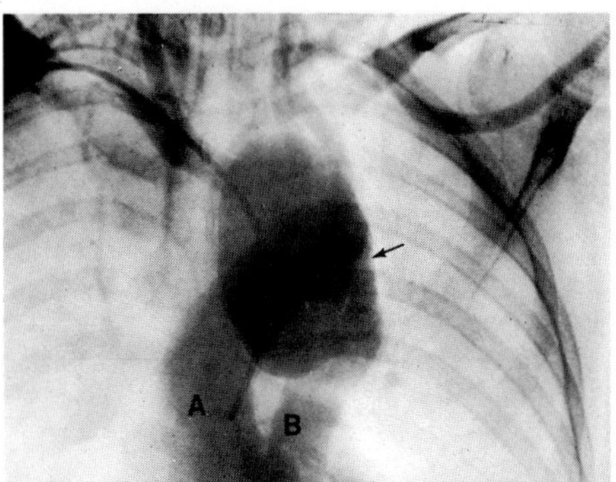

971c

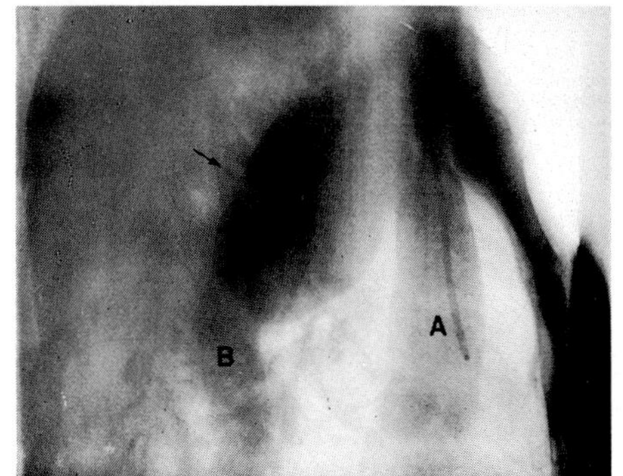

971a Rupture of the aortic isthmus with a **slow-growing pseudo-aneurysm**. This standard chest X-ray, taken three years after the subject was involved in a serious scooter accident, shows indirect signs of an aortic pseudo-aneurysm.

971b An angiogram (obtained by catheterisation of the right humeral artery) shows that the pseudo-aneurysm is located at the isthmus (→). A = ascending aorta, B = descending aorta.

971c Lateral view. Surgical wrapping. Recovery.

Rupture with intimal flap

When aortic rupture is incomplete, the flow of blood can raise and progressively detach a distal portion of intima. The flap can be of any length and is likely eventually to obstruct the lumen of the descending aorta. The clinical picture is one of *pseudocoarctation* (see **943, 944**) – high arterial pressure in the upper limbs, unequal pulses in the upper and lower limbs, ischaemia in the abdomen and below (with paraplegia and anuria) and, perhaps also, series of emboli in the subdiaphragmatic arteries. Rupture with intimal flap seems commonest in younger patients.

If the intima is calcified, a standard X-ray is adequate for diagnosis (see **970**, **975**).

The surgeon's task is first to reposition the intimal flap and then to restore normal circulation (see **973**).

972

Incomplete isthmic rupture with increasingly extensive and obstructive intimal flap **(pseudo-coarctation)**.

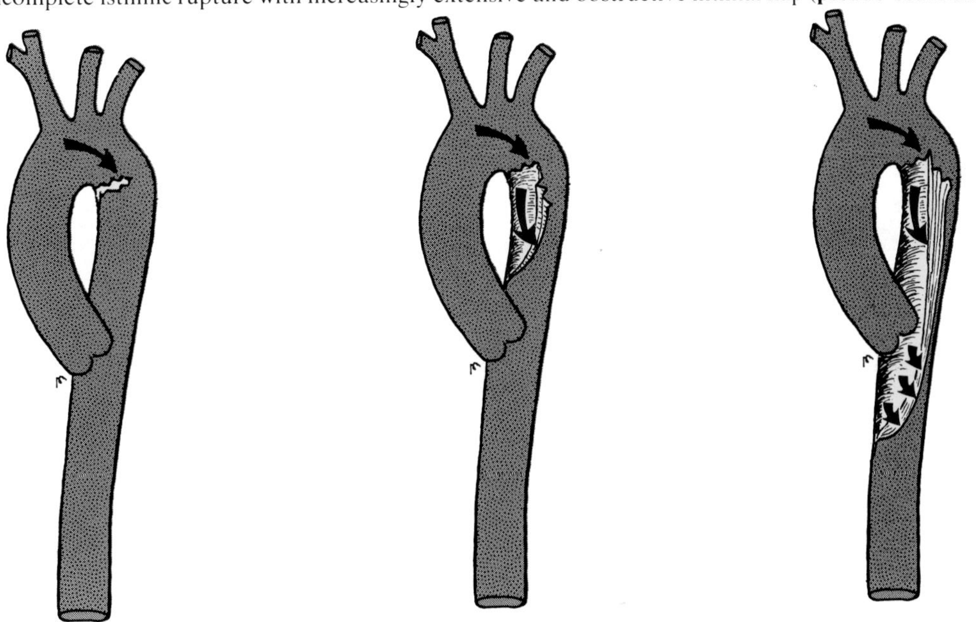

973 Repair of incomplete vascular rupture with **partial** intimal flap.

974

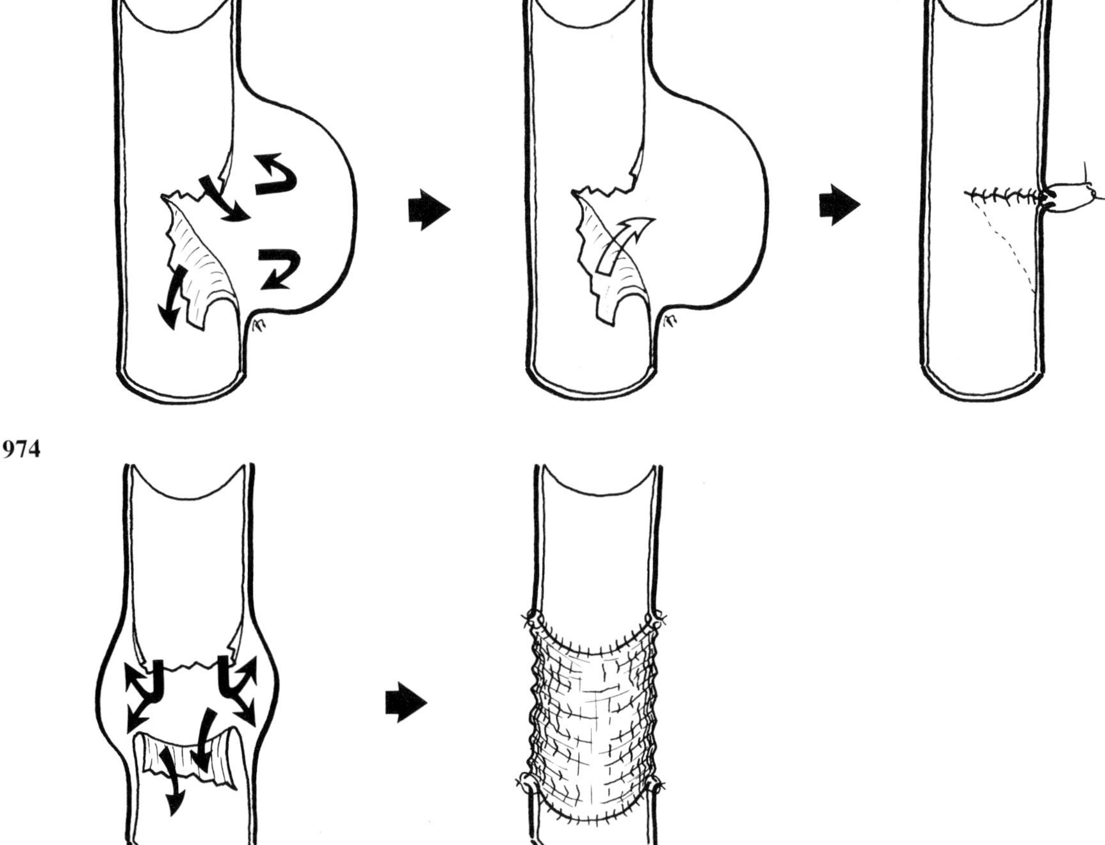

974 Incomplete vascular rupture with **circular** intimal flap repaired by resection and grafting.

975a

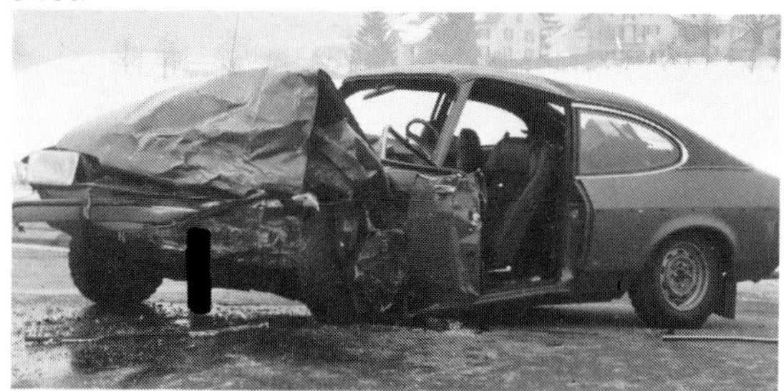

J.G. ♂ 77 yrs. 10 Feb. 1978.

975b

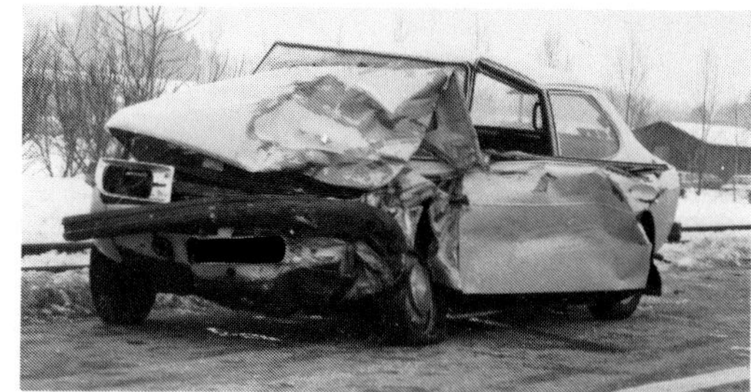

10 Feb. 1978

975c

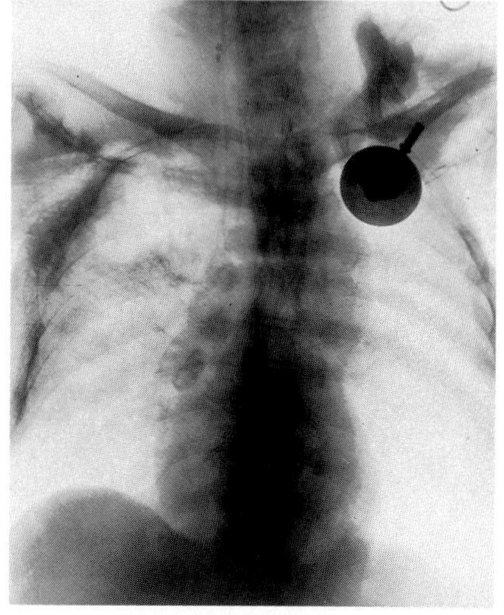

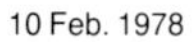

10 Feb. 1978

975d

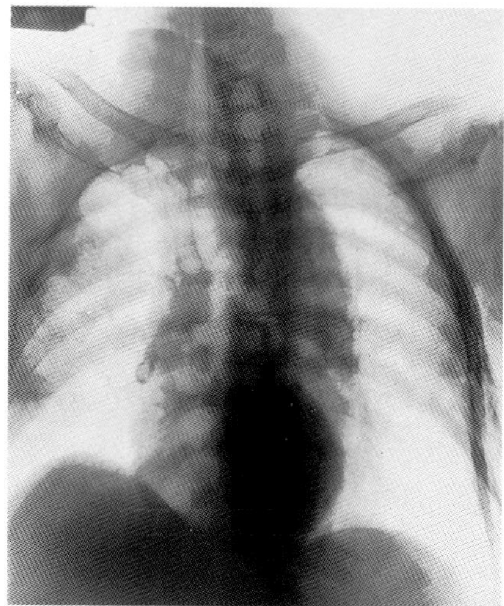

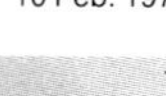

10 Feb. 1978

975e

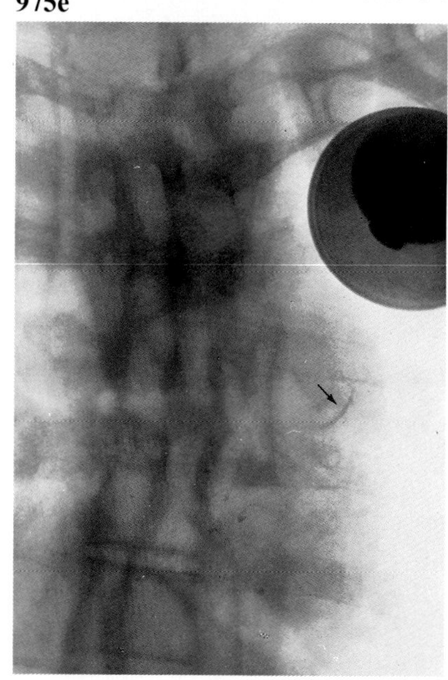

10 Feb. 1978

975f

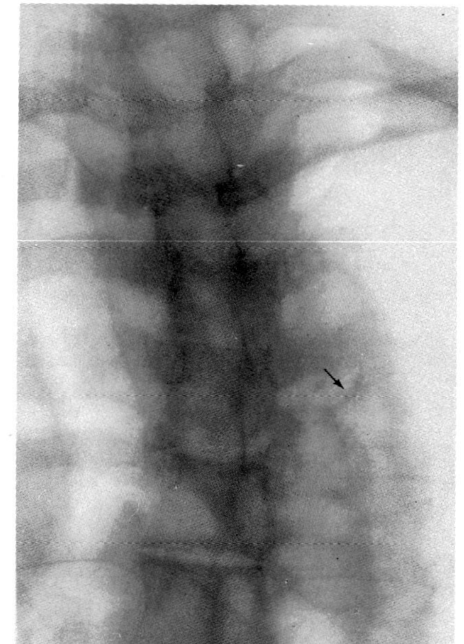

10 Feb. 1978

975g

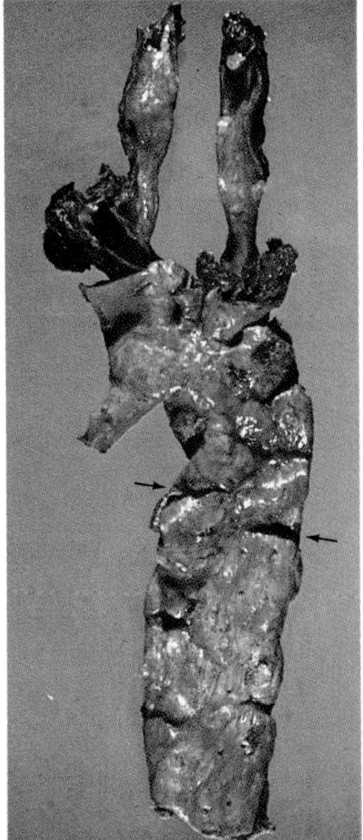

10 Feb. 1978

975h

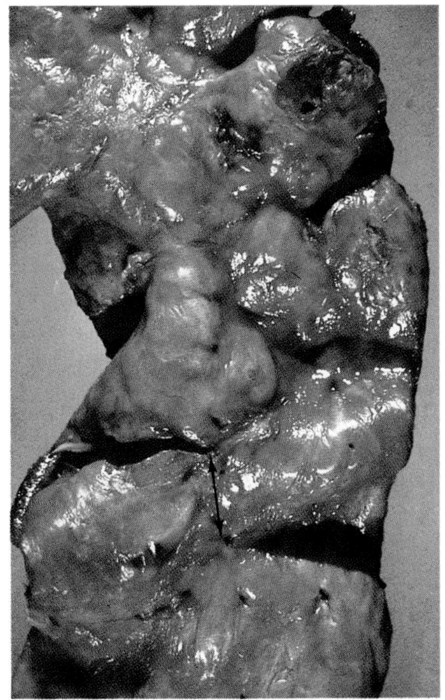

10 Feb. 1978

975i

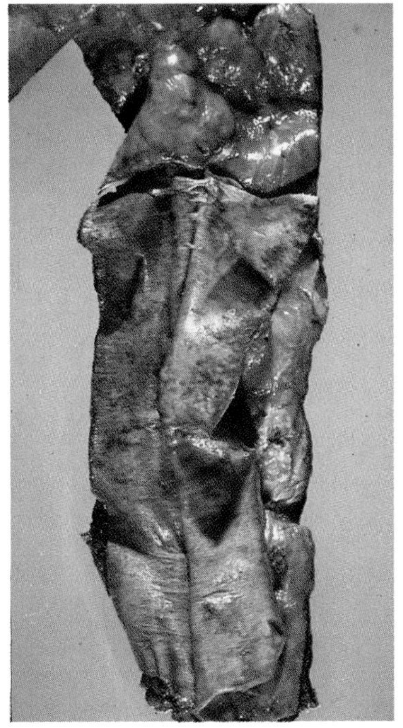

10 Feb. 1978

975a Isthmic rupture of the aorta with intimal flap. The driver of this car was involved in an almost head-on collision at 80 km/h . . .

975b . . . with this car travelling at about the same speed. Both drivers were difficult to free.

975c On admission, the patient displays an anterior flail chest with paradoxical motion over six ribs, and subcutaneous emphysema. The standard X-ray shows the upper mediastinum widened to the left and the trachea displaced to the right.

975d A few minutes later, the mid mediastinum appears to have widened; the left main-stem bronchus is clearly depressed.

975e A close-up of the aortic arch . . .

975f . . . shows dissociation of the calcified intimal and adventitial layers.

975g Death one hour after admission. Autopsy reveals a rupture of the aortic isthmus. (Institute of Pathology, Lausanne.)

975h Some 1 cm of the right wall is intact. Several atheromatous deposits are visible.

975i The blood stream has peeled away the intima along the full length of the descending aorta.

Surgical management

Vascular repair is now a common and safe procedure. Despite frequent and sometimes extensive associated injuries, aortic surgery for traumatic rupture is currently successful in 75% of cases. Many of these patients are young and in good general condition.

When repair is *early*, sequelae are uncommon.

However, large-scale studies have shown that **almost half of all aortic ruptures in patients surviving for more than a day are only diagnosed and treated after several weeks**.

Even so, late diagnosis and treatment are less common today than ten years ago when 70% to 75% of reported cases were treated after a lapse of more than three weeks. Today this figure has dropped to some 30%.

Haemostasis

When the aortic isthmus ruptures directly into the pleural cavity, the surgeon faces immense problems. The haemostasis necessary for end-to-end anastomosis is often impossible to achieve when the chest is open. Clamping of the aorta, especially when prolonged by the establishment of a by-pass, often fatally complicates the initial episode of deep shock. Indeed, those who survive are often anuric, paraplegic and cerebrally dead.

Experiments on cadavers and dogs have shown that haemostasis of a classically sited rupture can be effected by threading a Foley or Fogarty catheter through the left subclavian artery into the aortic arch. Once the tip of the catheter has reached the aortic arch, the cuff is inflated with about 3 ml of saline. In this way, the aorta is occluded above the rupture. Gentle traction on the catheter ensures that it does not occlude the ostium of the carotid or innominate arteries.

This procedure, which in no way hinders the actual process of repair, only takes a matter of minutes and can retrieve the most desperate situation. In many cases, it is a wise pre-operative precaution.

We tried it once during a thoracotomy on a patient whose aorta finally proved intact (see **924**). We found the technique easy, efficient and atraumatic; it gave rise to neither clotting nor embolism.

976

976 Percentages of **early and late** treatment (literature review).

977

BEFORE THORACOTOMY:

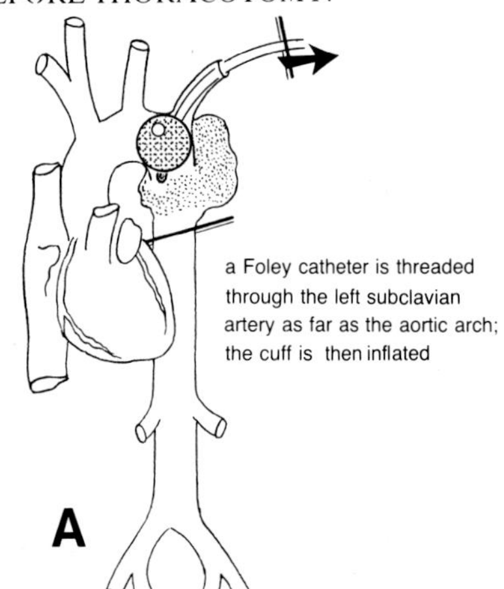

DURING THORACOTOMY:

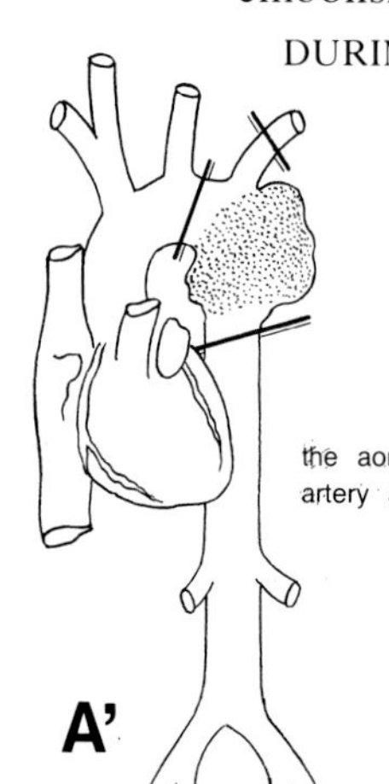

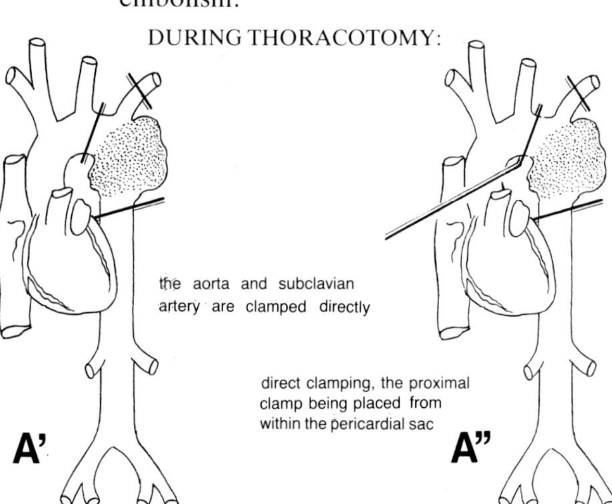

977 Temporary **haemostasis** of isthmic rupture of aorta

978a

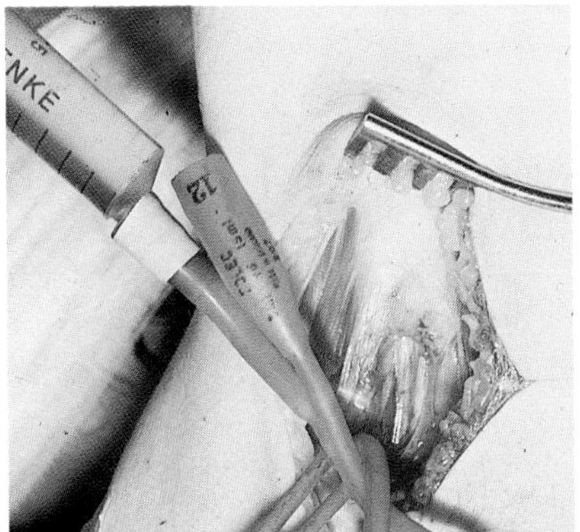

978a Emergency pre-operative haemostasis in cases of aortic or pseudo-aneurysmal rupture into the pleural cavity. The photograph shows a Foley (it could be a Fogarty) catheter inserted about 12cm into the proximal portion of the left axillary artery.

978b The blood stream inevitably draws the catheter towards the distal part of the aortic arch, and sometimes even into the pseudo-aneurysm itself – as in this autopsy photograph where the tip of the catheter lies 17cm from the axillary incision.

978c The injection of 3ml of saline into the cuff inflates it to a diameter corresponding to that of the aortic isthmus in a man of average build.

978b

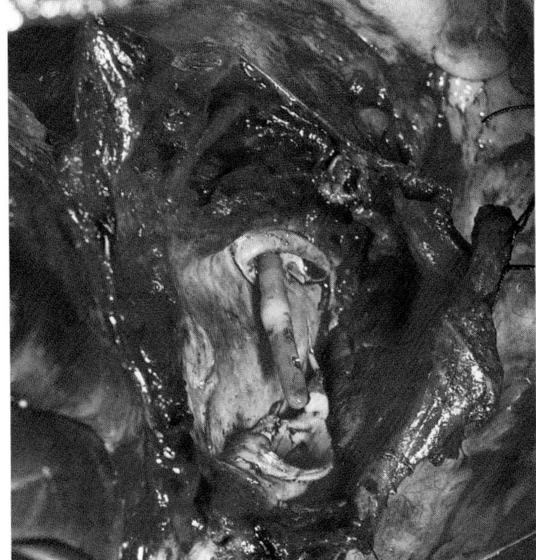

978c

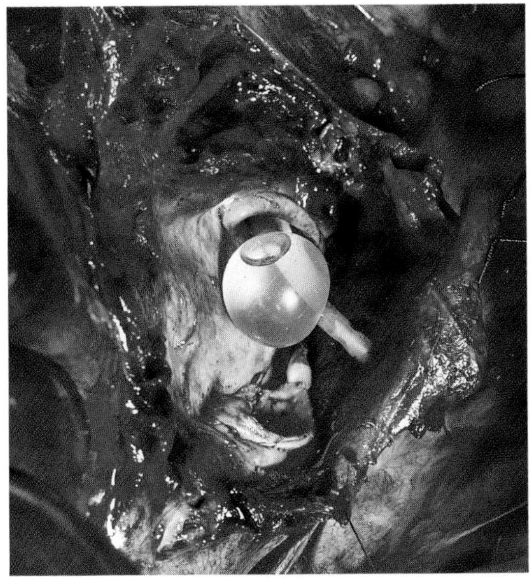

978d

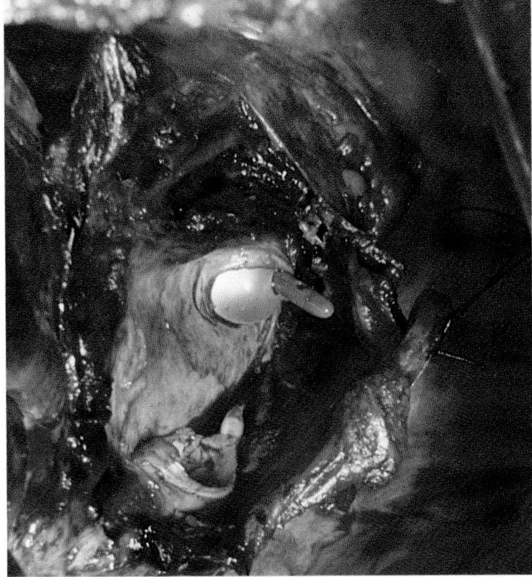

978e The aortic arch of the same patient seen through an anterior incision in its lesser curvature after excision of the ascending aorta. It will be noted that the haemostatic cuff obstructs the origin of neither the left carotid (B) nor the innominate artery (C); it is also sufficiently far from the rupture (A) not to interfere with repair.

978e

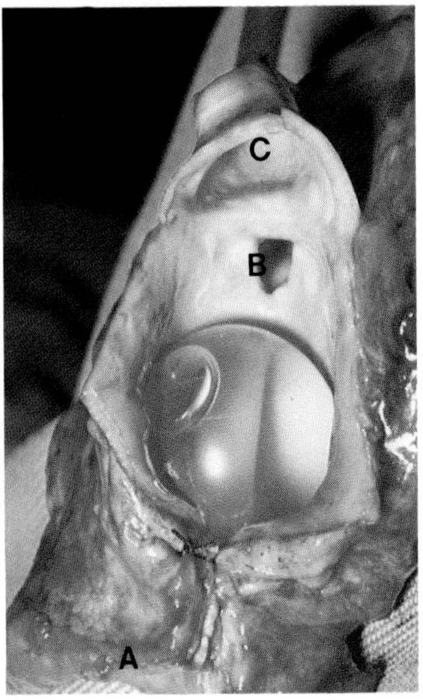

978d In practice, the cuff is inflated before it enters the pseudo-aneurysm; it is then withdrawn until it lies at the ostium of the left subclavian artery. With the aorta occluded, there is no risk of haemorrhage during repair. The cuff in this photograph is not yet in place; it will be withdrawn a further 3cm.

978f

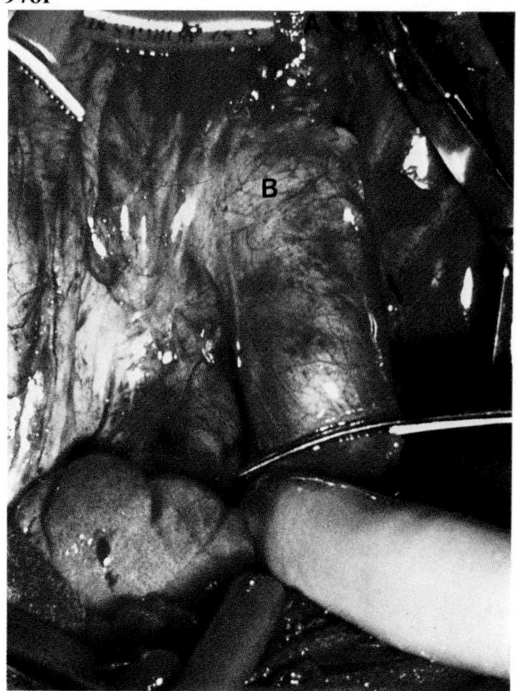

978f Haemostatic efficacy of Foley catheter in live dog. The catheter (A) has been introduced into the subclavian artery and the cuff inflated inside the aortic arch (B). The isthmus is then severed . . .

978g . . . 2cm (→) below the inflated cuff (B) to simulate traumatic rupture; there is no haemorrhage. The distal portion of the aorta (C) has been cannulated, but this is not strictly necessary.

978h The respective positions of the haemostatic cuff and the repaired aortic isthmus.

978g

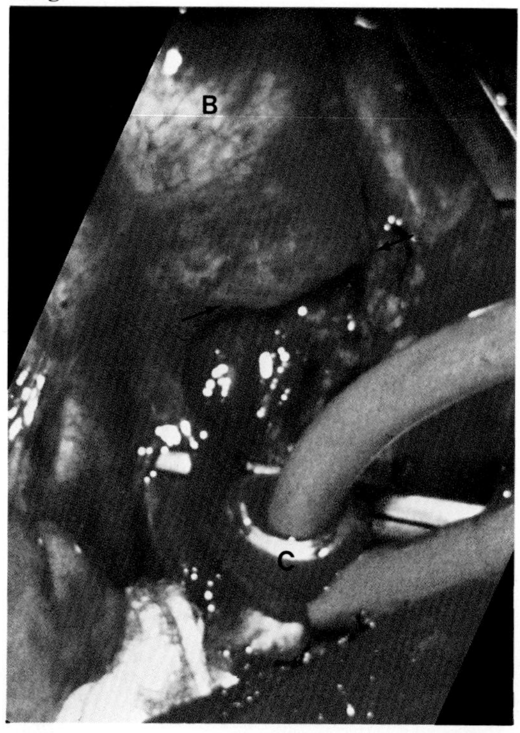

978h

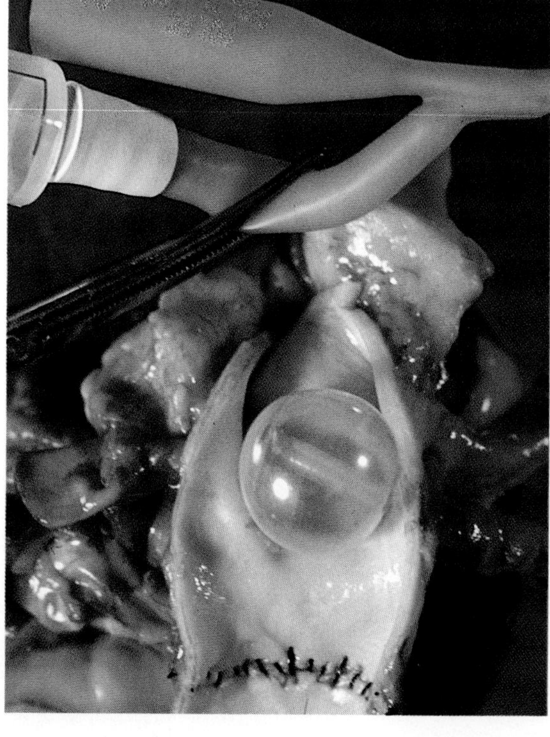

Accessory techniques

If prolonged, clamping of the aorta frequently results in paraplegia, anuria or acute cardiac failure. These difficulties can be obviated:

1. by rapid end-to-end suturing with direct clamping (see **977** A, A′, A″);
2. by the temporary insertion of a protective by-pass (see **979** B, B′, B″);
3. by placing the patient in extracorporeal circulation with or without an oxygenator (see **980** C, C′, C″).

The first of these three methods (direct suturing with simple clamping) is usually preferred. The use of an internal by-pass causes a delay and can lead to complications – clotting or embolism, for example. The third method (extracorporeal circulation with or without an oxgenator) is almost always contra-indicated because it requires heparin. Clearly, this would aggravate any haemorrhagic extrathoracic injuries (rupture of an abdominal viscus, fracture of the pelvis, etc.).

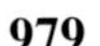

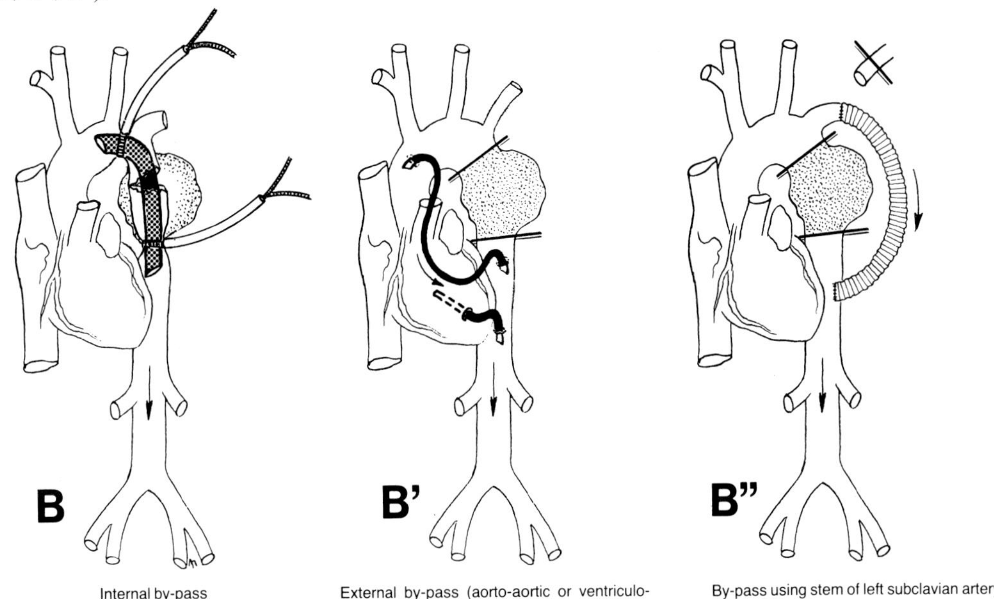

Internal by-pass

External by-pass (aorto-aortic or ventriculo-aortic)

By-pass using stem of left subclavian artery

979 The use of a protective **aortic by-pass** during repair is optional and may be risky.

980

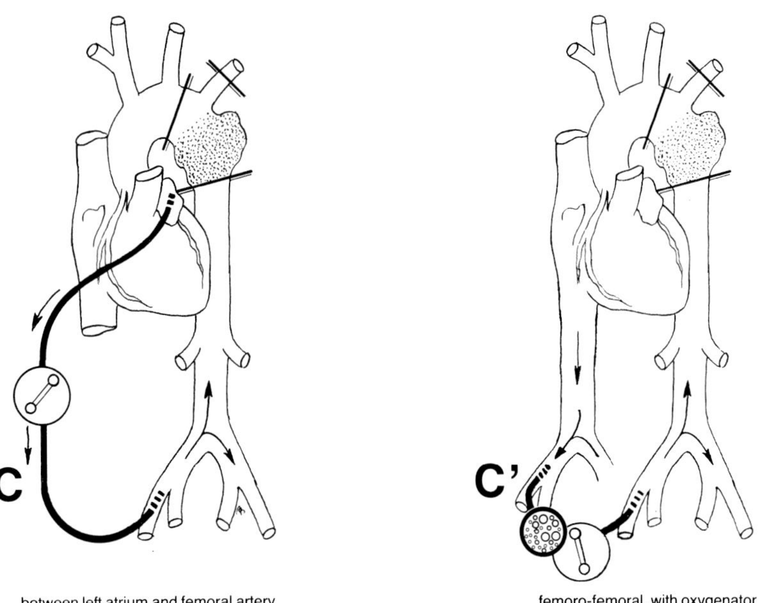

between left atrium and femoral artery

femoro-femoral, with oxygenator

980 Repair under protection of **extracorporeal circulation** (basically inadvisable because of the heparin required)

Procedures

Rupture of the aorta is so formidable an injury and so frequently accompanied by other severe injuries, that the current surgical success rate of 75% in certain large hospitals is quite remarkable.

In all instances and at any phase, surgery is indicated.

Any fresh rupture, whether with an acute or a chronic fast-growing pseudo-aneurysm, requires immediate repair. Successful repair was once quite outstandingly achieved in the emergency room when, despite cardiac arrest, a patient with an exsanguinating rupture was operated on without asepsis; a full recovery was achieved without complications or sequelae.

When the situation is precarious, an angiogram is a waste of time. In these circumstances, even if the suspected rupture does not exist, a left thoracotomy performed immediately can do little harm; if, on the other hand, it does exist, inaction simply invites a fatal outcome.

It is often a wise prophylactic step to introduce a Foley catheter into the aorta through the left subclavian artery (see **977**); this manoeuvre can be done as the chest is being opened. The thoracotomy should be through the fourth left intercostal space. Once haemostasis has been achieved, the extremities of the rupture should be examined and then sutured end-to-end or, if they have retracted, joined with a dacron graft. Repair is not difficult provided no by-pass is attempted; the occlusion time should be between 15 and 30 minutes. Various types of by-pass not only prolong clamping, but also seem to increase the incidence of anoxic complications in the spinal cord and kidneys. For both of these reasons, by-passes have been discarded by most surgeons.

With a **chronic, slow-growing pseudo-aneurysm**, planned intervention is possible. Direct end-to-end anastamosis or, more often, insertion of a dacron graft can be achieved with simple clamping or under the protection of a shunt; the aorta is usually not occluded for more than 20 to 40 minutes.

Repair of total rupture of aortic isthmus (through left thoracotomy)

981

1. The rupture seen after evacuation of the haemothorax (photographs taken at autopsy); (see **969**)

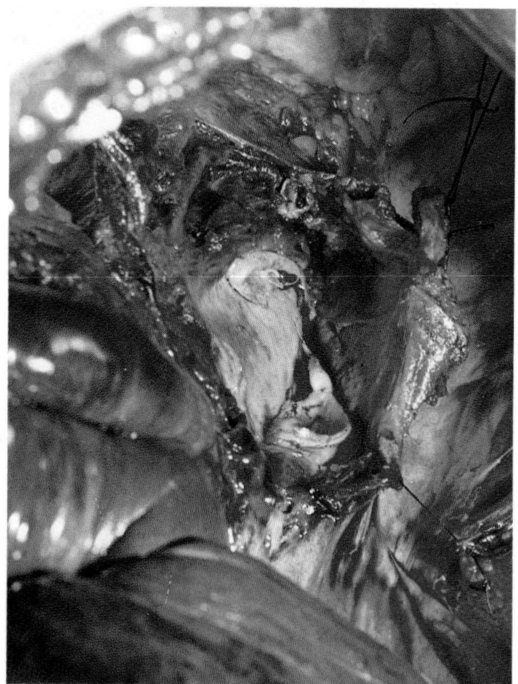

G.D. ♂ 36 yrs. 14 Feb. 1976

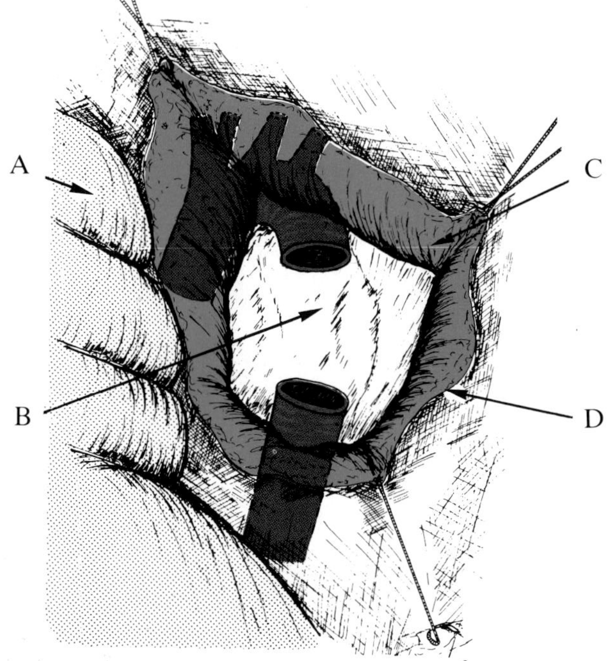

A. Left lung pushed aside

B. Complete rupture of the isthmus. The extremities have separated to leave a hiatus of 5 cm

C. Organised mediastinal haematoma, usually designated 'pseudo-aneurysm'

D. 15 cm tear in the mediastinal pleura

2. **Haemostasis** achieved with a Foley (12) catheter. The catheter is introduced through the left subclavian artery and kept under slight traction.

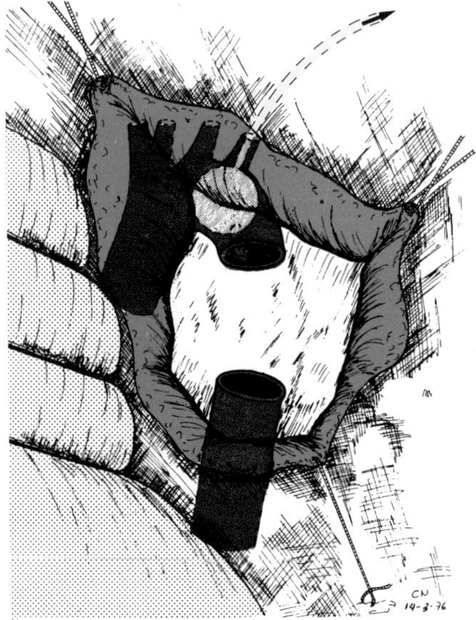

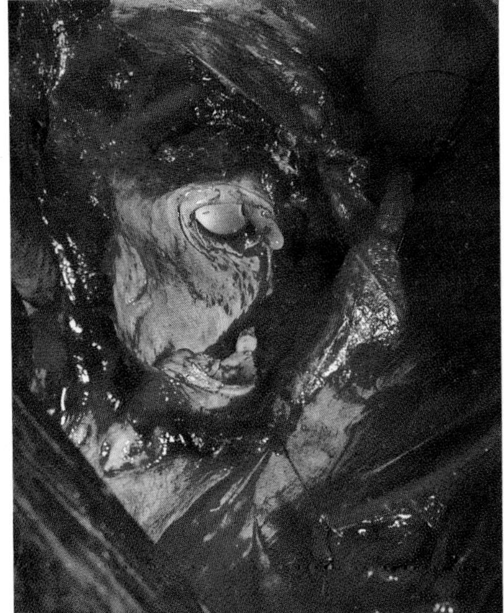

3. **Direct end-to-end anastomosis**.

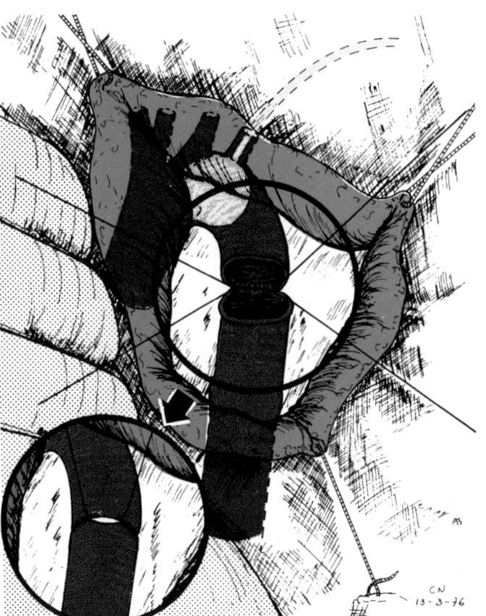

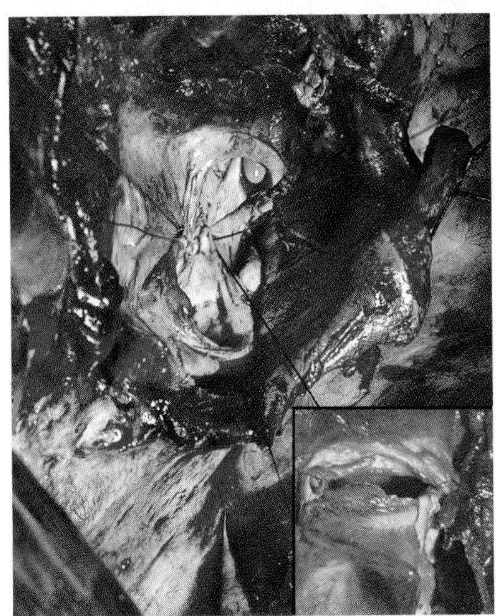

4. **Alternative**: interposition of a synthetic **graft** to prevent excessive traction on the sutures; a graft can be used also to replace an excised segment or to solve the problem of a friable aortic wall.

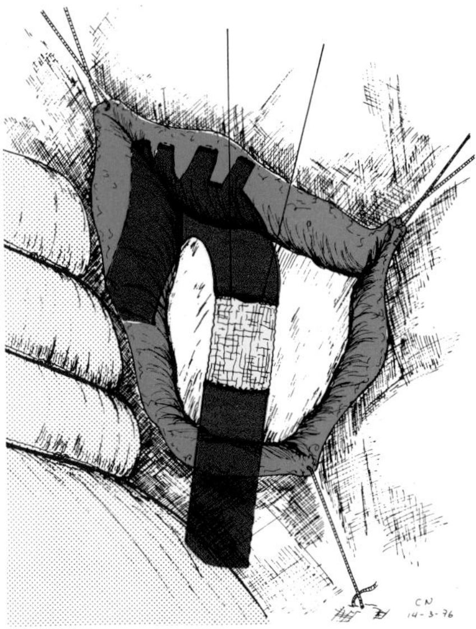

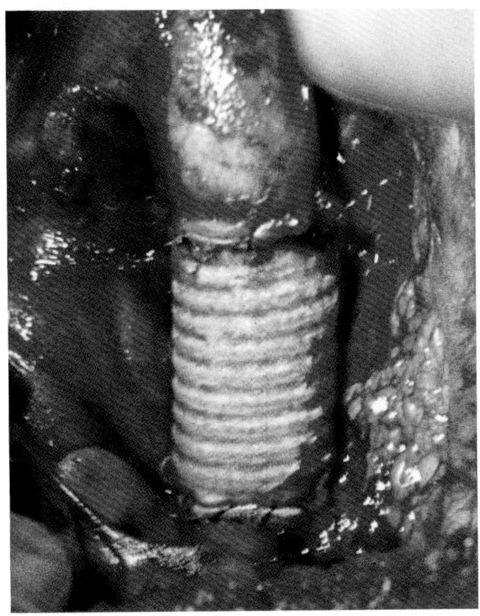

982

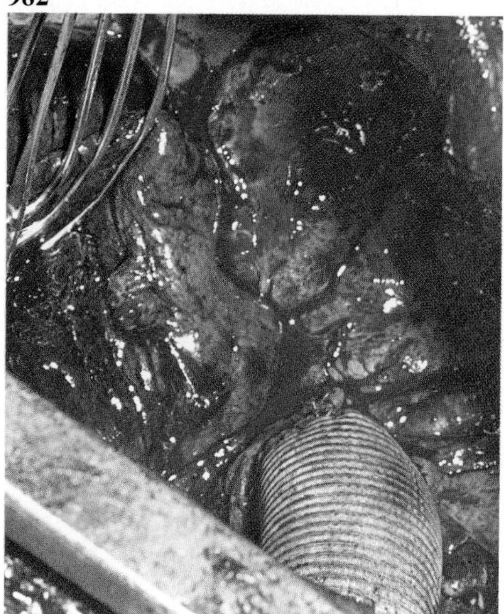

C.C. ♂ 58 yrs. 3 May 1976

982 Reconstruction of aorta with dacron graft after excision of a 9-year-old post-traumatic pseudo-aneurysm. Recovery. (See **971**.)

983a

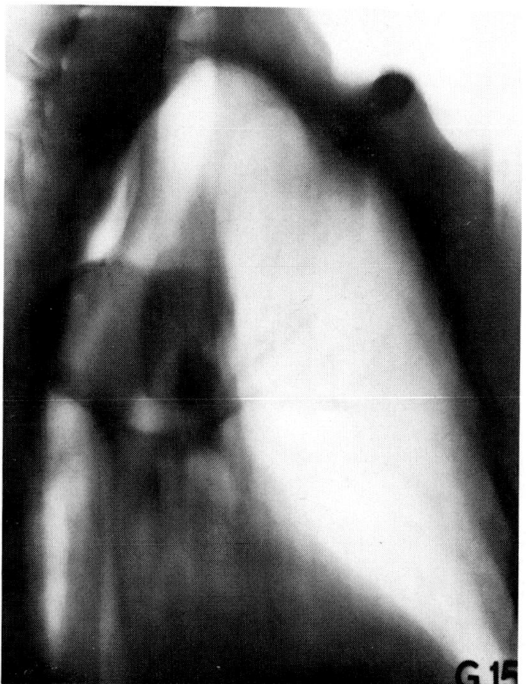

C.J. ♂ 38 yrs. 16 June 1959

983a Direct suture without excision of 11-year-old pseudo-aneurysm. The calcified pseudo-aneurysm extends posteriorly and to the left.

983b

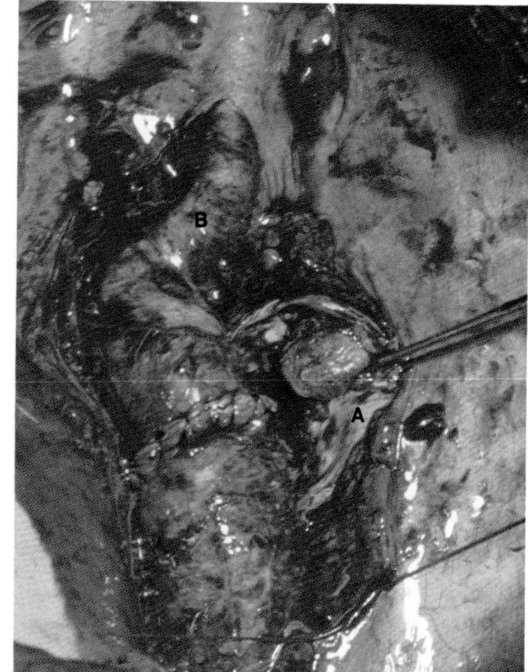

27 Nov. 1959

983b The rupture has been sutured directly. The wall of the pseudo-aneurysm (A) is held in forceps; an organised clot can be seen. The dissection of the subclavian artery (B) underlines the close relationship between this injury and isthmic rupture.

Complications

984a H.E. ♂ 32 yrs. 27 May 1967

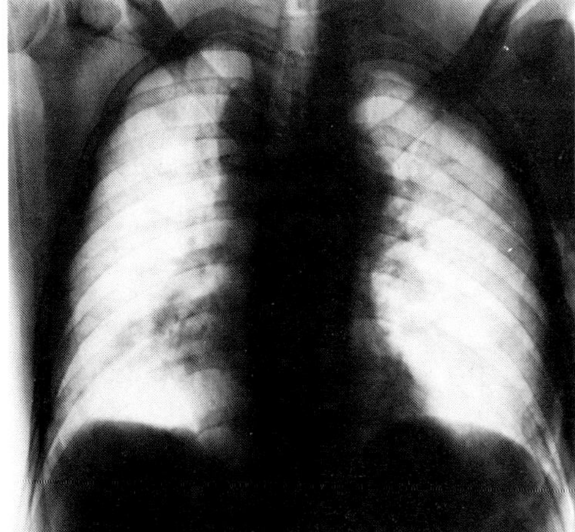

984a Successful surgical repair of an aortic rupture is usually followed by a **prompt recovery free of complications or sequelae**. This X-ray was obtained half an hour after the subject was involved in a 100km/h motorcycle accident. There is no haemothorax, but there is an apical cap sign and the mediastinum is clearly widened. Aortic repair. Recovery.

984b

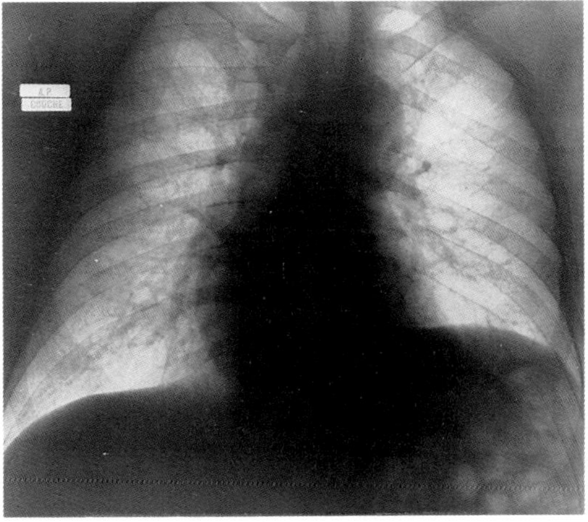

1975

984b Eight years later. The rupture of the aorta has produced no sequelae, but the torn left phrenic nerve has resulted in a paralysed hemidiaphragm.

985a

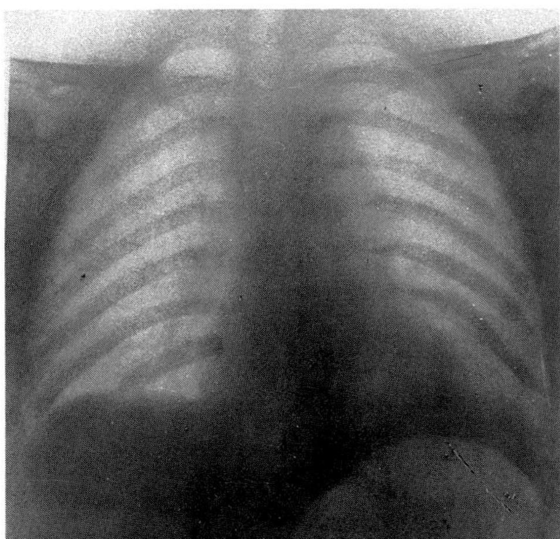

F.J. ♂ 19 yrs. 16 Oct. 1965

985a **Cerebral sequelae** after emergency repair of an aortic rupture. The widening of the mediastinum . . .

985b . . . increases by the hour. Angiography; left thoracotomy. The rupture is found to be total, and the proximal stump of the aorta shattered. Direct repair.

985c Four days after the operation, the mediastinum has returned to normal dimensions. Persistent psychoorganic disturbances are due perhaps in part to cerebral contusion, but probably have been aggravated by the shock and the clamping of the aorta.

985b

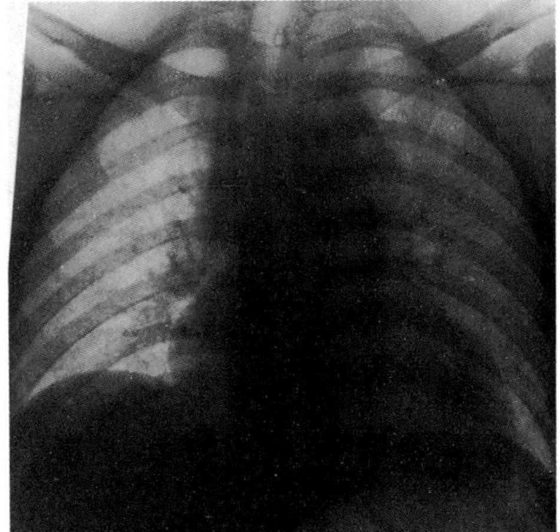

16 Oct. 1965

985c

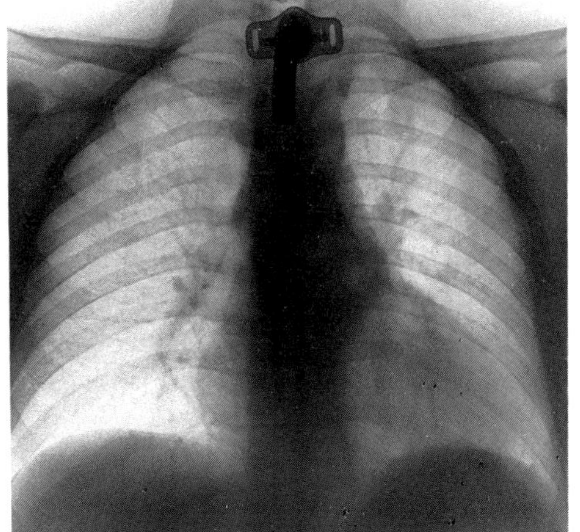

20 Oct. 1965

986a

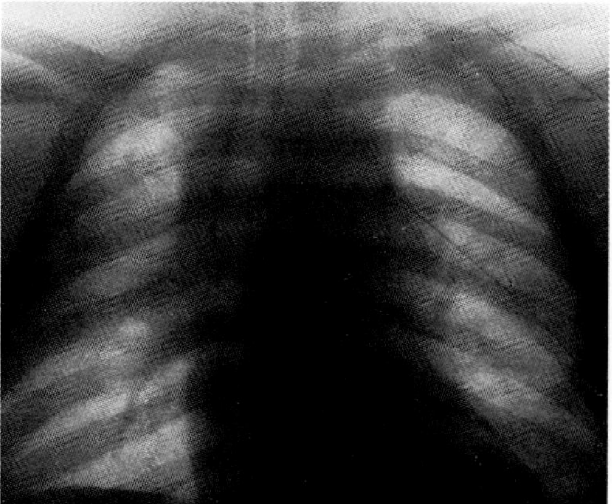

B.J. ♂ 23 yrs. 6 Feb. 1971

986b

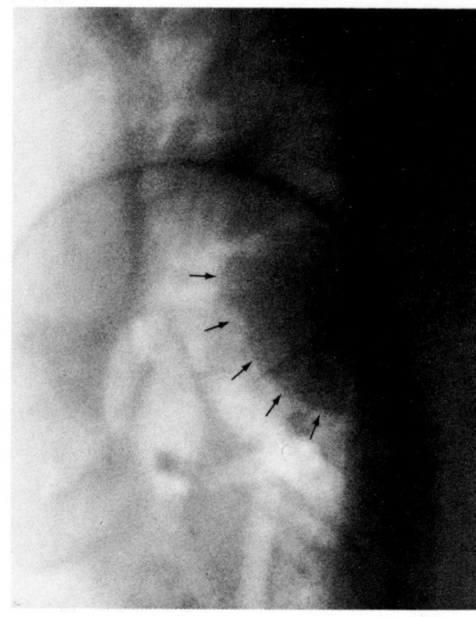

6 Feb. 1971

986c

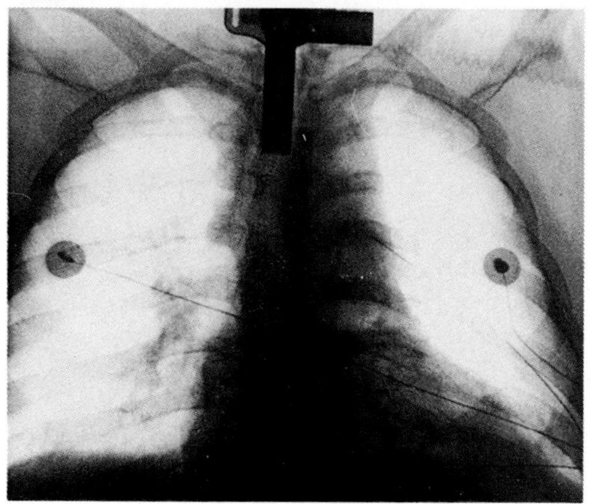

10 Feb. 1971

986a Postoperative paraplegia and anuria after repair of the aorta. The admission X-ray shows a widened mediastinum.

986b An angiogram reveals a classic rupture of the aortic isthmus (→). Left thoracotomy; end-to-end aortic anastomosis under extracorporeal circulation.

986c Four days later, the patient is paraplegic and anuric. Death despite a 'successful' operation.

In centres where the injury is routinely sought, the **hospital mortality** of aortic rupture has been reduced to 25%, despite frequently severe and extensive associated injuries. Considering the strength of the aortic wall and the relative youth of the majority of patients (their average age is 38 years), a survival rate of 75% is not altogether surprising.

However, in many hospitals regularly receiving road accident casualties, mortality among patients with aortic rupture is much higher. In our own department, we estimate that about half of all patients are beyond help on arrival.

So, taking into account all types of hospital, it seems likely that overall mortality is considerably higher than 25%.

987 **Hospital** deaths from aortic rupture (in our material, $n = 41$)
Overall hospital mortality of aortic rupture is 69%.

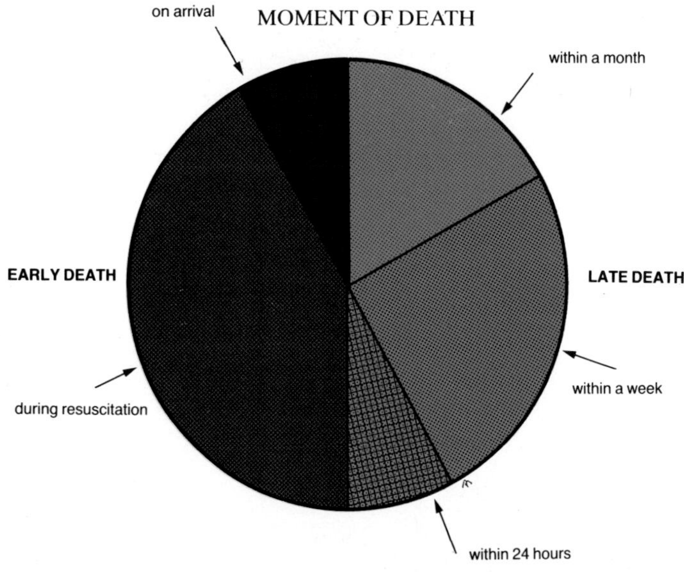

Deaths due specifically to aortic rupture amount to **54%**; the remaining 15% die from accompanying injuries or from some other cause.

Other types of aortic trauma

Most ruptures to the aorta involve the isthmus or the ascending aorta. Exceptionally, a complicated mechanism ruptures the aortic arch and sometimes also tears a major supra-aortic vessel or cardiac valve.

Injuries of this type occur when traction on the major vessels coincides with a direct blow to the chest. They are nearly always irretrievable.

Cases of isolated aortic valve rupture have been described occasionally. Heart failure is rapid but sometimes surgery has been successful (see **887, 888**).

Dissection or transection of the aorta at the level of or below the diaphragm is also very rare, and poses difficult diagnostic problems.

Finally, damage can be of iatrogenic origin; clearly, each such case is different.

However atypical the injury, surgical repair should be attempted whenever possible.

988

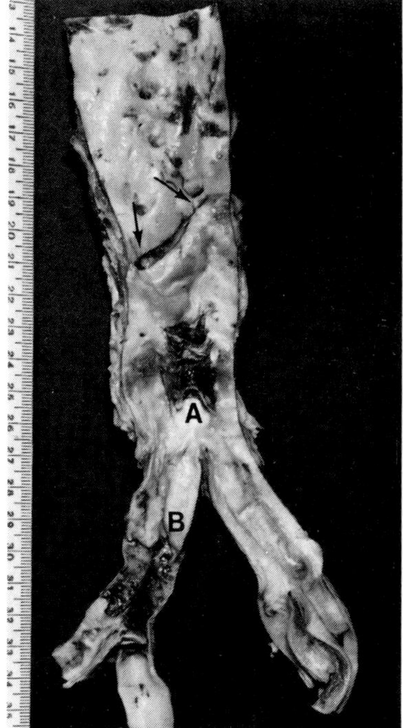

L.F. ♀ 72 yrs. 24 Aug. 1961

988 Isolated rupture of abdominal aorta, probably due to a direct blow to the abdomen, in a patient who died a week after throwing herself out of a window. The intimal and medial layers (→) were completely sectioned 1 cm below the renal arteries. Part of the resultant thrombus slid into the right common iliac artery (B), but its bulk stopped at the bifurcation (A). A number of thrombi were removed by peripheral disobstruction, but clotting recurred. The rupture and saddle-embolus were only discovered at autopsy.

989a

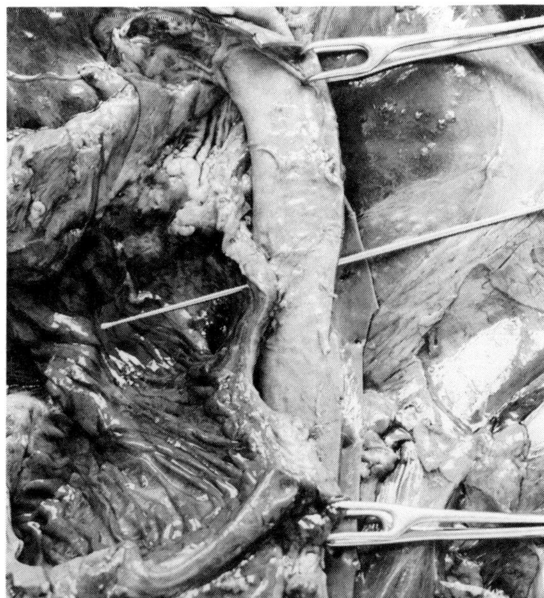

989b

K.C. ♂ 58 yrs. 7 Mar. 1959

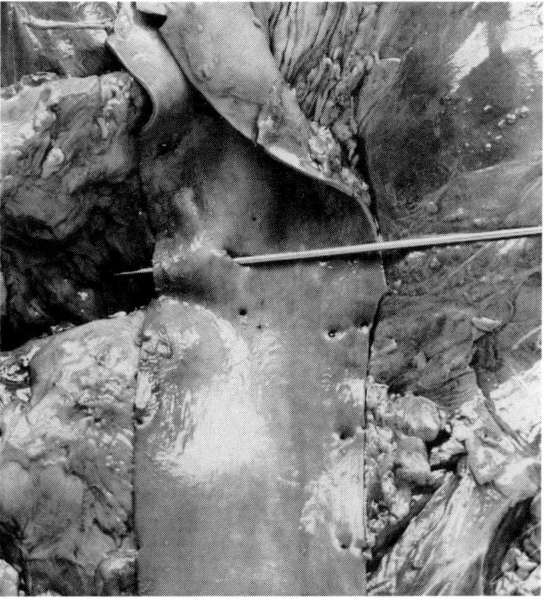

7 Mar. 1959

989a Iatrogenic oesophago-aortic fistula. A total gastrectomy for cancer was followed by an oesophago-jejunostomy. The patient died several weeks later from massive haematemasis and melaena.

989b Autopsy revealed that the perforation of the aorta into the oesophagel lumen occurred just above the anastomosis (blunt probe). Though the injury was known to be of iatrogenic origin, its precise mechanism could not be established (perforation due to a suture?). (Institute of Pathology, Lausanne.)

Injuries to the supra-aortic vessels

The following categories can be distinguished:
1. vascular contusion,
2. incomplete rupture,
3. complete, partial or total rupture and disinsertion,
4. gradual erosion from without (by a tracheostomy tube for instance). (See **750, 789-793, 996**.)

Injuries to the supra-aortic vessels are rare, amounting to only 1.8% of all severe thoracic injuries.

990 **Vascular damage by blunt trauma**.

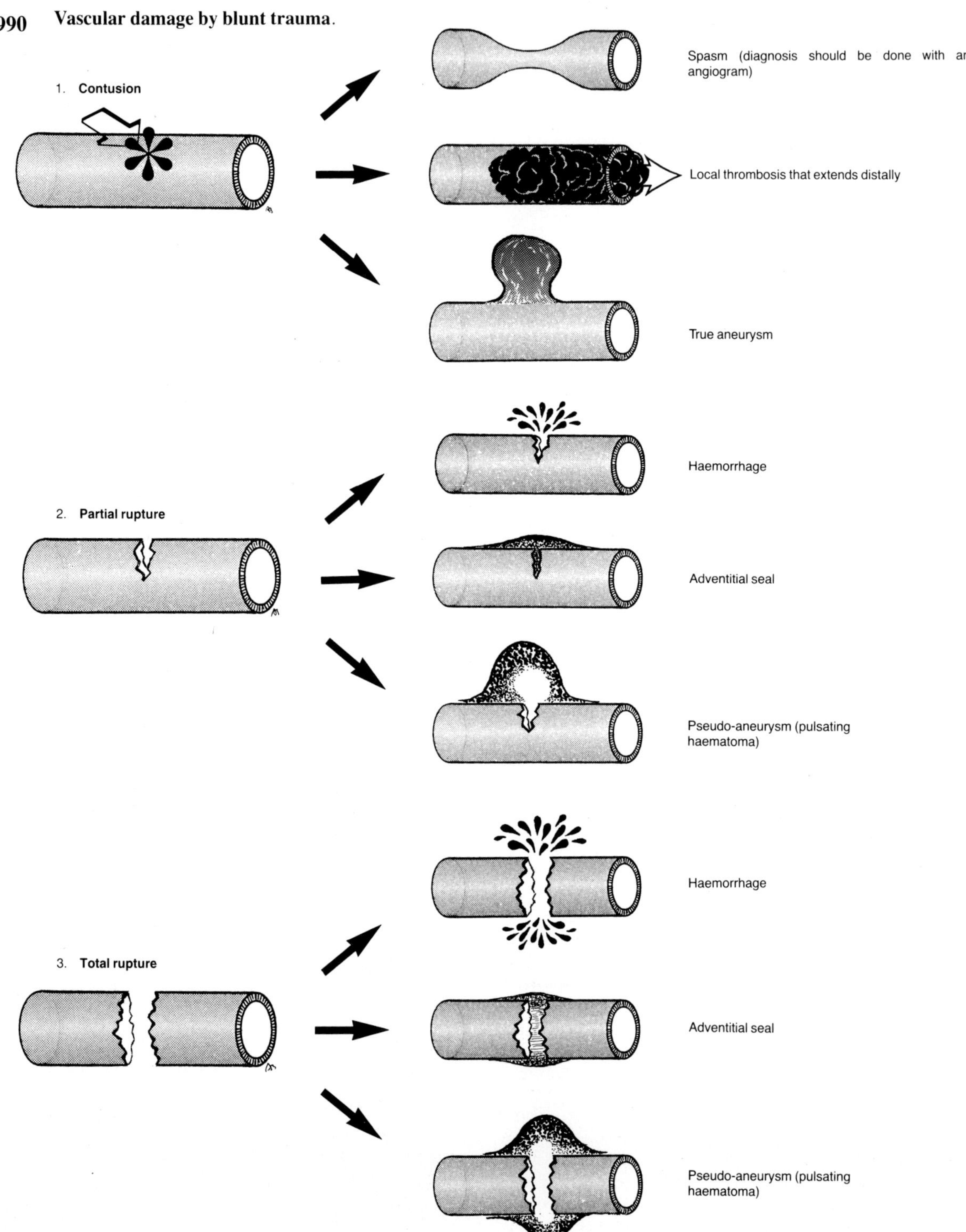

Injuries to the supra-aortic vessels can result in:
- severe **haemorrhage**, in the case of a rupture that opens into the pleural cavity,
- distal **ischaemia**,
- and possibly also a **vascular steal syndrome** (see **1001**).

Most injuries to the supra-aortic vessels are clearly symptomatic.

It ought to be relatively easy, therefore, to establish diagnosis and also to define the part played by associated injuries. However, theory being confounded by practice, late diagnosis is common.

991a

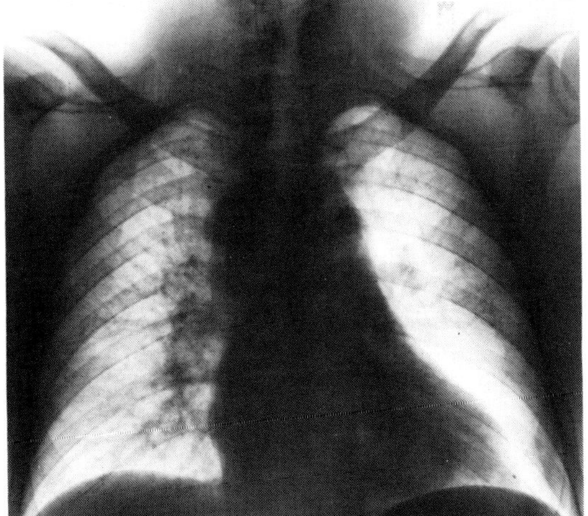

P.A. ♂ 31 yrs. 7 Aug. 1973

991a Unconfirmed suspicion of disinsertion of right subclavian artery. The upper mediastinum seems widened to the right . . .

991b

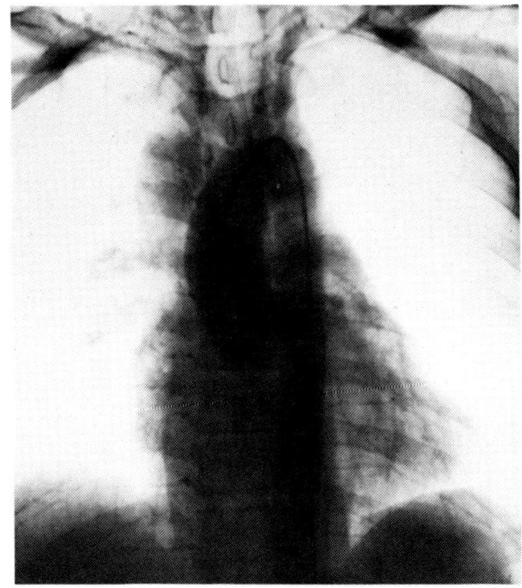

7 Aug. 1973

991b . . . but an emergency angiography confutes suspicion of a vascular injury.

992

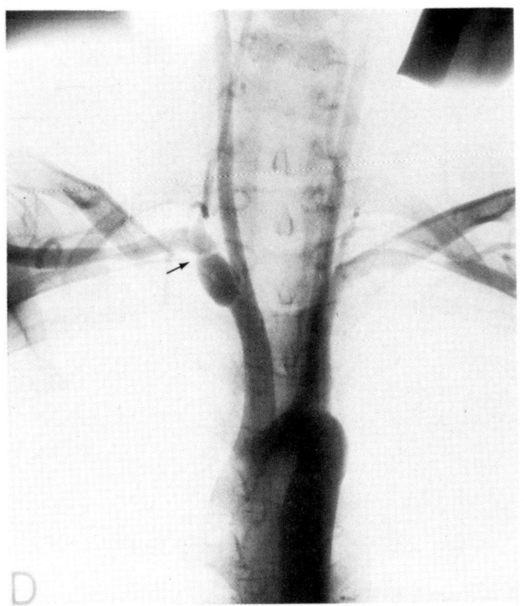

D.J.–C. ♂ 24 yrs. 8 Jan. 1965

992 Partial rupture of right subclavian artery (→) with chronic but stable pseudo-aneurysm after an impact against the steering wheel. The patient was treated conservatively because peripheral perfusion soon returned. Although his condition remained stable, surgery was indicated.

993

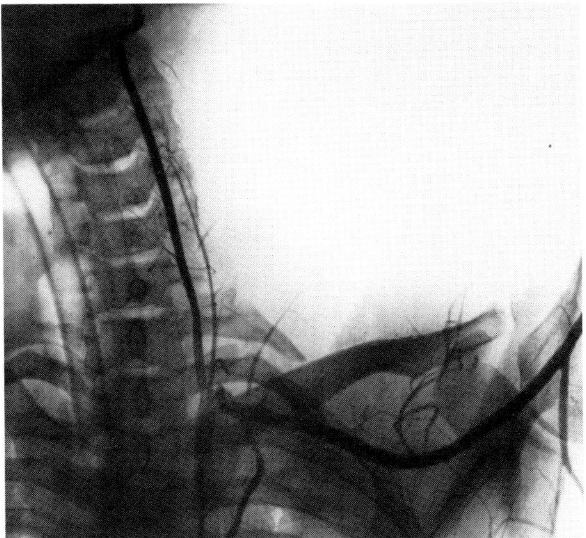

C.J.–C. ♂ 23 yrs. 23 June 1971

993 Partial tear of left subclavian artery at the level of the scalenus muscle, just after the origin of the vertebral artery (selective angiogram).
N.B. *The first rib is fractured* (see Volume I, **314**).

994a

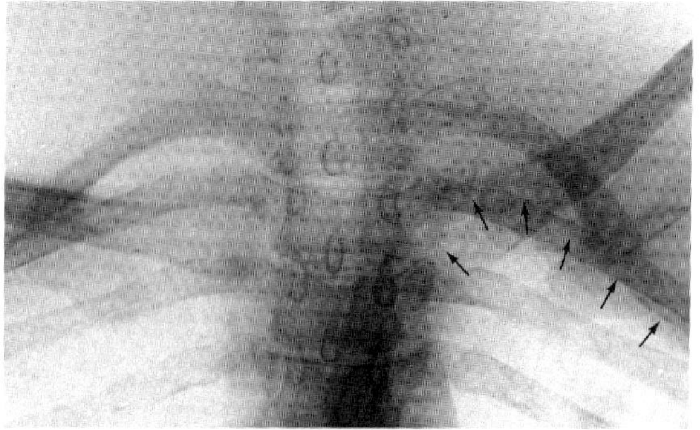

P.A. ♂ 20 yrs. 11 Sep. 1968

994a Total rupture of left subclavian artery with injuries to left brachial plexus and phrenic nerve. Motorcyclist who hit a tree at 100 km/h. The admission X-ray shows the extrapleural apical cap sign (→).

994b

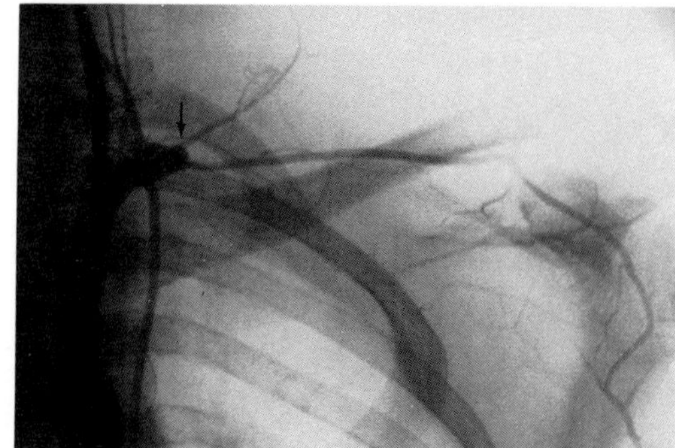

11 Sep. 1968

994b An angiogram reveals a rupture of the subclavian artery.

995a

B.M. ♂ 29 yrs. 20 May 1970

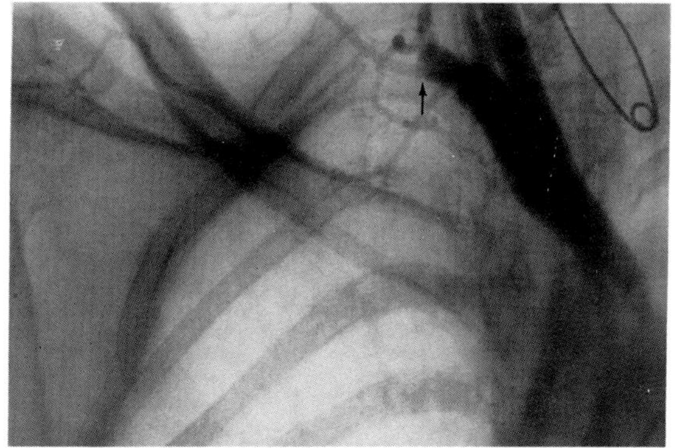

995a Initially undetected rupture of right subclavian artery (→). This angiogram was obtained 16 days after traumatic thrombosis of the right subclavian artery just beyond its bifurcation with the carotid. The patient's forearm is already gangrenous.

995b

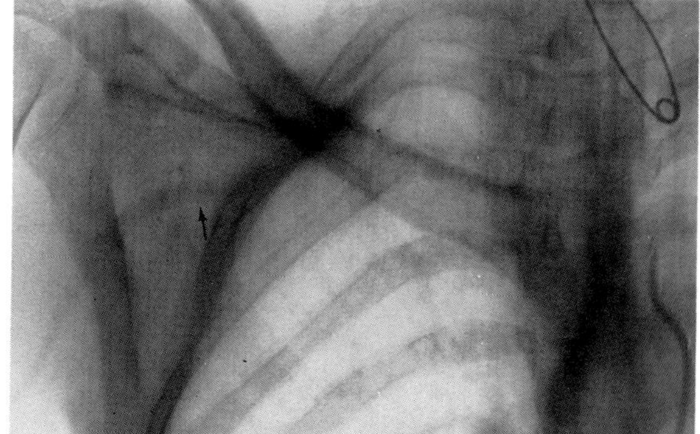

20 May 1970

995b After a delay, dye eventually impregnates the axillary artery through the collaterals.

995c

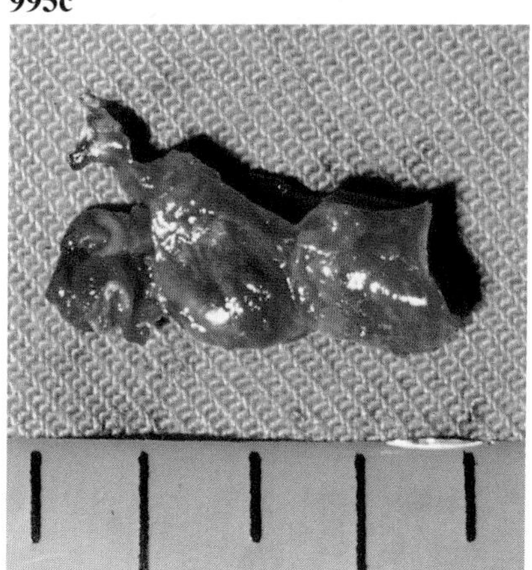

26 May 1970

995c The contused, thrombotic zone of the subclavian artery is resected . . .

995d

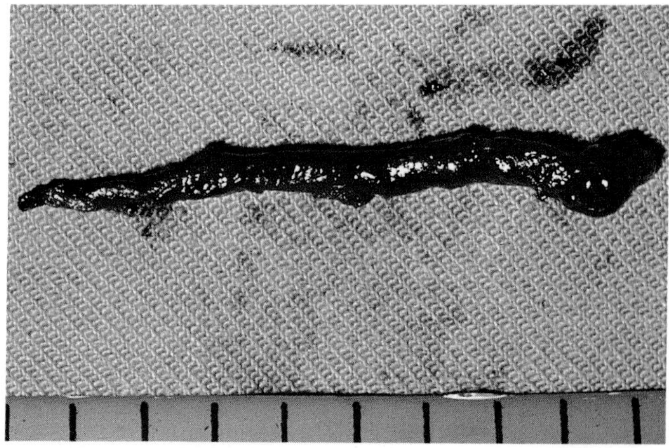

26 May 1970

995d . . . and the distal artery disobstructed. Intervention is too late to avoid amputation.

996

996 Erosion of innominate or right carotid artery by **tracheostomy tube** occurs either:

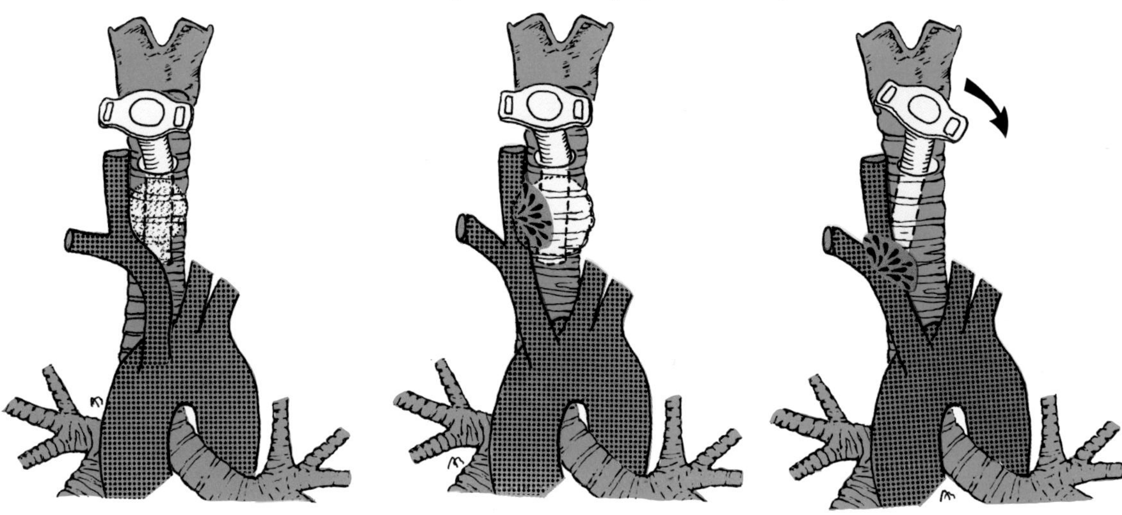

because the innominate artery takes an unusual course,

or because the cuff is over-inflated (see **788, 790, 997**)

or because the tube twists out of position (see **783**)

997

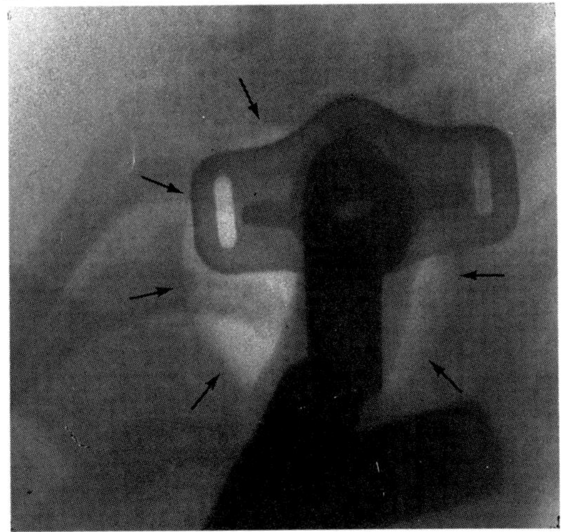

C.J.–J. ♂ 21 yrs. 17 Feb. 1972

997 Erosion of innominate artery by tracheostomy tube. The tetraplegic patient has been under controlled ventilation for 2 weeks. Extreme over-inflation of the cuff (→) of the tracheostomy tube has already caused tracheal necrosis. Some 14 weeks later, the innominate artery ruptures into the trachea, causing an instantly fatal haemorrhage.

998

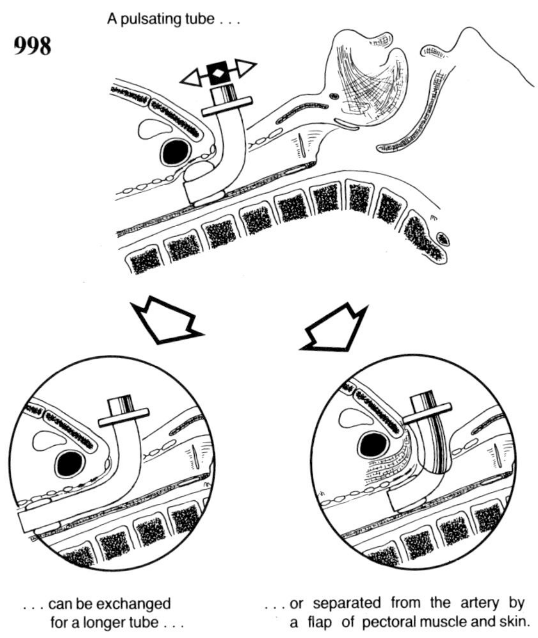

998 Prophylaxis of tracheo-arterial fistulisation by tracheostomy cannula.

Types of accident

Injuries to the supra-aortic vessels most commonly occur as a result of road accidents.

Type of accident	Incidence (n = 36)
Car accident	50%
Motorcycle accident	17%
Crush injury	11%
Fall from a height	5%
Others (e.g. erosion by a tracheostomy tube)	17%
Total	100%

Biomechanics

Vascular injury at the thoracic outlet is the result of compression by the scalene muscles combined with traction during violent movements of the head, neck, chest and arms. Injury usually consists of contusion with thrombosis.

An impact simultaneously contorting the chest and extending the cervical column is likely to avulse the major branches of the aorta. Complete disinsertion from the aortic arch has been reported, but it is generally the innominate artery or one of the subclavians that ruptures. If several supra-aortic vessels tear at the same time, the victim is unlikely to survive.

999

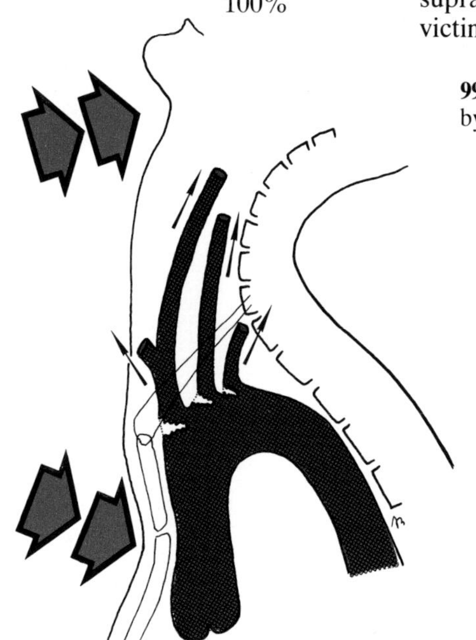

999 Avulsion of major supra-aortic vessels by extension of neck during deceleration.

N.B. These same tears can be produced by over-extension of the shoulder and arm. Such cases usually entail damage to the brachial plexus.

Localisation

1000

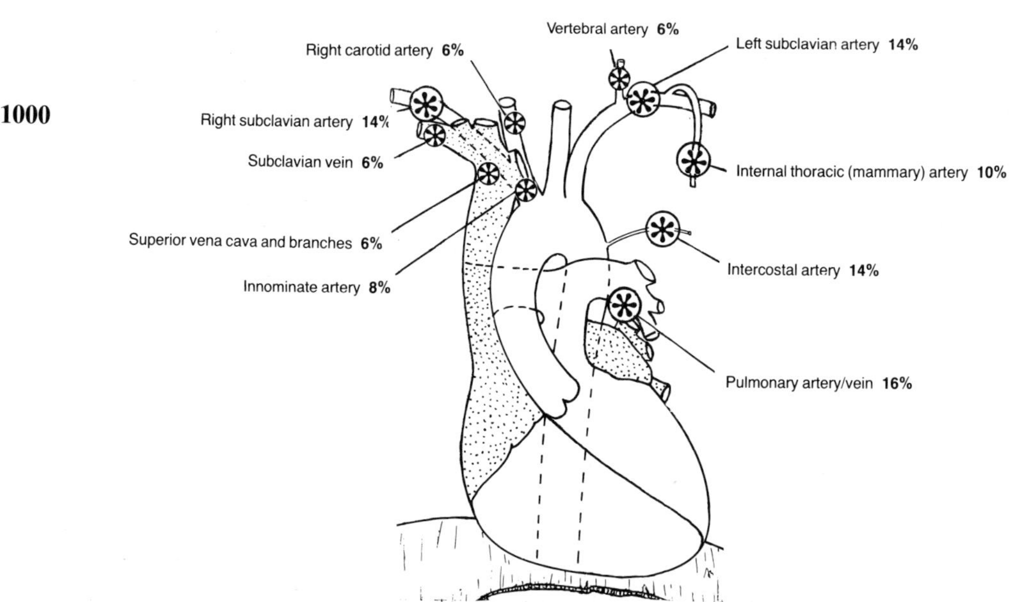

1000 Localisation of injuries to major thoracic vessels (excluding ruptures and wounds of the aorta). (n = 36)

Subclavian steal syndrome

Though rare, the **subclavian steal syndrome** after an injury is well defined clinically. When the proximal part of the subclavian artery is obstructed, its distal portion is vascularised through the carotid artery and Willis' circle, and through a reversed flow in the vertebral artery.

The symptoms of this condition are (1) cerebral or cerebellar ischaemia when the arm muscles are used and (2) ischaemia of the arm itself when the neck is extended, flexed or rotated sufficiently to occlude the vertebral artery.

The subclavian steal syndrome can arise from both open and blunt trauma: a *perforated subclavian artery* can become completely occluded (by acute thrombosis following contusion, by rupture-dislocation, by an intimal flap or by the retention of a bullet within the arterial lumen).

The symptoms of a subclavian steal syndrome following a *blunt trauma* are usually experienced remote from the site of injury. This makes diagnosis difficult.

1001

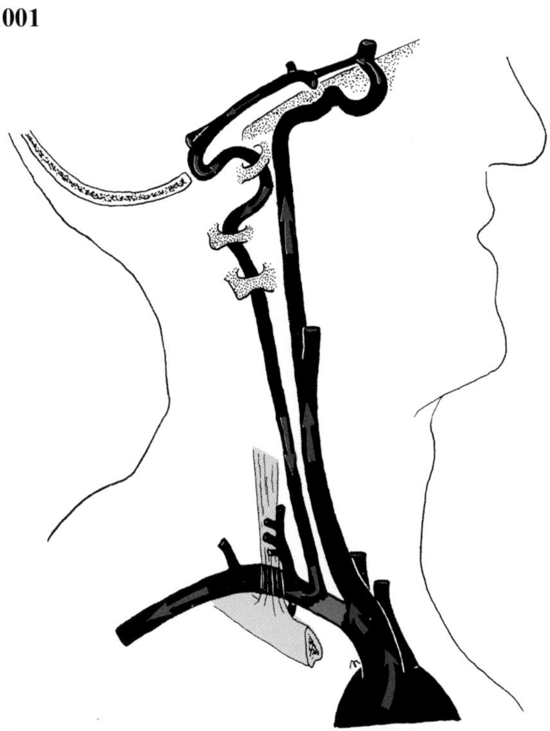

1001 Course of blood stream when proximal segment of **right** subclavian artery is obstructed. The likely result is a **subclavian steal syndrome**.

As long as it is not necessary to restore the normal anatomy, the subclavian steal syndrome can be managed surgically through a simple cervical or cervicomediastinal incision. These incisions have several advantages: (1) vascular repair is straightforward, (2) there is little risk of damage to the phrenic or recurrent laryngeal nerves and (3) later re-intervention in case of thrombosis or of a late pseudo-aneurysm is relatively easy.

1002

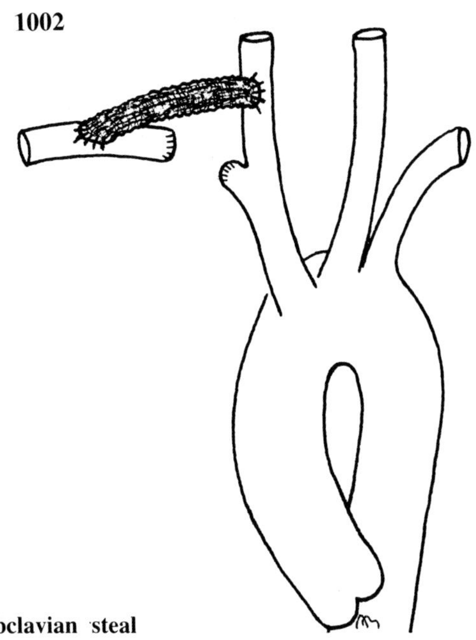

1002 Surgical repair of right subclavian steal syndrome. Interposition of a vascular graft.

1003a

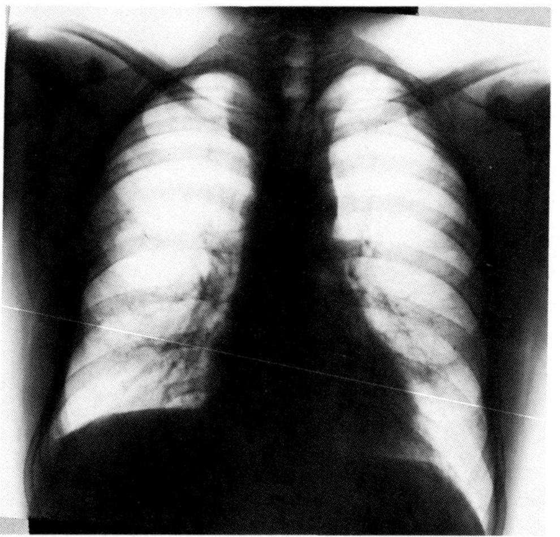

T.M. ♂ 27 yrs. 11 Nov. 1975

1003b

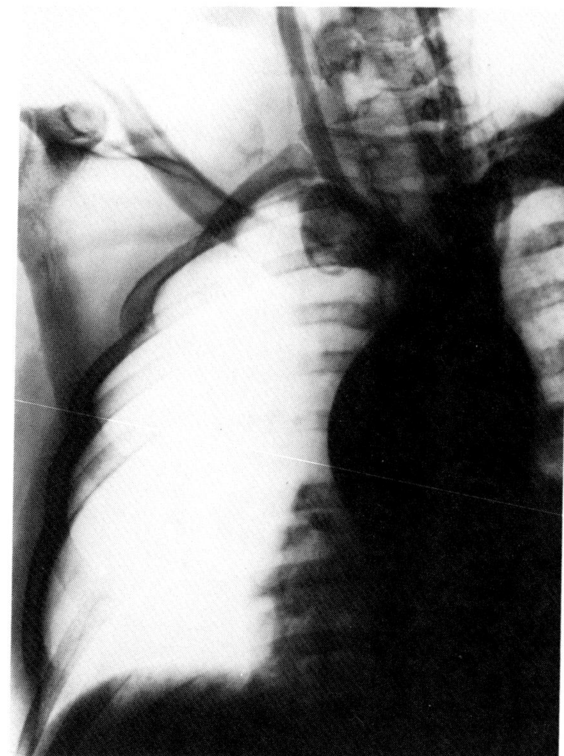

Nov. 1975

1003c

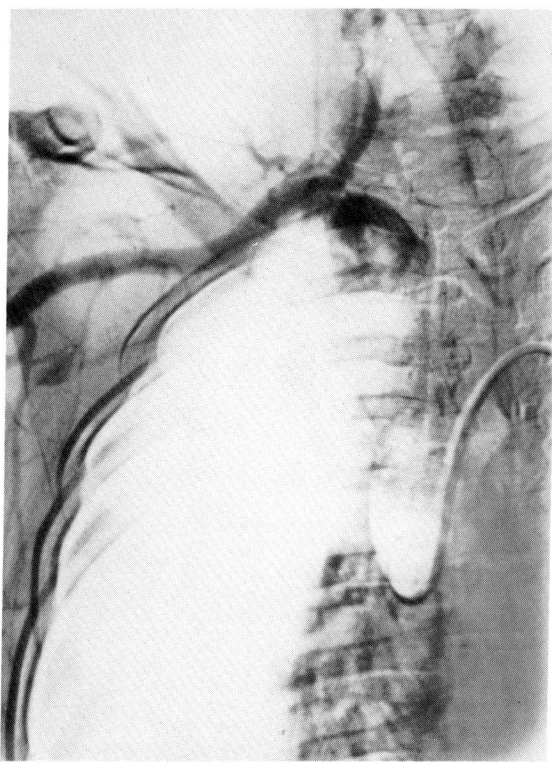

Nov. 1975

1003d

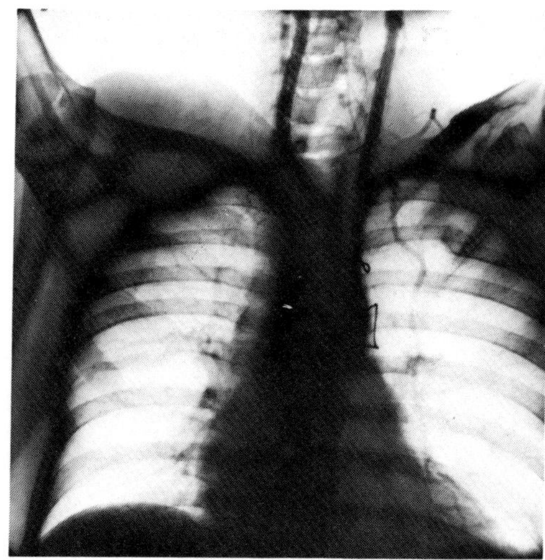

July 1978

1003a Pseudo-aneurysm and subclavian steal syndrome following rupture of right subclavian artery. The upper mediastinum is widened to the right, 5 months after an undiagnosed rupture of the right subclavian artery (see **826**).

1003b An angiogram shows an aneurysm at the origin of the right subclavian artery; the right carotid artery is soon impregnated.

1003c The rupture of the subclavian is complete, so the distal portion can only be vascularised by a reversed flow that enters the vertebral artery through Willis' circle. The patient typically experiences vertigo and lipothymia. The aneurysm is excised through a median sternotomy. The continuity of the subclavian artery is restored in situ by means of a vascular graft. (Prof. A.Senn, Berne.)

1003d The right recurrent nerve is paralysed but otherwise, recovery is complete.

1004

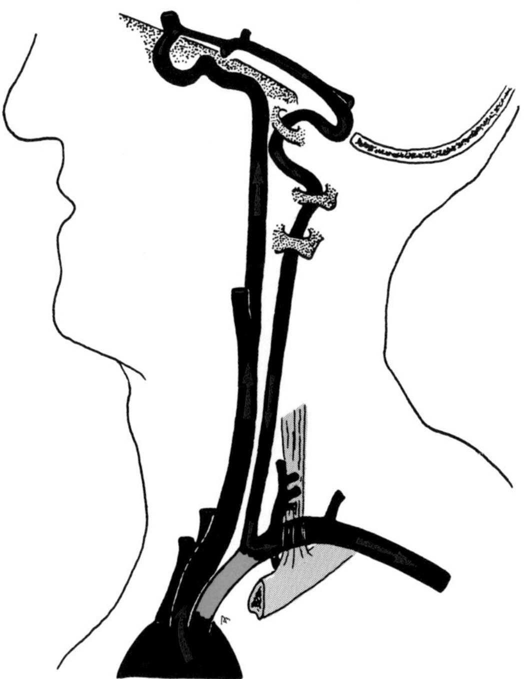

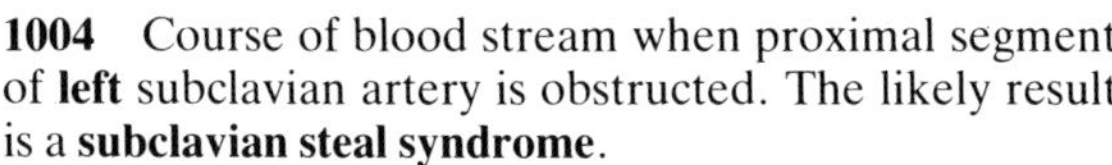

1004 Course of blood stream when proximal segment of **left** subclavian artery is obstructed. The likely result is a **subclavian steal syndrome**.

1005

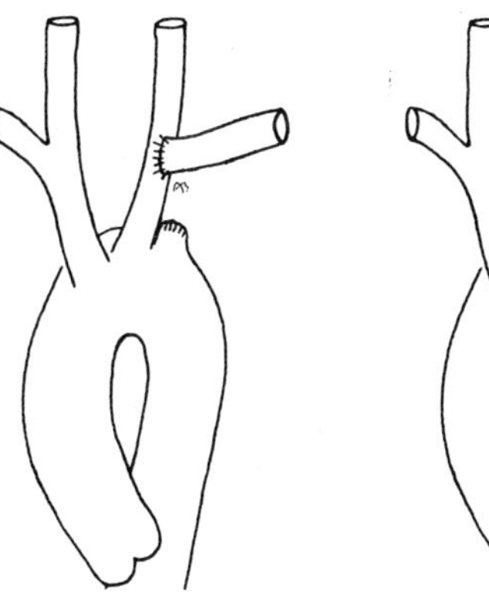

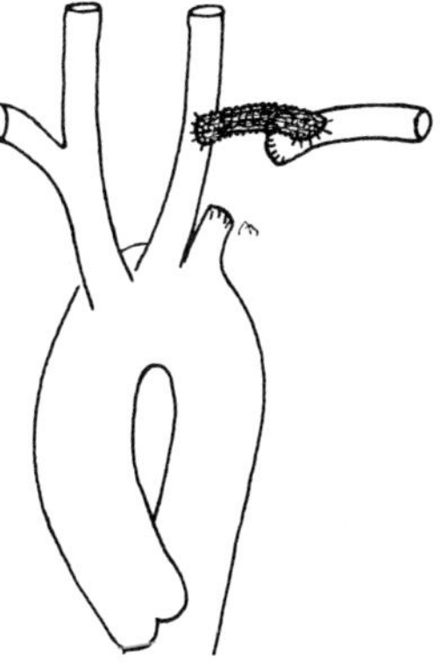

Proximal closure and distal reimplantation

Interposition of vascular graft

A protective carotid shunt is often necessary during the operation.

1005 Surgical repair of left subclavian steal syndrome.

Associated injuries

1006

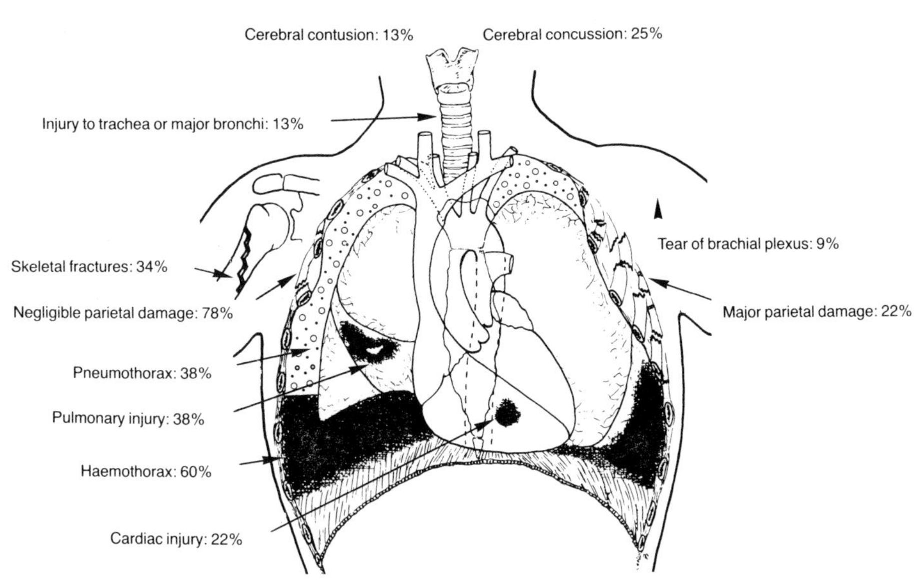

1006 Injuries associated with trauma of the great thoracic vessels (excluding aorta) (in our material)

Surgical management

Disinsertion of the major thoracic vessels from the aortic arch is difficult to diagnose and in most cases irretrievable. The approach is complex and repair intricate. A review of the literature gives a survival rate of 80%, but we feel that this figure is probably only based on favourable cases.

For the majority of more distal vascular injuries (extrathoracic injuries in particular), the post-operative prognosis is excellent.

In our cases, **mortality** of casualties with an injury to a supra-aortic vessel is **41%**; **death is directly due to the vascular damage** in **9%** of cases. The remaining 32% die from one or several associated injuries.

1007

1007 Surgical approaches for repair of major supra-aortic vessels.

1008 Rupture of **innominate artery repaired** under protection of temporary right carotid by-pass.

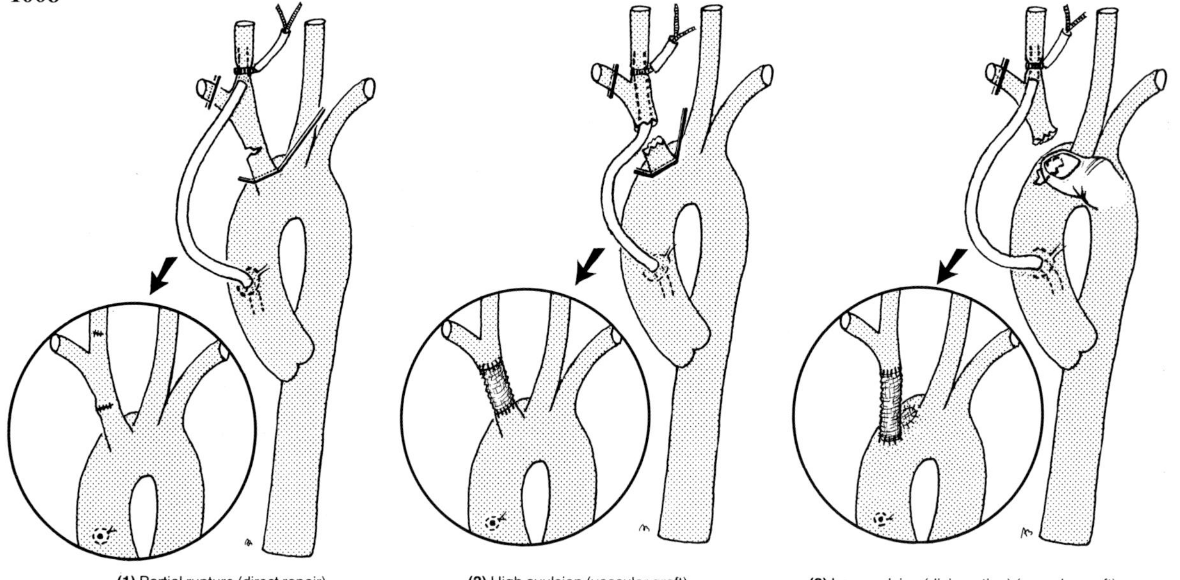

Open wounds of the thoracic vessels (see also Volume I, chapter 3)

In war-time, open wounds of the thoracic aorta and its major branches are rare. During the Vietnam war, for example, less than 1% of all arterial wounds involved the aorta or its intra-thoracic branches.

In peace-time, damage to major vessels is more common because most chest wounds are inflicted in murder or suicide attempts.

Low velocity bullets hitting a major vessel can remain trapped within the lumen rather than pass cleanly through. The result, as with projectiles that penetrate one of the cardiac cavities, is an embolus (see page 123) that lodges either in a branch of the pulmonary artery, or in a branch of the aorta (most often the left common iliac artery). Indeed, it is not unusual for a bullet penetrating the ascending aorta to be removed a few days later from the femoral artery.

Some wounds of the major vessels lead to arteriovenous fistulas with their characteristic symptoms and signs.

If the haemorrhage from a wound of a pulmonary artery is not massive, intercostal tube drainage is often sufficient. If uncontrollable bleeding indicates surgery, the damaged artery can be ligated without trouble. In the case of a venous injury, parenchymal excision is unavoidable since ligation would only cause infarction.

1009

1009 Wounds of major thoracic vessels.

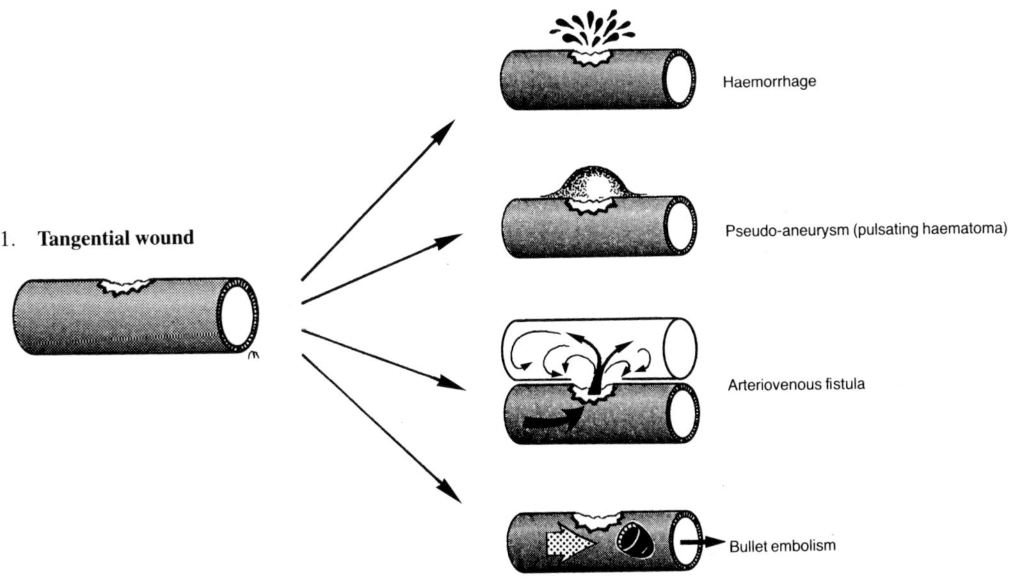

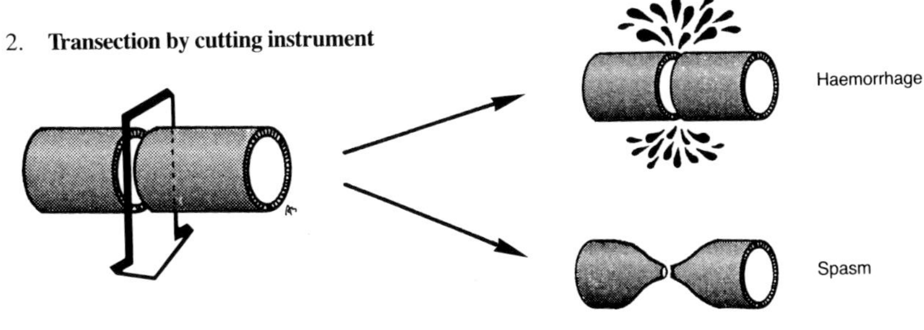

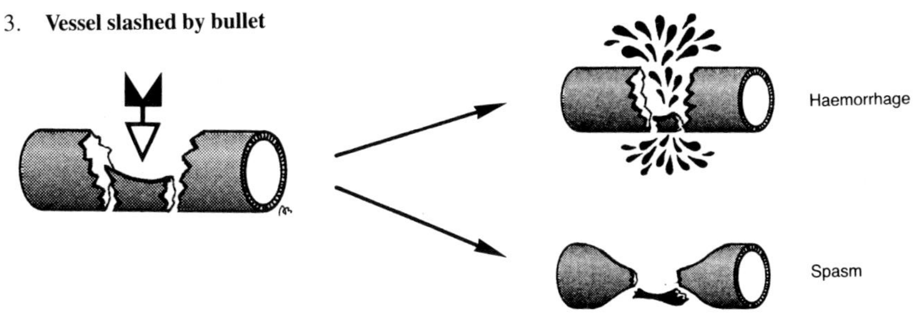

1010

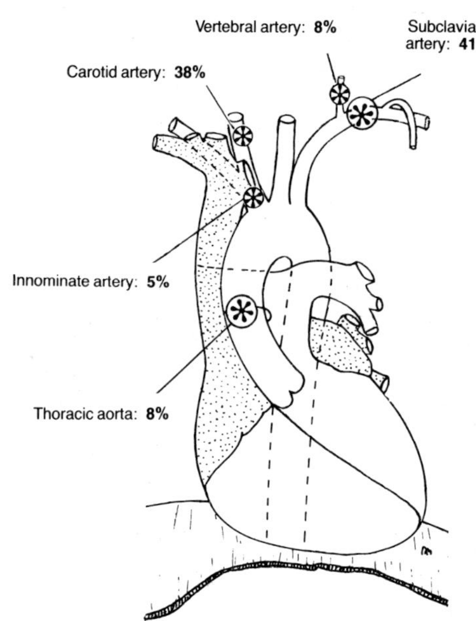

1010 Localisation of peace-time wounds of aorta and major supra-aorta vessels. (Literature review.)

The discrepancy between civilian and military statistics for open wounds to the thoracic vessels is due probably to the greater deliberation and accuracy of armed attacks during peace-time.

Early mortality is high: 90% of major vascular wounds are fatal within the hour – in other words, before most victims reach hospital.

Provided intervention is swift, there is about a 50% chance of successful repair.

In general, direct suturing under digital haemostasis is sufficient; otherwise a dacron patch or graft may be required sometimes. In some instances, it is prudent to support the sutures with a sliver of dacron felt.

The earlier treatment is effected, the better, particularly if haemorrhage is serious. External haemorrhage is an obvious surgical indication: temporary haemostasis can be achieved by manual pressure. In cases of haemorrhage into one of the pleural cavities, counteracting shock is the first priority; locating the wound and determining the approach should follow.

Their anatomical proximity makes the trachea, oesophagus and heart particularly prone to damage when the major thoracic vessels are wounded.

Associated injuries – whether cardiac, pulmonary or extrathoracic – have a great bearing on the prognosis.

1011

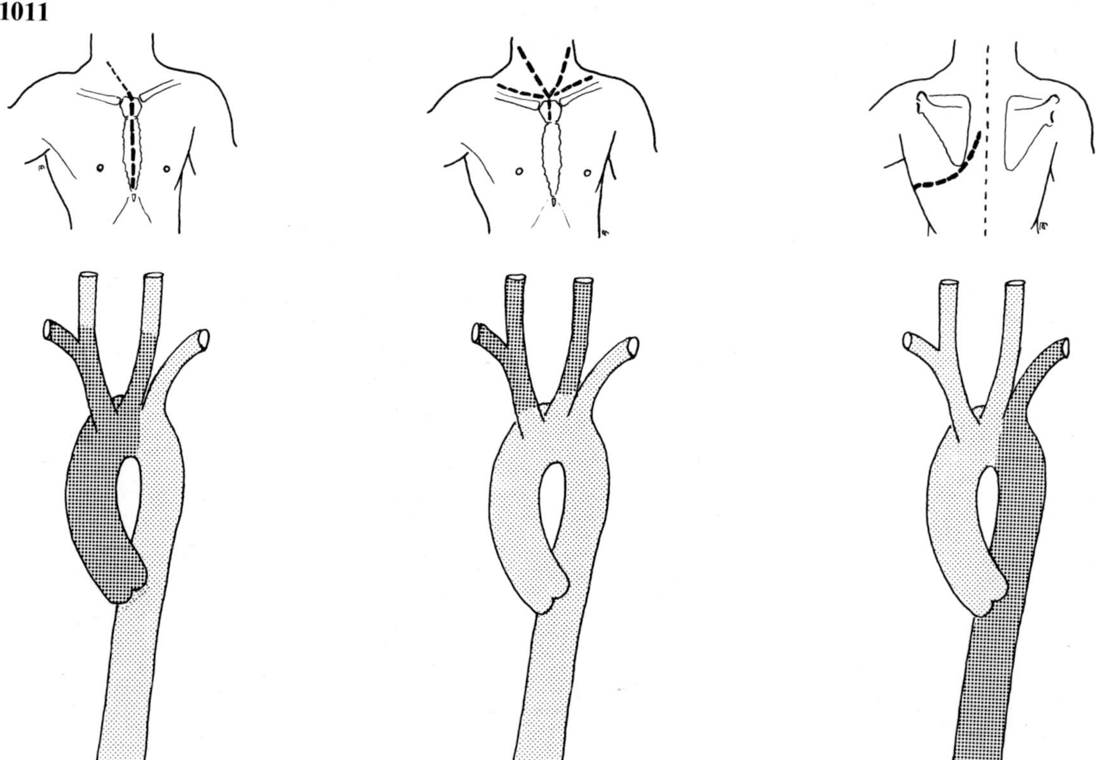

1011 Approaches for repair of wounds of aorta and major supra-aortic vessels

1012

An overall assessment should be made as soon as the most profusely bleeding wounds have been repaired. Particular attention should be paid to the adjacent cardiovascular structures:
- right ventricle and atrium,
- pulmonary artery,
- superior vena cava and left innominate vein,
- supra-aortic arteries.

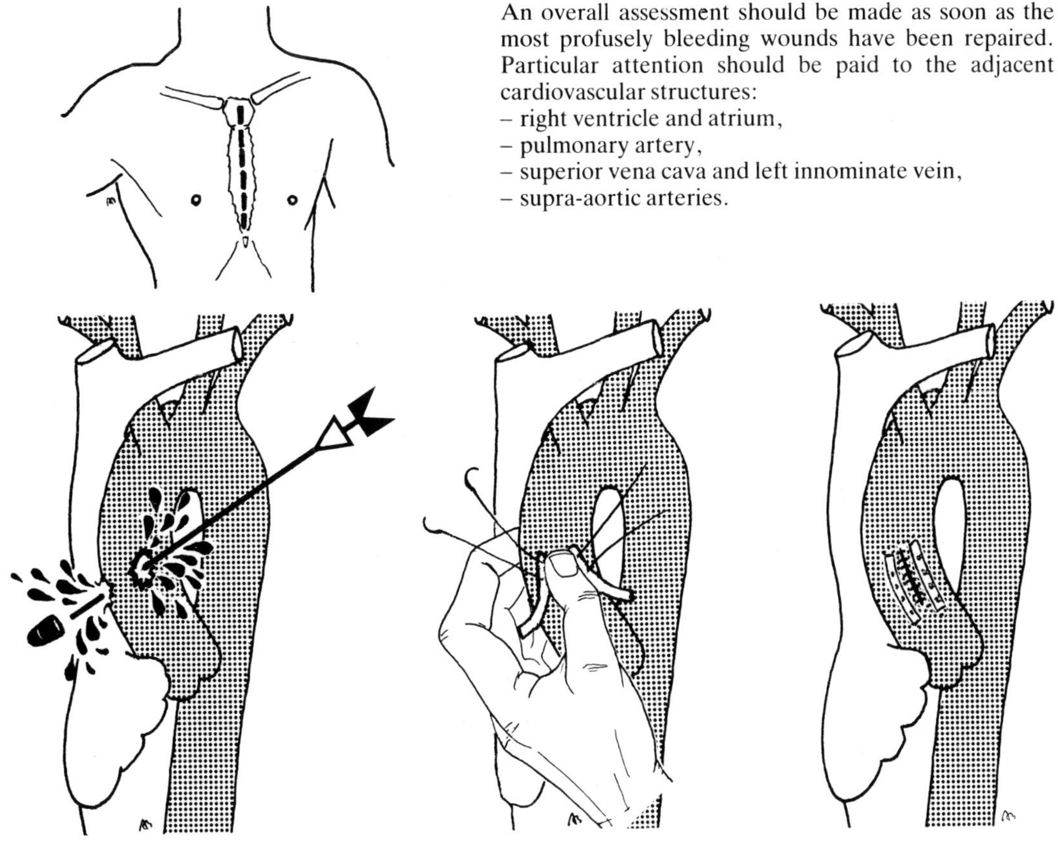

1012 Direct repair of **wound of mediastinal vessel** (the ascending aorta, for instance)

1013

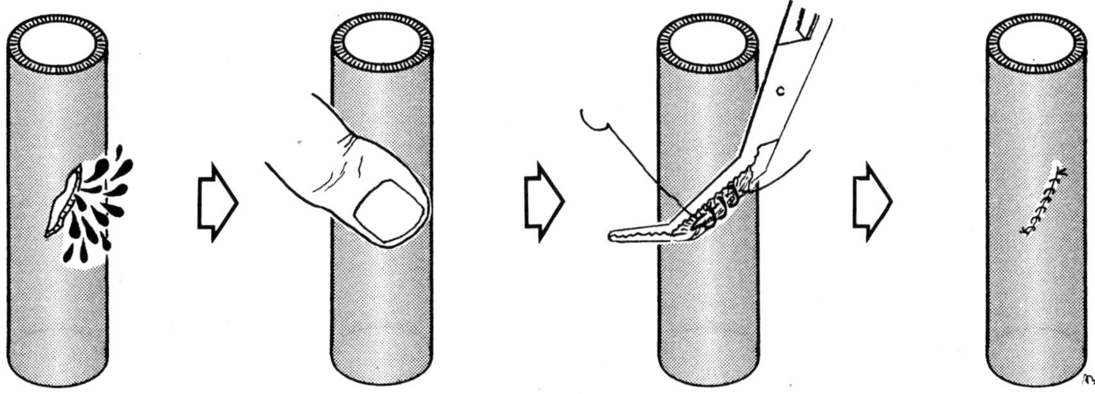

1013 Closure of **vascular wound**

1014

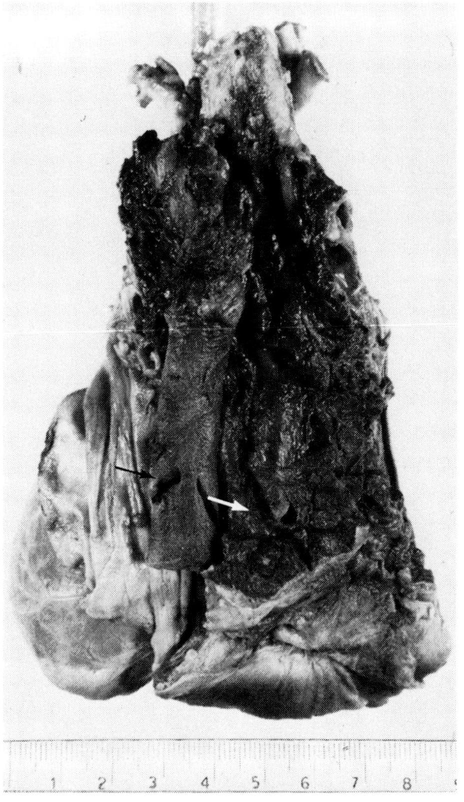

F.A.–S. ♀ 9 yrs. 18 April 1972

1014 Wound of descending aorta (←). The wound, inflicted by a bread knife, led to a haemomediastinum and a massive left haemothorax. The victim died within minutes. (See **893**).

1016

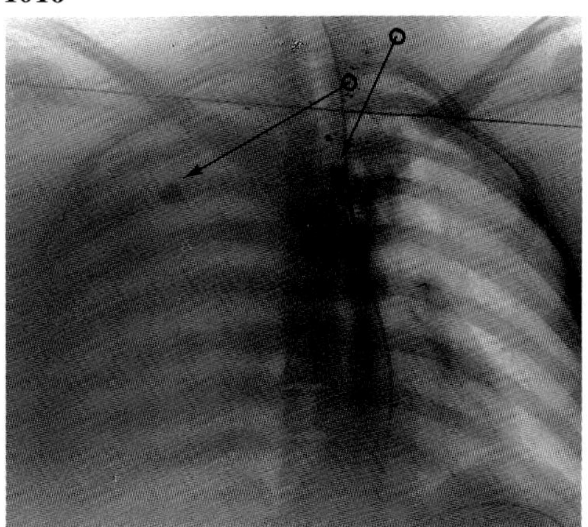

P.M. ♀ 32 yrs. 21 April 1976

1016 Gunshot wounds to innominate artery, trachea and oesophagus. Two low velocity lead bullets (both retained) entered the chest on a left-to-right, downward trajectory. The ruptured innominate artery has produced a 3000ml haemothorax. Survival, 1 hour. (See Volume I, **231, 247, 248.**)

1015

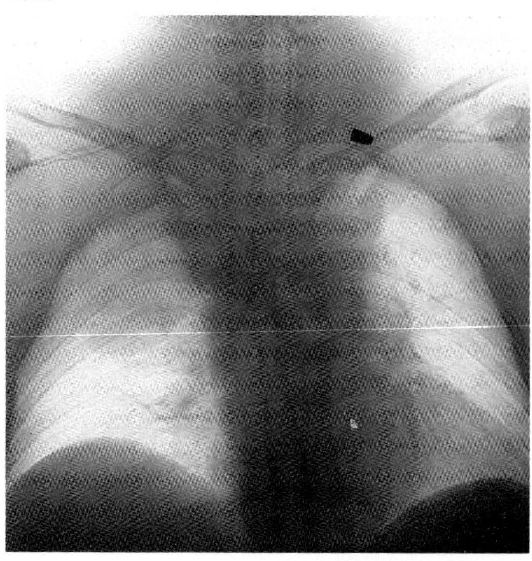

K.A. ♂ 54 yrs. 17 May 1970

1015 Gunshot wound to right carotid artery and jugular vein. The bullet is lodged in the left pleural apex. A bilateral apical extrapleural cap sign is particularly visible on the right. (See **1261** and Volume I, **256**.)

Iatrogenic arterial wounds usually consist of accidental puncture during the insertion of a central venous line. Unless there has been a serious technical error, the wound is rarely significant.

1017

1017 Complications arising from **puncture** (at thoracic outlet) of supra-aortic arteries

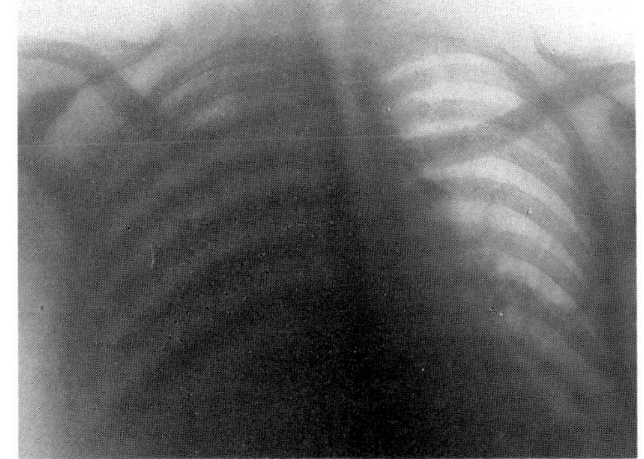

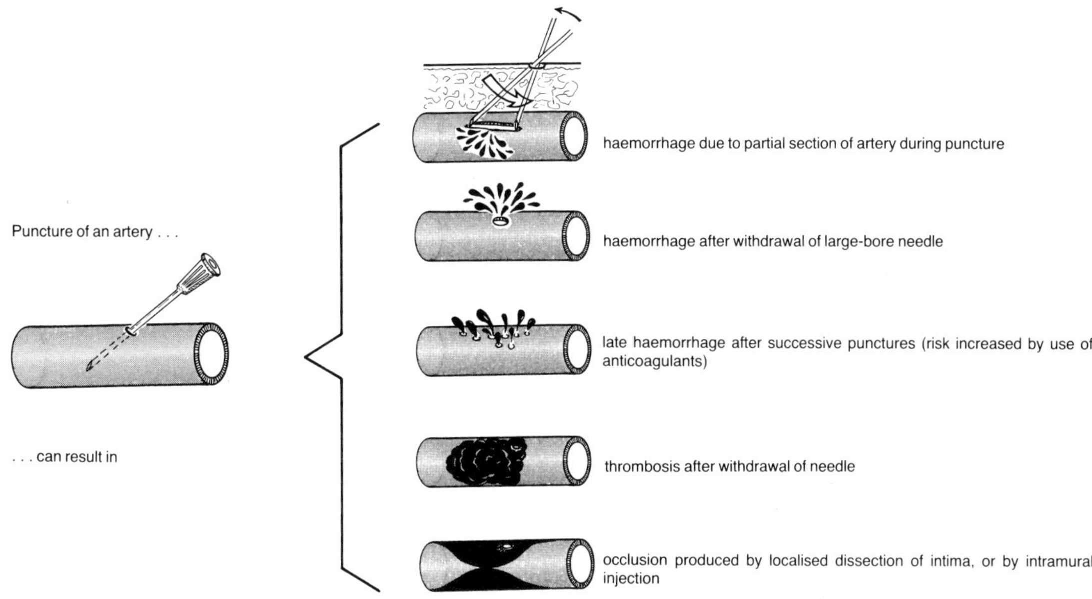

1018

L.M. ♀ 41 yrs. 13 Mar. 1975

1018 Right haemothorax due to iatrogenic laceration of subclavian artery. Partial section of the subclavian artery by the intra-cath needle during catheterisation of the subclavian vein has produced a massive haemothorax (see Volume I, **113**).

1019a

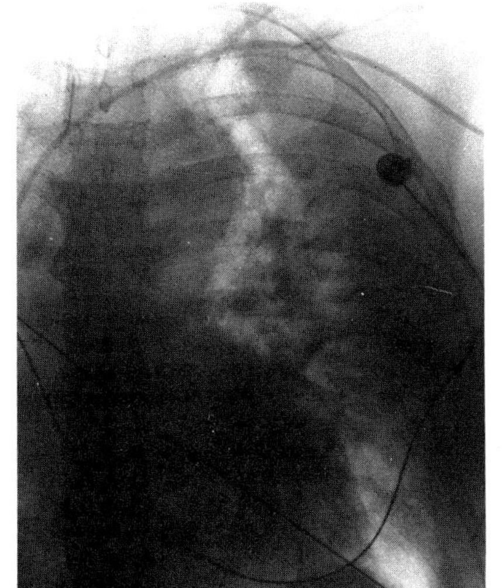

L.F. ♀ 60 yrs. 2 Oct. 1976

1019b

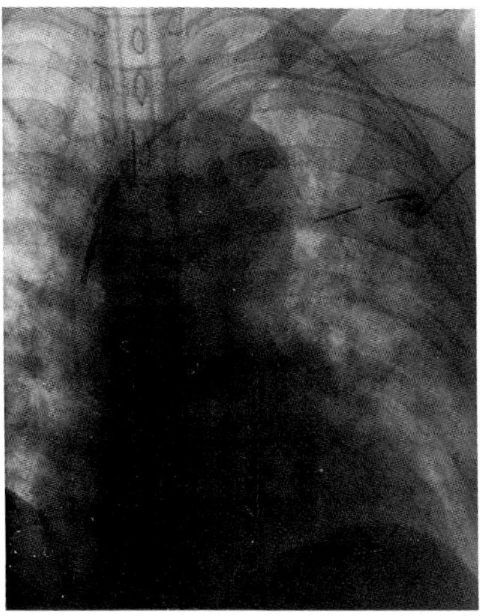

4 Oct. 1976

1019a Iatrogenic laceration of left subclavian artery. Attempted catheterisation of the left subclavian vein has led to an arterial laceration. A significant right haemothorax is aggravated by pre-existing clotting disorders.

1019b Recovery after pleural drainage.

10 Trauma of the diaphragm

1020

Anatomy

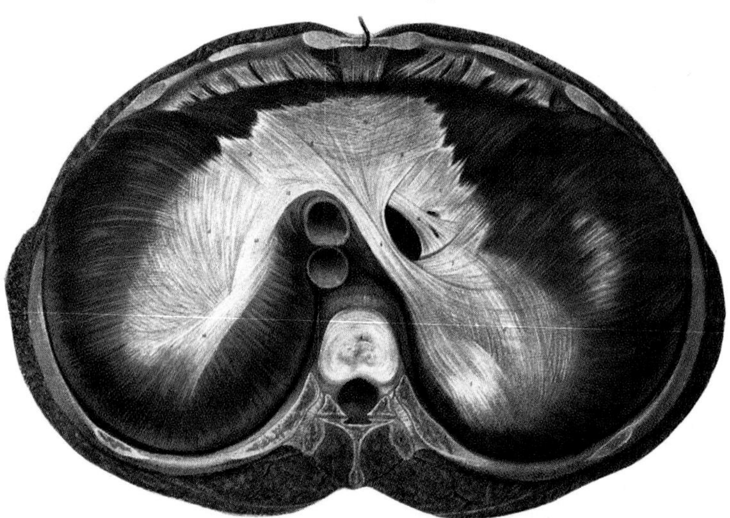

1020 Diaphragm seen from above (Bourgery, 1867). (See **1106.**)

1021 Diaphragm seen from below (Bourgery, 1867).

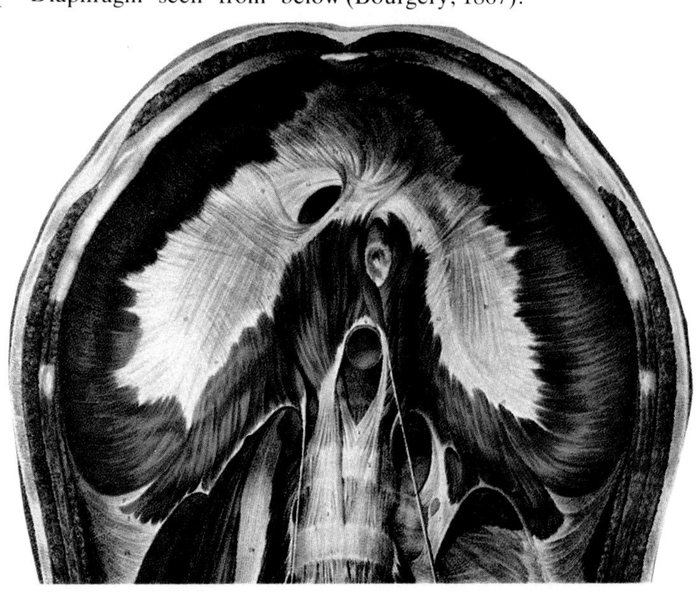

1022 **Types and incidences** of diaphragmatic injuries (in our material, $n = 138$).

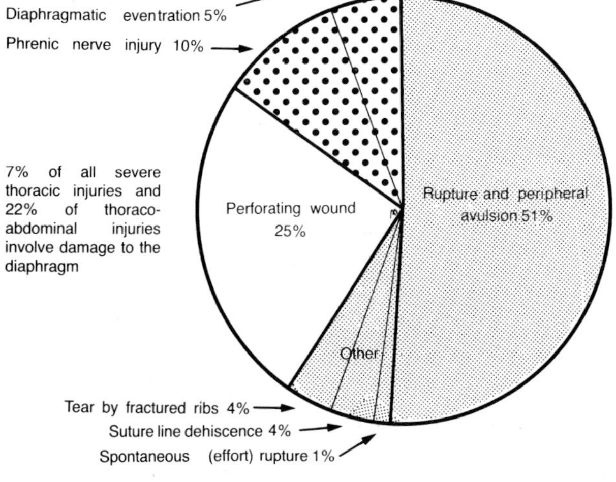

Incidence

Injuries of the diaphragm have become more frequent in recent years: today, 7% of all severe thoracic injuries, and 22% of all thoraco-abdominal injuries involve damage to the diaphragm. Diaphragmatic injuries are life-threatening unless diagnosed and treated early.

A severe blow to the lower thorax and upper abdomen (one third of all thoracic injuries) can cause massive intrathoracic or intra-abdominal haemorrhage. While shock is easily diagnosed and treated, diaphragmatic injury is far less obvious. It is often difficult to detect on early X-rays and in many cases, there is little external sign of damage. The type of accident and the nature of the associated injuries often form the only basis for suspicion.

About a third of diaphragmatic injuries are diagnosed only after 3 years (the delay ranges from nine days to 28 years). In our service over the past 10 years, diagnosis has been made immediately, or within a few days, in all instances.

Most diaphragmatic injuries are sustained by males involved in violent accidents. The average age of our patients is 38 years (3 to 82).

1023

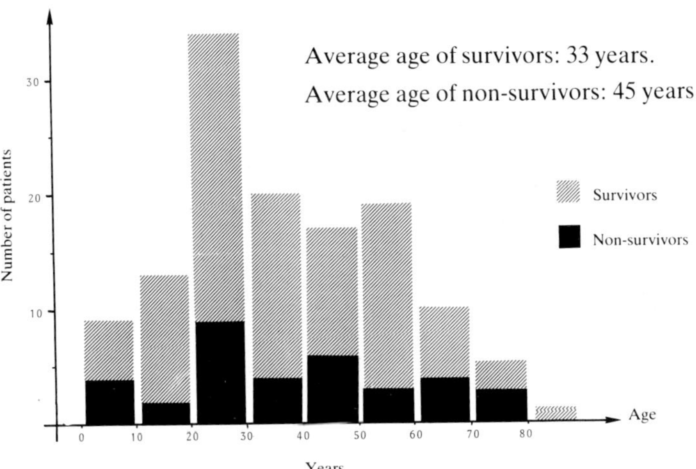

1023 Age distribution of patients with diaphragmatic injuries (n = 138).

The cause of injury is:	*Incidence*
– car accident	35%
– other road accident	15%
– explosion, fall or crush-injury	20%
– murder or suicide attempt	22%
– other	8%
	100%

Its localisation is:	
– left	77%
– right	20%
– bilateral	3%
	100%

The predominance of injuries to the left hemidiaphragm is explained (1) by the biodynamics of blunt diaphragmatic trauma (see **1034, 1035, 1039**), and (2) by the fact that most open wounds to the diaphragm are sustained in murder and suicide attempts aimed at the heart.

Tears by fractured ribs and peripheral avulsions are evenly distributed.

General management

Approaches

No hard and fast rules can be laid down. However, recent trauma of the left hemidiaphragm and anterior perforation of the right hemidiaphragm are best managed, in general, through laparotomy. Diaphragmatic repair is relatively easy, and associated abdominal injuries are accessible at the same time.

Thoracotomy should be avoided whenever possible since it aggravates existing damage. Nonetheless, old or strangulated herniae, suture dehiscence, and large ruptures of the right hemidiaphragm are best managed through the chest.

When a combined, sub- and supradiaphragmatic approach is required, it is well to begin with the abdominal operation.

1024

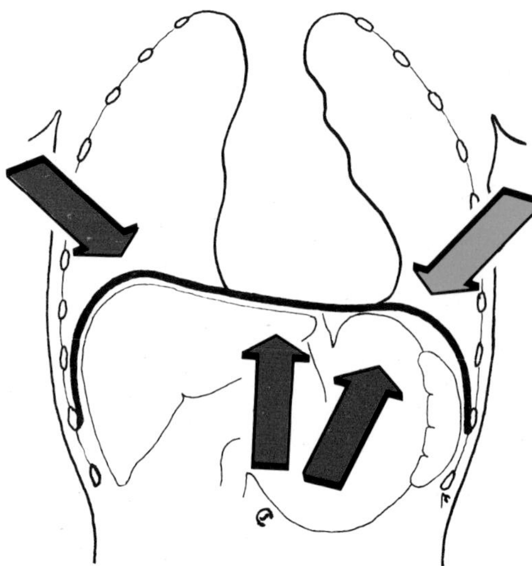

Right thoracotomy
- rupture of right hemidiaphragm
- associated lateral rupture of right pericardial wall
- right-sided perforating wounds (though not anterior wounds)

Laparotomy
- early diagnosed rupture of left hemidiaphragm
- rupture of pericardium and central diaphragm
- probable injuries to abdominal viscera
- perforating wounds of left hemidiaphragm and of anterior part of right hemidiaphragm

Left thoracotomy
- late diagnosed rupture of left hemidiaphragm
- dehiscence of suture line
- strangulated traumatic herniae
- associated lateral rupture of left pericardial wall

1024 Approaches to injuries of diaphragm (for wounds, see Volume I, chapter 3).

1025

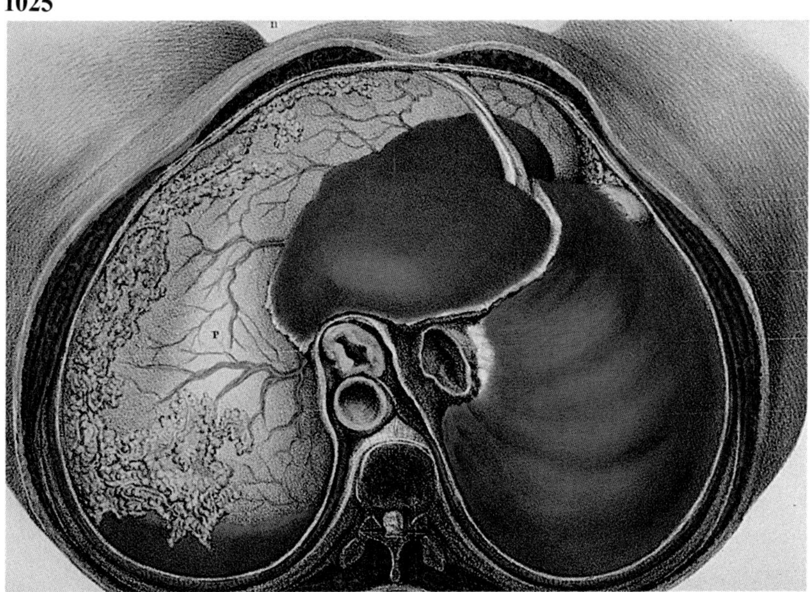

1025 Post-traumatic transdiaphragmatic herniation of subjacent organs is common. Three-quarters of left-sided ruptures lead to a gastrothorax, and two-thirds of right-sided ruptures to a hepatothorax. (The trunk seen from above, after excision of the diaphragm; Bourgery, 1867.)

Post-traumatic transdiaphragmatic herniation of abdominal organs (in our material, $n = 138$).

1026

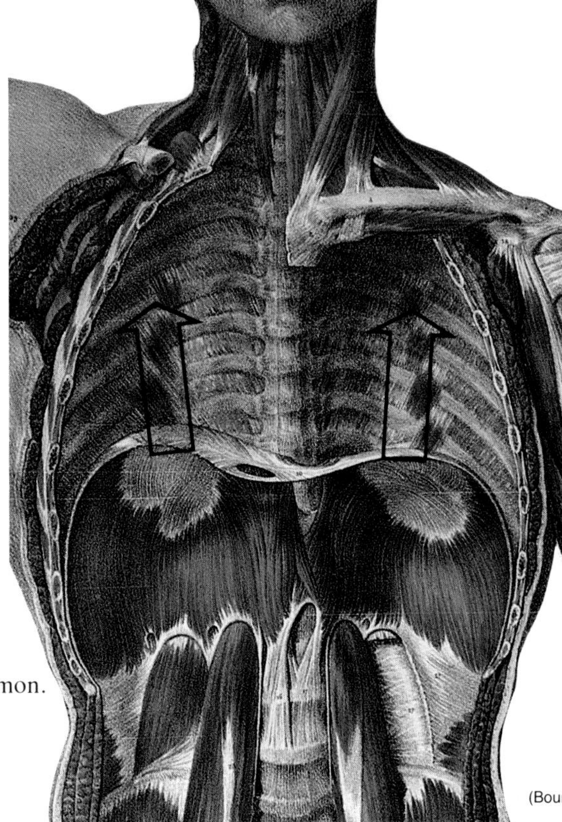

On the right:

Liver	54%
Colon	25%
Omentum	25%
Small bowel	8%
Blood	8%

On the left:

Stomach	76%
Colon	49%
Spleen	38%
Omentum	28%
Small bowel	25%
Blood	4%

Composite herniae are common.
N.B. The mobile viscera are herniated most frequently.

We have used the various approaches in the following proportions:

– laparotomy	36%
– laparotomy followed by thoracotomy	15%
– thoraco- phreno- laparotomy	7%
– thoracotomy	27%
	85%

In 7% of cases, the patient either was not operated on (phrenic nerve injury, minor eventration) or refused treatment. The remaining 8% of patients died before they could be brought to surgery.

Anaesthesia

The treatment of diaphragmatic injuries requires close co-operation between the anaesthetist and the surgeon. The patient should be prepared for surgery as quickly as possible. Aspiration of the stomach (see **1027, 1041c**) is often unsuccessful, but is nonetheless worth trying. Throughout the preparatory phase, the potential physiopathological repercussions of the diaphragmatic injury (see page 208) must be kept in mind.

Surgery should be preceded by resuscitatory measures to restore respiratory and cardiovascular equilibrium. It is important to: (1) drain any pleural effusion, (2) maximise oxygenation, (3) stabilise blood circulation (without using cardioplegic drugs or myocardial depressants), (4) check the acid-base balance of the blood, (5) check the water and electrolyte balance and (6) restore renal function if impaired.

In the case of a herniated abdominal viscus, the anaesthetic technique is clearly defined. The mediastinal shift caused by heavy or bulbous organs creates a highly unstable condition that is easily compromised during anaesthetisation. *Ventilatory assistance through a face mask* (which inevitably inflates the digestive system) and *positive pressure ventilation* through an endotracheal tube *must be avoided until the abdominal organs have been repositioned.* Far from aiding the reduction of the hernia, positive pressure ventilation aggravates the patient's condition by collapsing the pulmonary vessels. Intubation should be carried out without curarisation and the patient left in spontaneous respiration. Even during preparation for surgery, controlled ventilation, especially with PEEP, must be avoided since it further reduces cardiac output and can result in irreversible cardiac arrest (see page 208).

1027

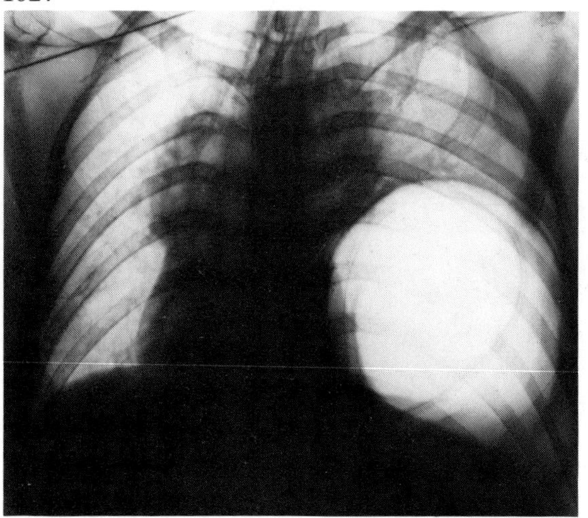

P.N.–A. ♀ 47 yrs. 20 May 1979

1027 After a large, transverse rupture, it may be possible occasionally to **decompress a gastrothorax through a nasogastric tube.**

Mortality

Mortality of diaphragmatic injuries
(in our material, n = 138)

	Mortality
Diaphragmatic rupture by blunt trauma or peripheral avulsion	35%
Effort (spontaneous) rupture	~0%
Dehiscence of the suture line	40%
Tear by fractured ribs	20%
Perforating wound	21%
Phrenic nerve injury	~0%
Eventration	17%

Overall mortality is 26% but, in 14% of cases, death was unrelated to the diaphragmatic injury.

Rupture of the diaphragm

Misleading radiological findings

1028a

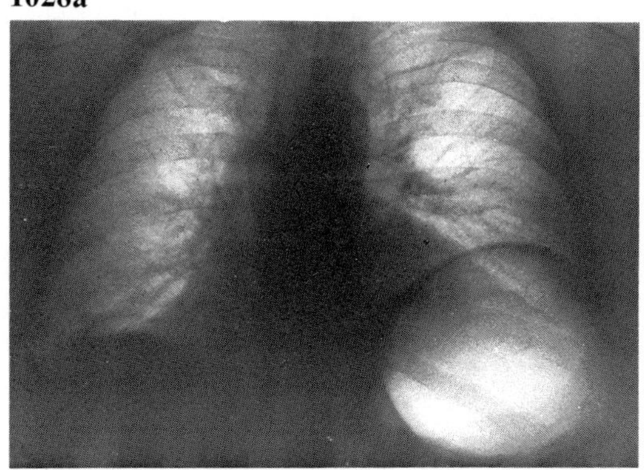

M.J.–L. ♂ 9 Feb. 1972

1028a **Acute gastric dilatation** masquerading as a gastrothorax in a semi-seated patient. There are no thoracic injuries and the diaphragm is intact.

1028b The same acute gastric dilatation is here seen on the standard abdominal X-ray.

Acute gastric dilatation often causes shock by compressing the inferior vena cava (as experimental studies suggest).

1028c Upright chest X-ray of the same subject with an empty stomach.

1028b

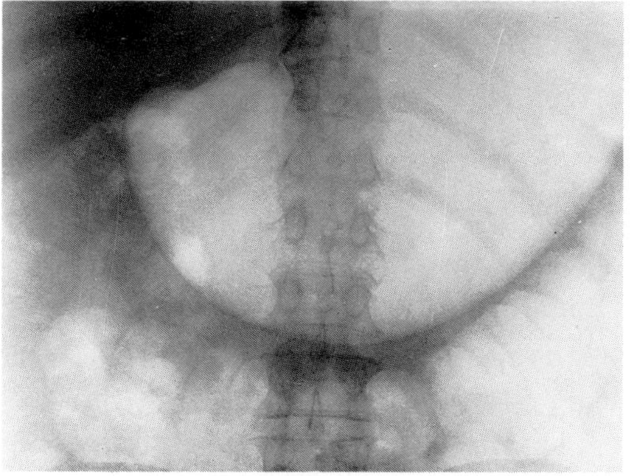

9 Feb. 1972

1028c

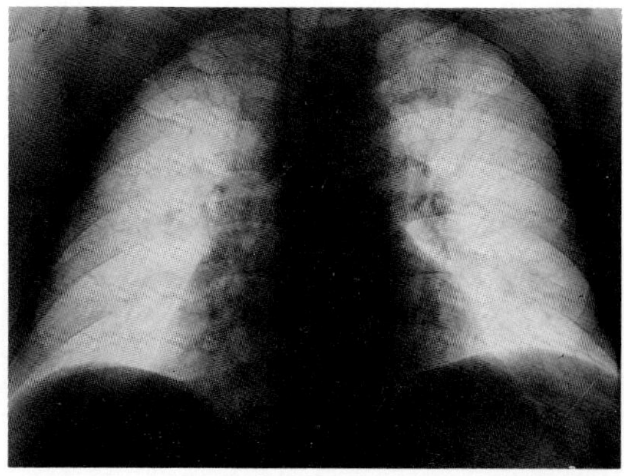

Diaphragmatic rupture is little different from other diaphragmatic injuries so far as sex ratio, type of accident, mechanism and average age are concerned (see **1022, 1023**). The average age of survivors is 33 years, and of those who die in hospital, 45 years.

It is well established that left-sided rupture is much more common than right-sided rupture; the ratio in our cases is 81% to 16%. Rarest of all is bilateral rupture (3% of our cases). Few victims of bilateral rupture reach hospital alive.

Mortality in diaphragmatic rupture is 46%. On admission, most patients are anoxic, comatose and in deep shock; death usually intervenes within the first two days.

1029a

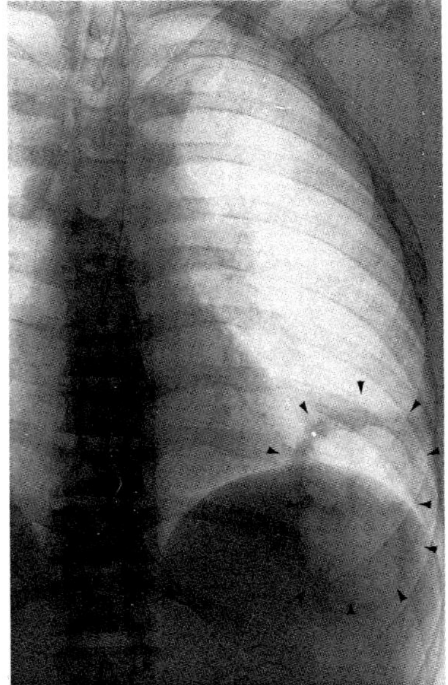

M.C. ♂ 20 yrs. 5 Oct. 1977.

1029a Lingular abscess masquerading as a gastrothorax in a motorcyclist who fell at high-speed without sustaining thoracic damage. The comatose patient has a cerebral haematoma and requires artificial ventilation. He is febrile and his expectorations are purulent. A polycyclic cyst-like cavity suggests a diaphragmatic rupture with an incipient gastro- or colothorax.

1029b

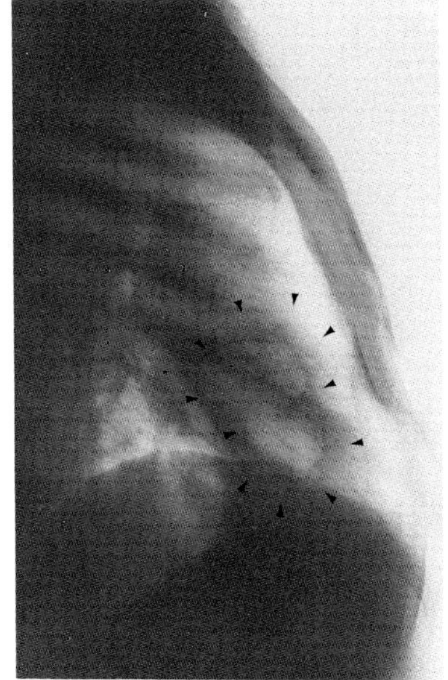

5 Oct. 1977

1029b A lateral view X-ray shows the 'cyst' to be a lingular abscess, probably caused by anaerobic germs. The blurred appearance is typical.

1029c

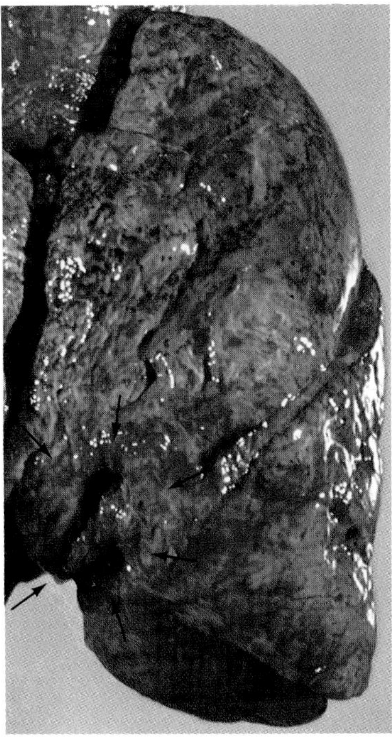

Oct. 1977

1029c The patient died subsequently from a metastatic cerebral abscess. Autopsy reveals that the lingular abscess (→) perforated the visceral pleura; it is surrounded by localised fibrinous pleurisy.

1030

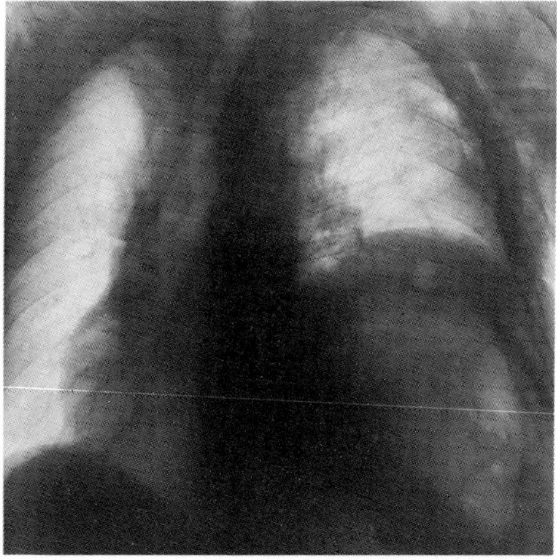

R.J. ♂ 70 yrs. 20 Dec. 1965

1030 Relaxation of diaphragm misdiagnosed as compressive gastrothorax. The 70-year-old patient has a flail chest with paradoxical motion. An emergency thoracotomy performed on suspicion of rupture reveals a relaxed diaphragm. Death.

1031

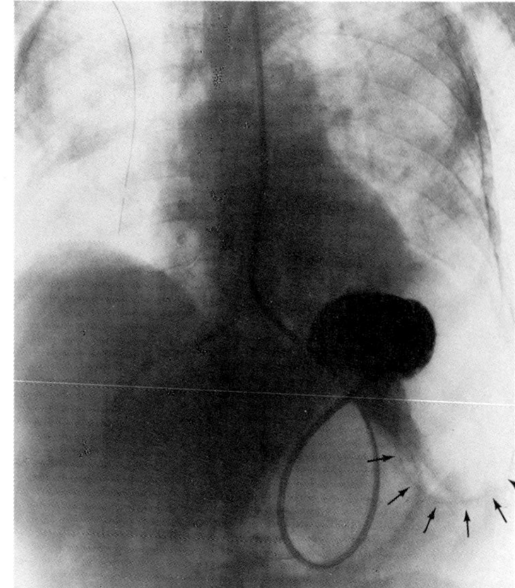

G.H. ♂ 66 yrs. 17 July 1973

1031 Pseudo-gastrothorax caused by inversion of diaphragm due to a localised tension pneumothorax. The stomach seems to have migrated above the diaphragm but, in fact, the anterior part of the left hemidiaphragm (→) is depressed below the gastric fundus which lies behind.

1032a

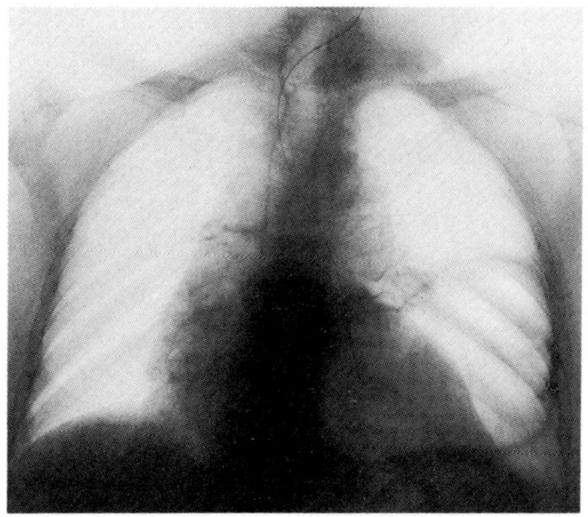

P.G. ♀ 88 yrs. 10 Jan. 1973

1032b

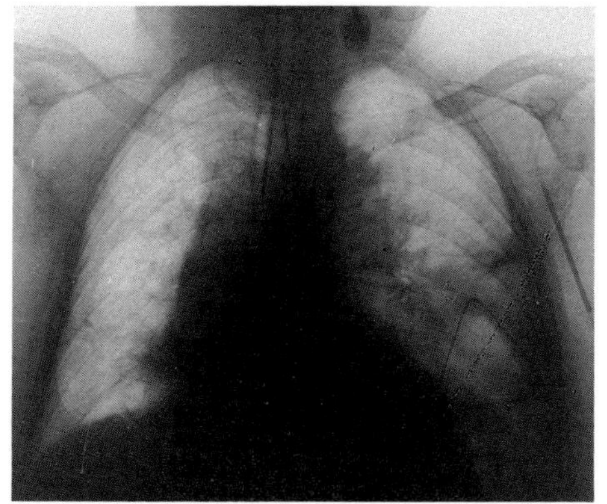

19 Jan. 1973

1032c

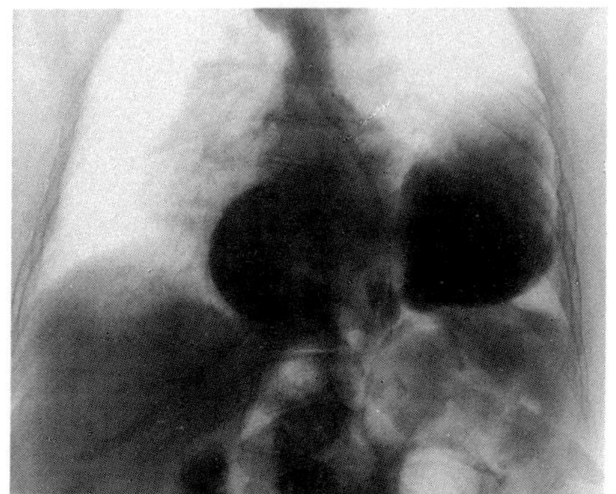

10 Feb. 1973

1032a Non-traumatic gastrothorax due to paraoesophageal hernia. The large air bubble in the lower thorax represents the stomach in chronic volvulus.

1032b The stomach has been emptied completely through a nasogastric tube. The tube is still in place.

1032c A barium study shows the inverted stomach.

1033a C.R. ♂ 53 yrs. 1 Mar. 1971

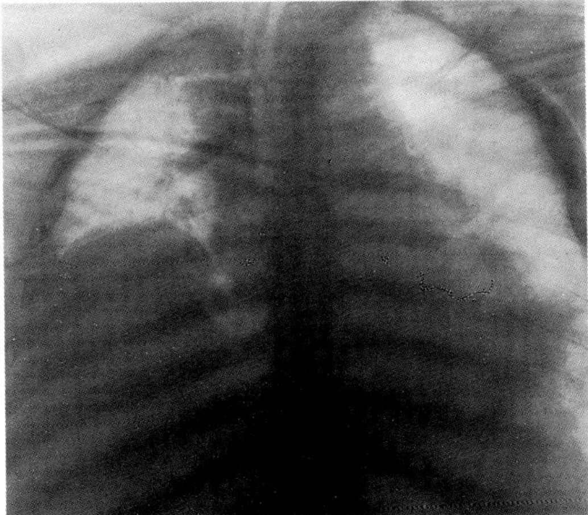

1033b 28 April 1972

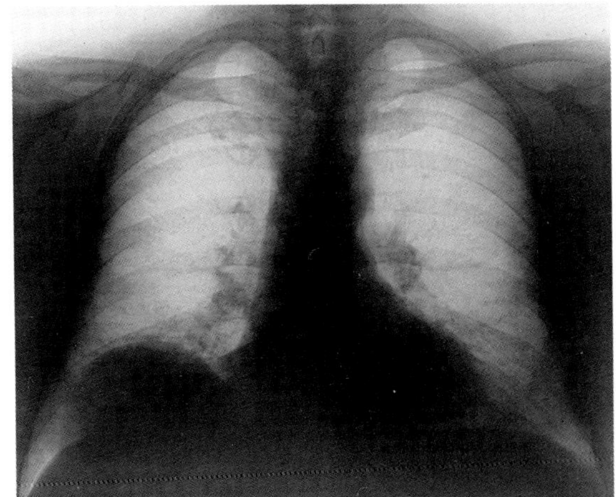

1033a Relaxation of right hemidiaphragm misdiagnosed as post-traumatic hepatothorax. A poor quality X-ray taken on the admission of a multiple-injury patient suggests a diaphragmatic rupture with herniation of the liver. A right thoracotomy shows the diaphragm to be intact, but locally relaxed. **1033b** The localised relaxation can be seen clearly on this later film, taken with the subject in deep inspiration.

Biomechanics

The diaphragm is more or less tensed according to the phase of respiration. Rupture occurs under the combined, though not necessarily simultaneous, effect of two mechanisms:

1. A sudden increase in tension, usually caused by a shock wave following a violent impact to the abdomen or lower thorax. The abdomen behaves as a liquid container in which the full force of the impact is transmitted (according to Pascal's law) to all parts of the cavity. The force exerted on the diaphragm is accentuated by the momentary deformation of its unsupported portion (see **1034, 1035**).
2. Localised traction due to the deformation of the lower thorax (see **1036, 1037**).

One or other of the two mechanisms sometimes predominates as, for example, in abdomino-thoracic compressions or crush-injuries of the chest.

The mechanism of injury – combined with the youth and bodily suppleness of many victims – explains why in 30% of cases there is no skeletal damage to the rib-cage. Moreover, the biomechanical similarity between diaphragmatic rupture and aortic rupture (see **935 to 938**) explains why the two injuries may be associated.

1034

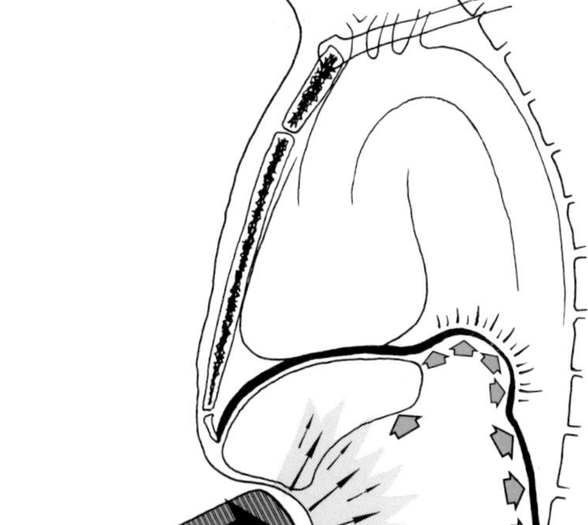

1034 Biomechanism of blunt diaphragmatic rupture from high abdominal impact. Lateral view.

1035

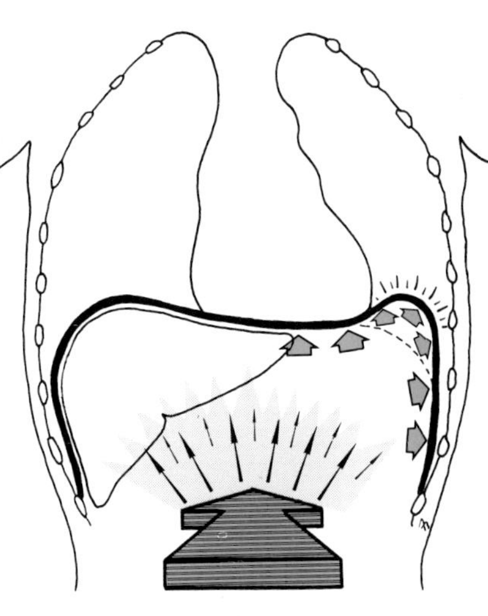

1035 Anterior view.

1036

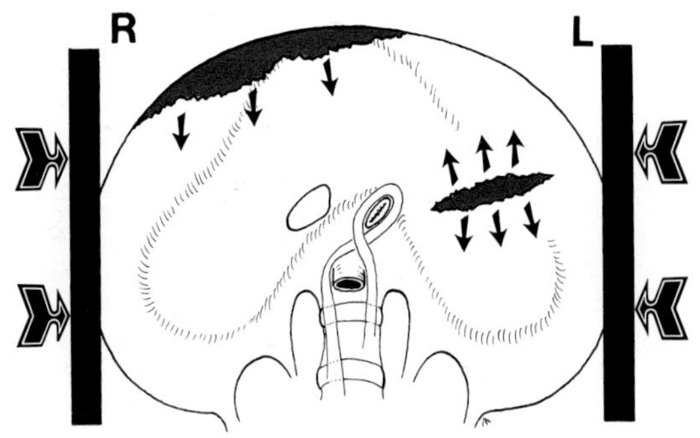

1036 Blunt diaphragmatic rupture (or peripheral avulsion) (1) **Transverse rupture** by lateral deformation.

(Lung contusion is commonly associated.)

1037

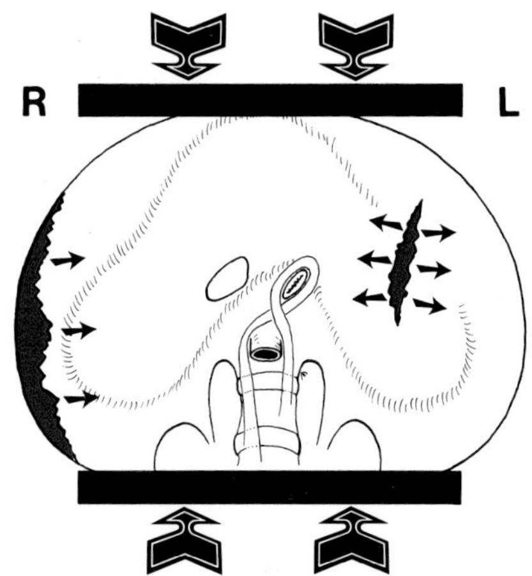

1037 (2) **Sagittal rupture** by antero-posterior deformation.

(Mediastinal injury is commonly associated.)

1038a

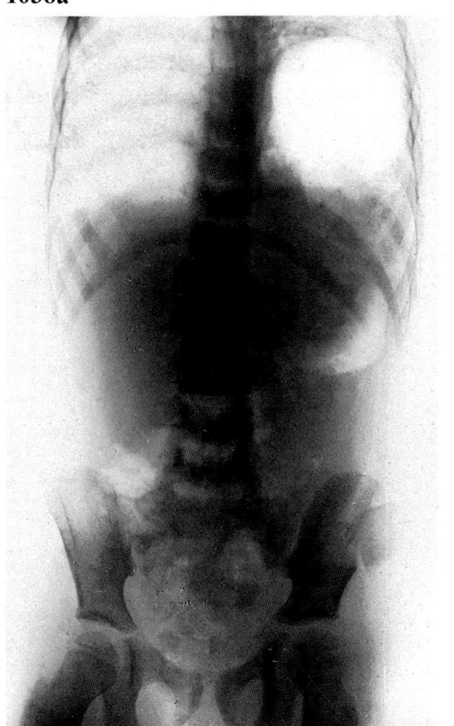

1038b

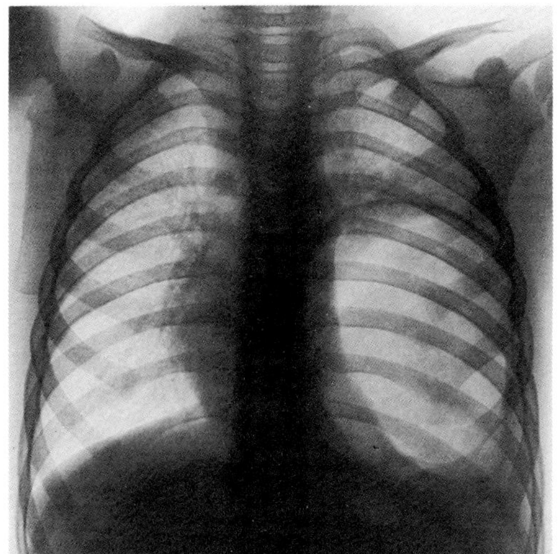

1038a Sagittal rupture of the diaphragm results from anteroposterior compression. This little girl sustained multiple fractures of the pelvis (left Voillemier and iliac wing fractures) when crushed under the wheel of a lorry.

1038b Tension gastrothorax (also visible on **1038a**).

1038c

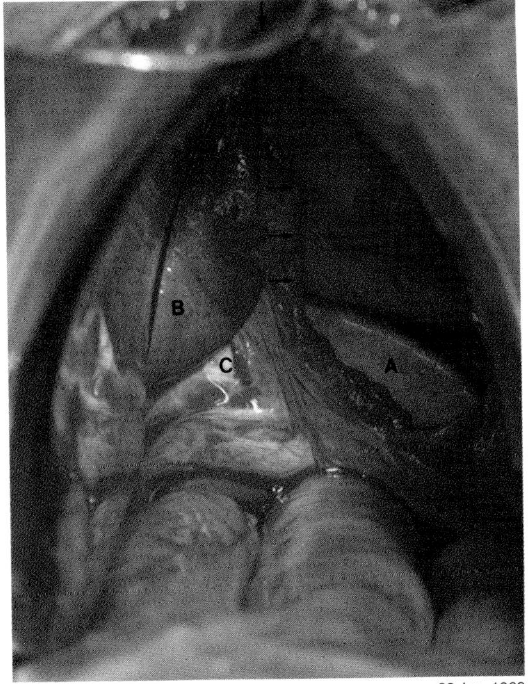

1038d

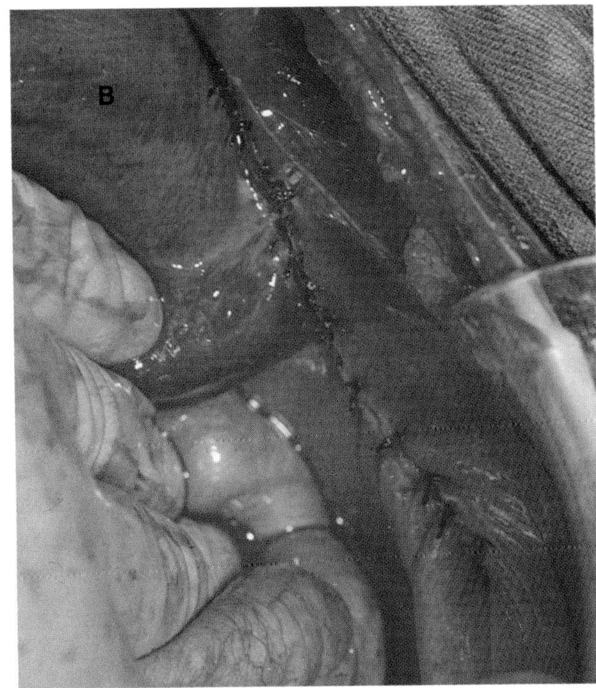

1038e

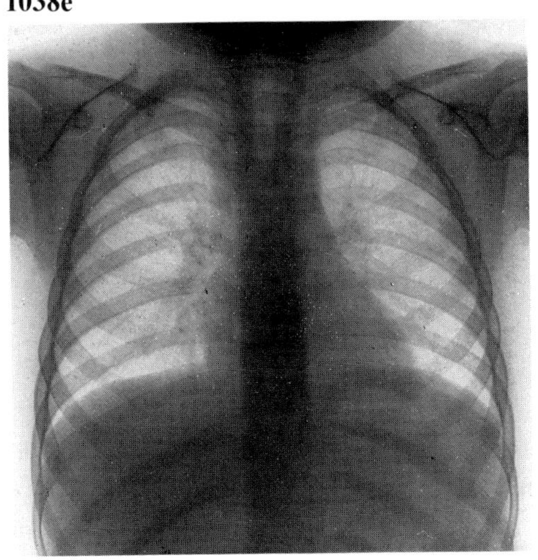

1038c The sagittal rupture (→) seen through a laparotomy after the reduction of the stomach. The partly atelectatic lower lobe of the left lung (A), the left lobe of the liver (B), the tendinous portion of the diaphragm (C) and the xiphoid appendix (→) are all visible.

1038d The repaired diaphragm.

1038e Recovery.

1039

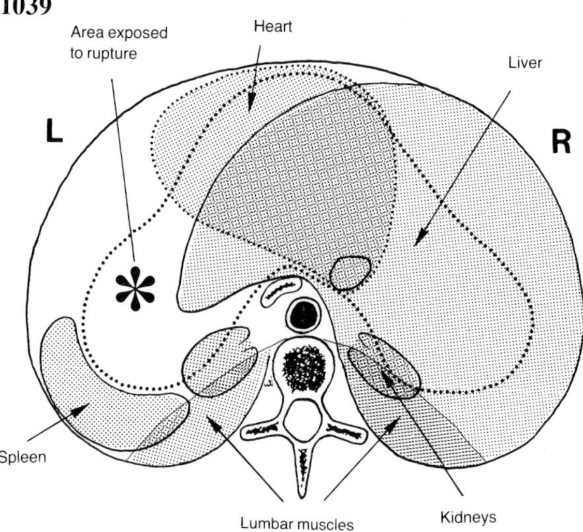

1039 Areas where the diaphragm is supported above and/or below by adjacent organs (superior view).

1040

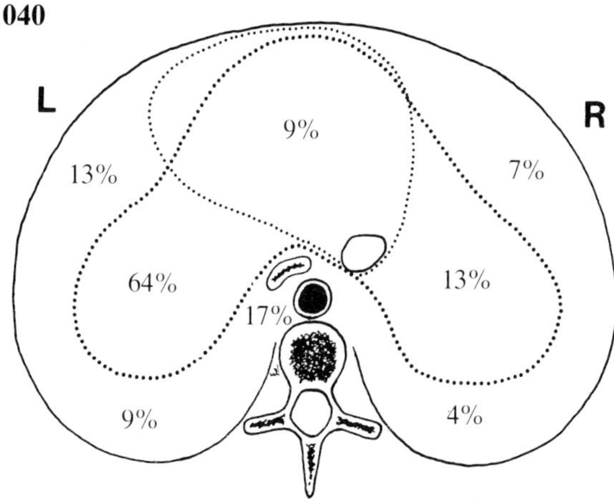

IN 70% OF CASES, DAMAGE IS CONFINED TO A SINGLE AREA.

1040 Incidence of diaphragmatic rupture in 8 different anatomical areas (in our material, $n = 74$).

The direction of the main axis of a diaphragmatic rupture indicates whether the impact was frontal, lateral or oblique. This index in turn indicates the likely associated injuries. A frontal impact commonly produces a mediastinal injury, and a lateral impact often causes lung contusion (see Volume I, **300**)

Both hemidiaphragms are supported above and below by adjacent organs (see **1020**, **1021** and **1025**, **1026**). The only unsupported portion is the apex of the left hemidiaphragm; it is here that rupture most often occurs.

Peripheral avulsions and tears by fractured ribs, on the other hand, are usually the direct result of extensive parietal damage. Incidence is the same on either side (see page 227).

The incidence of the various types of trauma – rupture, tear and avulsion – is different in each of the 8 anatomical areas where damage to the diaphragm can occur.

- 2 *vaults* (left and right),
- 4 areas of *peripheral* attachment (anterior and posterior, left and right),
- the *oesophageal* hiatus,
- the *central part of diaphragm and floor of the pericardium*.

The form of a rupture depends not only upon the violence and direction of the impact but also upon the position of the victim's body, his phase of respiration, and the state of repletion of his digestive organs at the moment of impact.

Whether a rupture is short or long (from 3 to 30cm) its edges are always flaccid, irregular and bloody. What is most important from the point of view of repair is that most ruptures are linear rather than star-shaped (see **1038c, 1091b**).

1041a

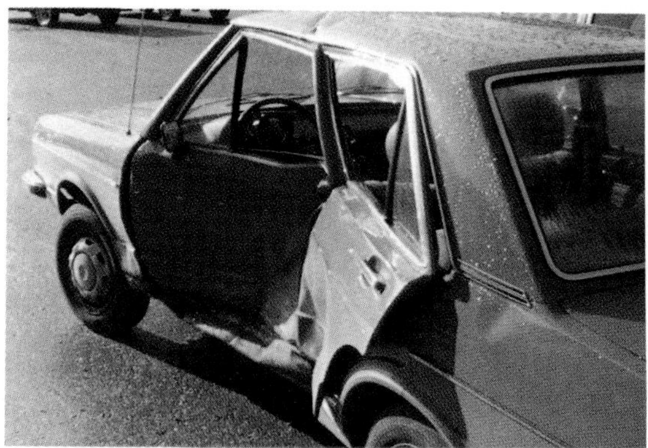

C.G. ♂ 59 yrs. 13 Nov. 1977

1041a Transverse rupture of the diaphragm results from lateral deformation of the lower thorax. The driver of this car was struck heavily on the left hypochondrium . . .

1041b

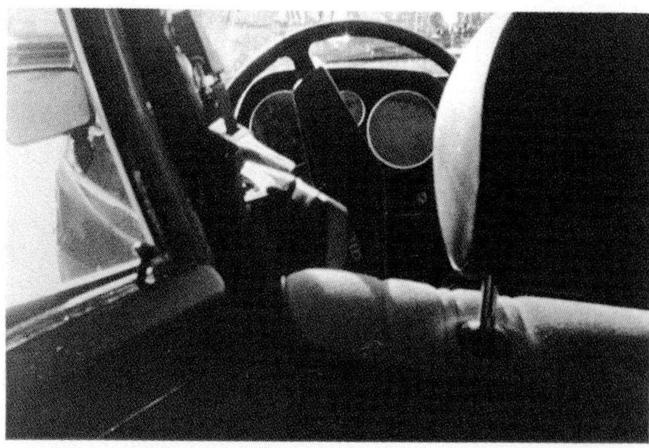

13 Nov. 1977

1041b . . . when his vehicle was hit by another car travelling at about 80km/h.

1041c

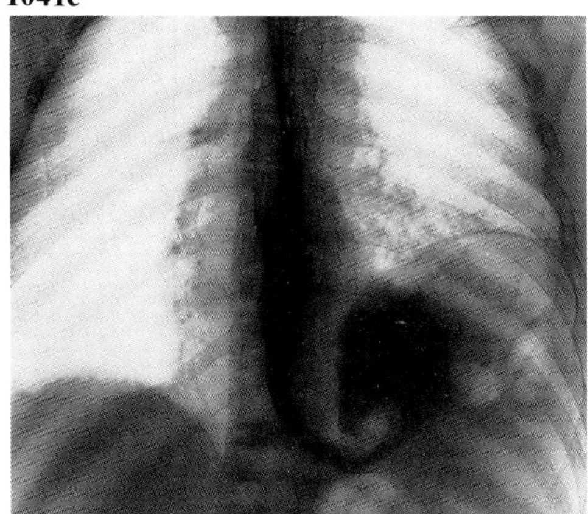

13 Nov. 1977

1041d

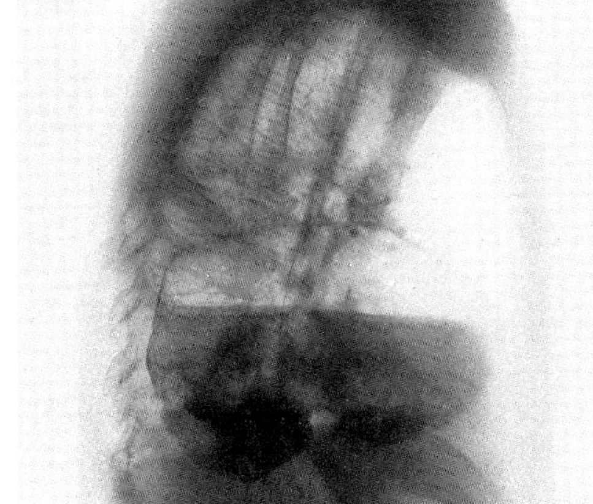

13 Nov. 1977

1041e

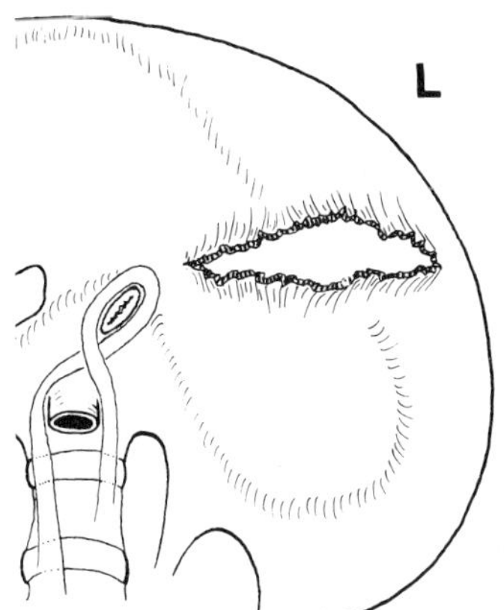

1041c The result was an 8 cm transverse rupture of the left hemidiaphragm.
N.B. The nasogastric tube extends into the herniated stomach.

1041d The (intact) spleen and omentum were also herniated. Laparotomy, repair. Recovery.

1041e The rupture represented diagramatically.

1042a

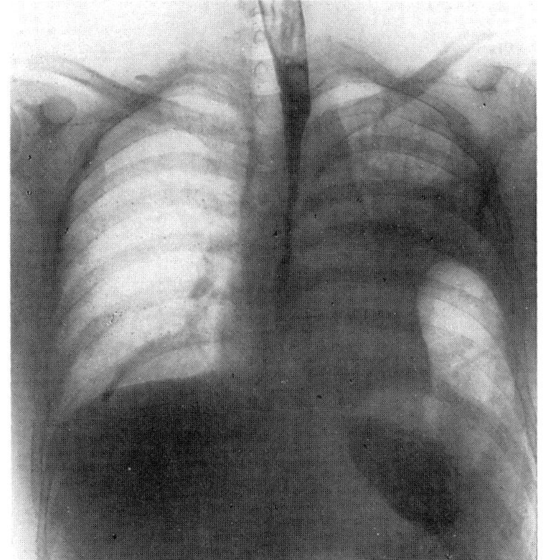

P.M. ♂ 25 yrs. 20 Oct. 1966

1042a Can the diaphragm be ruptured by a blast-injury, as in this case of transdiaphragmatic herniation of the colon in a miner exposed to a fire-damp explosion? The injury could be the result of a secondary impact.

1042b

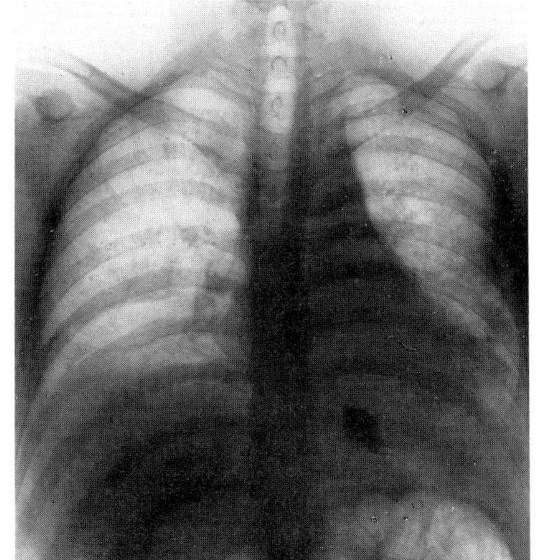

21 Oct. 1966

1042b Repair was effected through a laparotomy. Postoperative X-ray.

Associated injuries

Severe thoraco-abdominal injuries usually comprise a complex of lesions with involved physio-pathological repercussions. Cause and effect, and the order of priorities to be adopted in examination and/or treatment are often difficult to determine.

Certain combinations of injury are particularly life-threatening: the following simplified classification is intended as a guide-line for the preliminary examination of patients with injuries to the diaphragm.

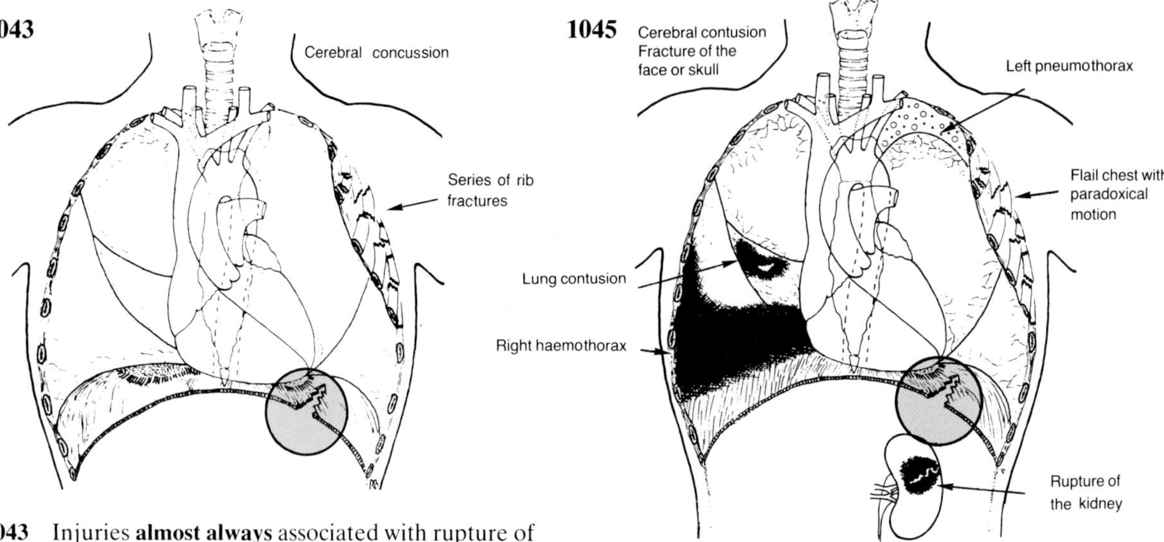

1043 Injuries **almost always** associated with rupture of diaphragm (in *over half* of our cases; $n = 74$).

1045 Injuries **sometimes** associated with rupture of diaphragm (in a *tenth to a quarter* of our cases).

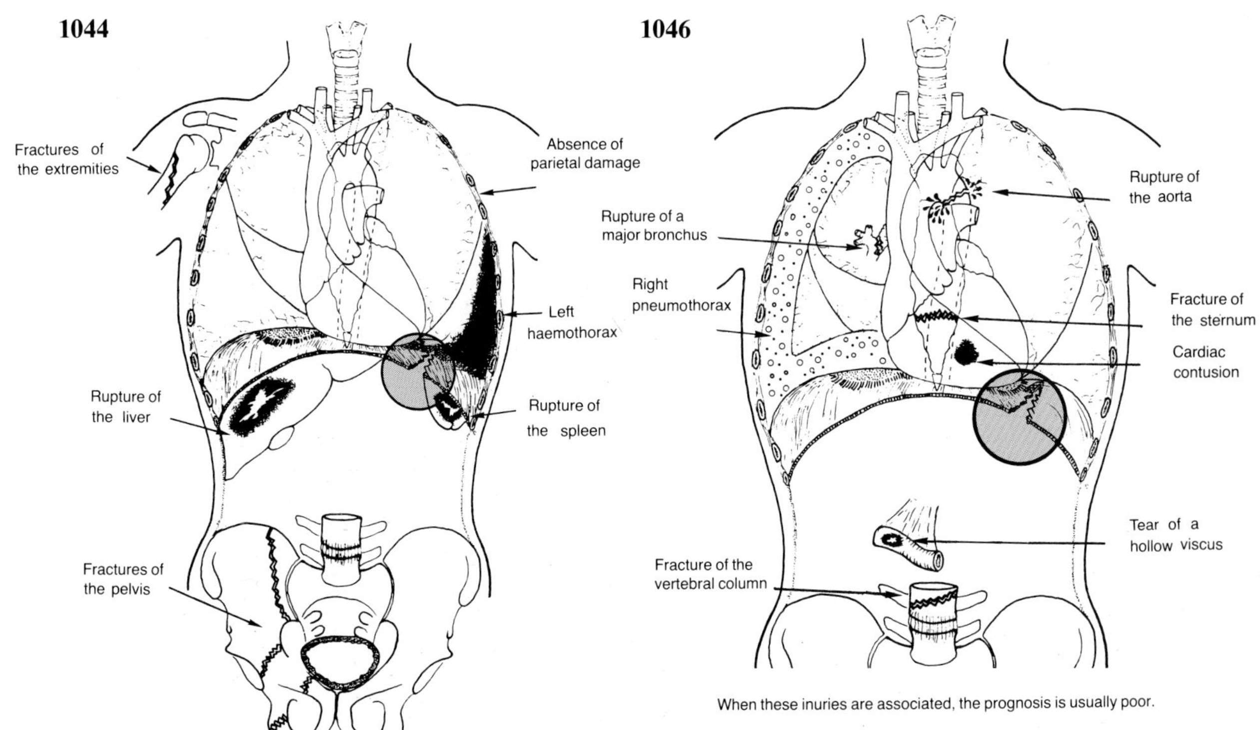

1044 Injuries **often** associated with rupture of diaphragm (in a *quarter to half* of our cases)

1046 Injuries **rarely** associated with rupture of diaphragm.

1047a

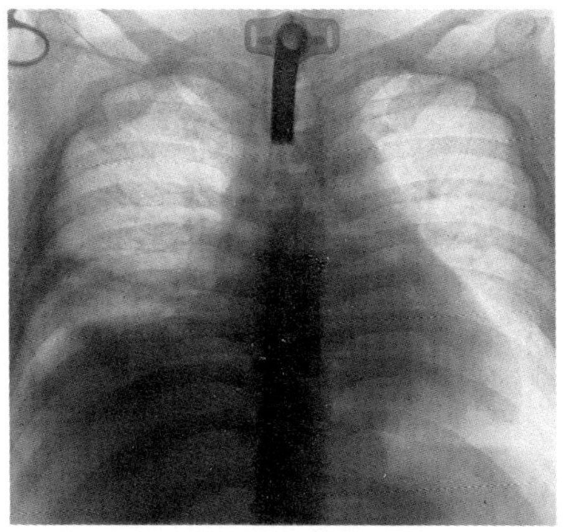

V.W. ♂ 41 yrs. 20 July 1966

1047a Rupture of the diaphragm with **laceration of the liver**. Initial X-ray of a car driver who drove into a pylon. Transfer to the University Hospital 4 days after the accident.

1047b A thoraco-phreno-laparotomy shows the liver to be directly in contact with the lung. There are several lacerations: the visible apical laceration is superficial but continues to bleed. Haemostasis.

1047c The liver is re-positioned into the abdomen.

1047d Repair of the 25cm longitudinal breach in the diaphragm. Recovery.

1047b **1047c** **1047d**

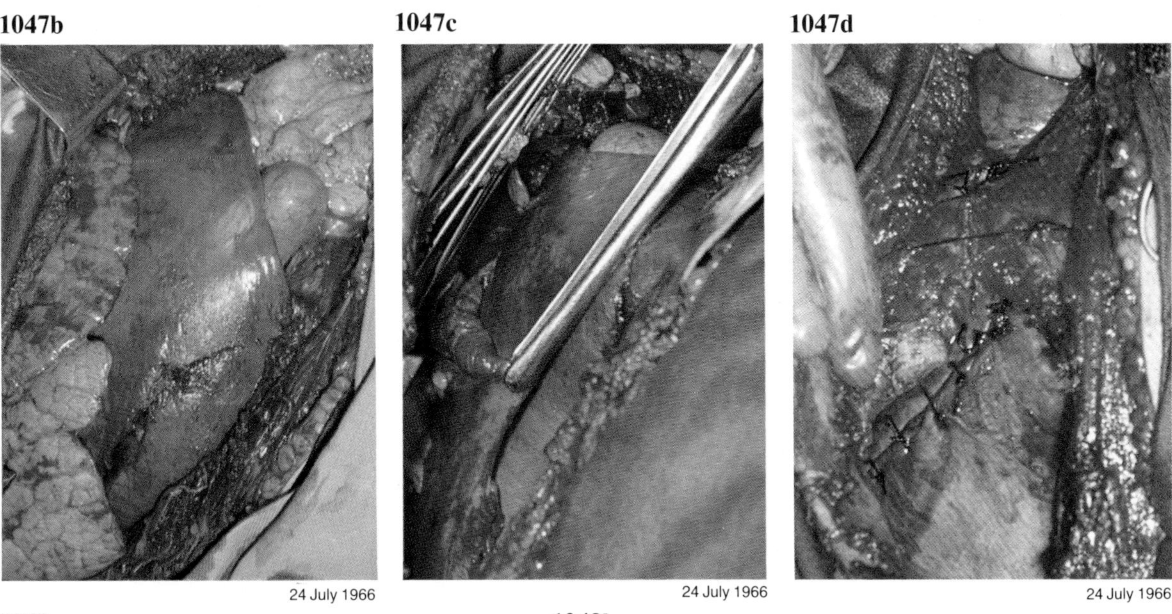

24 July 1966 24 July 1966 24 July 1966

1048a

B.M. ♀ 52 yrs. 14 Mar. 1966

1048a Rupture of the diaphragm with **minor parietal damage to the thorax**. (2 rib fractures). The initial supine X-ray shows a diffuse opacity in the lower left lung field.

1048b

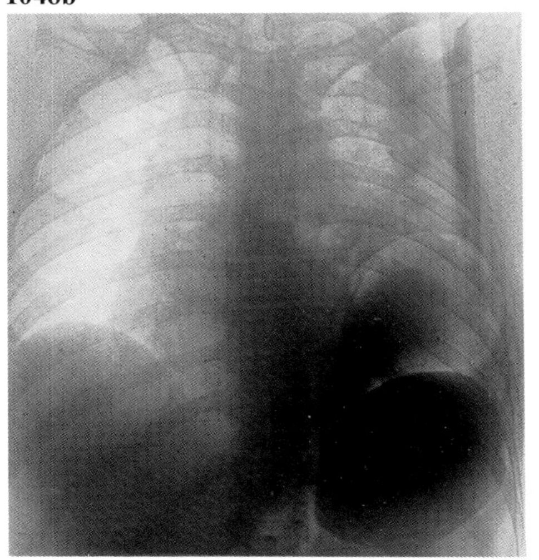

14 Mar. 1966

1048b A contrast study reveals a gastrothorax.

1049a

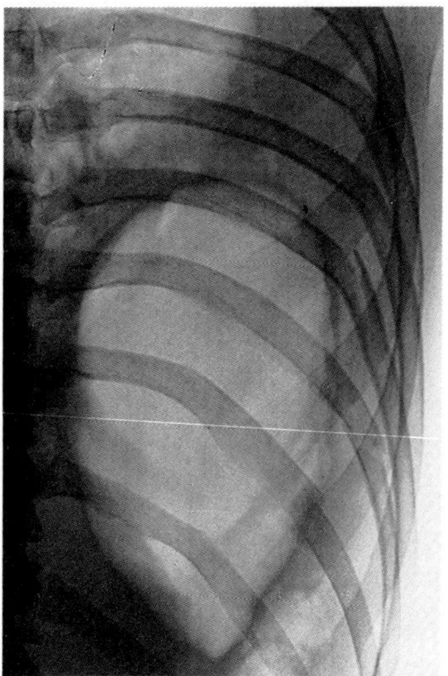

F.W. ♂ 27 yrs. 21 May 1970

1049b

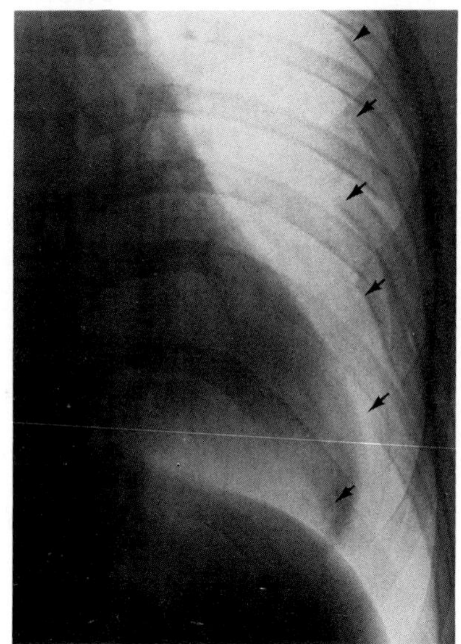

21 May 1970

1049c

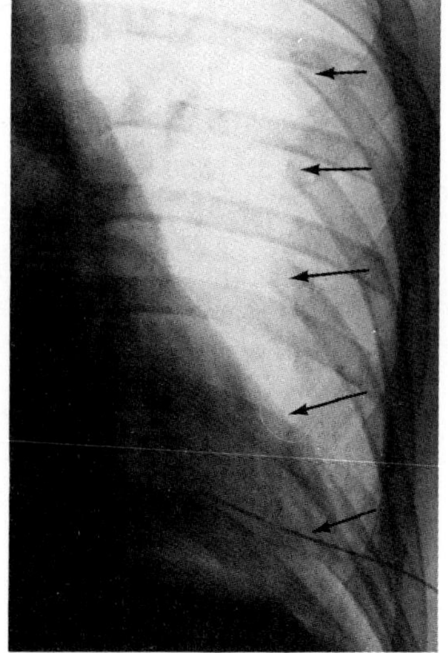

23 May 1970

1049a Long peripheral avulsion with a lower left **flail chest** with paradoxical motion.

1049b The abdominal viscera are replaced and the diaphragm closed (through a laparotomy). The resultant dislocation of the costal fractures converts the flail chest with paradoxical motion into a stove-in chest.

1049c The fractures dislocate further and consolidate. Recovery without noticeable sequelae (see Volume I, **326**).

1050a

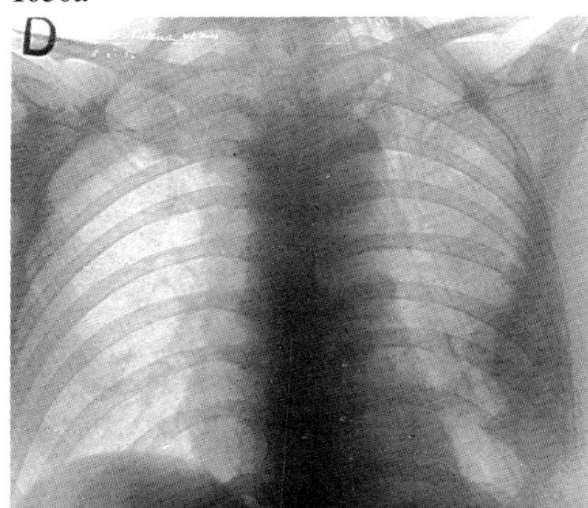

R.V. ♀ 42 yrs. 15 Nov. 1956

1050b

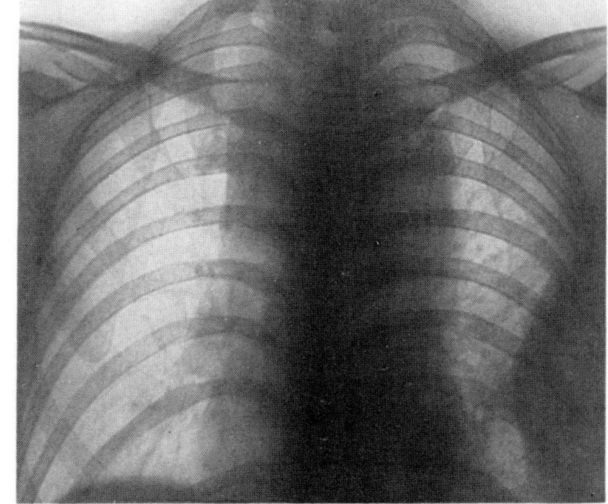

26 Nov. 1956

1050c

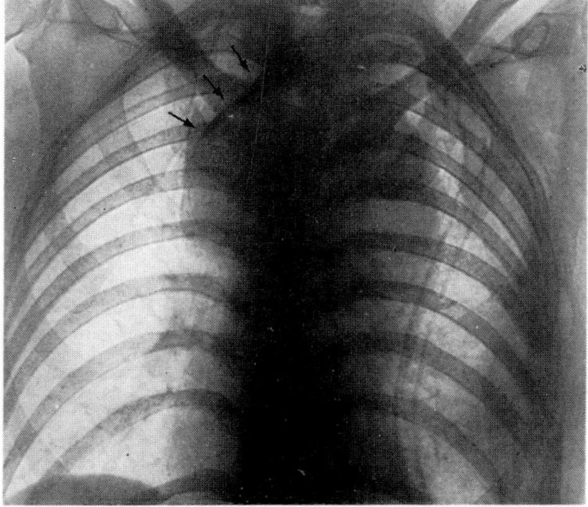

29 Nov. 1956

1050a Rupture of the diaphragm with an aortic rupture and a **fast-growing pseudo-aneurysm**. An emergency thoracotomy to repair a rupture of the left hemidiaphragm reveals an unsuspected aortic rupture. The aorta cannot be repaired, however, since surgery of major vessels is still in its infancy (1956). (See **942**.)

1050b A pseudo-aneurysm develops rapidly.

1050c It depresses the left main-stem bronchus and displaces the oesophagus to the right (→). Twenty-seven days later, it ruptures into the left pleural cavity causing immediate death.

1051a

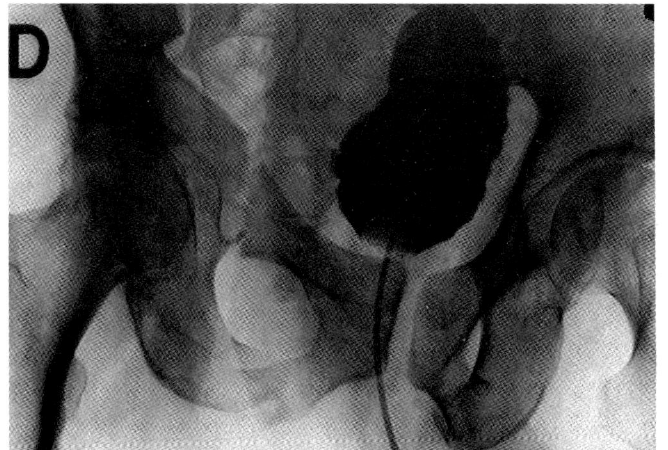

C.F. ♂ 62 yrs. 26 Mar. 1972

1051c

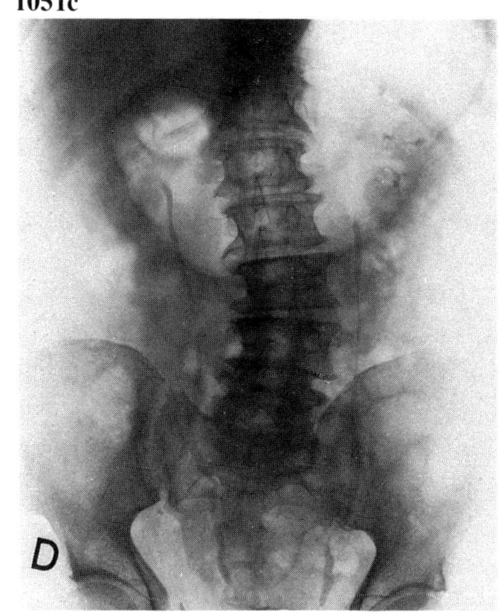

28 Mar. 1972

1051b

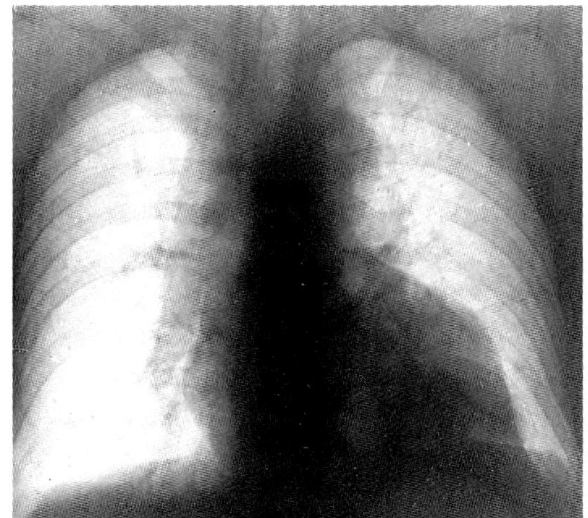

26 Mar. 1972

1051d

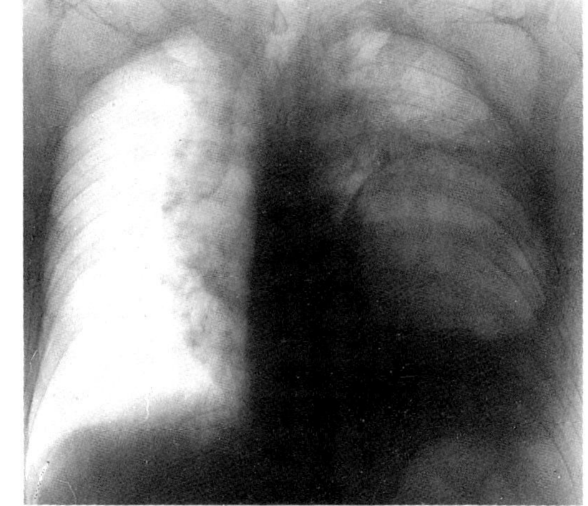

28 Mar. 1972

1051a Rupture of the diaphragm with **pelvic fractures** following a crush-injury to the abdomen and pelvis. The 4 ischio-ilio-pubic rami are fractured and there is a retroperitoneal haematoma displacing the bladder.

1051b The initial chest X-ray is considered normal.

1051c Aerophagy (during intravenous urography) leads to acute gastric dilatation . . .

1051d . . . and a massive tension gastrothorax that reveals the rupture of diaphragm. Intubation. Reversible cardiac arrest as positive pressure ventilation is initiated. Laparotomy, repair. Death 22 days later from gastric stress ulcers.

1052

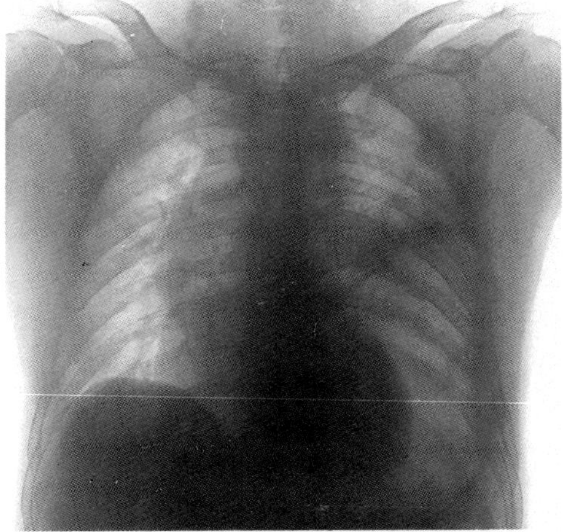

S.M. ♂ 58 yrs. 15 May 1958

1052 Rupture of the diaphragm with a **pulmonary laceration**. Transdiaphragmatic herniation of the stomach, spleen, colon and greater omentum coincides with a left pneumothorax due to a pulmonary laceration. The diaphragm is repaired through a thoracotomy. Death 2 days later.

1053

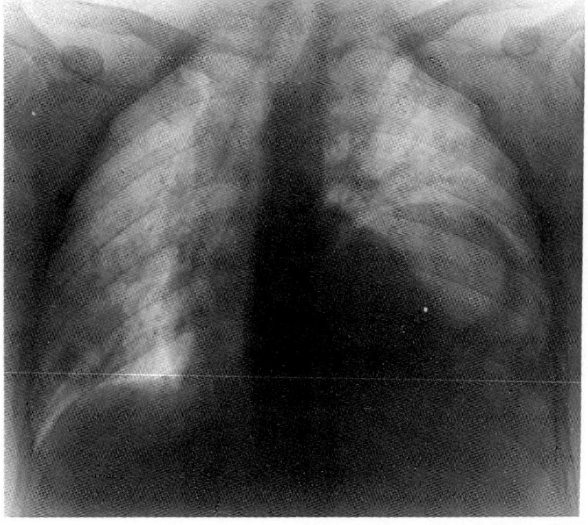

H.J.–D. ♂ 24 yrs. 23 Aug. 1966

1053 Rupture of the diaphragm with pulmonary **contusion and an intrapulmonary haematoma**. This supine X-ray reveals a tension gastrothorax and a cavitary opacity in the lower lobe of the right lung. The diaphragm is sutured through a laparotomy and the pulmonary haematoma is treated conservatively. Recovery.

1054

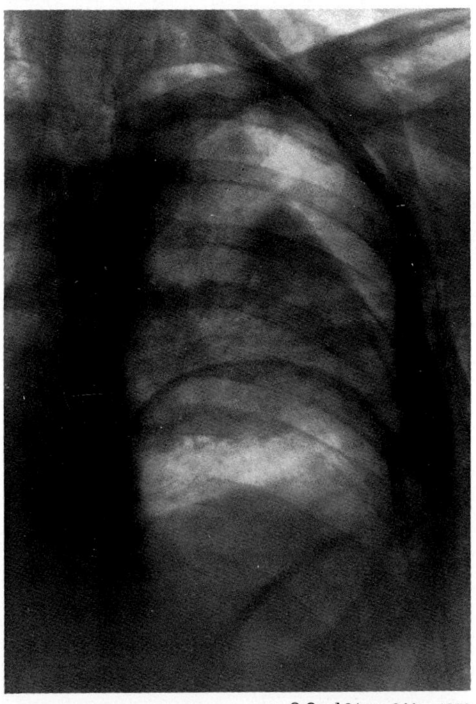

G.G. ♂ 24 yrs. 8 Mar. 1973

1054 Left pneumothorax accompanying a tension gastrothorax.

1055

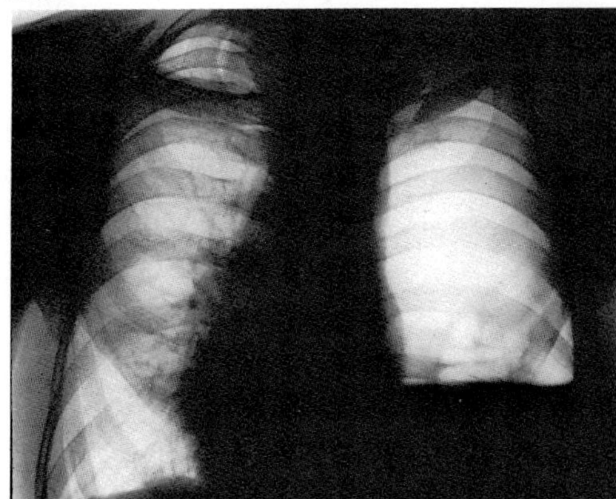

Z.G. ♂ 6 Nov. 1930

1055 Tension left pneumothorax accompanying a moderate colothorax.

Rupture of the left hemidiaphragm

Rupture of the left hemidiaphragm accompanies 4% of all severe thoracic injuries, and 11% of thoraco-abdominal injuries.

The average age of our patients is 42 years (ranging from 4 to 82 years). Four out of five are in shock on admission.

1056 Localisation, extent and direction of left-sided rupture and/or avulsion (seen from above). (n = 59)

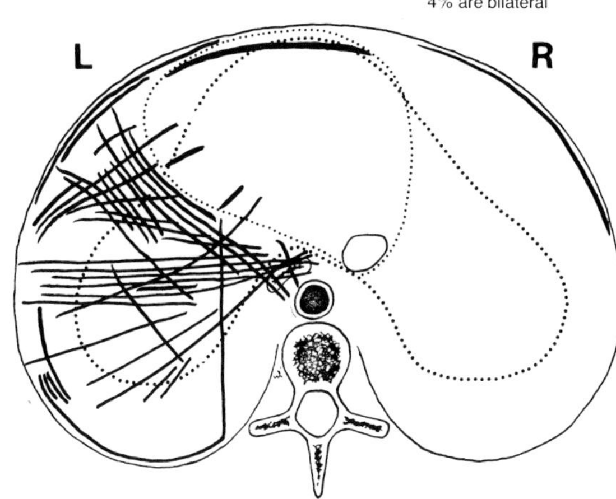

1057 Two-layer suturing of ruptured left hemidiaphragm through laparotomy.

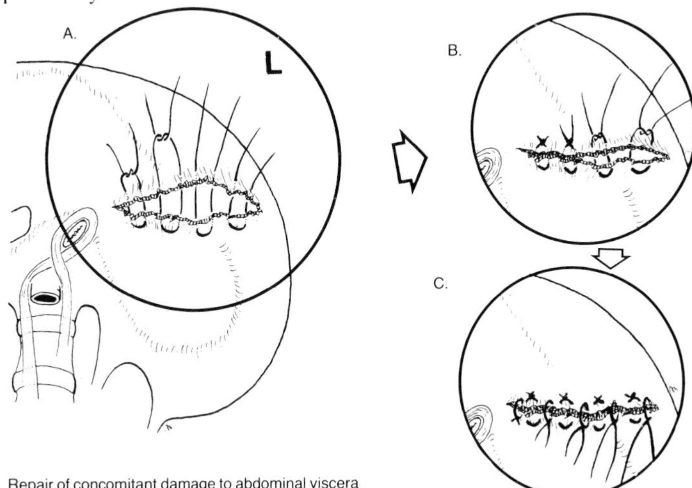

A. Repair of concomitant damage to abdominal viscera
B. Toilet and drainage of the left pleural cavity, with examination of the pericardium
C. Two-layer suturing (vicryl)

The types of accident are as follows:

		Incidence
road accident		75%
car	54%	
(motor) cycle	11%	
pedestrian	10%	
crush-injury		10%
fall from a height		9%
violent blow or explosion		6%

Rupture is:
- transverse (frontal impact) in 50% of our cases,
- sagittal (lateral impact) in 31% of our cases,
- oblique (oblique impact) in 19% of our cases (see **1036, 1037**).

Neither the direction nor the localisation of a rupture has any bearing on its prognosis. The direction, however, does give some indication of possible associated injuries (see Volume I, **300**).

Diagnosis is basically a matter of X-ray – either a standard chest X-ray or an oesophagogastric contrast study; if the initial film is negative, fresh films should be taken at least once a day until a definite diagnosis is possible. Rupture of the diaphragm should be routinely suspected in any multiple injury patient who presents the typical associated injuries.

Most recent ruptures of the left hemidiaphragm can be sutured through laparotomy (see **1024**). Laparotomy not only provides for solid, two-layer repair of the diaphragm but also gives access to damaged abdominal viscera (see **1043** to **1046**). The alternative thoracic approach aggravates chest damage and makes anaesthetisation more hazardous.

Mortality of left diaphragmatic rupture in our cases is 36%.

Death is attributable to the diaphragmatic injury in 17% of cases (directly in 7%, indirectly in 10%) and to some other cause in 19% of cases.

Gastrothorax

1058

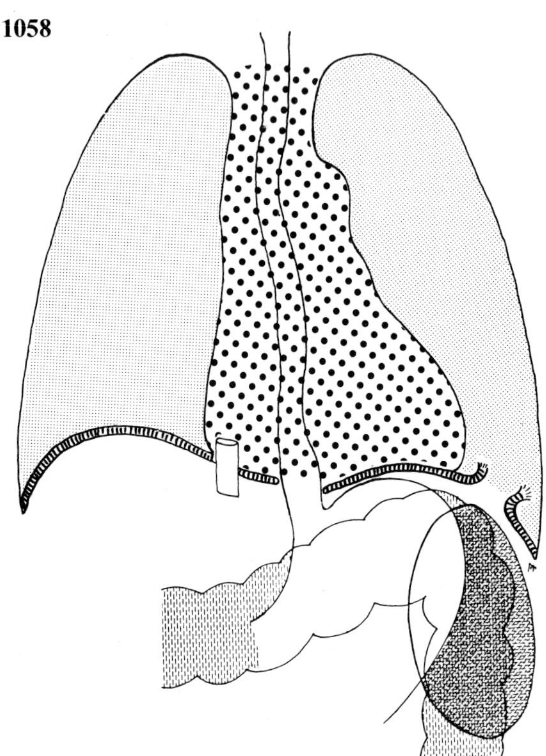

1058 **Rupture of the left hemidiaphragm without herniation of abdominal viscera.**

1059

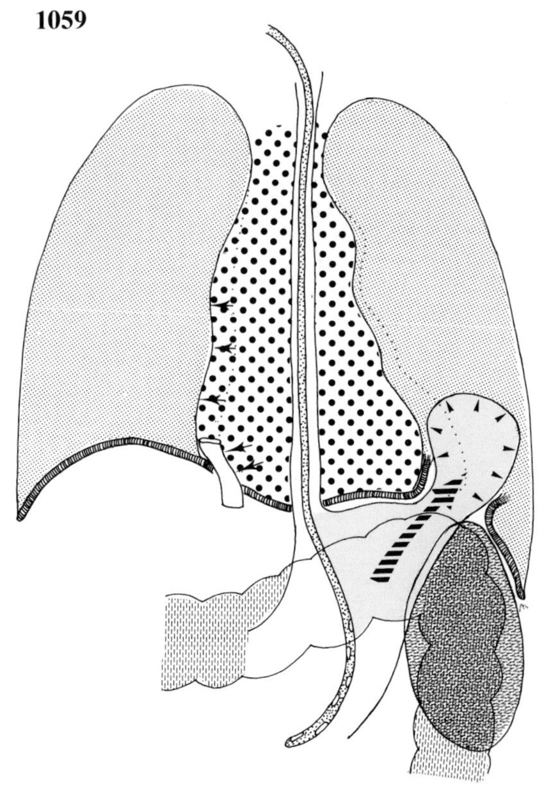

1059 **Moderate gastrothorax.**

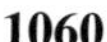

1060

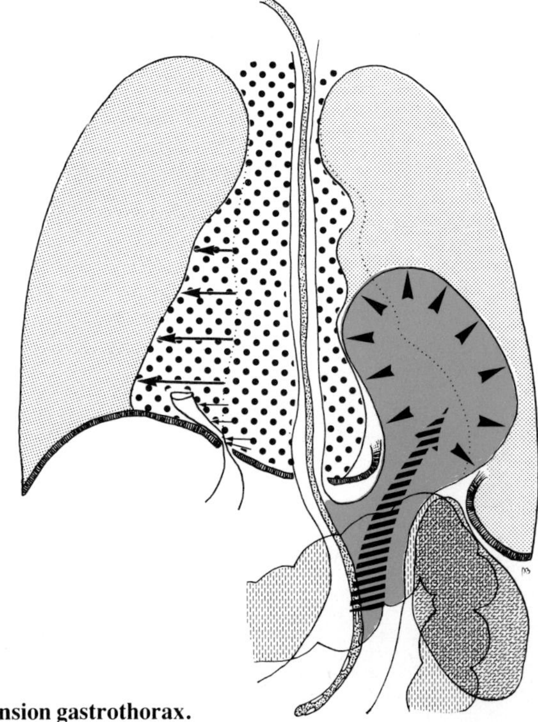

1060 **Tension gastrothorax.**

1061a

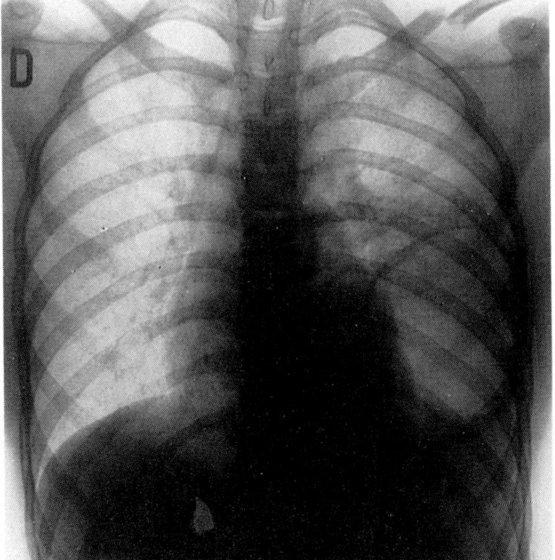

C.A. ♀ 15 yrs. 2 Aug. 1974

1061a Uncomplicated left gastrothorax accompanied by fractures of the clavicle and pelvis. The supine X-ray shows no mediastinal shift.
(Dr A. Keller, Payerne.)

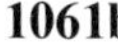

1061b

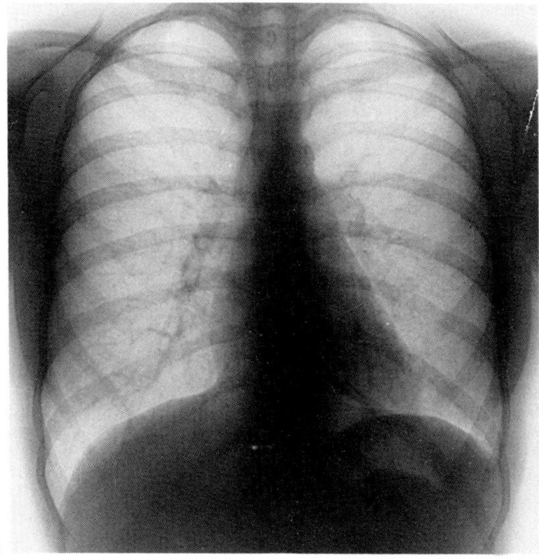

27 Aug. 1975

1061b Diaphragmatic repair. Recovery. Long-term follow-up.

1062

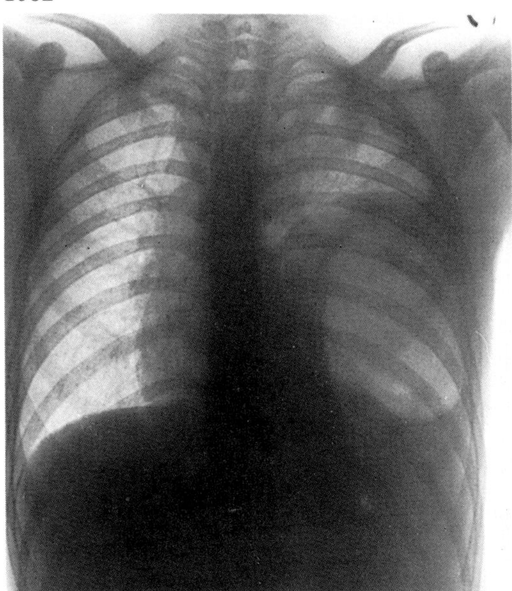

C.D. ♂ 11 yrs. 7 Oct. 1959

1062 Left gastrothorax accompanied by colothorax in a child crushed under the wheels of a cart.

In 76% of cases, rupture of the left hemidiaphragm is accompanied by a gastric hernia into the thorax (see **1026**).

In 38% of cases, the gastrothorax is initially uncomplicated; in 36%, it is already compressive on admission; in 2%, late strangulation occurs.

Undetected gastrothorax nearly always becomes compressive and seriously life-threatening. The build-up in pressure – the result of an intricate physiopathological mechanism – is usually swift and unforeseen. Resuscitatory efforts are inevitably harmful (see page 208).

In some cases, herniation causes immediate respiratory distress. In others, sudden herniation occurs later after an episode of agitation, coughing, vomiting, hiccoughing, sneezing or defecation. The pressure gradient between the abdomen and the thorax varies between 7 and 20cm of water during normal respiration, but it may rise to 100cm of water during deep breathing or coughing, and to over 240cm of water during vomiting. Although, as far as we know, there are no corroborating experimental data, it seems likely that the gradient is still higher during trauma.

Physiopathological consequences of intrathoracic gastric herniation

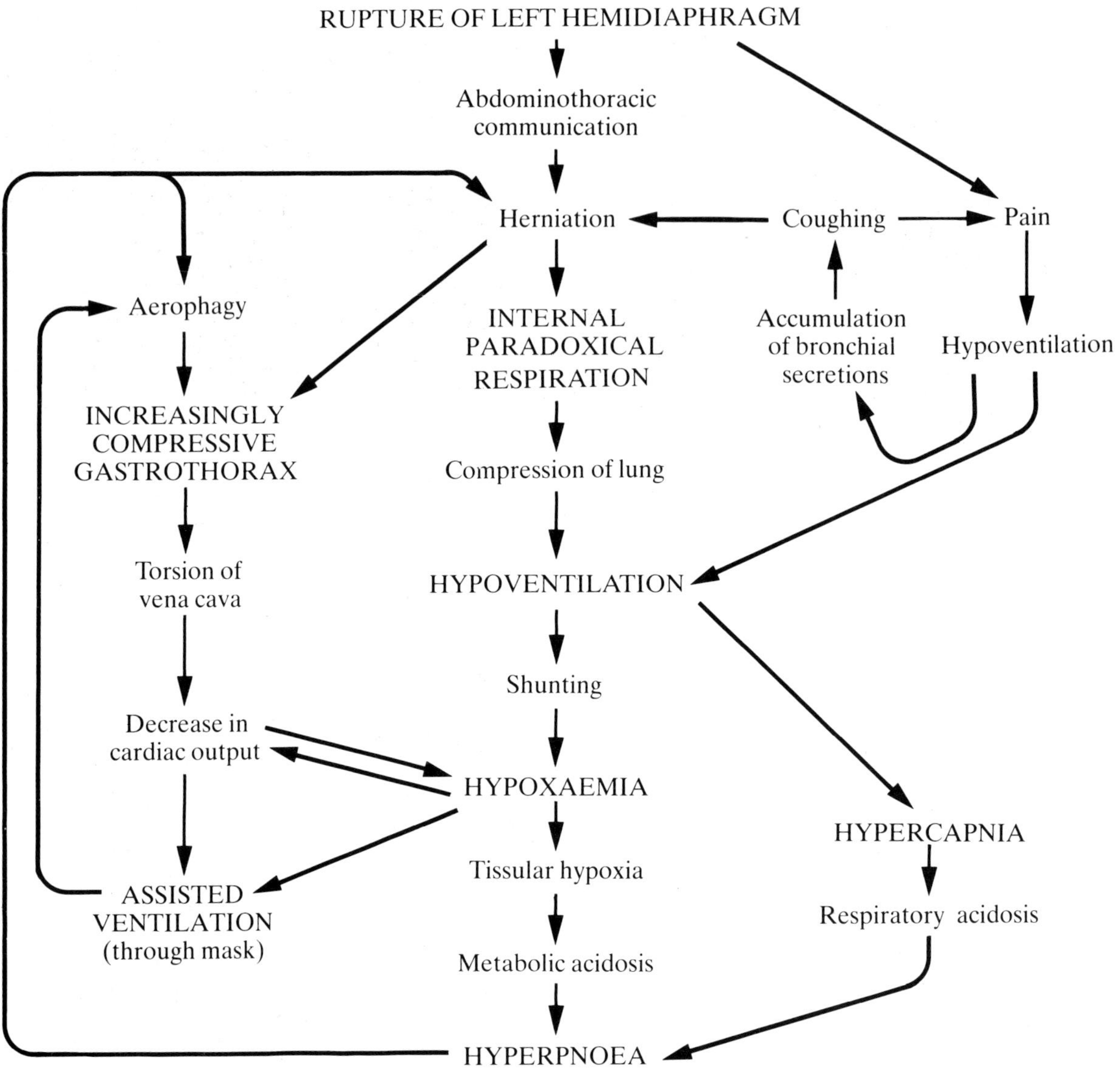

Tension gastrothorax has the same basic clinical manifestations as tension pneumothorax (see Volume I, page 260). However, certain additional factors make it even more dangerous.

Its immediate repercussions are:

- arteriovenous shunting in collapsed pulmonary territory; this hinders haematosis;
- mediastinal shift that hampers venous return and reduces cardiac output;
- acid-base imbalance due to partial strangulation of the herniated digestive organs.

These physiopathological disturbances are often complicated by accompanying injuries to the brain (contusion, coma), abdominal viscera (hypovolaemic shock) or extremities (fat embolism after multiple fractures).

Only rarely (see **1027, 1041c**) is it possible to decompress tension gastrothorax through a nasogastric tube. In general, the diaphragmatic crura remain intact and create an angle which the tube cannot negotiate (see **1059**).

Fibroscopic decompression of gastrothorax is not to be recommended; the preliminary oesophagogastric insufflation inevitably aggravates the hernia.

In an extreme case or in the absence of the necessary surgical facilities, a massively compressive gastrothorax could be drained (immediately before anaesthetisation) through anterolateral transthoracic puncture with a large-bore needle or a pleural catheter.

1063a

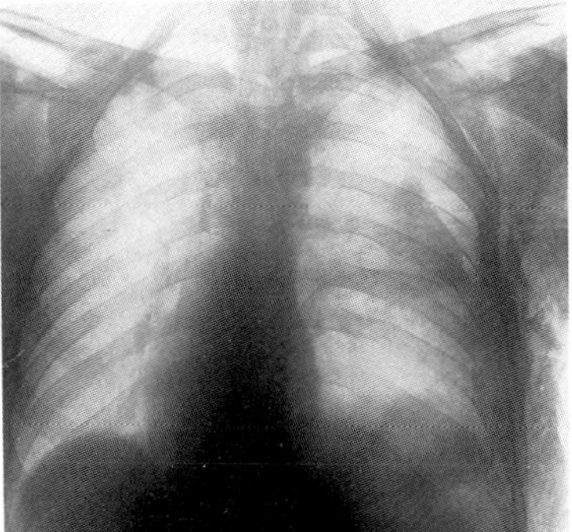

G.G. ♂ 24 yrs. 8 Mar. 1973

1063a Gaseous tension gastrothorax in the driver of a car hit by a train. The diaphragm and the left pericardial wall have ruptured. A tension gastrothorax displaces the mediastinum.

1063b

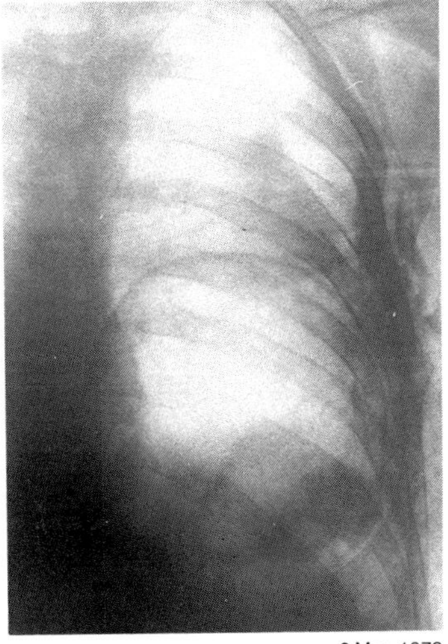

8 Mar. 1973

1063b The gastrothorax in close-up.

1063c

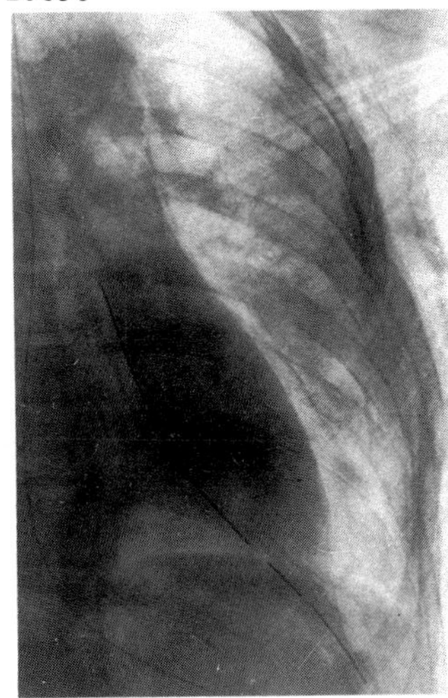

8 Mar. 1973

1063c Laparotomy: reduction of the stomach, splenectomy for a ruptured spleen, and closure of the left hemidiaphragm. The postoperative film shows mediastinal emphysema due to a pulmonary laceration which will have to be sutured through a thoracotomy 5 days later.

1064a

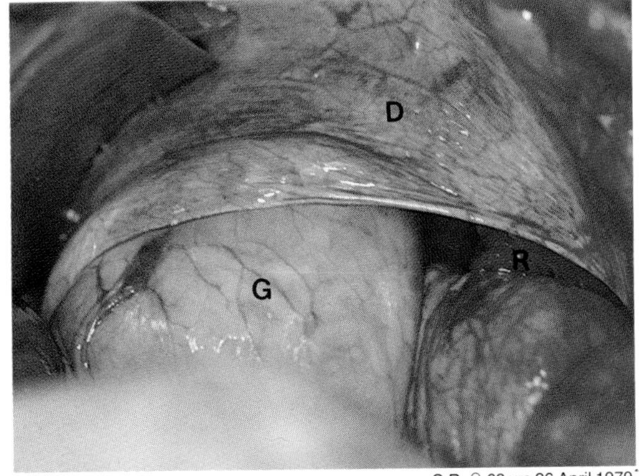

C.R. ♀ 63 yrs 26 April 1979

1064b

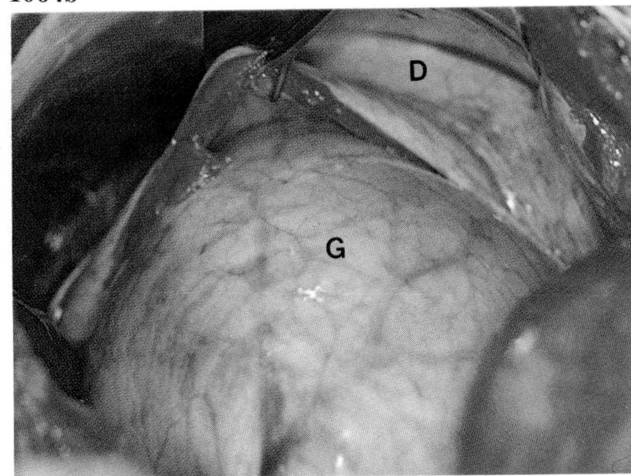

1064a-d Tension gastrothorax (G) seen through laparotomy during repositioning of the stomach. The rupture of diaphragm (D) is transverse. Spleen (R) is slightly injured.

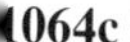

1064c

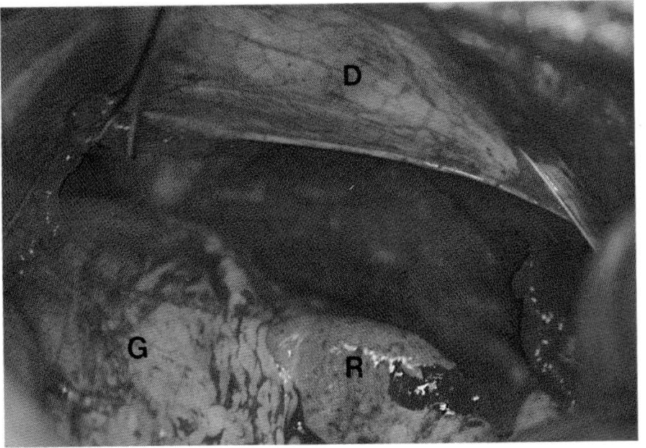

1064d

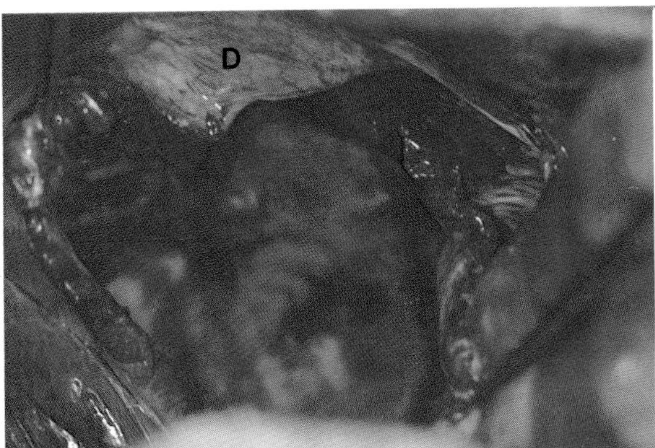

1065a

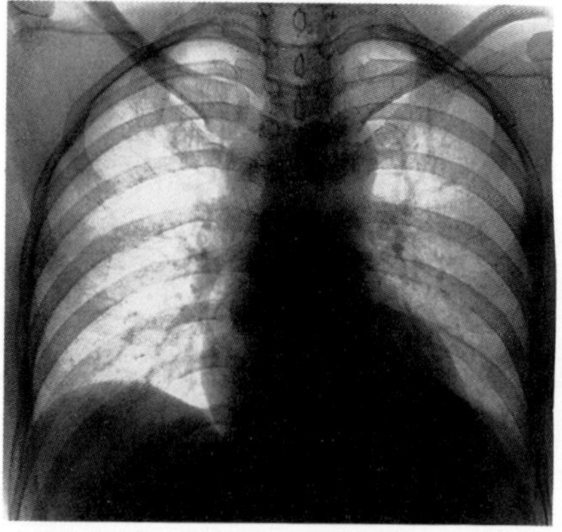

G.S. ♂ 31 yrs. 10 Jan. 1976

1065b

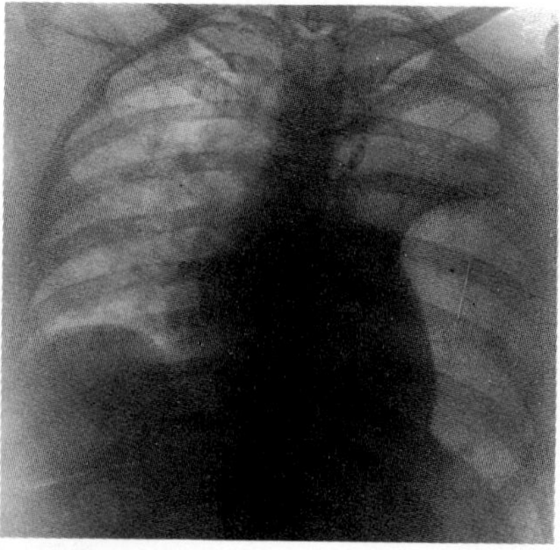

13 Jan. 1976

1065a Sudden gastrothorax on removal of Levin tube. Admission X-ray. The pelvis is fractured. (Dr M. Rigo, Monthey.)

1065b Removal of the Levin tube 3 days later is followed by acute gastric dilatation and transdiaphragmatic herniation of the stomach. Respiratory distress. Laparotomy, reduction and diaphragmatic repair. Recovery. (See also **1051**.)

1066a

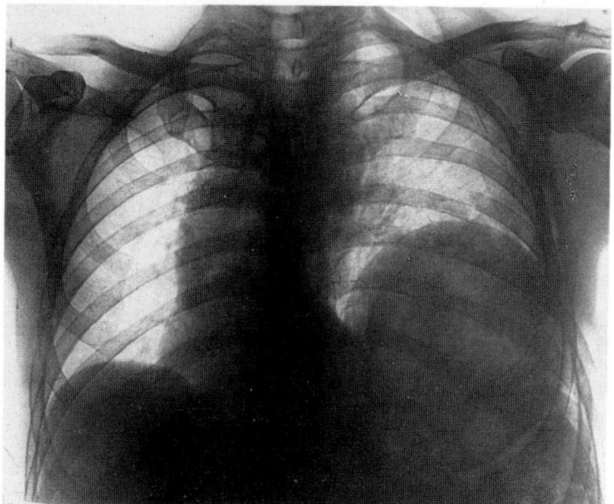

R.C. ♂ 53 yrs 17 Sep. 1961

1066b

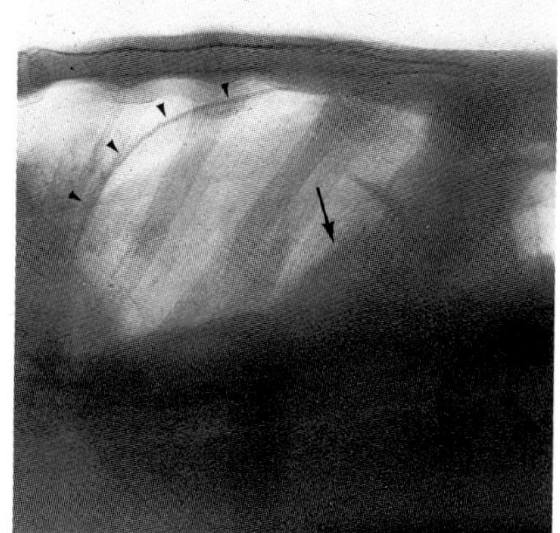

18 Sep. 1961

1066c

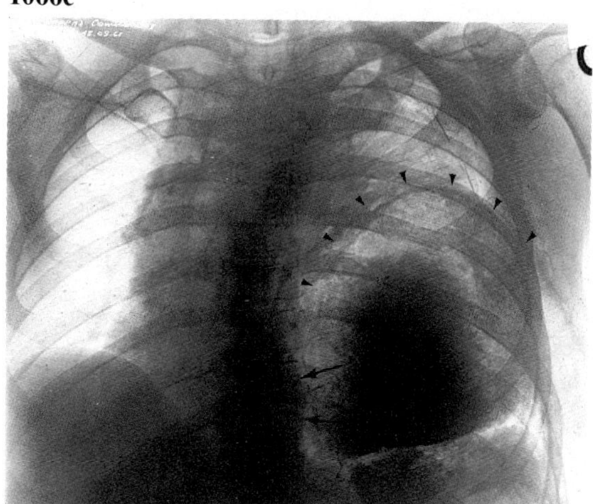

18 Sep. 1961

1066d

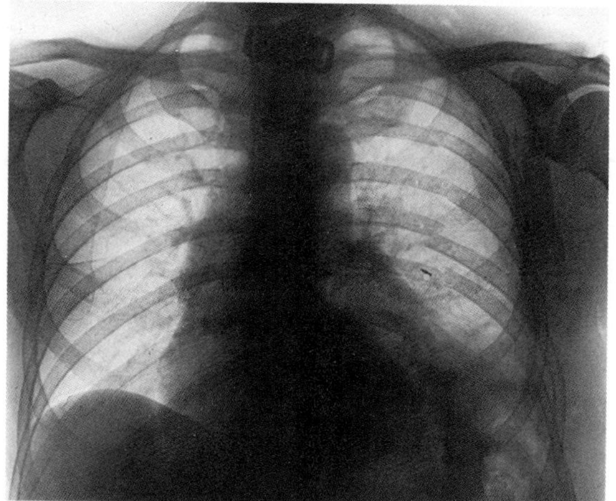

26 Sep. 1961

1066a Liquid tension gastrothorax. Supine X-ray. Rightward displacement of the mediastinum hampers venous return in the inferior vena cava.

1066b Lateral supine view: the stomach (→) is in contact with the anterior thoracic wall. The heart (**→**) is depressed.

1066c Contrast study: dye does not fully diffuse in the stomach because the patient is still in the supine position. → show the actual limit of the intrathoracic portion of the stomach. The heart (**→**) is further depressed.

1066d Left thoracotomy, repair. Recovery.

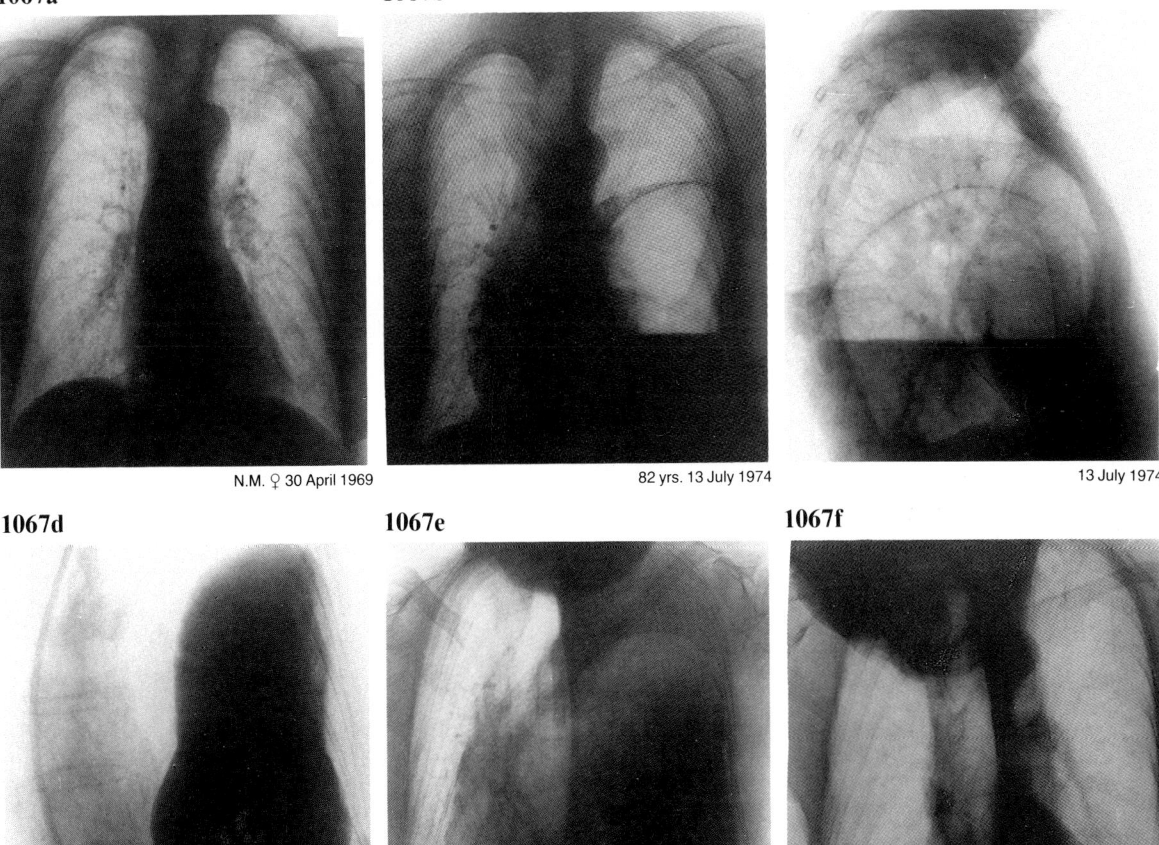

1067a — N.M. ♀ 30 April 1969

1067b — 82 yrs. 13 July 1974

1067c — 13 July 1974

1067d — 13 July 1974

1067e — 15 July 1974

1067f — 30 July 1974

1067a Late diagnosis of tension gastrothorax in an 82-year-old woman. Before the accident, the chest is normal.

1067b The patient was the passenger in a car accident. An impact to her right side ruptures the left hemi-diaphragm, causing a gastrothorax. Upright anterior view . . .

1067c . . . and lateral view.

1067d Corroborative contrast study.

1067e Volvulus of the stomach increases over the next 2 days.

1067f Laparotomy 3 days after the accident. Reduction of the stomach and closure of the diaphragm. Recovery.

Colothorax

In our experience, 49% of ruptures of the left hemidiaphragm lead to herniation of the colon. The length of intestine that migrates into the thorax varies.

Tension colothorax occurs in 2% of cases.

1068

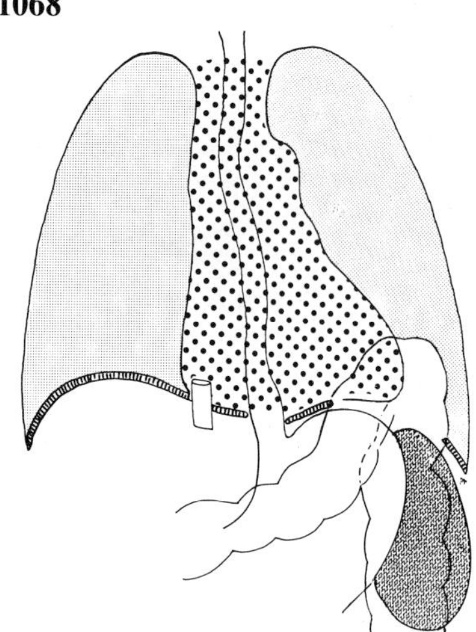

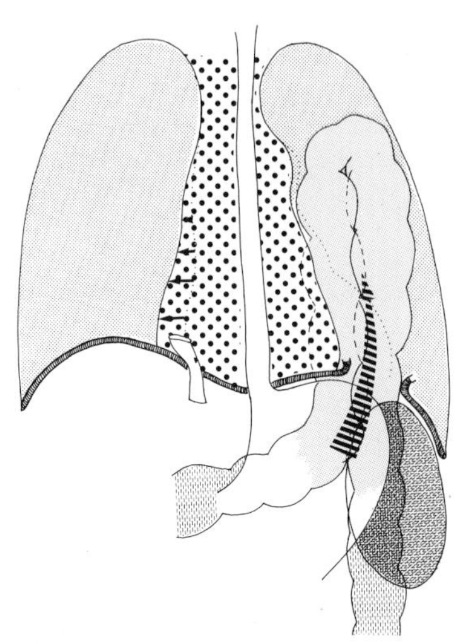

1070

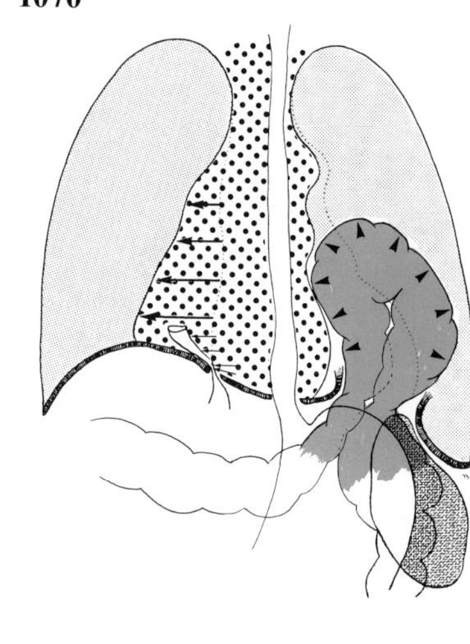

1068 **Moderate left colothorax.**

1069 **Massive left colothorax.**

1070 **Tension left colothorax.**

1071

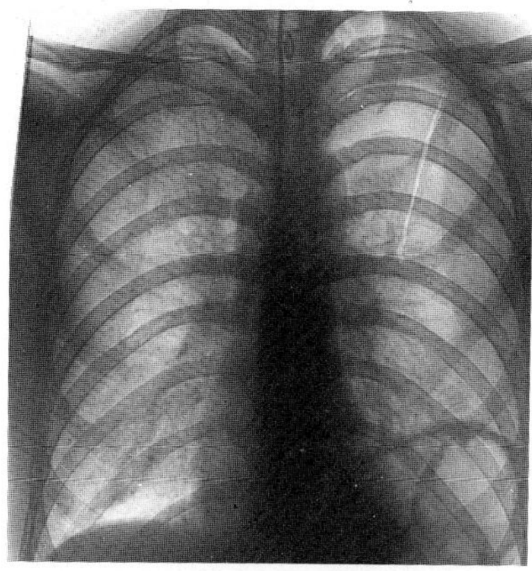

G.A. ♂ 23 yrs. 21 May 1951

1071 **Moderate left colothorax with pneumothorax**.

1072

H.M. ♀ 72 yrs. 6 Sep. 1967

1072 **Large left colothorax**. Standard X-ray.

1073

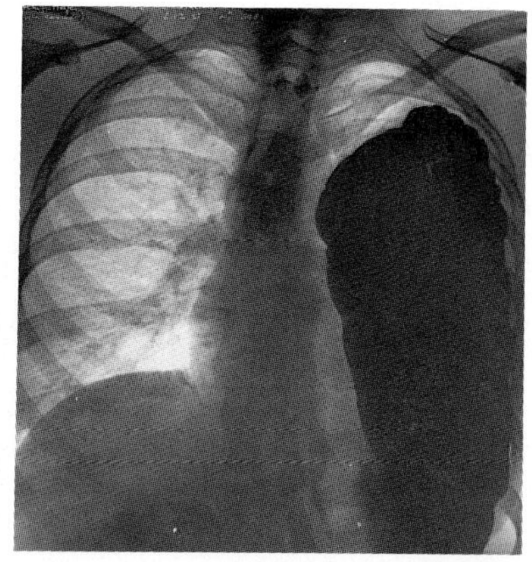

M.Y. ♀ 27 yrs. 6 Dec. 1957

1073 Undetected **massive left colothorax** well tolerated for 1½ years. Left thoracotomy for reduction and repair (see **1125** and Volume I, **73**).

1074a

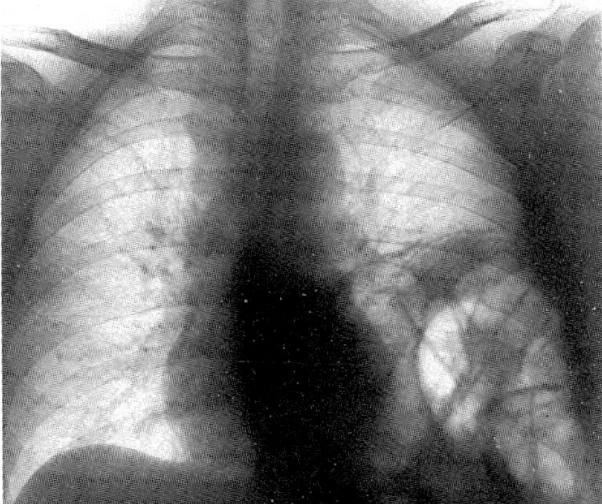

D.A. ♂ 46 yrs. 29 Aug. 1968

1074a Colothorax and herniation of small intestine in a farmer crushed under a tractor. Rupture of the left hemidiaphragm with herniation of the splenic flexure of the colon and of the small bowel.

1074b

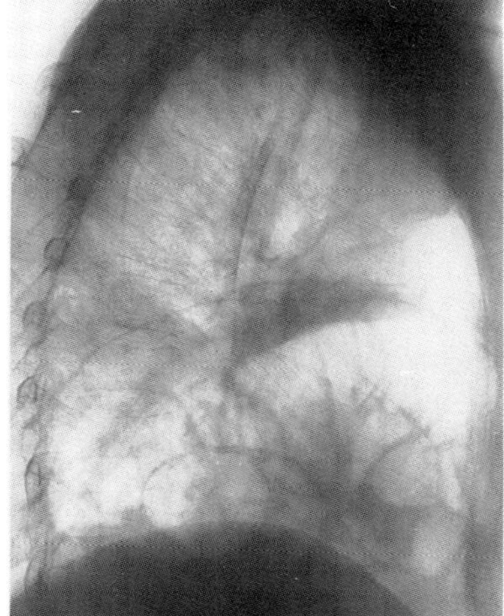

29 Aug. 1968

1074b Lateral X-ray. There is no gastrothorax because of a Billroth II type gastric resection performed 8 years previously.

1075a

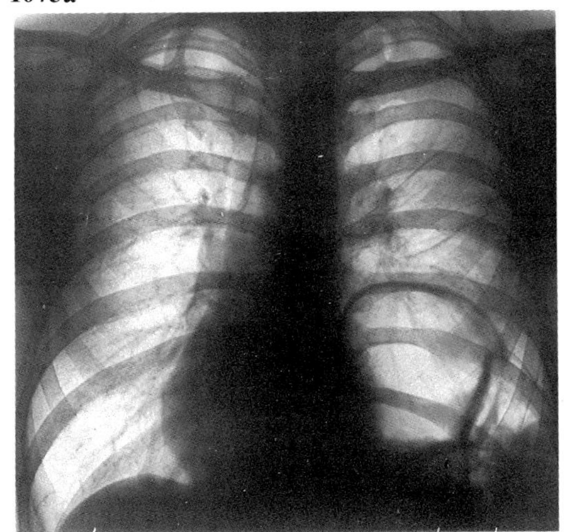

G.M. ♂ 26 yrs. 23 May 1944

1075a Tension left colothorax due to violent compression between the buffers of two railway carriages. The mediastinum is displaced to the right. The patient recovered but the diaphragmatic rupture passed unnoticed. Nine years later, in another hospital, the rupture was recognised but not repaired.

1075b X-ray 26 years after the accident.

1075c Lateral X-ray. For barium enema, see Volume I, **60**. Thoracotomy, repair. Recovery.

1075b

3 Feb. 1970

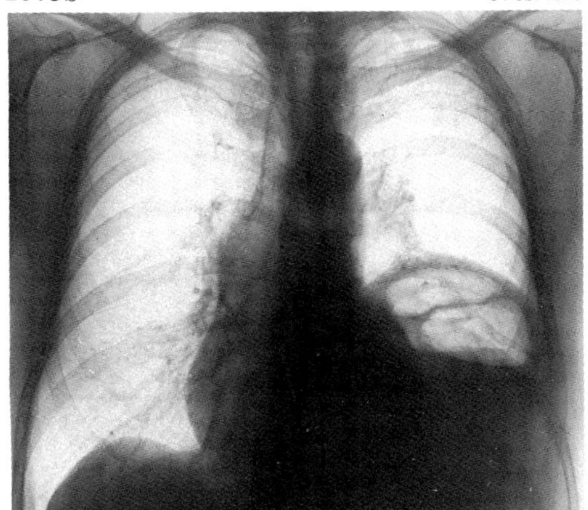

1075c

3 Feb. 1970

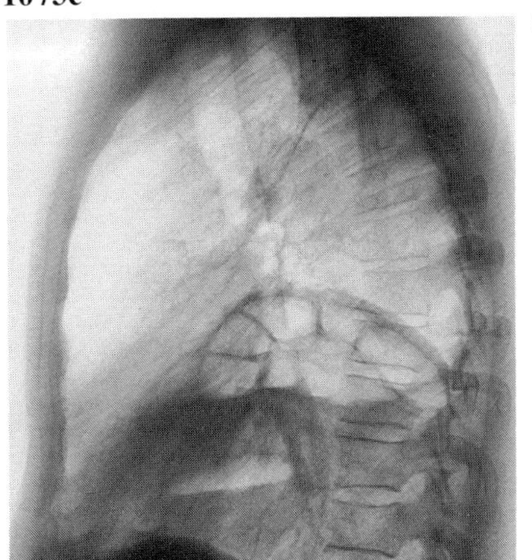

Splenothorax

According to our figures, 38% of large ruptures and peripheral avulsions of the left hemidiaphragm result in combined herniation of the stomach and spleen.

In half of these cases, the spleen remained intact (see **1078** and Volume I, **366b**). In the other half it burst, either as a result of the impact or of direct laceration by a fractured rib (see **1080, 1085**). The resultant haemothorax ranged from slight to severe (see **1079**).

Surgery is often the only way of establishing diagnosis. The surgical indication usually consists of:

- an output of blood through the drainage system of more than 300 ml per hour;
- the swift recurrence of the haemothorax if and when the drain becomes blocked;
- residual thoracic opacities after initially successful drainage (partial clotting or herniation of digestive organs);
- an associated gastrothorax (see Volume I, **362**).

Sometimes the spleen ruptures within the abdomen and bleeds into the thorax through a small tear in the diaphragm (a tear caused by a fractured rib, for example) (see **1121**). This possibility is often neglected (see Volume I, page 279), but is worth keeping in mind (see **1087** and Volume I, **571**).

1076 Tension left spleno-gastrothorax.

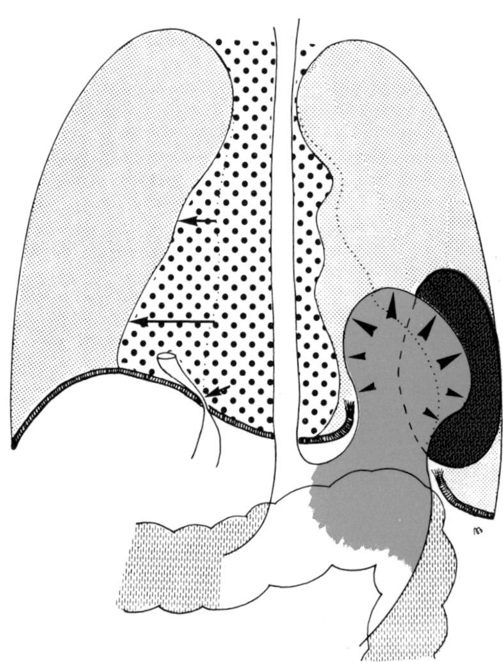

1077 Tension left spleno-gastrothorax with haemothorax due to rupture or laceration of spleen.

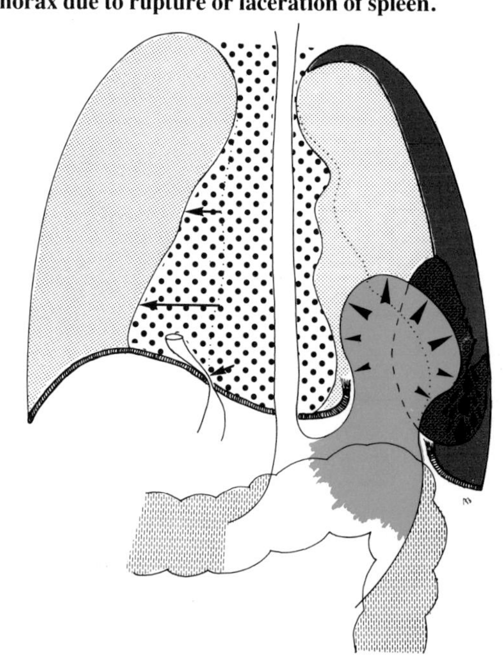

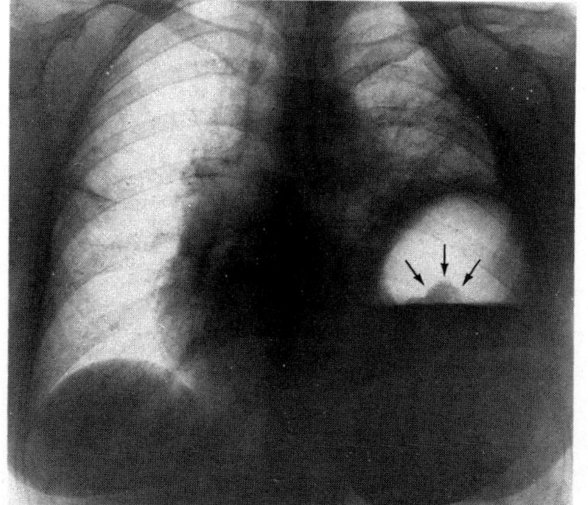

1078

1078 Thoracic herniation of intact spleen. The apex of the spleen (→) can be seen through a tension gastrothorax. There is no haemothorax. Laparotomy, repair. Recovery.

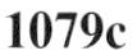

1079a

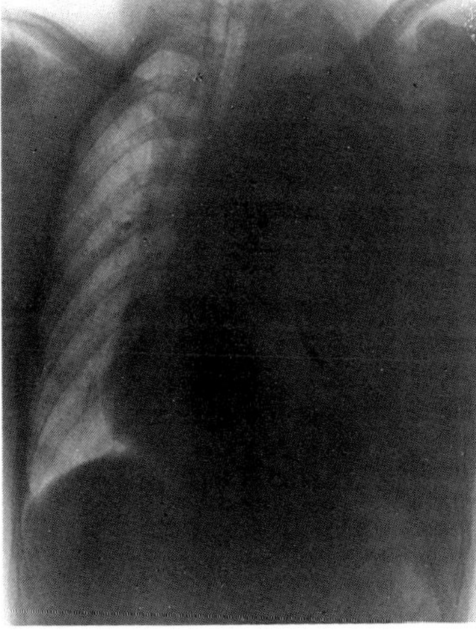

M.G. ♂ 20 yrs. 16 July 1972

1079b

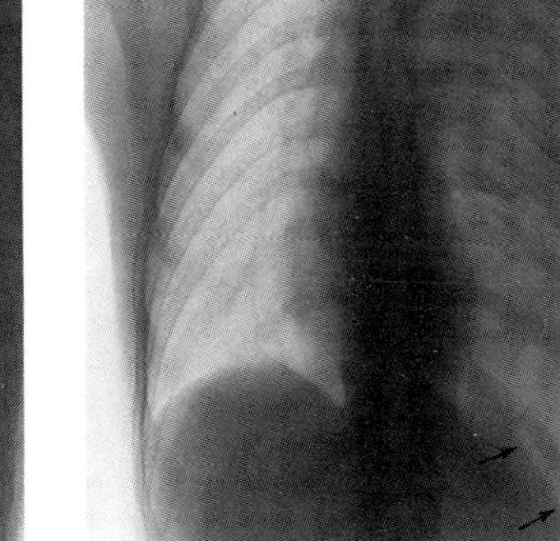

16 July 1972

1079c

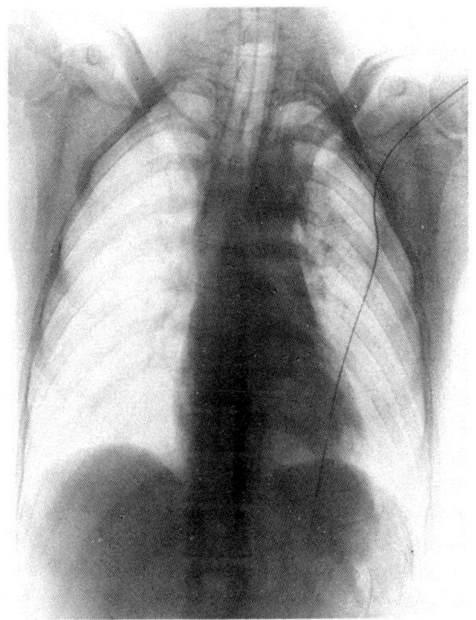

16 July 1972

1079d

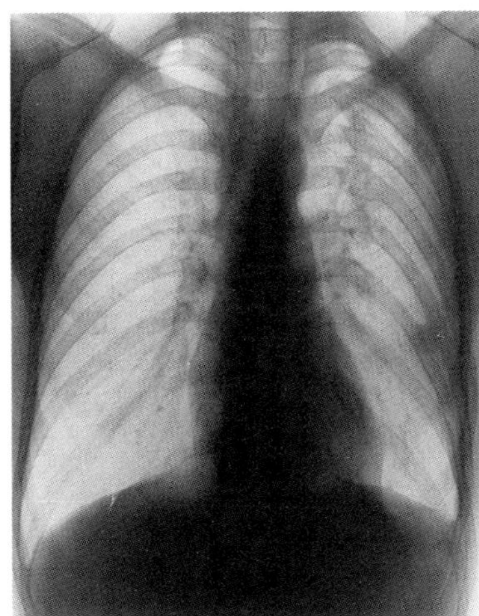

12 Oct. 1973

1079a Thoracic herniation of ruptured spleen. Admission X-ray of a car driver thrown from his car at high speed. There is a massive left haemothorax.

1079b The slight displacement of the mediastinum persists after drainage of the haemothorax. The opacities in the left lower chest are due to an intestinal hernia. The left hemidiaphragm is inverted (→).

1079c Emergency laparotomy: palpation of the thoracic viscera reveals no damage; splenectomy; closure of the diaphragm; drainage of a pancreatic contusion. Recovery.

1079d Long-term follow-up.

1080

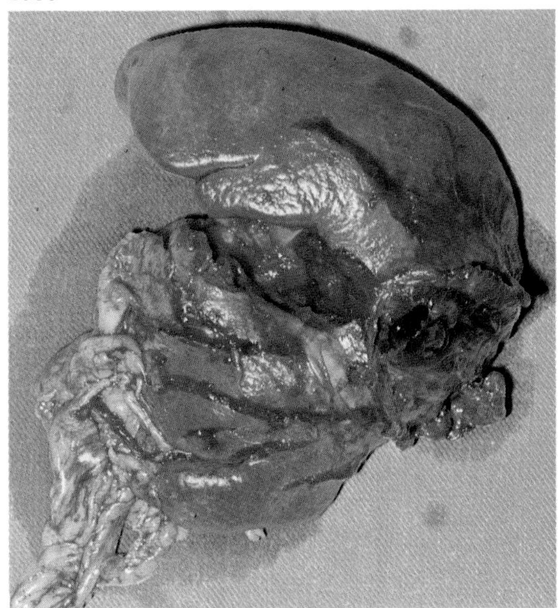

W.S. ♂ 23 yrs. 6 June 1968

1080 Diaphragmatic rupture with multiple direct lacerations of spleen by fractured ribs. A splenectomy was performed three weeks after the trauma. The main laceration is sealed by blood clots but several others remain open (see **1085**).

Composite herniae

Composite herniae are frequently encountered. In many cases the hernia is large and under tension. The standard diagnostic and therapeutic dicta are applicable (see page 205).

1081

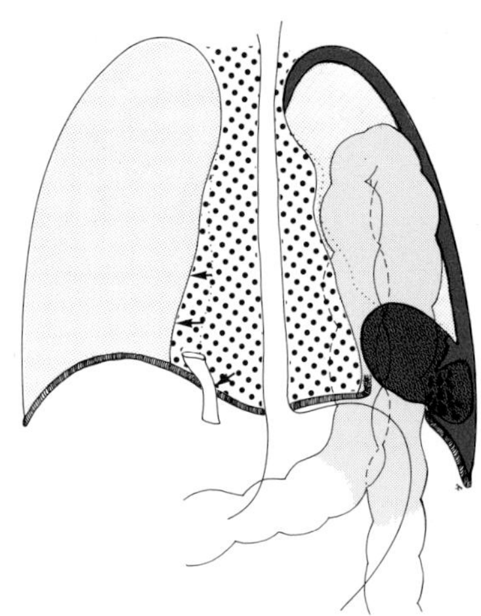

1082

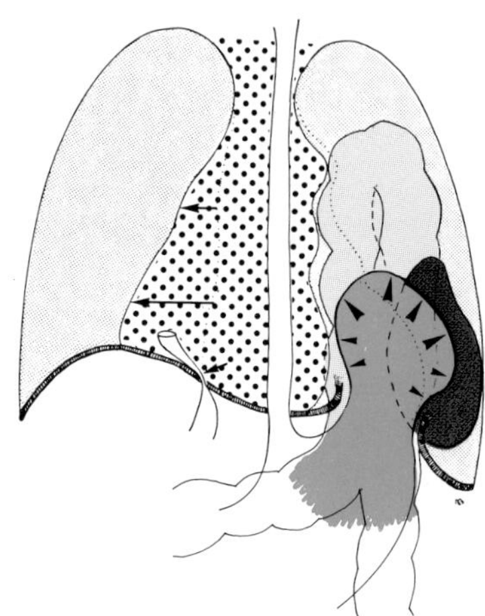

1083

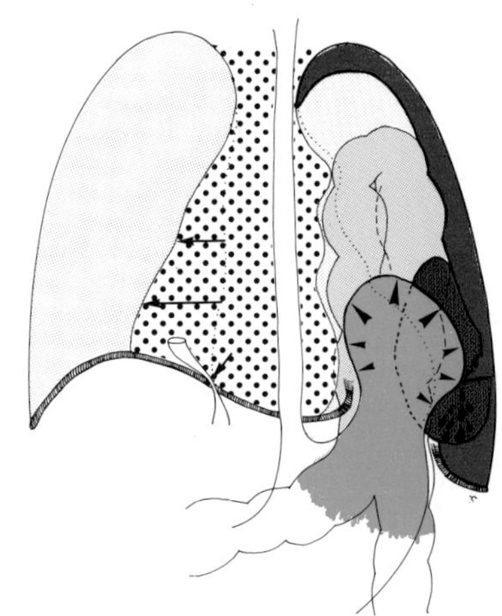

1081 Left spleno-colothorax with haemothorax due to rupture of spleen.

1082 Tension left colo-spleno-gastrothorax.

1083 Tension left colo-spleno-gastrothorax with haemothorax due to rupture of spleen.

1084

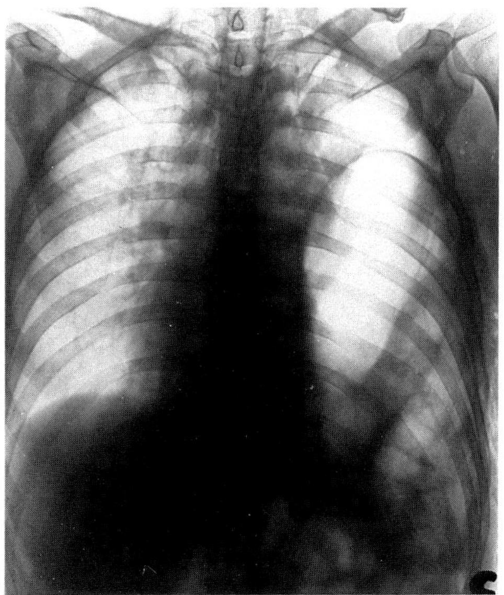

T.E. ♂ 44 yrs. 16 Nov. 1958

1084 Traumatic herniation of stomach, colon, spleen, small bowel and omentum in a mountaineer who fell on to rocks. Death from severe multiple injuries 12 days after the diaphragm was closed through a thoracotomy. *N.B. Today, an abdominal approach would have been preferred.*

1085a

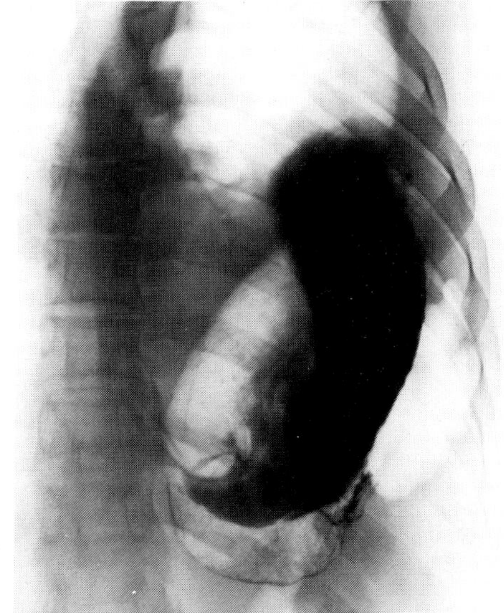

W.S. ♂ 23 yrs. 25 May 1968

1085a Rupture of left hemidiaphragm with composite herniae that passed undetected for 3 weeks. Contrast study 5 days after a serious car accident. The gastrothorax (with volvulus) is not recognised.

1085b 25 May 1968

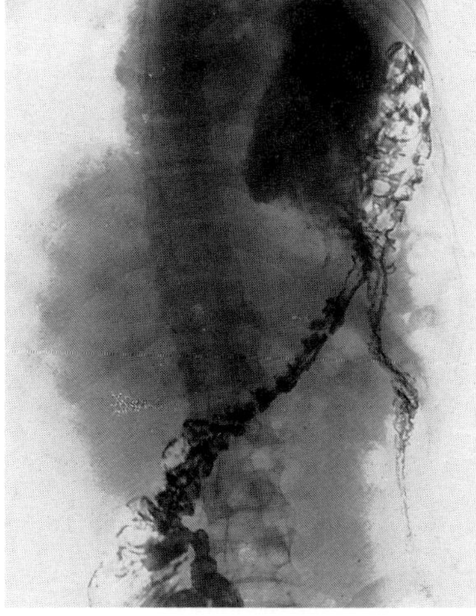

1085c

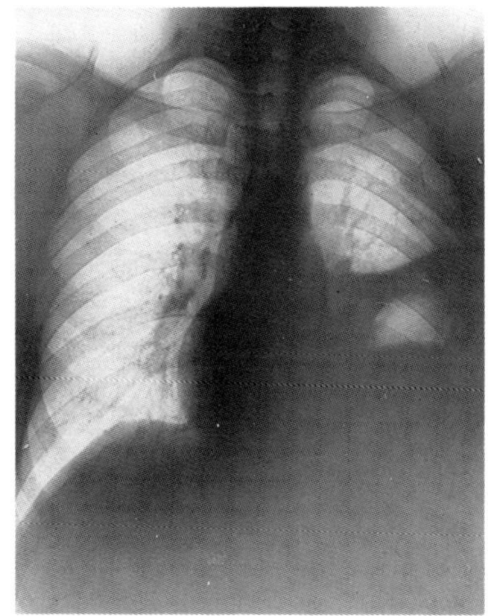

1 June 1968

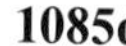

1085d

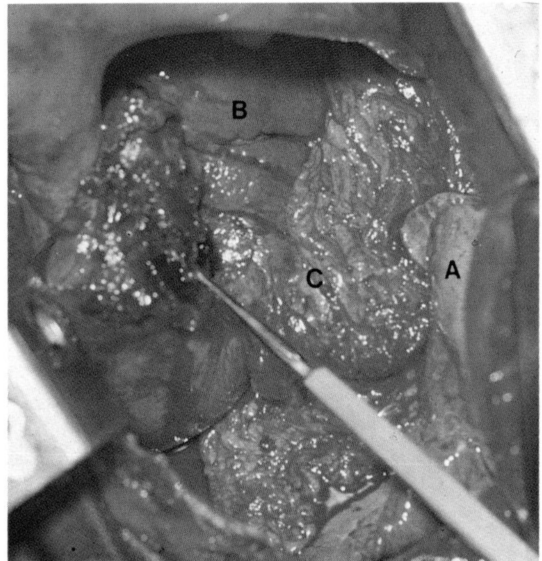

6 June 1968

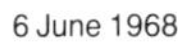

1085b A simultaneous barium enema study is made.

1085c Standard, upright X-ray 12 days after the accident.

1085d Thoracotomy 3 weeks later. The lung (A) is displaced by the spleen (B) and omentum (C). The spleen displays several lacerations; the largest (dissector) is sealed by a clot (see **1080**).

1085e Further exploration exposes the small bowel (D), the stomach (E) and the colon (F). The left lobe of the liver (G) is visible through the diaphragmatic rupture (→).

1085f The rupture after reduction of the abdominal viscera.

1085e

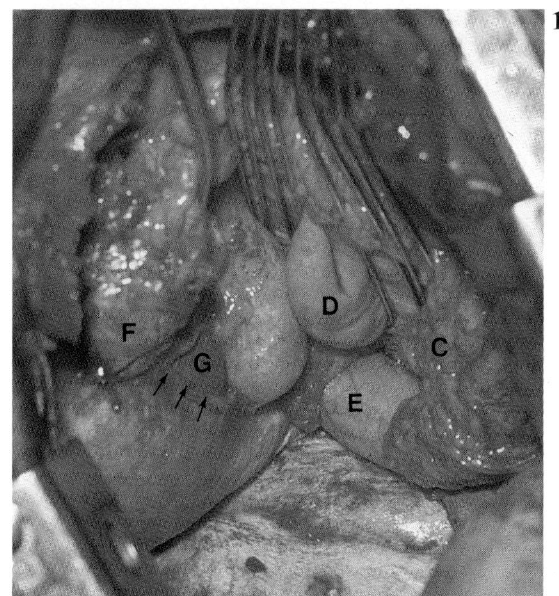

6 June 1968

1085f

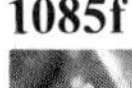

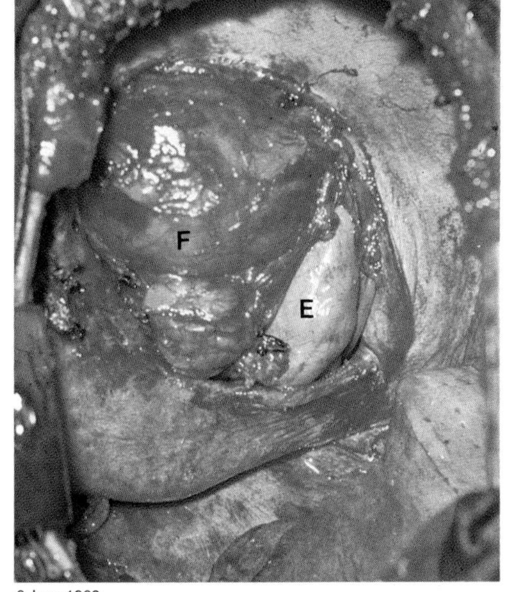

6 June 1968

Transdiaphragmatic haemothorax

Unless there are obvious abdominal signs, transdiaphragmatic haemothorax is usually only diagnosed on surgery.

According to our observations, 4% of diaphragmatic ruptures, many of them tears from fractured ribs, give rise to a transdiaphragmatic haemothorax (see **1085, 1087, 1121** and Volume I, **571**).

Surgical repair is easiest through an abdominal approach. The need for careful pleural toilet and drainage sometimes poses problems.

1086

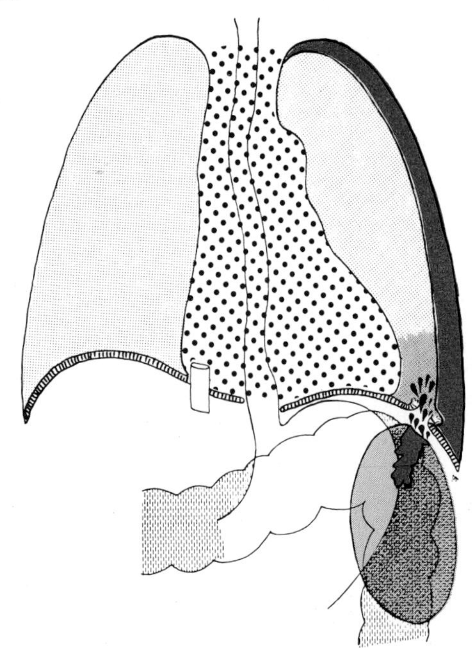

1086 Left haemothorax due to rupture of spleen and diaphragm, or to transdiaphragmatic laceration of spleen.

1087a

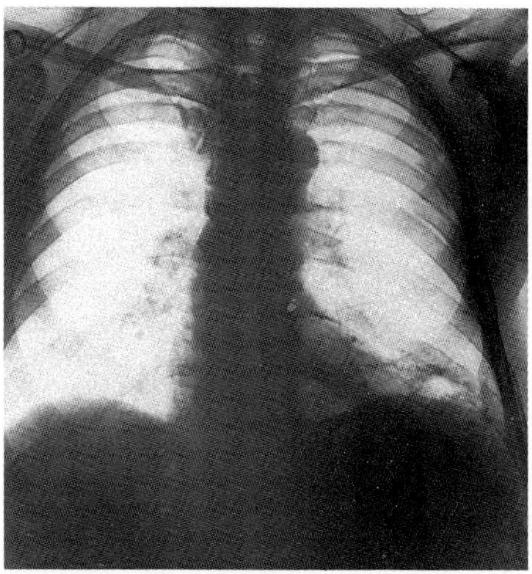

H.J. ♂ 62 yrs. 5 July 1973

1087b

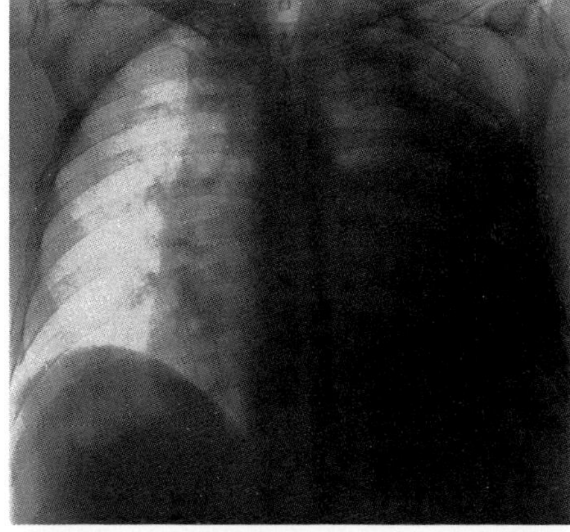

10 July 1973

1087c

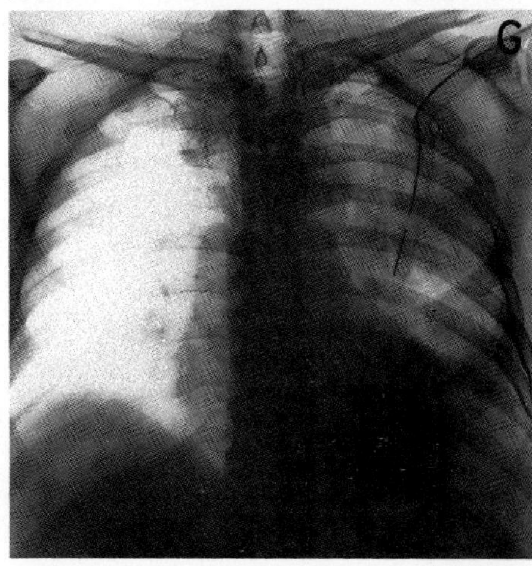

10 July 1973

1087a Transdiaphragmatic haemothorax after a rupture of the diaphragm. The patient was crushed against a wall by a cart.

1087b Shock develops due to a 1500 ml haemothorax.

1087c The haemothorax is partially evacuated by intercostal drainage.

1087d

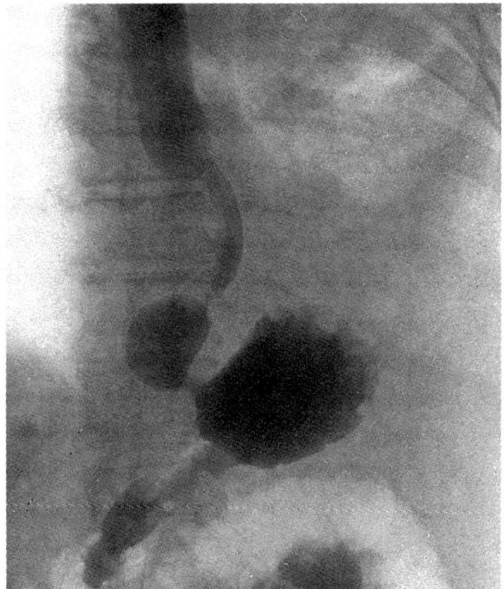

1087d A contrast study shows that the stomach is still within the abdomen. A laparotomy reveals that the haemothorax was entirely attributable to a ruptured spleen. Splenectomy, pleural toilet, drainage, and closure of the diaphragm. Recovery.

Rupture of the right hemidiaphragm

Right-sided rupture of the diaphragm (0.8% of thoracic and 2.3% of thoraco-abdominal injuries is five times less frequent than left-sided rupture (see **1040**). The epidemiology is the same on both sides. There is one noteworthy difference, however. Although right-sided rupture is generally the result of a more violent accident, shock is often very much less significant.

Half of all right diaphragmatic injuries are treated late because diagnosis is often difficult.

1088

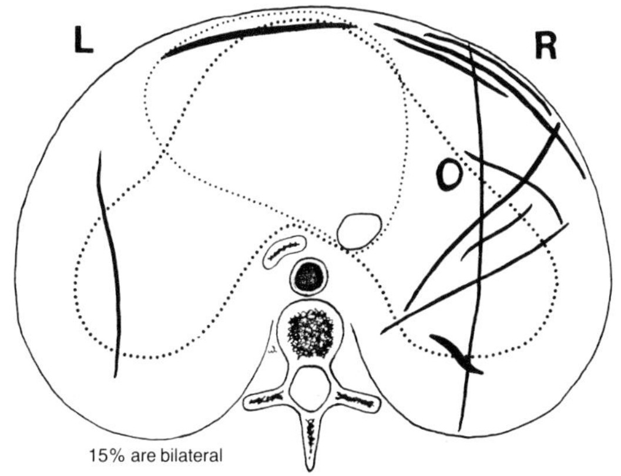

1088 Localisation, extent and direction of right-sided rupture (n = 13)

Rupture of the right hemidiaphragm is usually best approached through thoracotomy, though anterior peripheral avulsion is sometimes most easily managed through laparotomy. Some patients require a combined approach: two-thirds have at least one haemorrhagic injury to an abdominal viscus, and 70% have a laceration of a thoracic viscus (see **1024, 1043 to 1046**).

1089

1089 Two-layer suturing of right hemidiaphragm through thoracotomy.

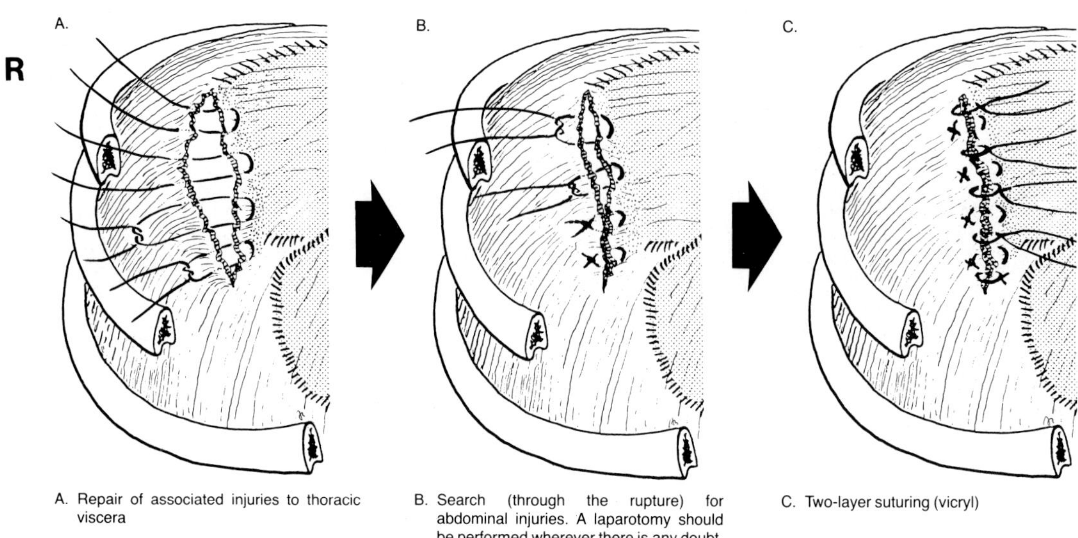

A. Repair of associated injuries to thoracic viscera

B. Search (through the rupture) for abdominal injuries. A laparotomy should be performed wherever there is any doubt

C. Two-layer suturing (vicryl)

Right-sided rupture is more serious than left-sided rupture and mortality is higher. In our material, mortality of right-sided rupture is 31%, death being directly attributable to the diaphragmatic injury in 16% of cases and indirectly to it in the remaining 15%.

Hepatothorax

In our experience, 54% of right-sided ruptures give rise to a hepatothorax (see **1047, 1110** and Volume I, **367, 569, 577**).

The extent of liver herniation is determined by the length of the diaphragmatic rupture: hepatothorax is complete in 46% of cases and partial or progressive in 8%.

Diagnosis on the basis of clinical examination is virtually impossible and the interpretation of X-rays is often difficult. A large opacity in the lower right thorax is more readily attributed to a haemothorax or to a pulmonary infarct than to a hepatothorax; an X-ray of the right hypochondrium showing intestinal air cannot be considered pathognomic. Diagnosis sometimes can be established through:

- a pneumoperitoneum,
- an angiogram,
- an intravenous cholecystogram (if the bladder opacifies),
- technetium liver scintigraphy,
- grey scale ultrasonography,
- computerised tomography.

Confirmation of a suspected hepatothorax is largely a matter of eliminating the other possibilities. A cryptogenic radiological opacity in the lower right lung requires circumspection: pleural tap on the easy assumption of a haemothorax can seriously damage herniated abdominal viscera.

Untreated, complete hepatothorax is very often fatal. Complications are quick to develop. Torsion of the pedicles occludes the inferior vena cava, causing progressive shock. The result is sometimes an acute Budd-Chiari syndrome (see opposite page). In cases of doubt, a short exploratory thoracotomy should be performed.

1090 Rupture of right hemidiaphragm with complete hepatothorax.

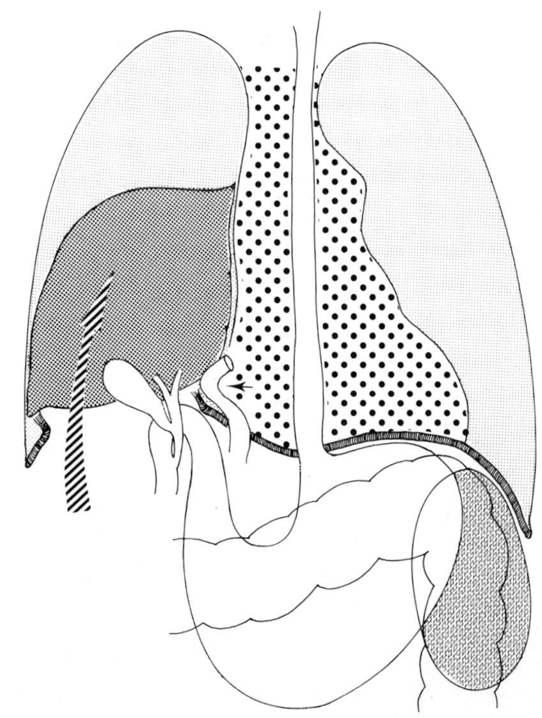

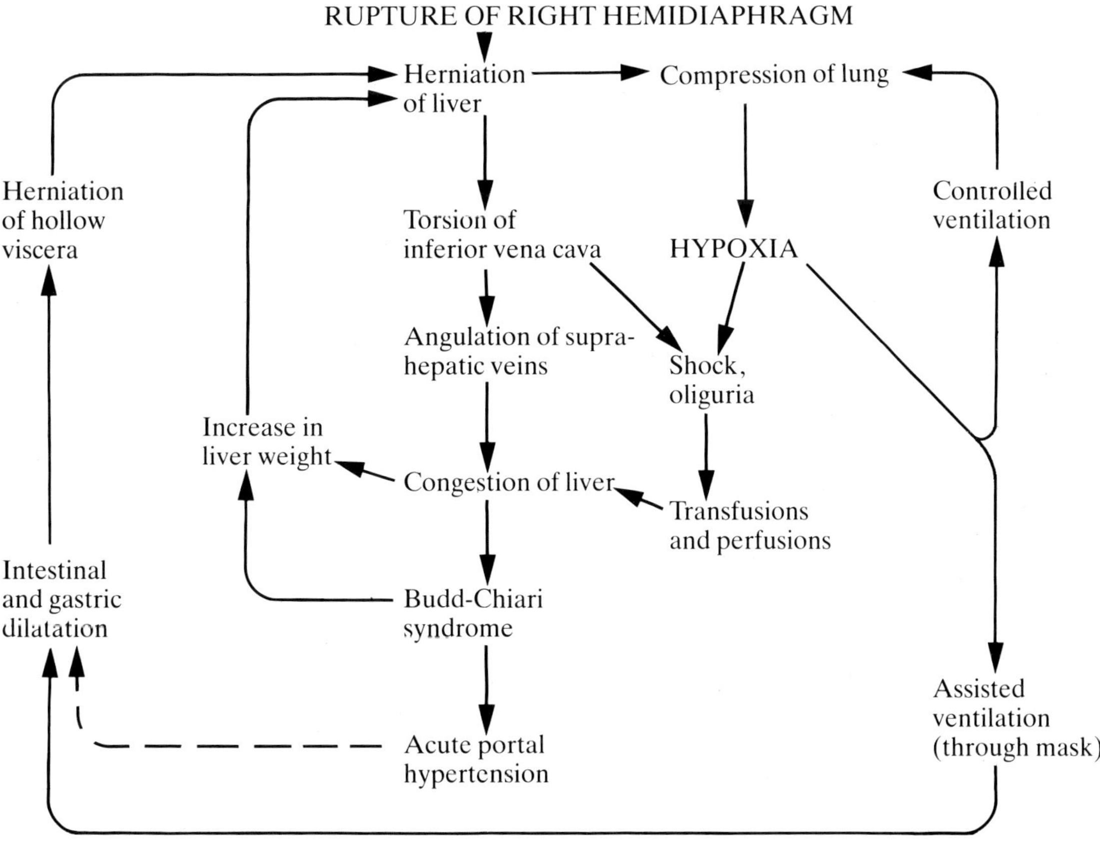

1091a

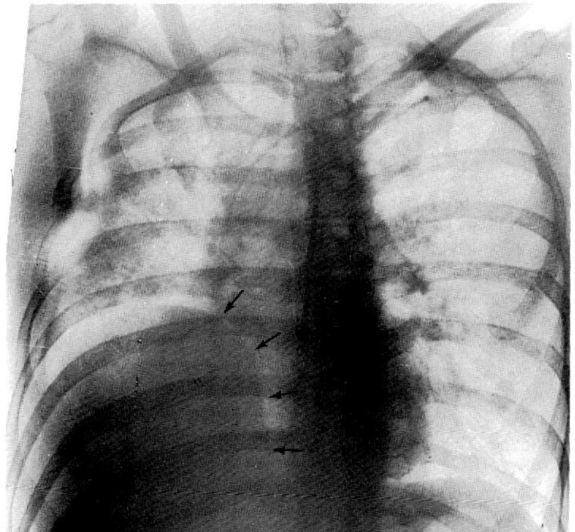

Z.Y. ♀ 43 yrs. 25 Sep. 1972

1091a Rupture of right hemidiaphragm with complete hepatothorax in a car passenger involved in a head-on collision. Associated injuries include fractures of the skull and pelvis. Thoracic damage is aggravated by an earlier Halsted procedure. The left edge of the hepatothorax is clearly visible (→) on the admission X-ray.

1091b

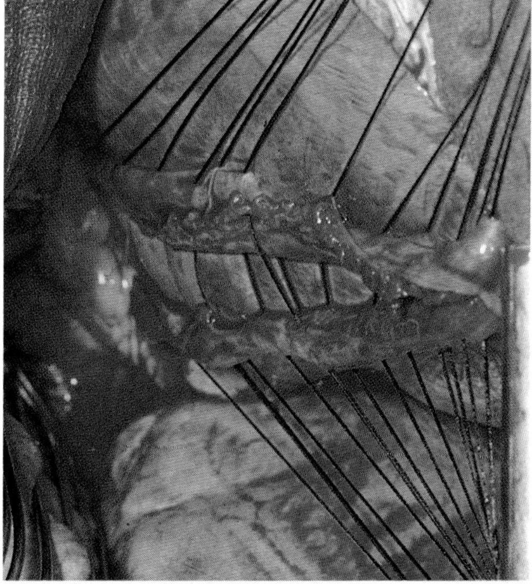

25 Sep. 1972

1091b Right thoracotomy to reposition the liver and close the diaphragm (the first layer of sutures is already in place). Recovery after severe post-operative complications.

1092a

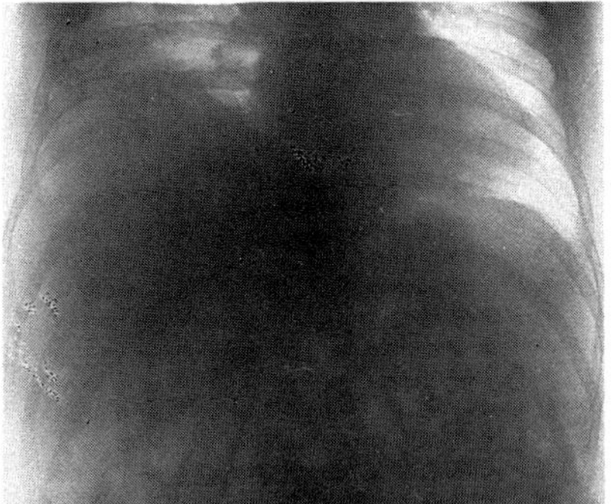

K.M. ♂ 35 yrs. 2 Feb. 1972

1092b

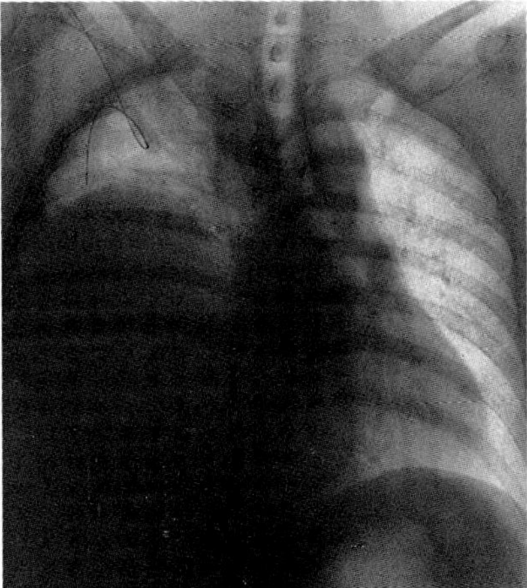

15 Feb. 1972

1092e

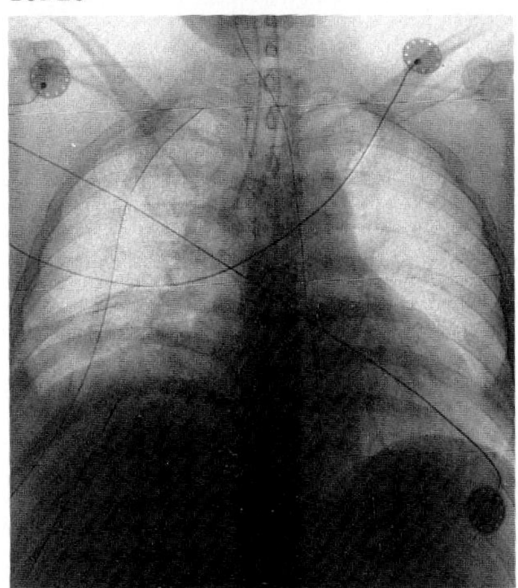

16 Feb. 1972

1092c

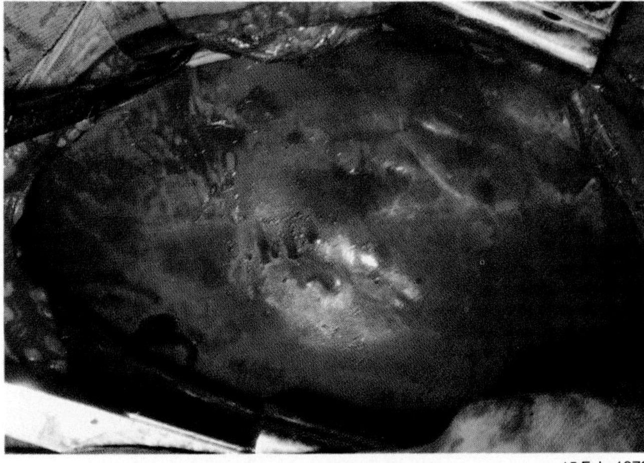

15 Feb. 1972

1092d

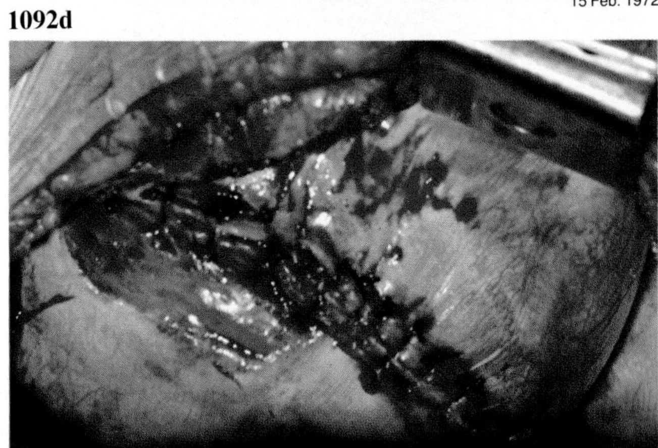

15 Feb. 1972

1092a Rupture of right hemidiaphragm with hepatothorax. Late diagnosis. Death. Car driver involved in a violent head-on collision. X-ray 2 days after admission shows a partial hepatothorax. Associated injuries include fractures of the pelvis and femur.

1092b Thirteen days later, the hepatothorax is total. However, the opacity in the right lung field is interpreted as a haemothorax; pleural puncture is repeatedly unsuccessful. Persistent shock leads to anuria, and peritoneal dialysis is required. Diagnosis is established 16 days after the accident when the dialysate emerges through the chest tube. Transfer to the University Hospital.

1092c A right thoracotomy reveals a complete hepatothorax with torsion of the inferior vena cava (the cause of shock). The apex of the liver displays several superficial cicatrized lacerations: significant liver laceration occurs very seldom in rupture of right hemidiaphragm.

1092d The liver is repositioned and the diaphragm closed.

1092e Anuria nevertheless persists postoperatively and the patient dies 2 days later from massive abdominal haemorrhage. Autopsy failed to elucidate the cause of haemorrhage and death was provisionally attributed to heparinisation.

Colothorax

The colon is often herniated in conjunction with the stomach and small bowel (see **1110**). It is herniated on its own only when the mesocolon is particularly long.

In our experience, 25% of right-sided diaphragmatic ruptures give rise to a colothorax. Strangulation is more common on the right than the left; it occurs in 5 to 8% of cases (see **1116**).

1093

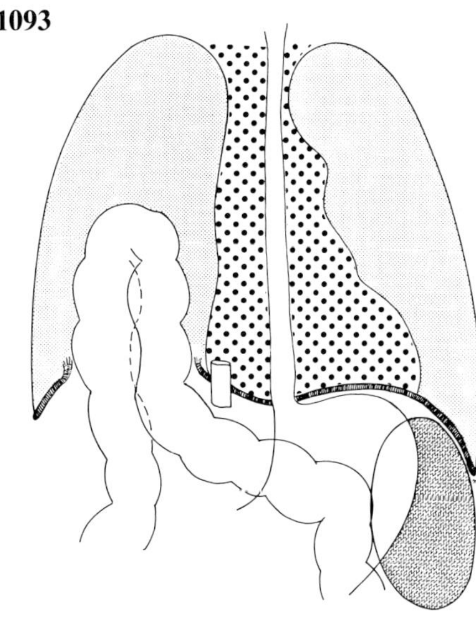

1094

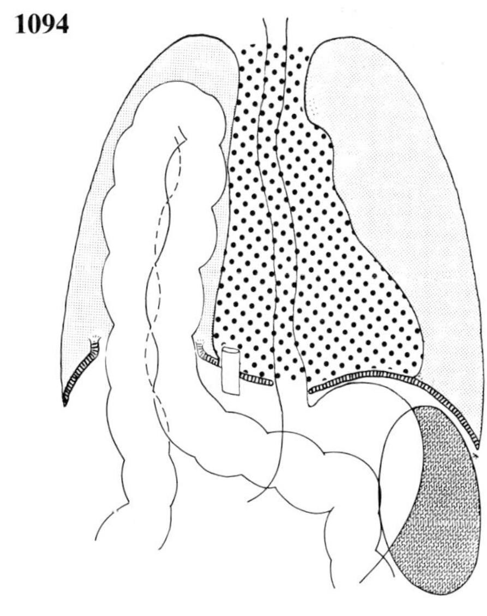

1095

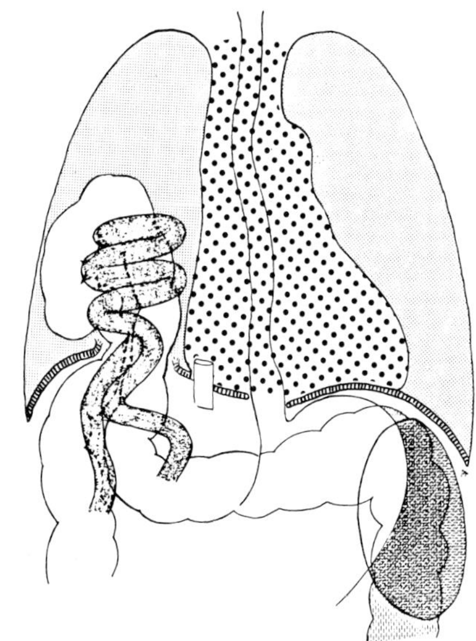

1096

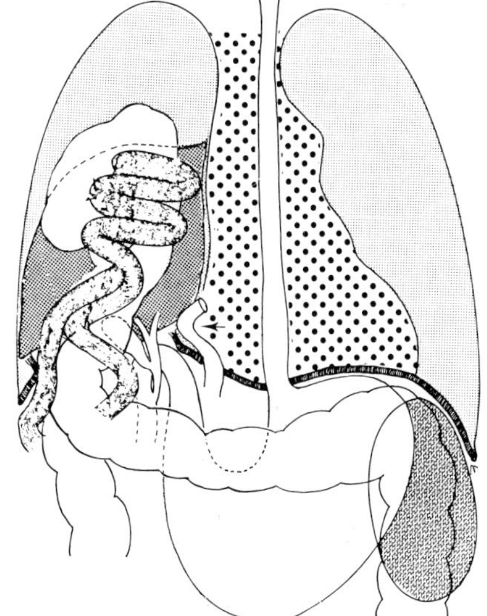

1093 Right colothorax.

1094 Massive right colothorax.

1095 Combined right herniation of colon and small bowel.

1096 Combined right herniation of liver, colon and small bowel.

1097

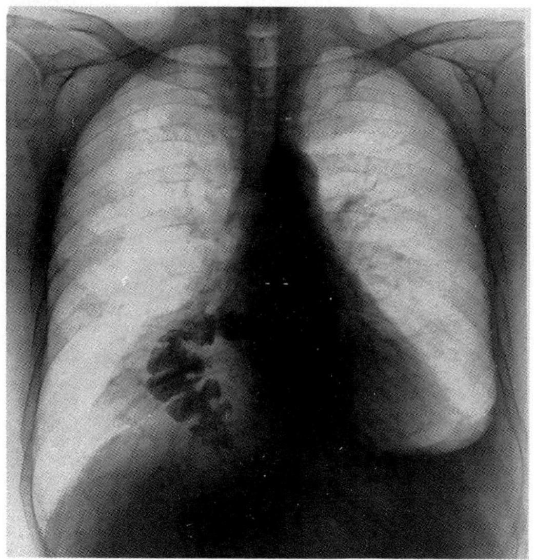

E.J.–L. ♂ 65 yrs. 21 Nov. 1973

1097 Moderate right colothorax in an osteoporotic patient under long-term corticoid treatment. Barium enema study obtained 9 years after an anterior right rupture of the diaphragm with herniation of the transverse colon. The patient initially was considered too fragile for surgery (see **1116**).

1098

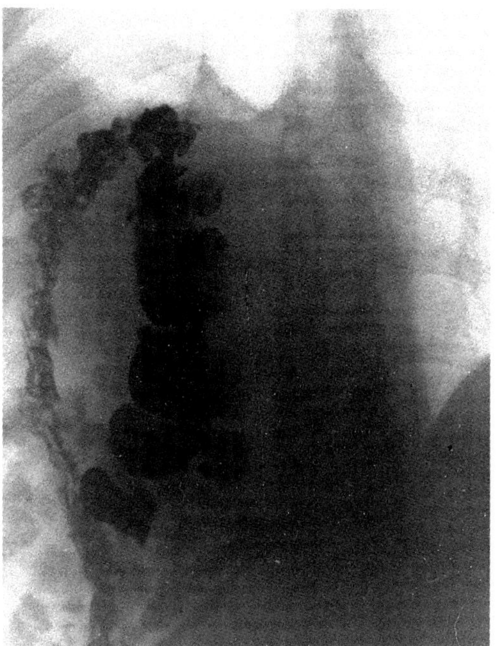

A.G. ♂ 34 yrs. 10 May 1968

1098 Barium study of a **massive right colothorax** after an effort rupture of the right diaphragm (see **1110**).

1099

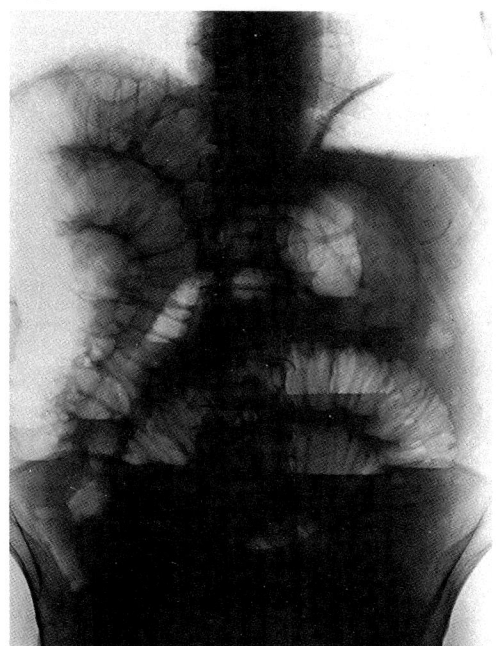

L.L. ♂ 67 yrs. 19 Dec. 1976

1099 Chilaiditi syndrome with interposition of intestine between liver and diaphragm. Because the mesentery is unusually long, the small intestine of this non-traumatised patient is in contact with the diaphragm above the liver. Even in the absence of ileus, rupture of the diaphragm could result in intestinal herniation.

Haemobiliothorax

Haemobiliothorax following blunt injury of the right diaphragm is rare. It is usually the result of a laceration of the diaphragm and liver by a fractured rib or large projectile (see **1102** and Volume I, **613**). The mixture of bile and blood usually clots and organises early. Difficult drainage is therefore an important diagnostic sign. Most cases require pleurectomy with decortication (see **1102f** and Volume I, **614**).

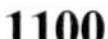

1100

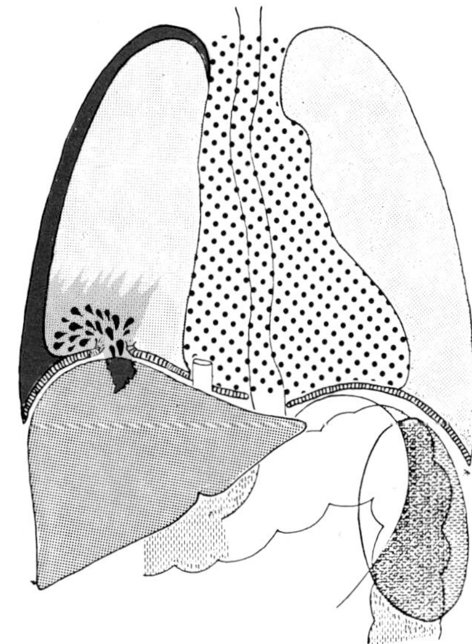

1100 Right haemobiliothorax by simultaneous rupture or laceration of diaphragm and liver.

1101

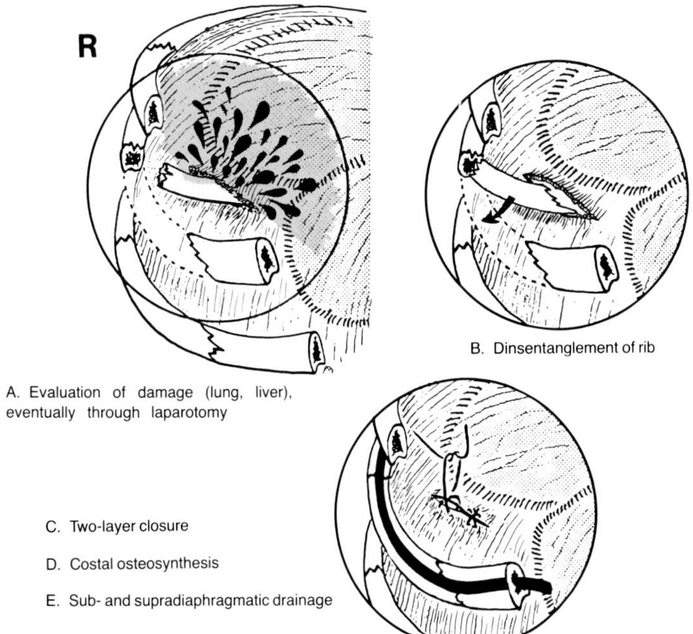

1101 Treatment of right-sided diaphragmatic **tear by fractured rib (haemobiliothorax of abdominal origin)**.

1102a

F.R. ♂ 44 yrs. 7 Jan. 1957

1102b

19 Feb. 1957

1102c

20 Feb. 1957

1102d

1 April 1957

1102e

3 May 1957

1102f

10 May 1957

1102g

1102h

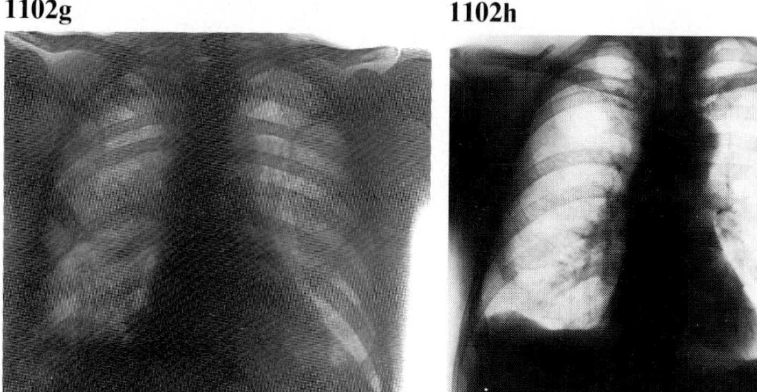

11 May 1957

13 Feb. 1965

1102f Right thoracotomy for decortication and pleurectomy. A diaphragmatic laceration is found and re paired. The specimen clearly shows the imprint of the ribs. Histological examination ultimately reveals fragments of hepatic parenchyma.

1102g Postoperative X-ray.

1102h Follow-up 8 years later.

1102a Massive organised haemobiliothorax due to laceration of liver and diaphragm. The patient is in respiratory distress 18 days after a violent impact to the right hemithorax.

1102b Repeated pleural puncture fails to evacuate the clotted haemothorax (clotted because of the presence of bile).

1102c Two months after the accident, the right lung is almost completely collapsed.

1102d Six weeks later, displacement of the mediastinum is less marked, but the haemothorax persists.

1102e Four-and-a-half months after the accident, the pleural cavity is loculate and contains a hydroaeric level.

Other types of diaphragmatic rupture

Peripheral avulsion

Peripheral avulsion is produced by the same mechanism as rupture. Its incidence (in proportion to other types of rupture) is 31% on the right and 12% on the left (see **1056, 1088**). It is most commonly found in patients with extensive parietal damage (see **1049**).

The high incidence of right-sided avulsion is perhaps explained by the fact that a violent impact to the liver tends to be dispersed to the periphery of the diaphragmatic leaf rather than concentrated at its vault.

Avulsion often extends over 25 or 30cm. On both right and left, the resultant hernia can be massive.

Repair is often difficult. The diaphragm must be reinserted (if possible in two layers) either to the intercostal muscles or with pericostal sutures. Internal fixation of the lower ribs and rib cartilages is sometimes necessary; the procedure is delicate, especially in the anterior region.

1103a

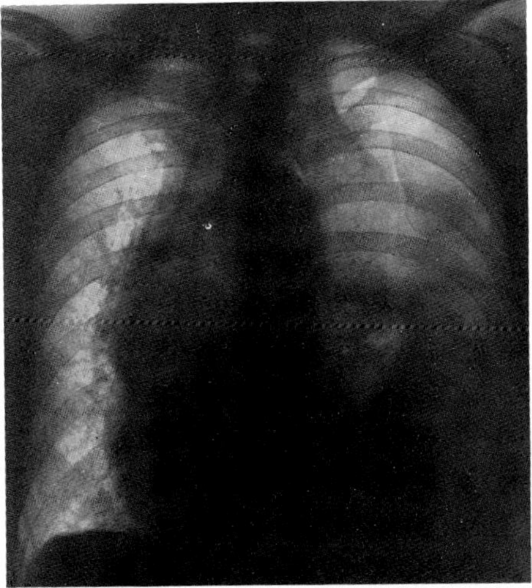

C.M. ♂ 71 yrs. 11 Feb. 1966

1103b

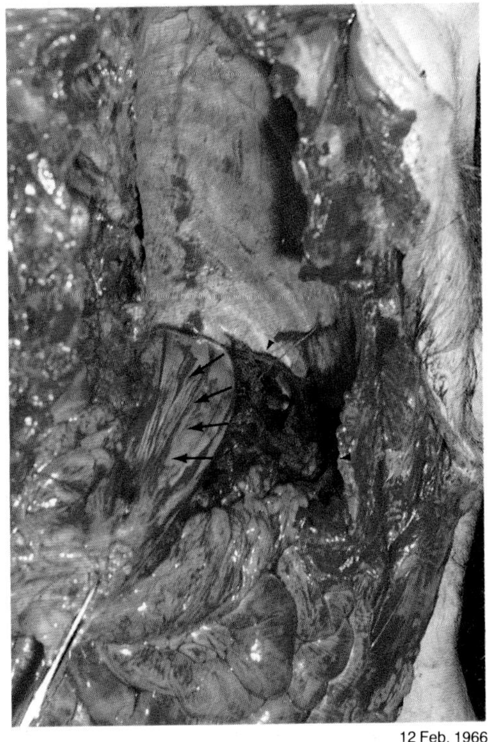

12 Feb. 1966

1103a Left anterior peripheral avulsion of diaphragm with a tension gastrothorax in the driver of a car thrown against the steering wheel in a head-on collision. The spleen has ruptured.

1103b Death 15 minutes after admission. Autopsy reveals an avulsion of the anterior left hemidiaphragm (→). The spleen is surrounded by a clotted haemoperitoneum.

1104

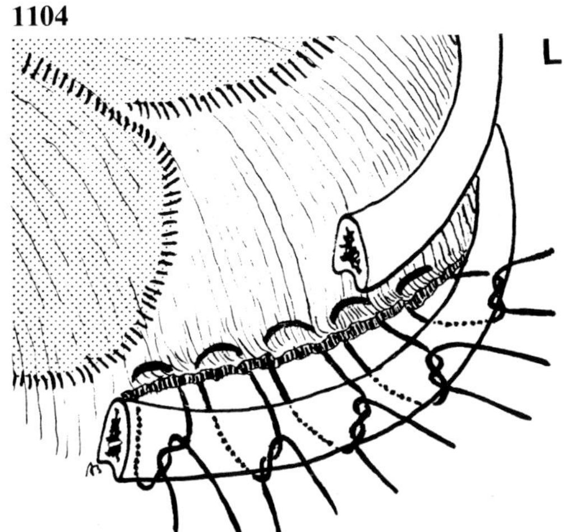

1104 Repair of left anterior peripheral avulsion (with vicryl pericostal sutures).

Rupture of crura

Rupture of the crura (17% of our cases) is a variant of left diaphragmatic rupture caused by a particularly violent impact. It is not known to occur in conjunction with right diaphragmatic rupture. Associated visceral injuries are often severe and the prognosis is poor.

Repair is as difficult through an abdominal as through a thoracic approach.

Some authorities argue that sliding hiatal hernia can result from trauma, giving examples to support their argument. In Lausanne, we have never had a case that definitely could be attributed to trauma. Perhaps the cases described would be better regarded as localised rupture of the diaphragmatic crura? In our experience, this type of injury is exceptional.

1105a

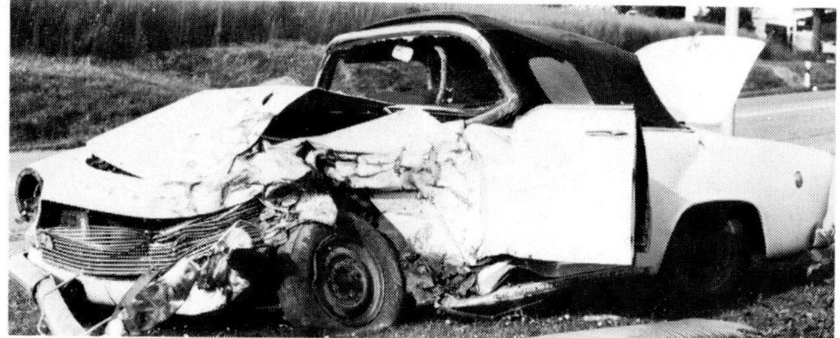

T.J. ♂ 45 yrs. 27 May 1973

1105b

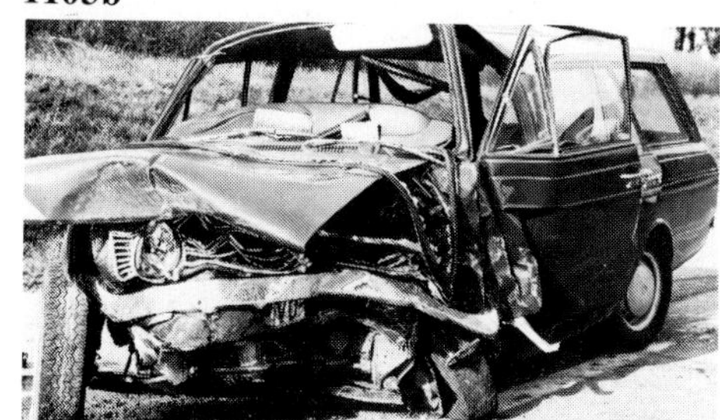

27 May 1973

1105c

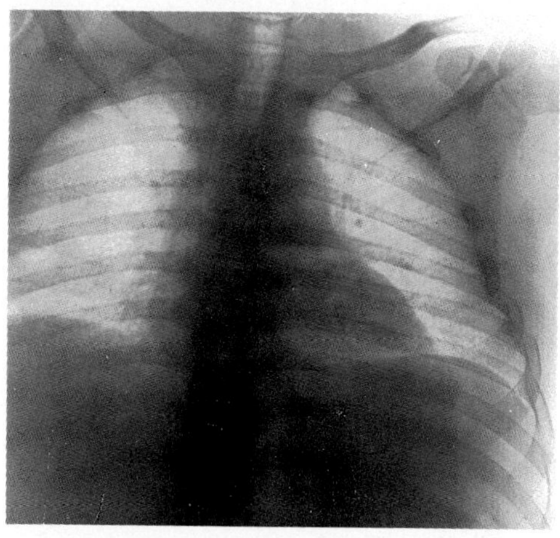

27 May 1973

1105d

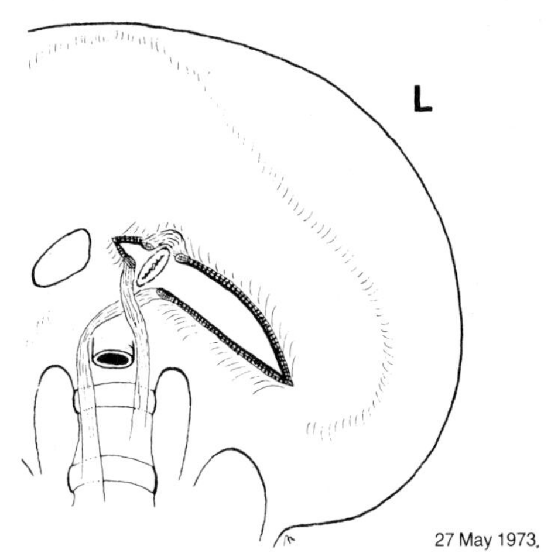

27 May 1973.

1105a **Rupture of left hemidiaphragm and crura**. The driver sustained multiple deceleration injuries in a violent head-on collision (from 11 o'clock).

1105b The two occupants of the other car were killed.

1105c The admission chest X-ray is normal. Laparotomy to counteract shock due to laceration of the liver.

1105d Diagramatic representation of the laparotomy findings: a 10cm oblique posterior rupture of the left hemidiaphragm encompassing the crura and oesophageal hiatus. Death 8 days after surgery.

Rupture of the pericardium and diaphragm

The pericardium ruptures simultaneously with the left hemidiaphragm in 6% of cases, and with the right hemidiaphragm in 8% of cases.

Lateral rupture of the pericardium – the result of an extremely violent impact – can lead to dislocation of the heart out of its natural cavity. Torsion of the major veins then rapidly reduces cardiac output. In many cases, the associated injuries are fatal in themselves.

Lateral rupture of the pericardium is often discovered by serendipity during emergency thoracotomy; in patients with severe associated injuries, it is frequently only noticed at autospy.

Rupture of the **pericardial floor** and tendinous centre of the diaphragm is rare (about 1% of all ruptures of the diaphragm). In most cases, the gradual herniation of the omentum and transverse colon causes sub-acute cardiac tamponade. Cardiac tamponade by abdominal viscera is less symptomatic than liquid tamponade but, given the weight and contents of the herniated organs, it nonetheless can be serious.

Rupture of the pericardial floor and tendinous centre of the diaphragm is usually long and anterior, close to the costal margin. Diagnosis is never easy. In most cases, herniation is so slow that the symptoms only become clear months or years later. Chronic tamponade can be well tolerated. Cases in which the heart is displaced into the abdomen are generally seen only at autopsy.

Lateral rupture of the pericardium is repaired through left or right thoracotomy. The pericardium is sutured to prevent dislocation of the heart and a small window left to obviate fluid tamponade.

Rupture of the tendinous portion of the *diaphragm and pericardial floor* requires upper laparotomy. Repair – consisting of reinsertion and two-layer suturing – is usually easy. Attempts to perform this operation through left, right or bilateral thoracotomy have failed.

1106

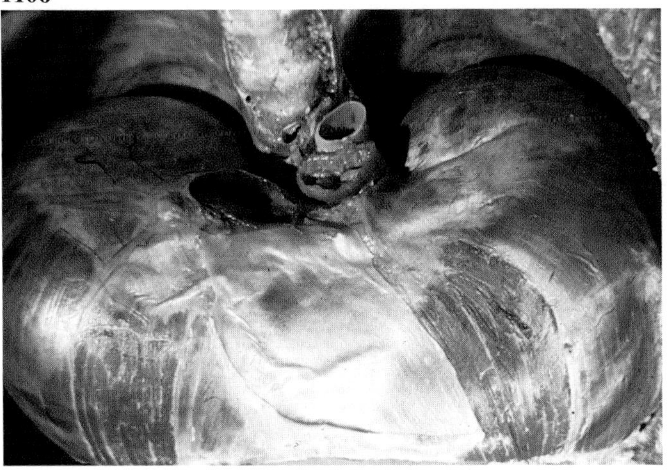

1106 The anatomical relationship between the tendinous portion of the diaphragm, the three hiatuses and the pericardial floor. (Prof. Stephan Kubik, Zürich.)

1107

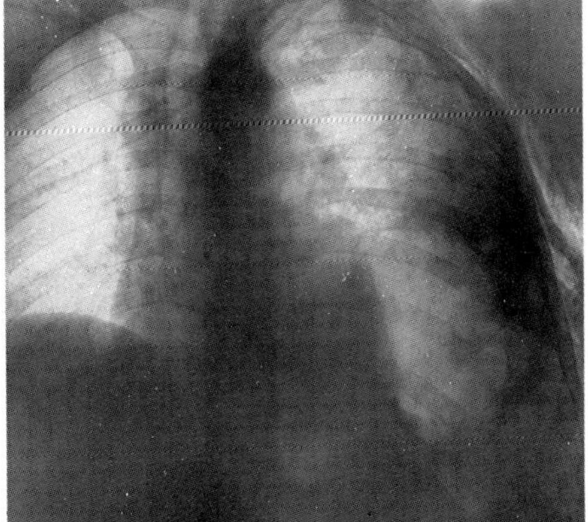

C.J.–D. ♂ 50 yrs. 14 Sep. 1971

1107 Discontinuous rupture of diaphragm and left pericardial wall. The stomach and spleen have been herniated through a large rupture of the diaphragm. The spleen has ruptured and bled into the chest. Laparotomy for splenectomy and repair of the diaphragm. Left thoracotomy for closure of the pericardial tear (which is vertical and lies 1.5cm in front of the phrenic nerve). Death 12 days later in anuria.

1108

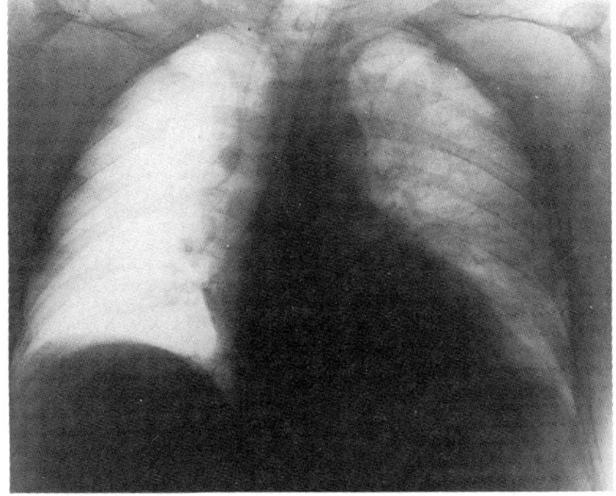

M.F. ♂ 59 yrs. 25 April 1974

1108 Simultaneous rupture of diaphragm and left pericardial wall in the driver of a car in collision with a lorry. Laparotomy shows shock to be due to a rupture of the spleen that has bled profusely into the peritoneum and thorax through a large tear in the diaphragm. Further exploration reveals a rupture of the pericardium in continuity with the diaphragmatic rupture. Repair, drainage. Recovery.

1109a

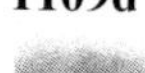

N.P. ♂ 69 yrs. 12 Oct. 1975

1109b

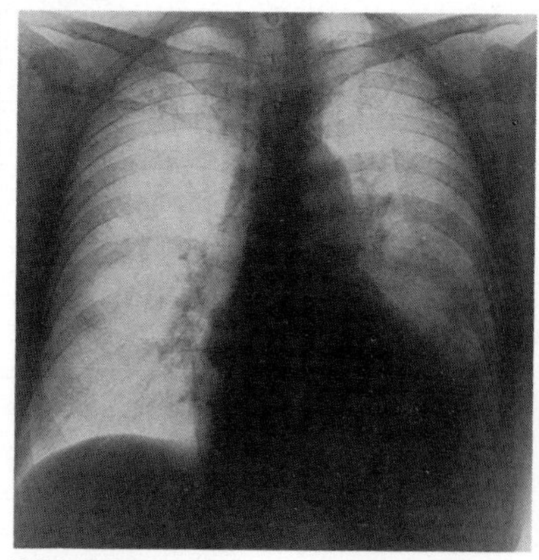

17 Oct. 1975

1109c

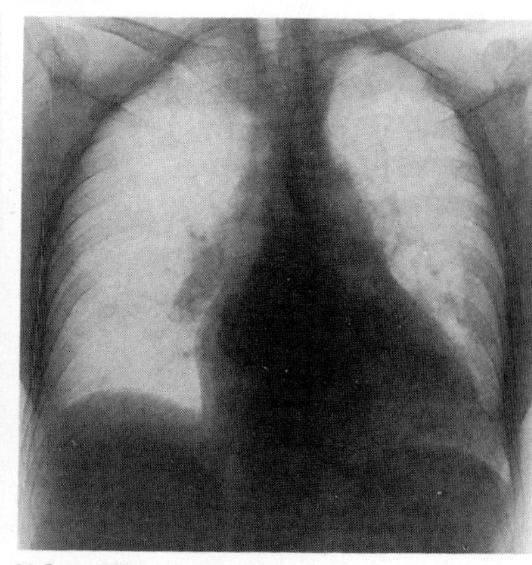

22 Oct. 1975

1109d

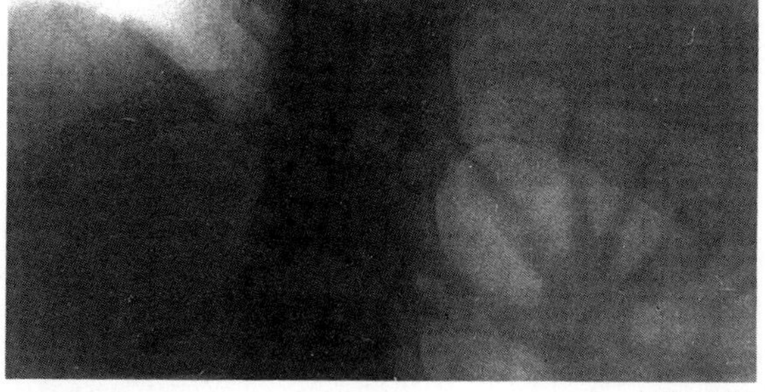

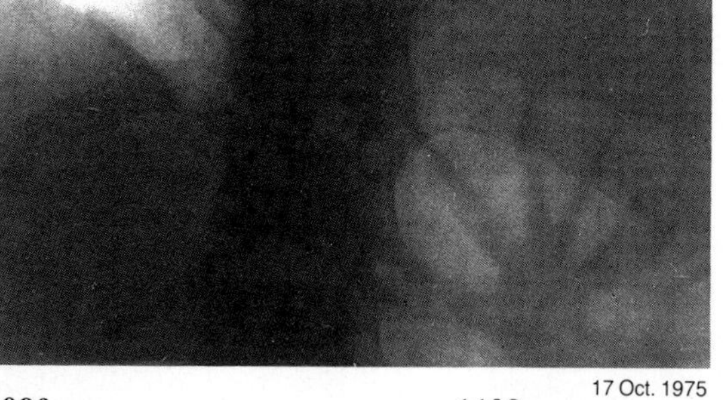

17 Oct. 1975

1109e

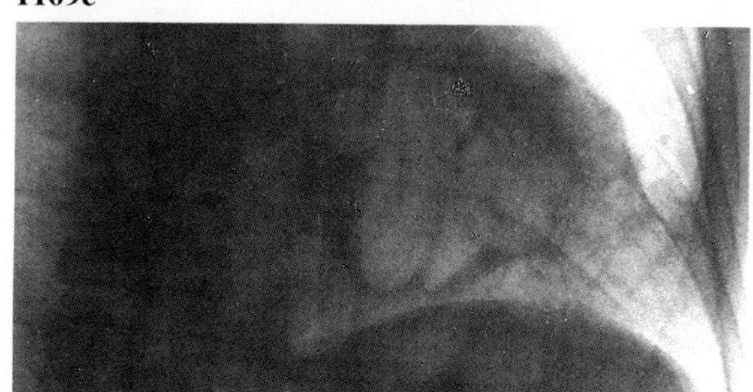

22 Oct. 1975

1109f

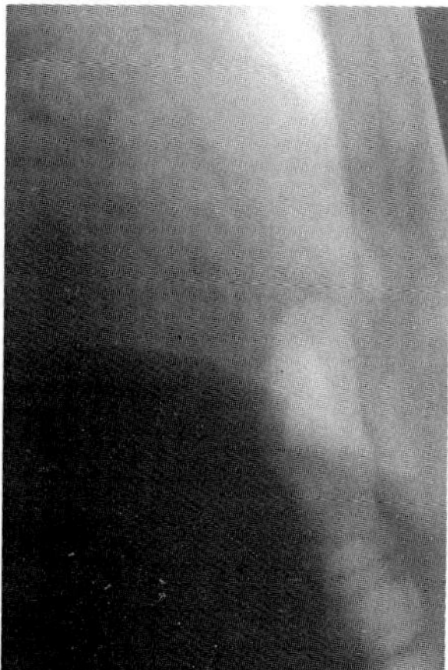

22 Oct. 1975

1109g

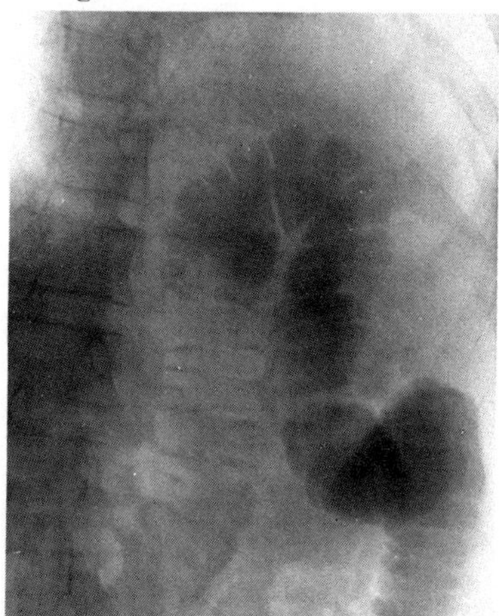

22 Oct. 1975

1109a Rupture of tendinous centre of diaphragm and of pericardial floor with subacute tamponade. The patient was driving this car when it was hit laterally by another car travelling at about 100 km/h.

1109b Five days after the accident, the left hemidiaphragm is obscured by a pleural effusion.

1109c The diaphragm can be seen again after pleural puncture of 600 ml of blood.

1109d Detail of the colic haustrations over the heart shadow before pleural puncture.

1109e The haustrations seen in relation to the diaphragm after pleural puncture.

1109f Lateral X-ray showing the colon above the anterior diaphragm, immediately behind the sternum.

1109g A barium enema study clearly evinces the transverse colon. Laparotomy reveals chronic cardiac tamponade due to the transdiaphragmatic herniation of the greater omentum and colon (see **840, 854** and Volume I, **71**). Repair. Recovery.

1109h

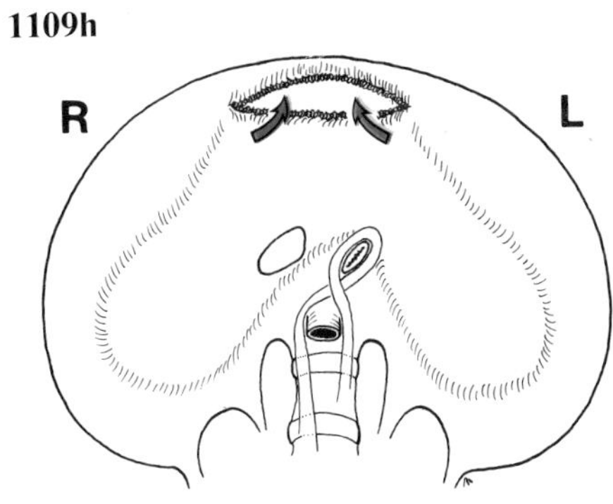

1109i

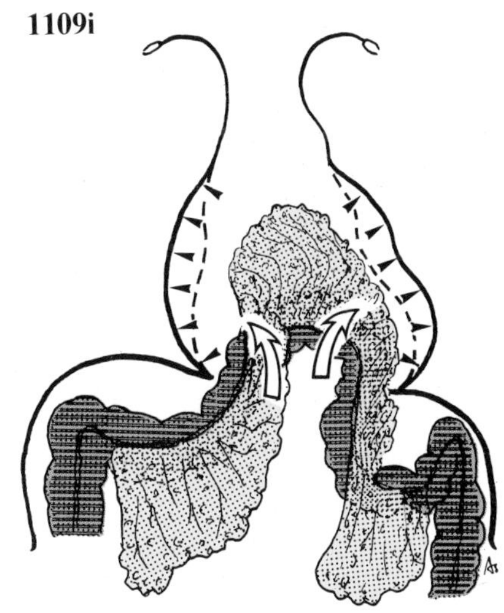

Effort (or 'spontaneous') rupture

Effort (or 'spontaneous') rupture of the diaphragm can occur on either side. It results from a sudden and brutal Valsalva manoeuvre during which the abdominal muscles exert extreme pressure on the diaphragm and lower thorax. Momentary lack of co-ordination during vigorous muscular activity – athletics, water polo, weight-lifting or even dancing – is the commonest cause. Occasional cases have been observed during delivery, violent vomiting, coughing and defecation.

Effort rupture (about 1% of all diaphragmatic ruptures) is especially difficult to diagnose on the right (see Volume I, **367, 577**). Inopportune exploratory pleural punctures are often attempted.

Rupture or sudden dehiscence of a diaphragmatic suture line will be discussed later (see **1124** to **1126**).

Treatment follows the classic surgical principles.

1110a A.G. ♂ 34 yrs. 29 April 1968

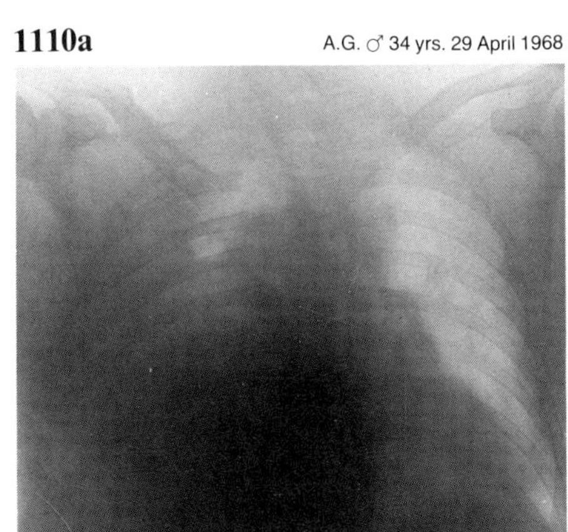

1110b 2 May 1968

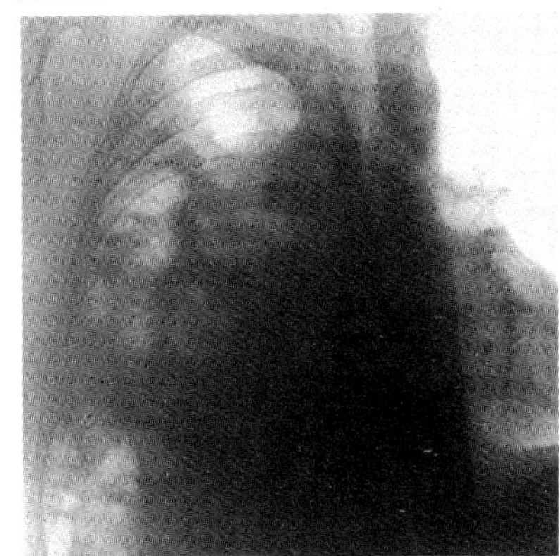

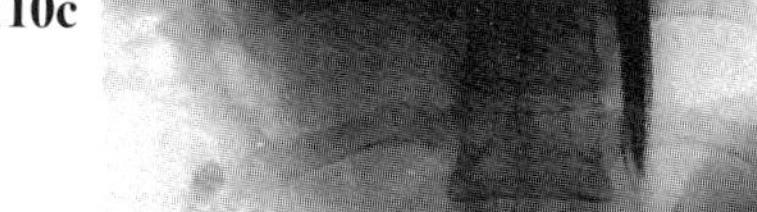

1110c 10 May 1968

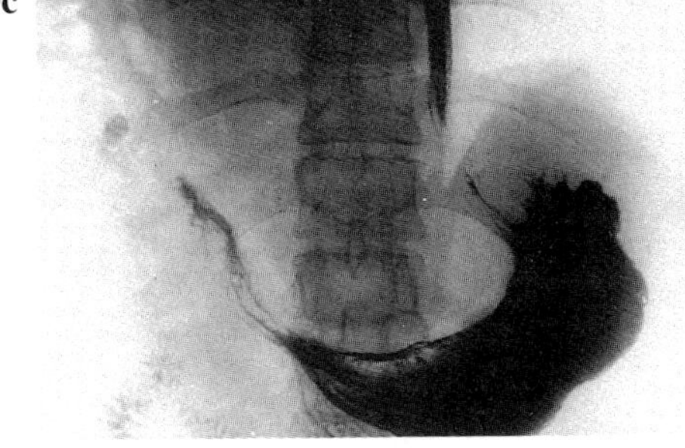

1110a Effort rupture of right hemidiaphragm with herniation of liver, colon and small bowel. X-ray obtained a few hours after surgery for a massive abdominal eventration. The abdomen was tightly bandaged after surgery. In the recovery room, the patient suddenly developed respiratory distress and began to cough violently. A pleural effusion is diagnosed from the X-ray, but puncture fails to find any fluid.

1110b The right pleural cavity is punctured several times over the next few days, but without success. Ventilation improves slightly (see Volume I, **367, 577**).

1110c Diaphragmatic rupture is finally diagnosed through a barium study. Thoracotomy 2 months later reveals a complete rupture of the right hemidiaphragm with herniation of the liver, right colon and small bowel. Reduction and closure of the diaphragm. Recovery.

Undiagnosed rupture of the diaphragm and late sequelae

One third of left-sided ruptures and *half* of right-sided ruptures pass undetected for several days. Some cases are not diagnosed for several years (the longest time lapse quoted in the literature is 44 years). One may deduce (1) that many doctors are unfamiliar with the X-ray appearance of left-sided rupture, both with and without herniation, and (2) that surgical exploration is still the only reliable means of establishing early diagnosis of right-sided rupture (see page 220).

One emergency team making a routine search for diaphragmatic rupture nevertheless diagnoses at least 75% of cases within 8 hours of admission.

As Ambroise Paré first pointed out, no rupture or wound of the diaphragm of any length ever cicatrizes spontaneously. An unrepaired rupture sometimes remains asymptomatic but, in most cases, there are elusive digestive and respiratory disturbances. The common symptoms and signs are pain in the shoulder, distension or immobility of the hemithorax, unilateral tympany (or dullness), muffled respiratory sounds, intestinal signs in the thorax, slight but recurrent effusions due to torsion of the epiploic fringe, and subileus or ileus. However, none of these signs is pathognomic or constant. The likelihood of **herniation and strangulation** increases the longer diagnosis is delayed.

Diagnosis rests on (1) any memory the patient may have of the accident (some patients require to be prompted), (2) any documents available on the exact circumstances of the accident and, above all, (3) standard X-rays and contrast studies (barium meal and enema, cholangiography and angiography).

Late repair of diaphragmatic rupture is best performed through thoracotomy since, after a certain time, the herniated abdominal organs tend to adhere to thoracic viscera (see **1024**). On both left and right, reduction is followed by two-layer suturing.

The prognosis is better for left-sided rupture (without ileus) than for right-sided rupture, especially after hepatothorax. In the case of a strangulated hernia, every effort should be made to obviate supra- and subdiaphragmatic septic complications.

1111a

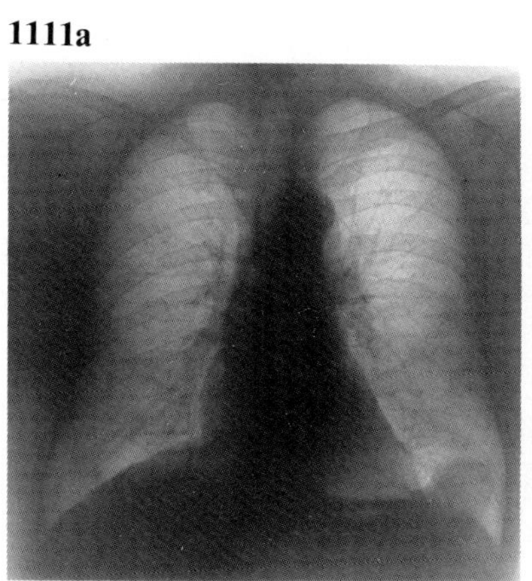

G.O. ♂ 53 yrs. 6 Dec. 1966

1111b

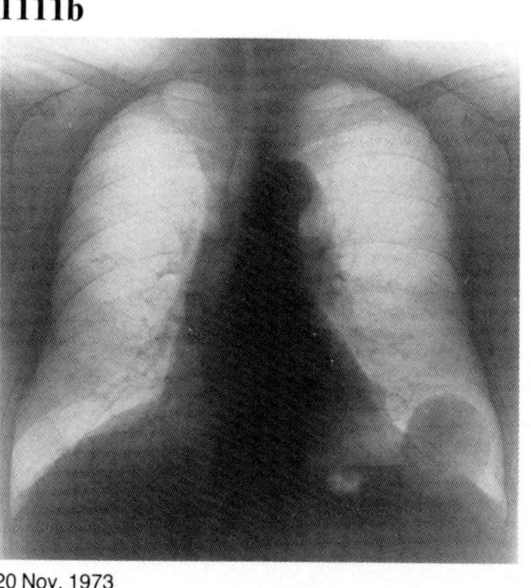

20 Nov. 1973

1111c

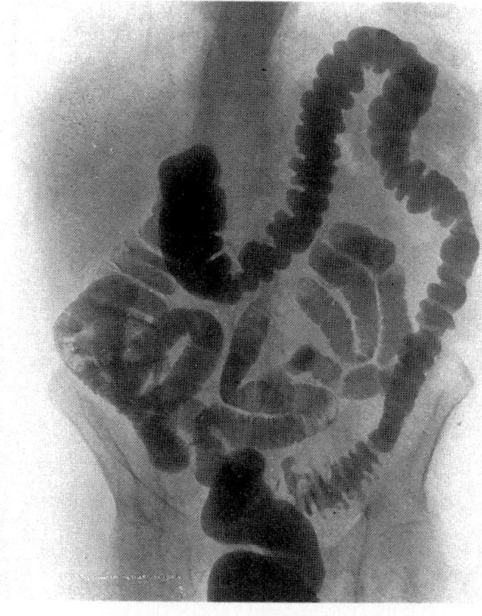

27 Nov. 1973

1111a Minor rupture of left hemidiaphragm, undetected for 13 years. Six years after violent contusion of the lower left thorax, a 'mushroom-like' opacity is noticed above the diaphragm.

1111b Seven years later – 13 years after the accident – the opacity is larger.

1111c The splenic flexure of the colon lies within the thorax. Thoracotomy, reduction and direct repair.

1112a

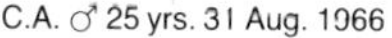

1112b

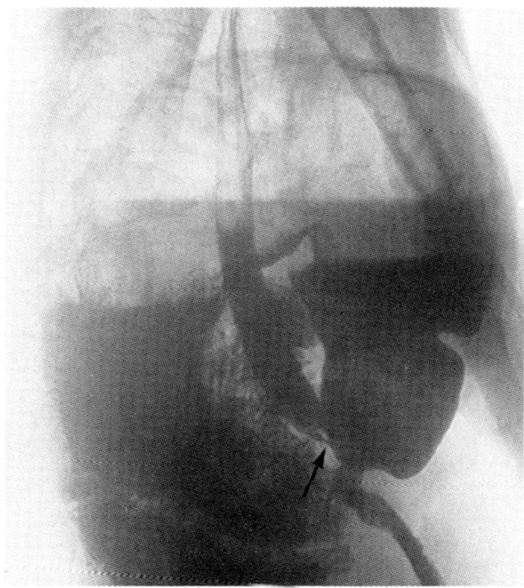

1112a Major rupture of left hemidiaphragm, undetected for 14 years. The stomach and transverse colon have migrated into the left hemithorax.

1112b Intrathoracic volvulus of the stomach with the cardia (→) and pylorus side by side. Thoracotomy, repair. Recovery.

Strangulated gastrothorax

A small rupture of the left hemidiaphragm can remain asymptomatic and radiologically inapparent for a long time. If the tear is median and behind the heart, part of the fundus may herniate. If the herniated stomach then distends, it can become strangulated by blockage of its venous return. Parietal oedema quickly gives way to ischaemia.

Strangulated gastrothorax produces no ileus and haematemesis occurs only if the strangulation suddenly and spontaneously reduces.

In its early stages, strangulated gastrothorax is as difficult to diagnose as strangulated para-oesophageal hiatal hernia. The two are very similar in radiological appearance.

The first symptom is excruciating pain which no sedative can ease. The radiological signs may only become clear several hours later. Diagnosis should be followed by immediate surgery.

The traumatic origin of strangulated gastrothorax is clear from the absence of a hernial sac (see **1114e**).

Repair is easiest through lower left thoracotomy; a short diaphragmatic incision is sometimes necessary to release the strangulated viscus without inflicting further damage. Closure of the diaphragm usually poses little problem.

1113

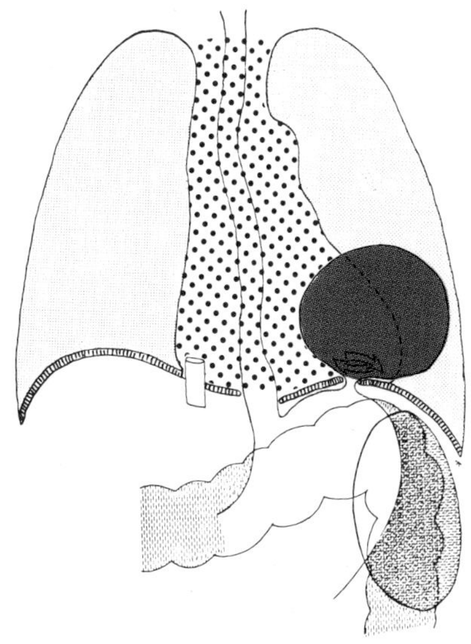

1113 Late strangulation of gastrothorax.

1114a

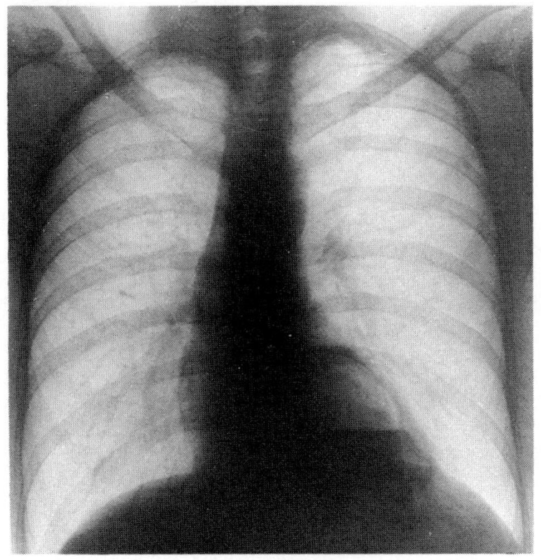

R.M. ♂ 35 yrs. 26 Feb. 1976

1114b

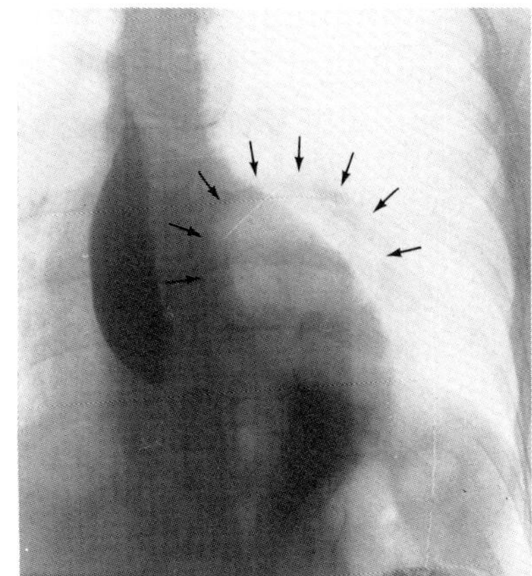

26 Feb. 1976

1114c

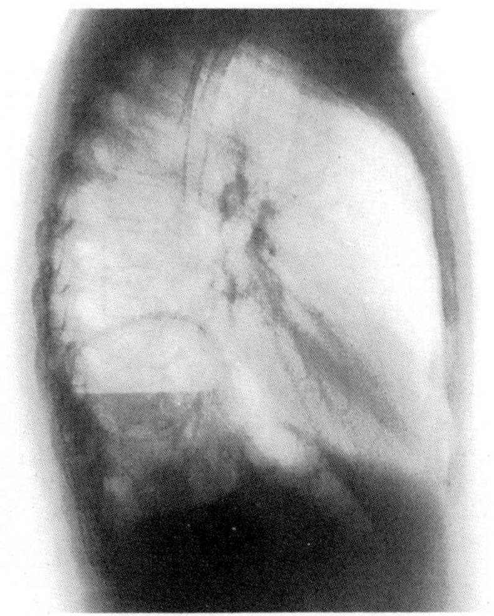

26 Feb. 1976

1114d

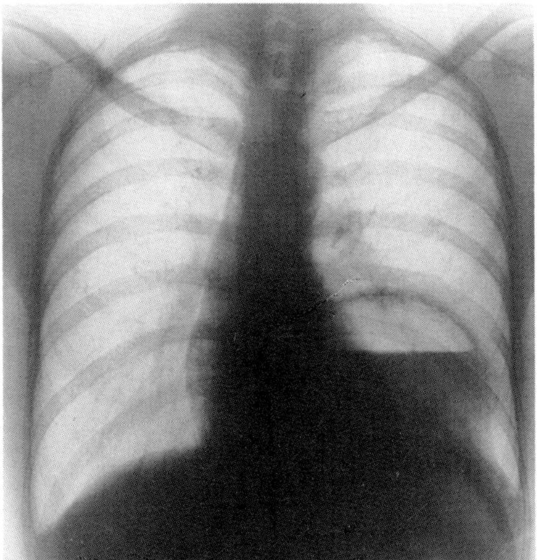

27 Feb. 1976

1114e

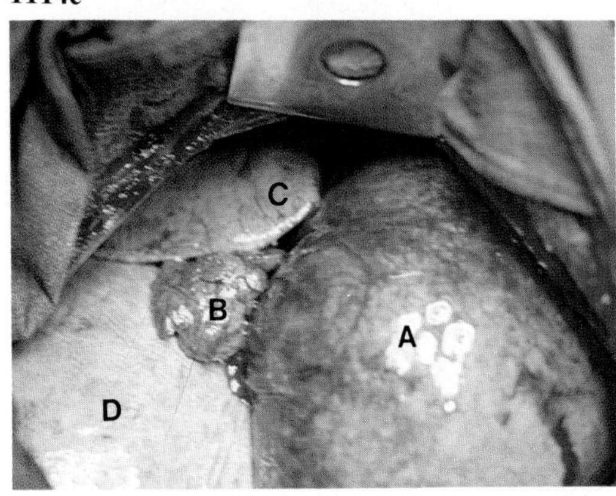

27 Feb. 1976

1114a Late strangulation of gastrothorax. Twelve years after deceleration against the steering wheel (unbelted driver in a head-on collision at 65km/h), the patient experienced sudden pain and respiratory difficulty. An infarct is suspected, but the admission X-ray is negative. Three days later, pain is excruciating and X-ray (above) shows a retrocardiac hydro-aeric level.

1114b Contrast study. Volvulus prevents the dye from entering the supradiaphragmatic portion of the stomach (→).

1114c The hernia lies in the posterior thorax.

1114d The hernia swells and strangulation increases. Pain is extreme.

1114e Transfer to University Hospital. Thoracotomy exposes the strangulated gastrothorax (A); ischaemia is severe. A small portion of the greater omentum is also exposed (B). Despite the absence of a pleuroperitoneal hernial sac (post-traumatic hernias never have a hernial sac), the abdominal viscera have not adhered to the lung (C). A 2cm rupture in the left hemidiaphragm (D) lies close to the oesophageal hiatus. The hernia will be reduced through a short incision enlarging the rupture. Repair of the diaphragm. Recovery.

Strangulated colothorax

A small rupture of the diaphragm can also lead to a strangulated colothorax or a strangulated hernia of the small bowel. The result is mechanical ileus. Both conditions are rare. The main danger is postoperative septic complication.

Whether on the left or right, the hernia is usually anterior; an abdominal approach is advisable.

1115

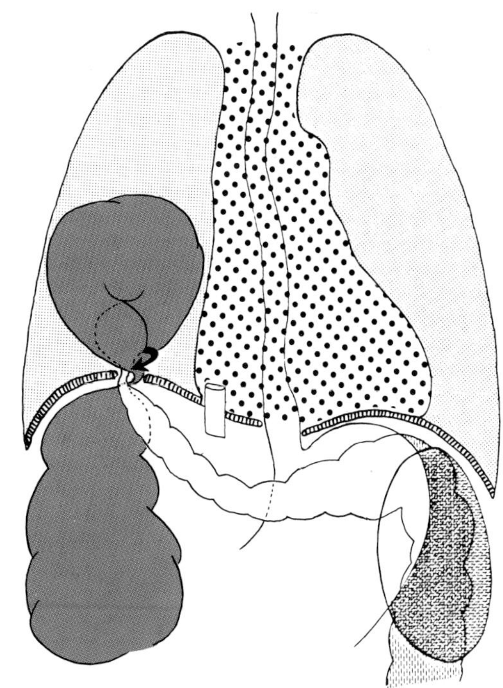

1115 Late strangulation of right colothorax.

1116a

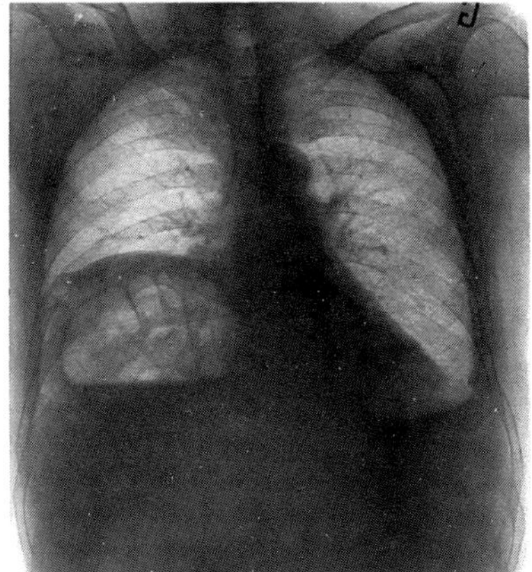

E. J.–L. ♂ 65 yrs. 28 Dec. 1973

1116a Late strangulation of right colothorax. A month after the diagnosis was made in another hospital (see **1097**) and 9 years after trauma, sudden strangulation of the herniated transverse colon causes ileus.

1116b

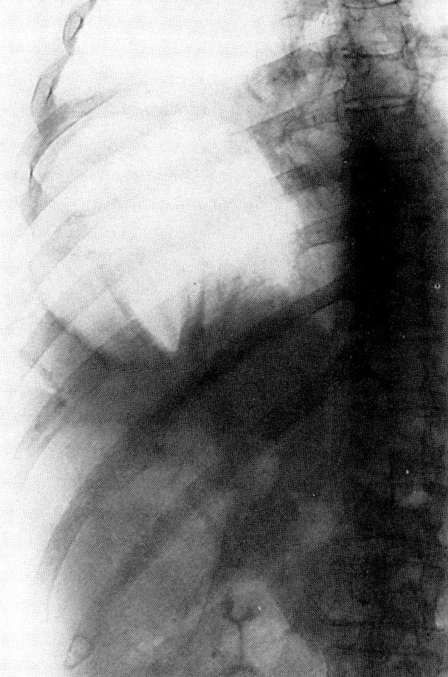

28 Dec. 1973

1116b Strangulation is aggravated by volvulus.

1116c

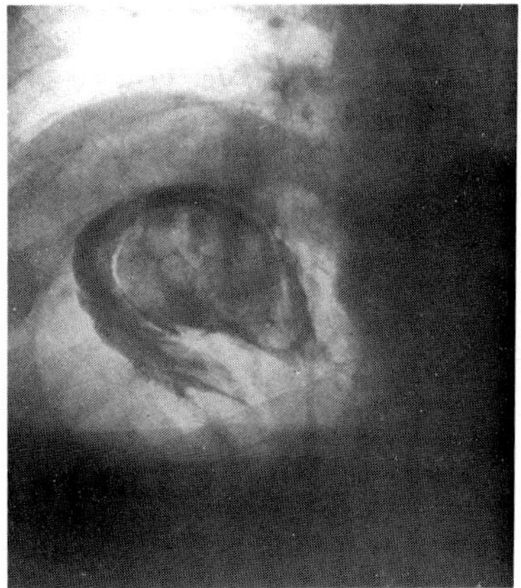

28 Dec. 1973

1116c A non-dilated portion of the colon has been dislocated also. Laparotomy, reduction and right hemicolectomy. Subsequent dehiscence of the ileocolostomy, stress ulcers and bronchopneumonia. Death.

Progressive hepatothorax

Depending upon the size of an unrecognised right-sided rupture, herniation of the liver is progressive or complete.

The physiopathological repercussions of complete hepatothorax depend upon the degree of respiratory and circulatory interference (see page 221).

Progressive herniation of the liver through a small rupture appears radiologically as a 'champagne cork' in the right lower thorax.

Both conditions require surgery.

1117a **1117b** **1117c**

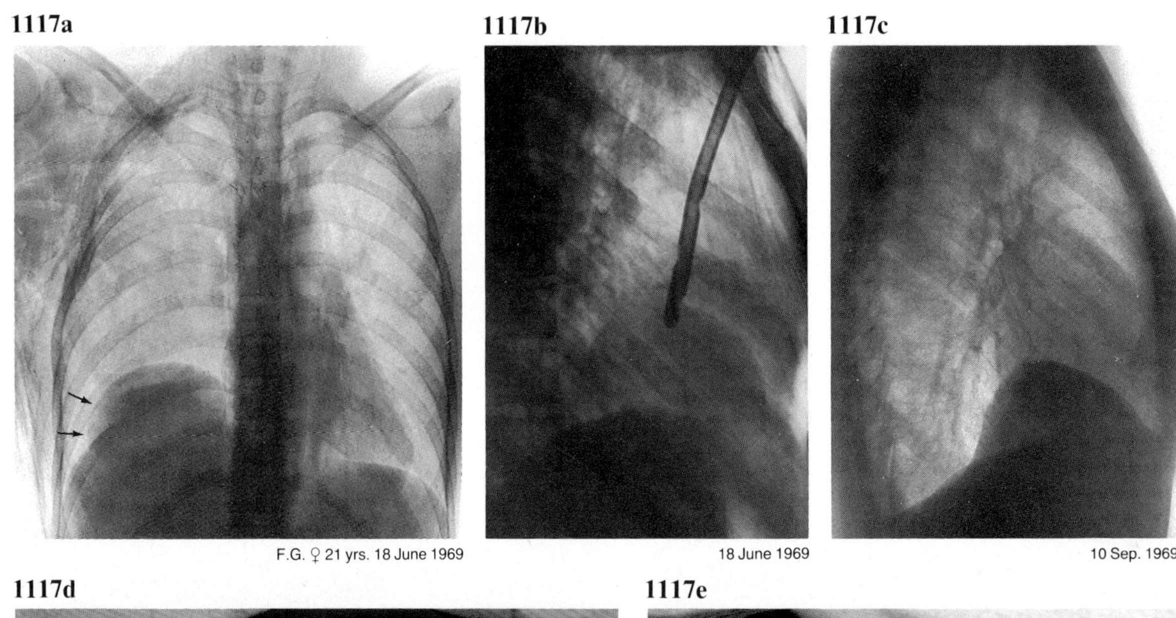

F.G. ♀ 21 yrs. 18 June 1969 · 18 June 1969 · 10 Sep. 1969

1117d **1117e**

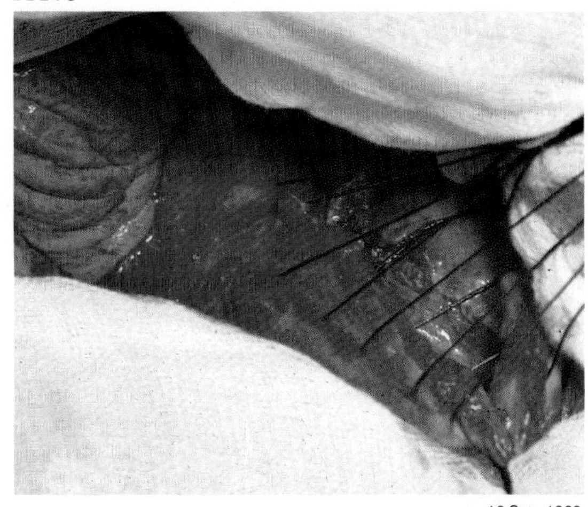

16 Sep. 1969 · 16 Sep. 1969

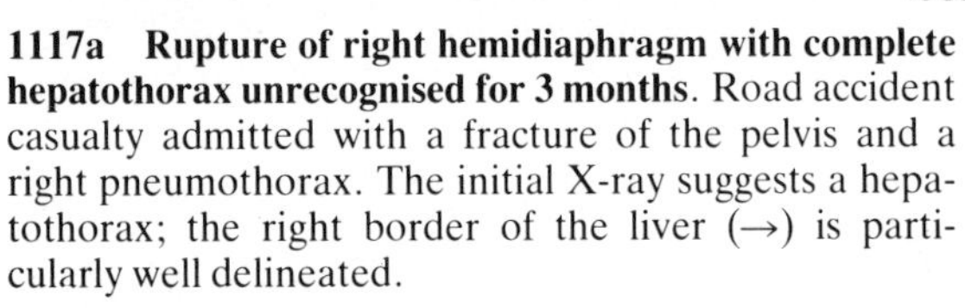

1117a Rupture of right hemidiaphragm with complete hepatothorax unrecognised for 3 months. Road accident casualty admitted with a fracture of the pelvis and a right pneumothorax. The initial X-ray suggests a hepatothorax; the right border of the liver (→) is particularly well delineated.

1117b The same opacity is visible on the lateral X-ray, but still passes undiagnosed.

1117c No change 3 months later.

1117d Thoracotomy exposes the rupture.

1117e Two-layer repair. Recovery.

1118

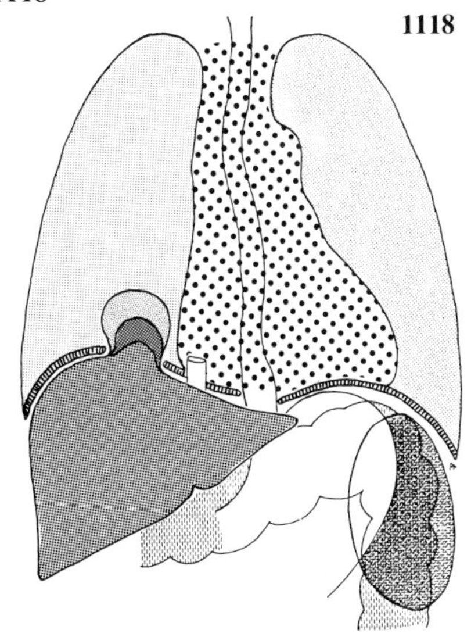

1118 Progressive hepatothorax.

1119a

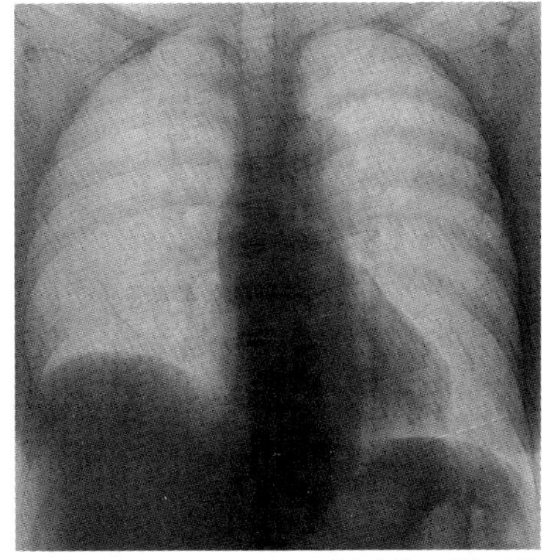

D.E. ♀ 48 yrs. 8 May 1960

1119b

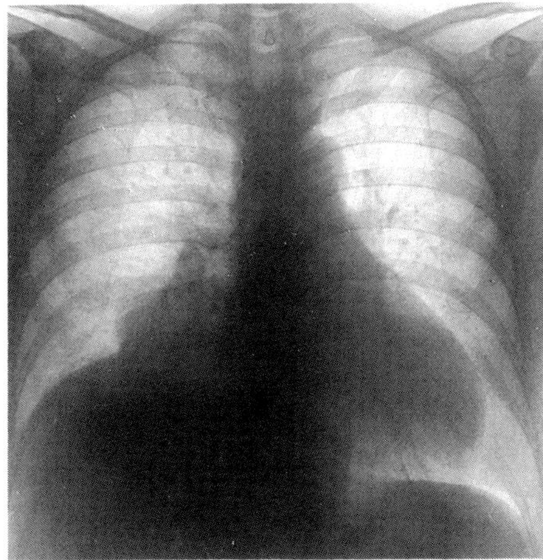

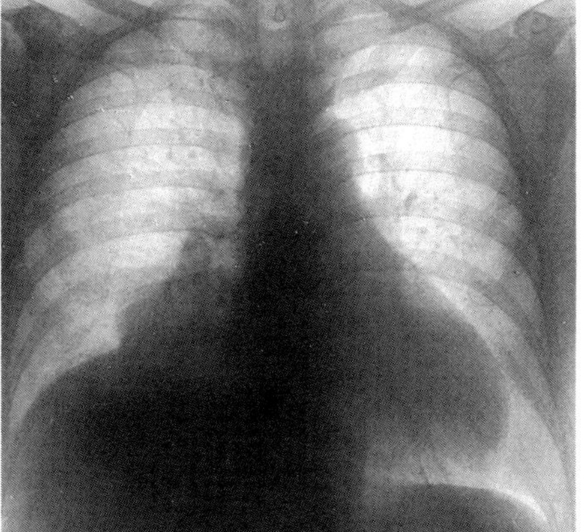

28 May 1960

1119c

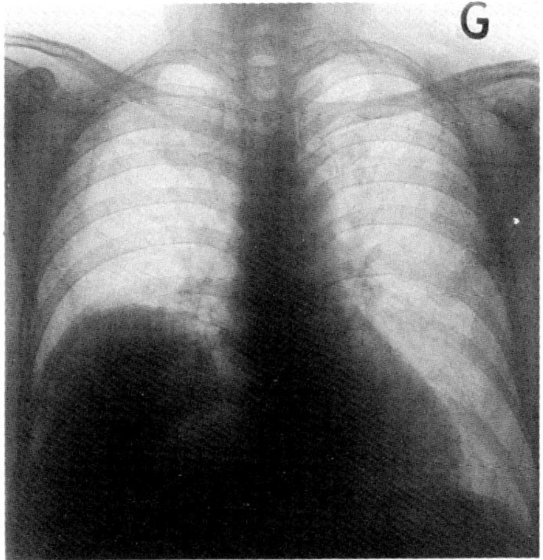

2 Nov. 1960

1119d

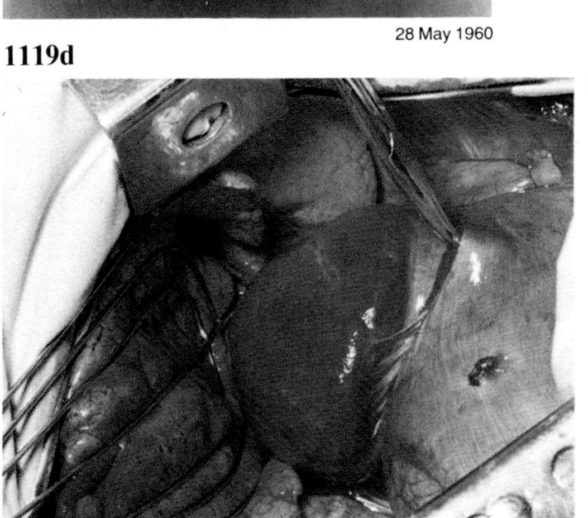

8 Nov. 1960

1119e

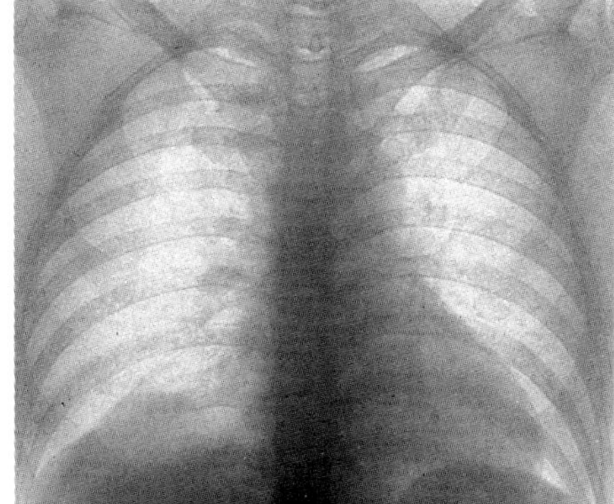

15 May 1965

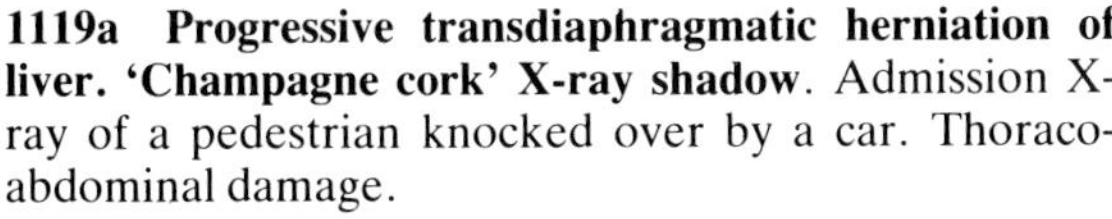

1119a Progressive transdiaphragmatic herniation of liver. 'Champagne cork' X-ray shadow. Admission X-ray of a pedestrian knocked over by a car. Thoraco-abdominal damage.

1119b X-ray 3 weeks later shows progressive herniation of the liver. The condition is asymptomatic.

1119c The undiagnosed hernia increases in size over the next 6 months.

1119d Thoracotomy 6 months after trauma. The fibrous borders of the diaphragmatic rupture slightly constrict the neck of the hernia, producing a 'champagne cork' shadow. Repair, recovery.

1119e Five-year follow-up.

Special diaphragmatic injuries

Tear by fractured ribs

The sharp extremities of fractured ribs can lacerate the diaphragm, puncturing the spleen (see **1080, 1085, 1121**), omentum (see **1122**), kidney (see Volume I, **163**), or liver (see **1101**).

About 8% of all diaphragmatic injuries involve tears by fractured ribs.

The laceration can be very small and, if there is no visceral damage, it is often only discovered later by serendipity (see **1122d**). The largest lacerations reach about 5 cm.

Tears of the spleen or kidney commonly result in haemoperitoneum, haemothorax or delayed renal infarction.

The surgical procedure for a laceration of this type is the same as for an open wound of the diaphragm – two-layer suturing after detailed evaluation of associated thoracic and abdominal damage. In order to examine the viscera in both cavities, one may have to enlarge the laceration. Internal fixation of the ribs can be performed with non-absorbable sutures or wire.

1120 A. Evaluation of damage (lung, kidney, spleen), possibly through laparotomy or incision of the diaphragm.
(haemothorax of abdominal origin)

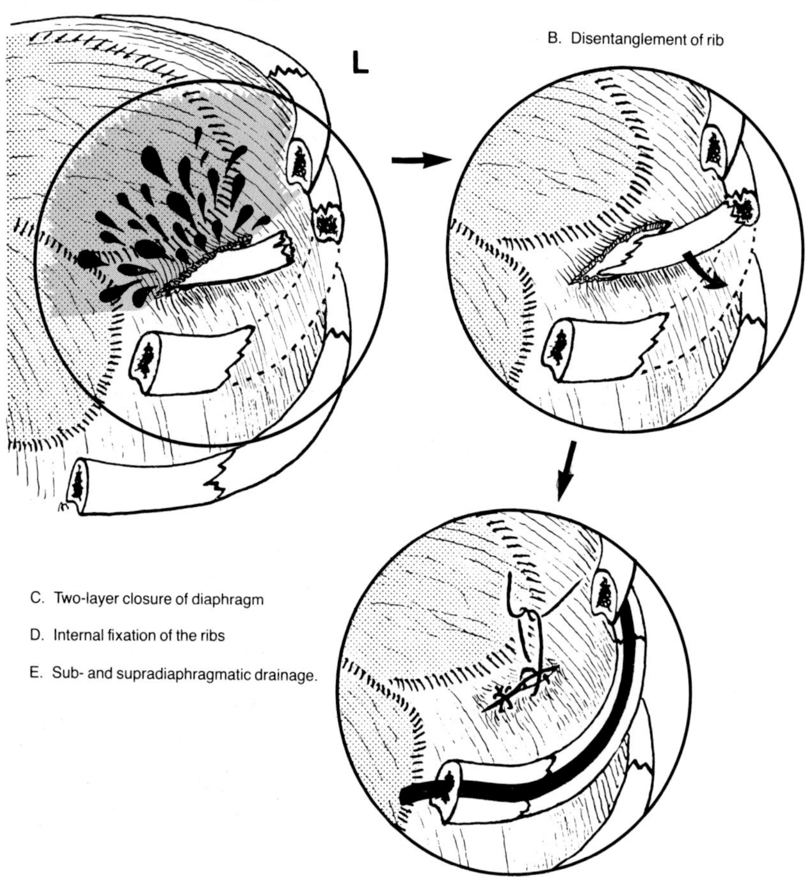

1120 Treatment of left-sided costal laceration of diaphragm.

1121a M.G. ♂ 45 yrs. 11 Jan. 1967

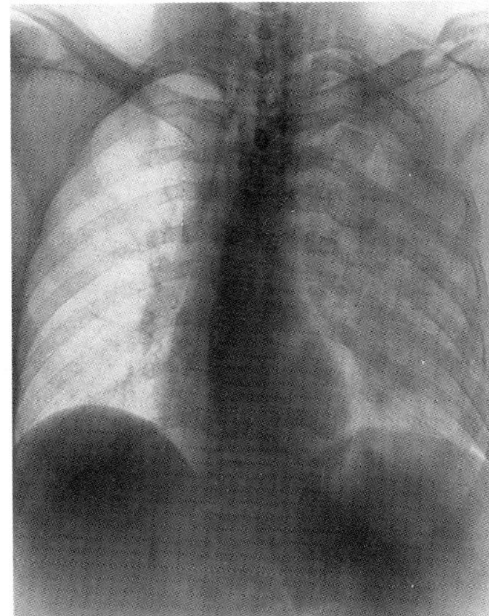

1121b 20 Jan. 1967

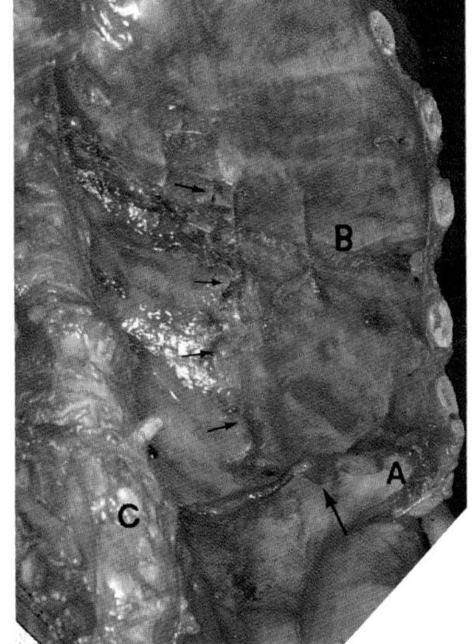

1121c 20 Jan. 1967

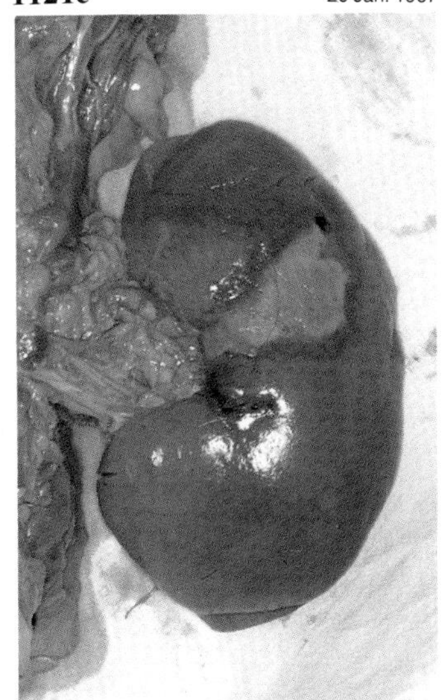

1121a Transdiaphragmatic laceration of spleen with haemothorax. The patient sustained multiple fractures of the left ribs when struck by a heavy door torn away by a passing train. A haemothorax develops rapidly. Thoracotomy 2 days later for uncontrolled pleural haemorrhage reveals that the haemothorax is of abdominal origin. The spleen is bleeding into the thorax through a posterior diaphragmatic laceration. Diaphragmatic incision: there is no haemoperitoneum; splenectomy. Death due to crush-syndrome.

1121b Autopsy reveals that the diaphragmatic laceration was the result of fracture-dislocation of 4 ribs (←). The insertion of the left hemidiaphragm (A), one of the perforations (←), the sutures closing the thoracotomy (B) and the vertebral column (C) are all visible.

1121c The lacerated upper part of the left kidney displays a white infarct.

1122a G.V. ♂ 67 yrs. 16 Nov. 1970

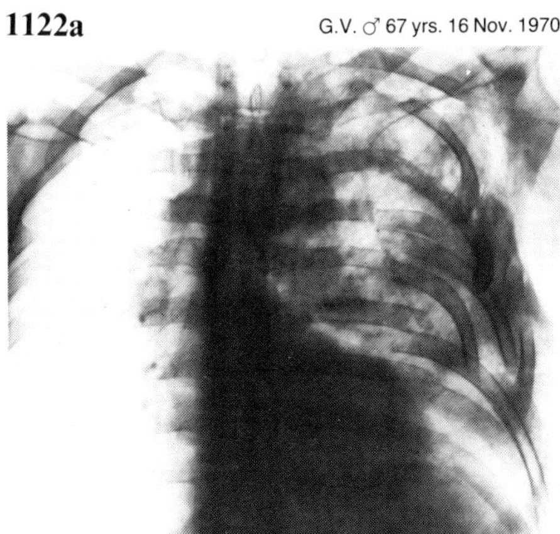

1122b 1 Dec. 1976

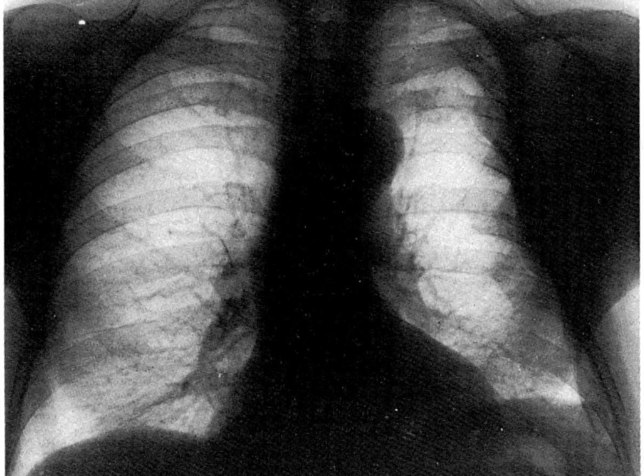

1122c 9 Dec. 1976

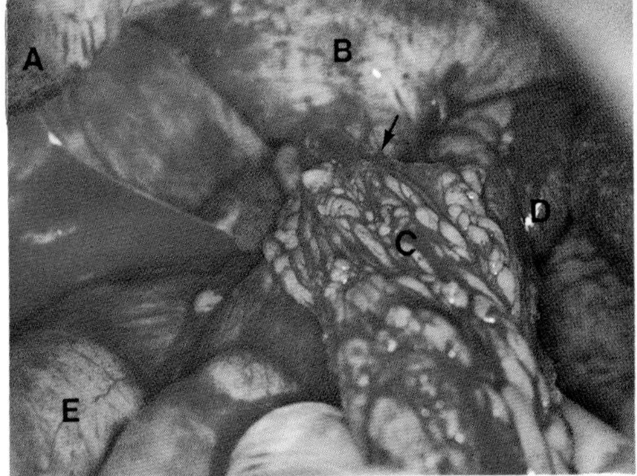

1122a Transdiaphragmatic puncture of omentum unrecognised for 6 years. Driver crushed in his car by the buffer of a locomotive. The initial X-ray shows a flail chest with fracture-dislocation of several ribs and a haemothorax. Drainage of the haemothorax. Contrast study for suspected diaphragmatic rupture: there is no gastrothorax.

1122b X-ray 6 years later, shortly before a laparotomy for an abdominal mass (which proves to be a gastric leiomyosarcoma).

1122c The laparotomy exposes the left lobe of the liver (A), a 1 cm laceration (→) of the left hemidiaphragm (B), the punctured omentum (C), the spleen (D) and the stomach (E). Reduction of the omentum, closure of the diaphragm. Recovery. (See Volume I, **340**).

N.B. The intruding rib missed the spleen by 1 cm.

Dehiscence of the suture line

Dehiscence of the suture line of a traumatic wound or of a surgical incision accounts for about 10% of diaphragmatic 'ruptures'.

Routine radioscopy should be carried out during the first two postoperative weeks to check for *early, total dehiscence*. Although strangulation is unlikely, repair is nonetheless urgent.

Late dehiscence is often dramatic. It can result from seemingly insignificant exertion, and commonly involves only part of the suture line. Herniated viscera are often strangulated. The clinical result is massive ileus.

X-ray evidence is unmistakable.

Both early and late dehiscence are repaired through a thoracic approach. Reduction of the herniated abdominal viscera is followed by careful two-layer suturing (see **1057, 1089**). The diaphragm is then allowed to cicatrize under cover of gastro-intestinal aspiration (through a Miller-Abbott or Dennis tube).

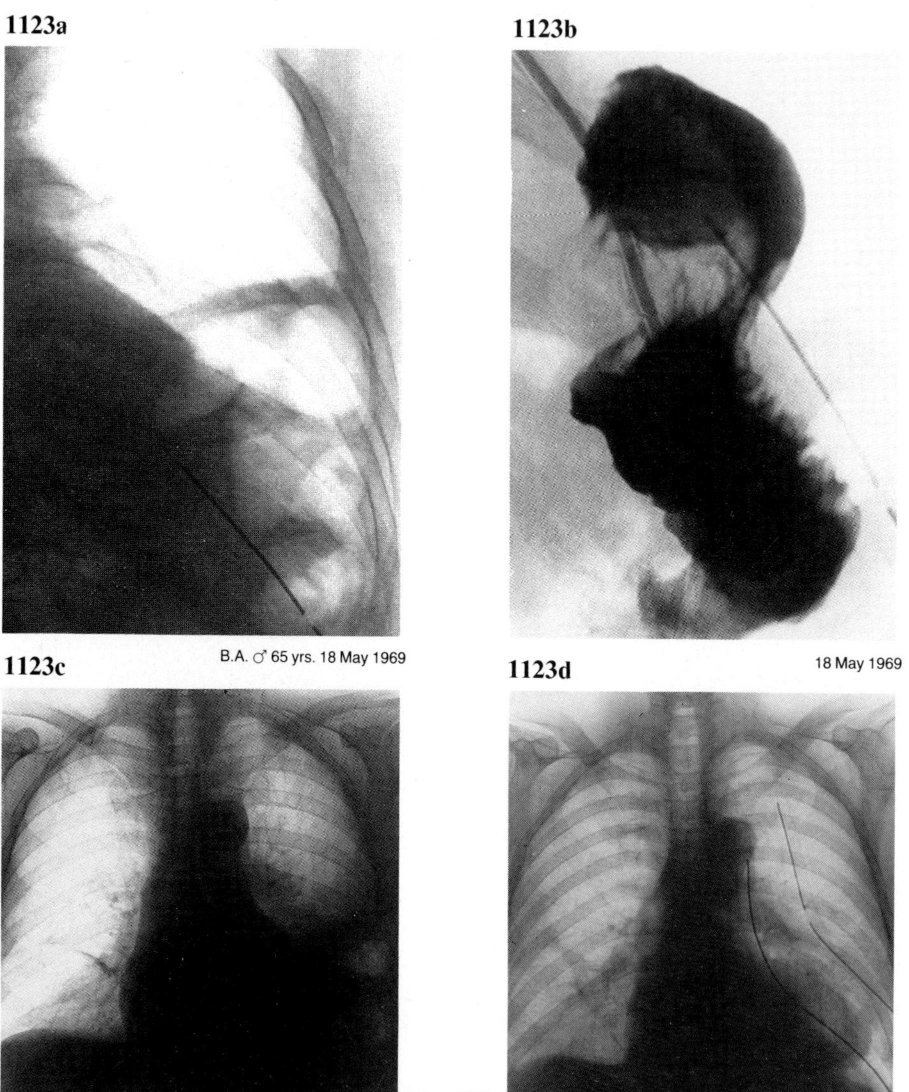

1123a Early dehiscence after surgical incision of diaphragm. The day after the repair (with Nissen fundoplication) of a transmural gastro-oesophageal laceration (Mallory-Weiss syndrome), the standard chest X-ray shows the small bowel in the left hemithorax

1123b A contrast study shows that part of the stomach has migrated into the thorax.

1123c Upright X-ray 15 days later. The diaphragm is repaired afresh through a combined thoracic and abdominal approach.

1123d Postoperative X-ray. Recovery.

1124a

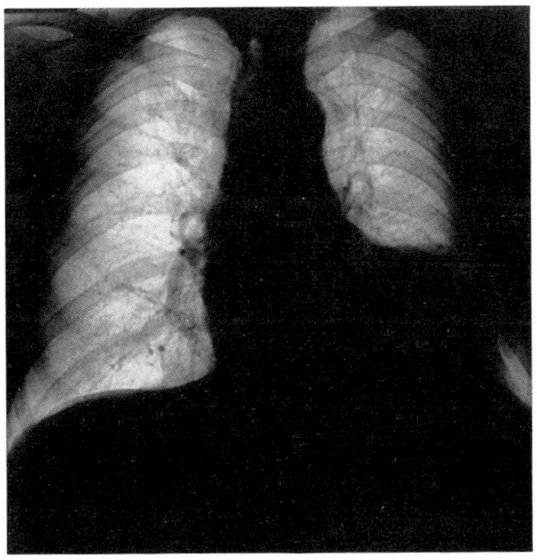

M.F. ♂ 61 yrs. 1 July 1976

1124c

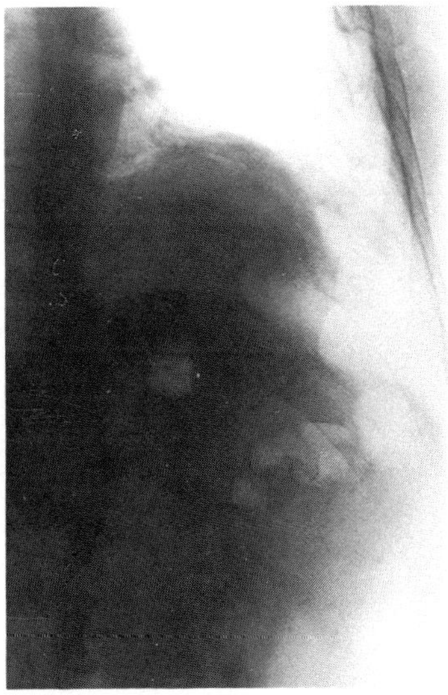

1 July 1976

1124d

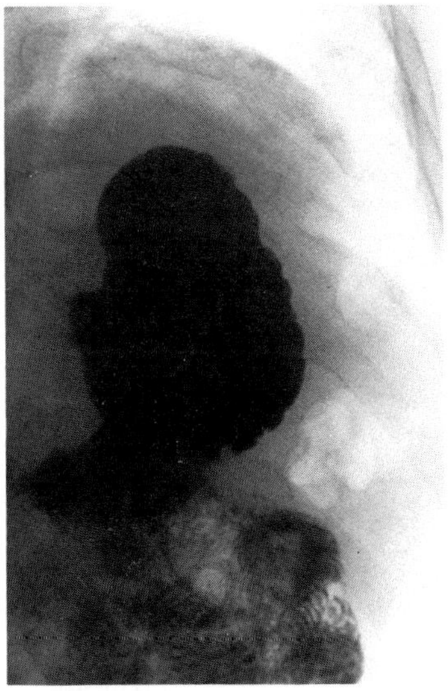

1 July 1976

1124b

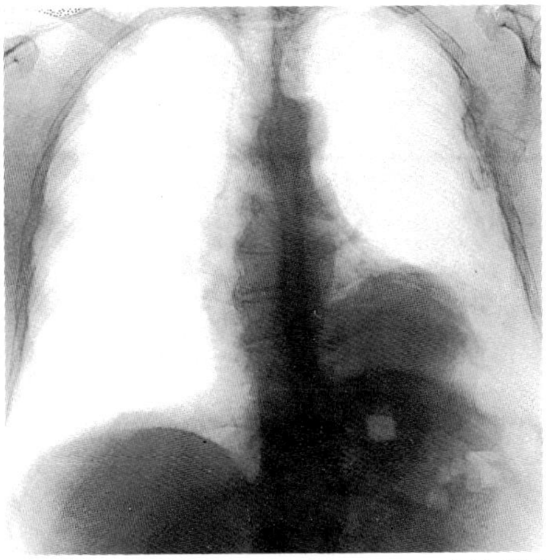

1 July 1976

1124e

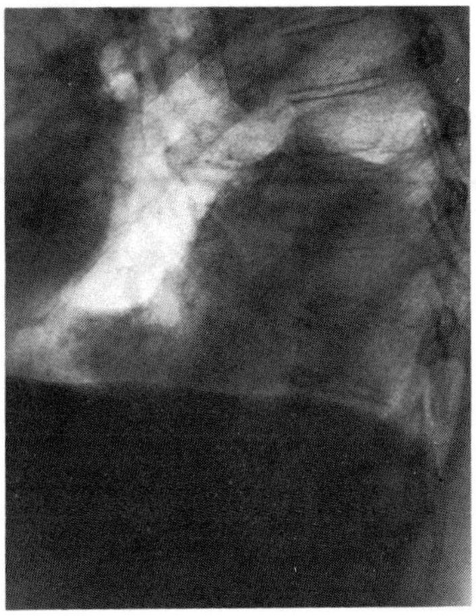

1 July 1976

1124f

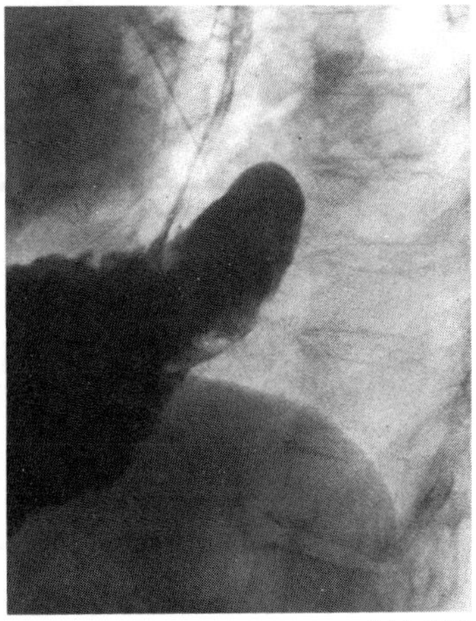

1 July 1976

1124a Dehiscence of suture line of diaphragmatic rupture. Conservative treatment. Standard upright X-ray 2 years after repair of the left hemidiaphragm and pericardium.

1124b An over-exposed X-ray suggests an iterative transdiaphragmatic hernia.

1124c Localised X-ray of the hernia.

1124d The position of the stomach.

1124e The hernia is posterior (lateral view).

1124f Barium study (lateral view). The injury causes neither inconvenience nor pain, and the patient refuses surgery.

1125a

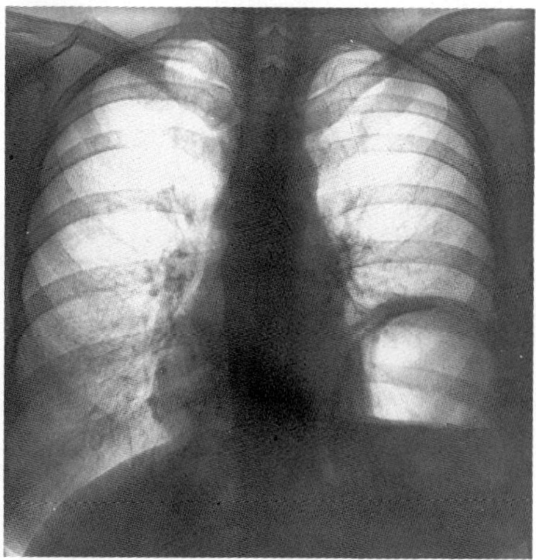

M.Y. ♀ 27 yrs. 20 Nov. 1964

1125b

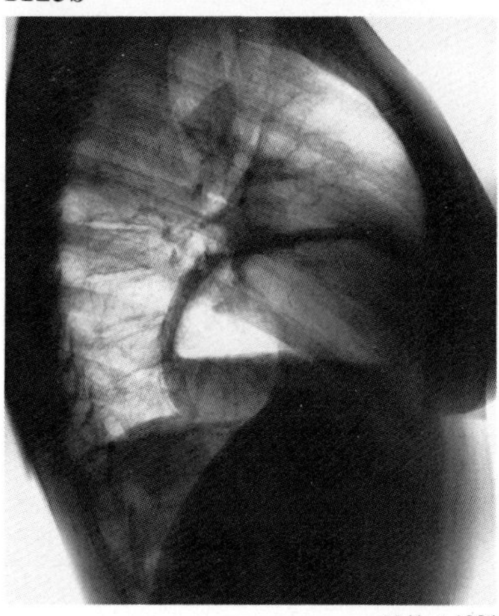

20 Nov. 1964

1125c

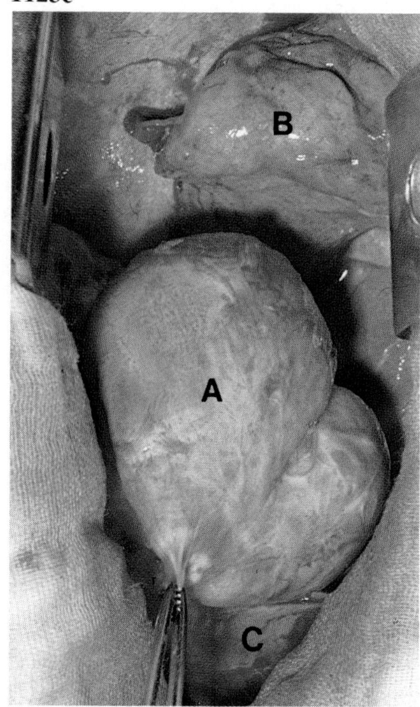

4 Dec. 1964

1125a Late dehiscence. Seven years after the initial left thoracotomy, dehiscence **of the suture line of a diaphragmatic rupture** results in the gradual herniation of the stomach (see **1073**).

1125b Volvulus of the supradiaphragmatic portion of the stomach.

1125c Thoracotomy reveals the stomach (A) in contact with the lower lobe of the left lung (B). Reduction and closure of the diaphragm (C). Recovery.

1126a

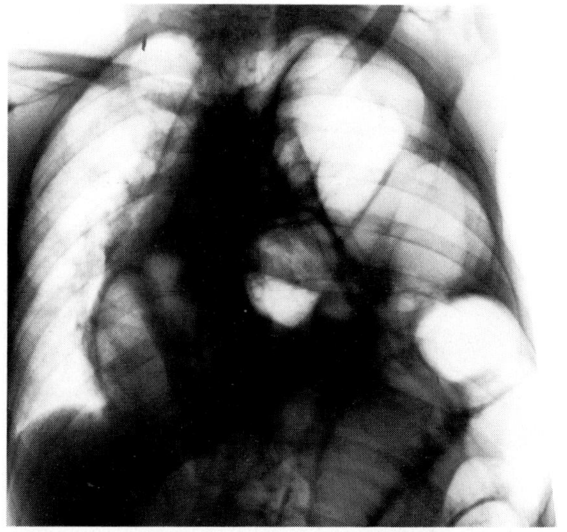

N.W. ♂ 53 yrs. 10 April 1970

1126a Late dehiscence with mechanical ileus. A year after the diaphragm was incised for a Nissen gastro-oesophageal fundoplication (through a left thoracotomy), the suture line suddenly dehisces. Herniation of the colon, small bowel and stomach results in massive mechanical ileus.

1126b

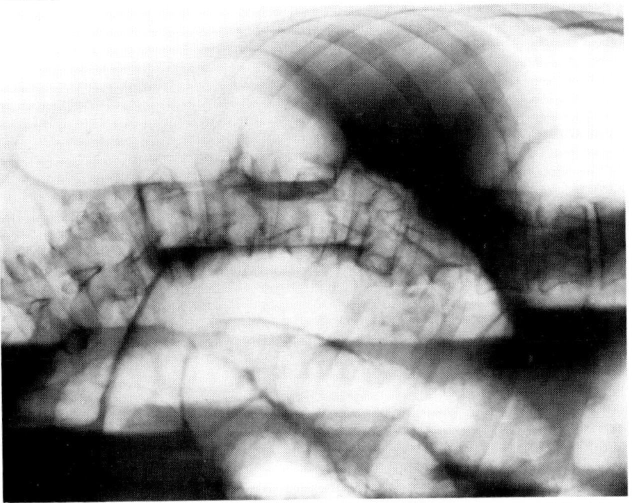

10 April 1970

1126b Ileus has severe abdominal repercussions.

1126c

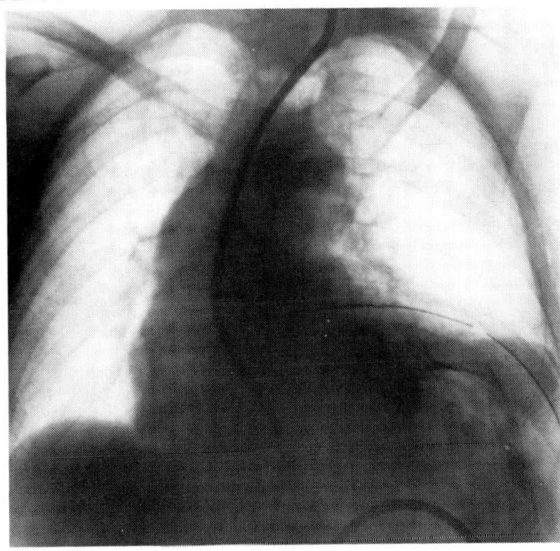

11 April 1970

1126c Left thoracotomy reveals a 5 cm opening in the diaphragm. Drainage and repositioning of the herniated viscera. Two-layer repair of the diaphragm. Recovery.

Post-traumatic relaxation

Phrenic nerve injury

In our experience, 11% of all diaphragmatic injuries involve damage to the phrenic nerve. Such damage can take the form of:

- *a primary tear* of the phrenic nerve or brachial plexus. This type of injury is often found in motorcyclists who have fallen or been struck violently on the shoulder. It is frequently associated with rupture or thrombosis of the subclavian or axillary vessels, and with fractures of the upper part of the thoracic cage. The resultant paralysis is almost irretrievable
- *primary section or contusion* of the thoracic portion of the phrenic nerve (knife or gunshot wound). Although this type of injury is again virtually irreparable, it is rarely the most serious injury that the patient presents
- *neurapraxia* resulting from irritation or contusion of the phrenic nerve in the neck or thorax (during resuscitation or the placement of a drain, for example). Short-lived (6 to 8 weeks) ventilatory disturbances are usually followed by a complete recovery.

Paralysis of a hemidiaphragm induces internal paradoxical motion; it is often accompanied by the accumulation of bronchial secretions or atelectasis.

1127a C.D. ♂ 54 yrs. 5 April 1966

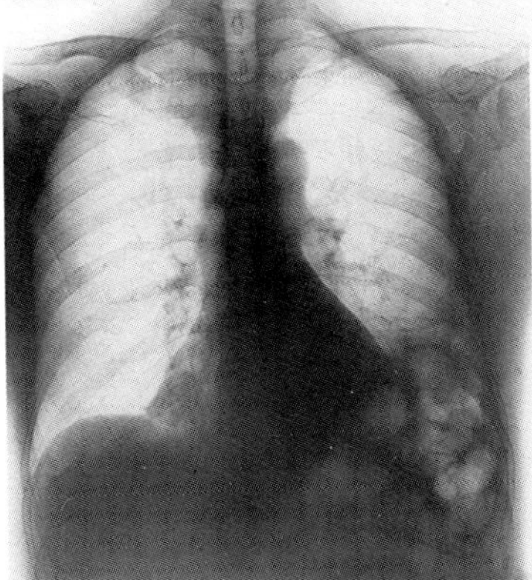

1127a Temporary post-traumatic neurapraxia of phrenic nerve. The film shows an 8 cm elevation of the left hemidiaphragm shortly after an injury to the upper left thorax with contusion of the shoulder in a patient with Recklinghausen's disease.

1127b 6 April 1966

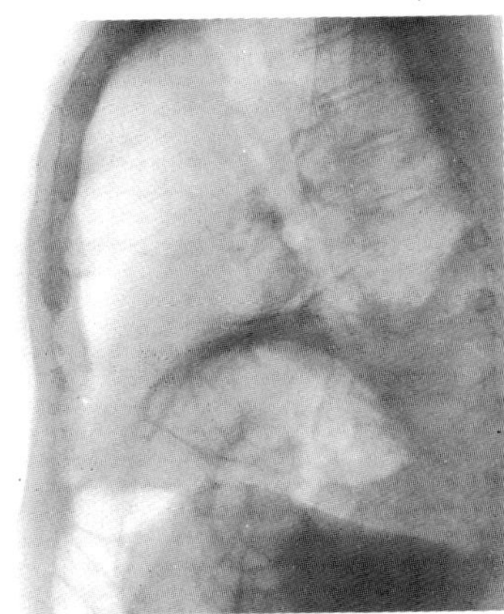

1127b Lateral X-ray deceptively suggests a rupture of the diaphragm with herniation of the small bowel and colon.

1127c 20 May 1966

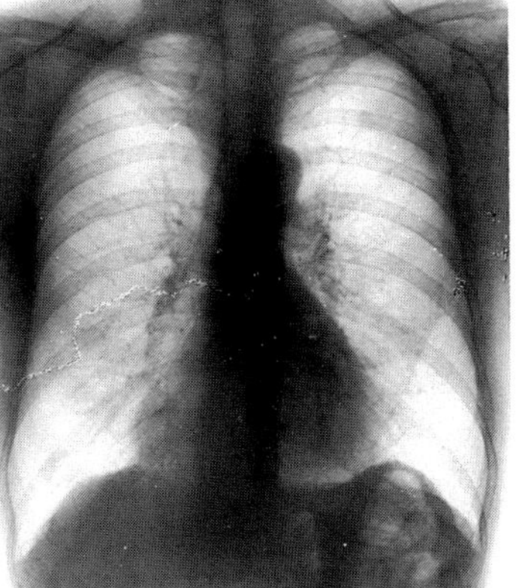

1127c Six weeks later, the phrenic neurapraxia has subsided.

1128a

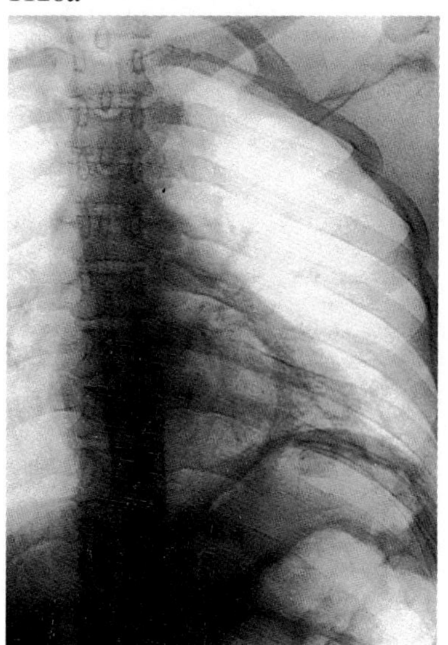

P.A. ♂ 20 yrs. 15 Sep. 1968

1128b

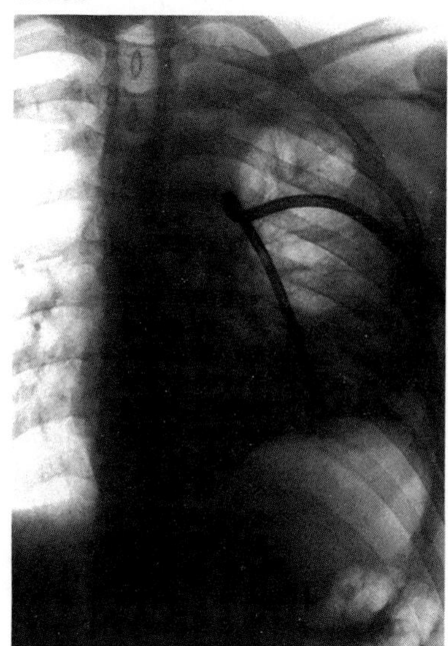

23 Sep. 1968

1128c

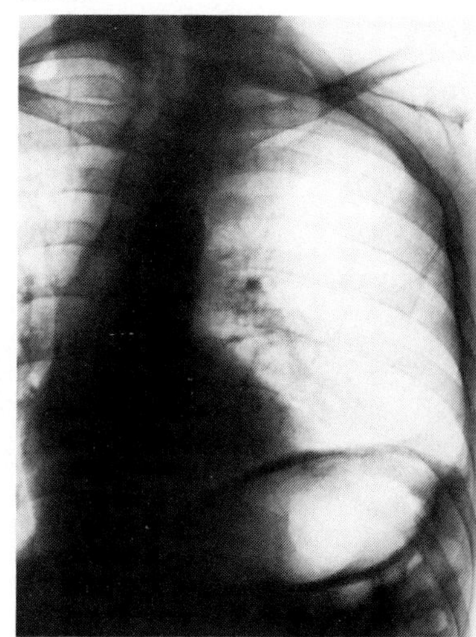

10 July 1978

1128a Paralysis of left hemidiaphragm by tear of phrenic nerve and brachial plexus in a motorcyclist who hit a tree at 100 km/h. He has already undergone a splenectomy, tamponade of a hepatic rupture, drainage of a contused pancreas and repair of an incomplete gastric tear. Four days after the accident, the left hemidiaphragm is relaxed and immobile.

1128b The paralysis is aggravated by a pleural effusion. The ill-ventilated lower lobe of the lung is atelectatic.

1128c Ten year follow-up.

1129a

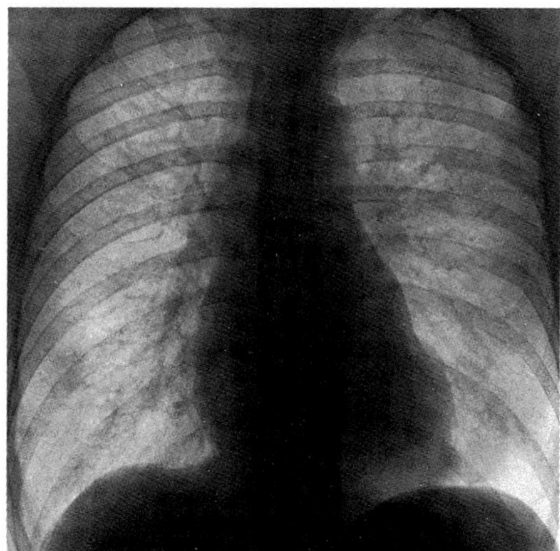

B.S. ♀ 29 yrs 4 July 1976

1129b

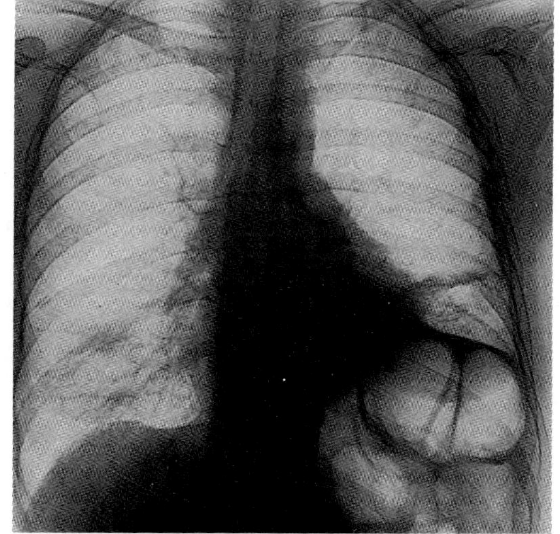

12 July 1976

1129a Iatrogenic phrenic nerve injury. The admission X-ray, one hour after a fall from the first floor, shows a left haemopneumothorax.

1129b The phrenic nerve is damaged by friction against a thoracic drain; paralysis (see Volume I, **464**) results in partial atelectasis of the left lower lobe.

1129c

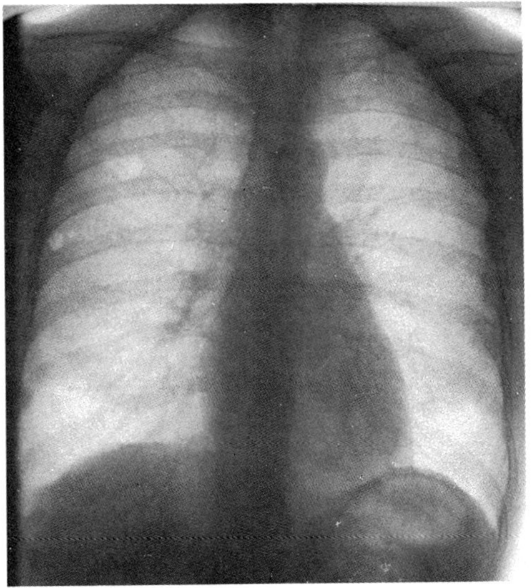

1129c Recovery without sequelae in 2 months.

Eventration

In most cases, diaphragmatic eventration is of non-traumatic origin but there are exceptions (see **1133**).

An eventration, noticed after a violent trauma, can be mistaken at X-ray for a transdiaphragmatic hernia; the confusion of the two can lead to unnecessary surgery (see **1132**). Deaths have been reported.

Diaphragmatic eventration causes internal paradoxical respiration. In combination with parietal damage, it commonly results in respiratory decompensation. Many cases require intubation with positive pressure ventilation; others demand surgical plication of the thinned portion of the diaphragm.

1130

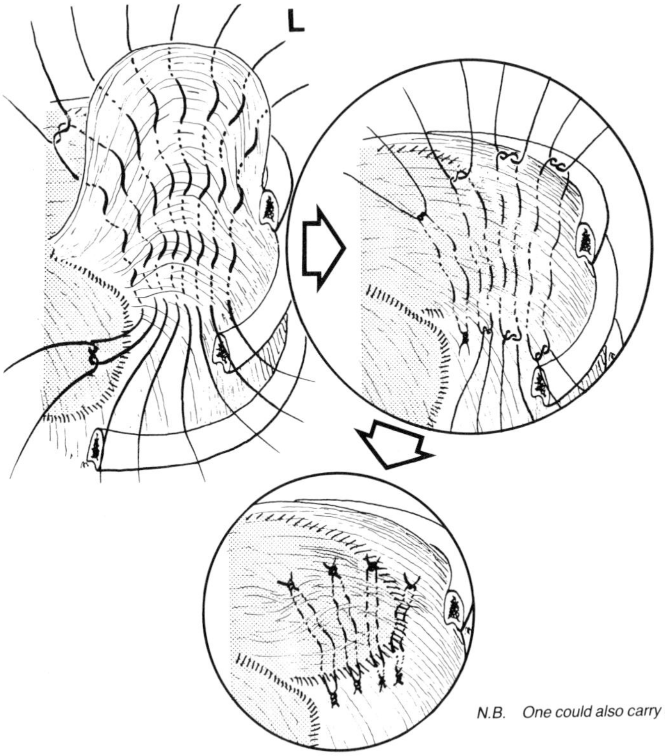

L

N.B. One could also carry on making up a 'waistcoat'.

1130 Thoracic approach to plicate large, left-sided diaphragmatic eventration.

1131

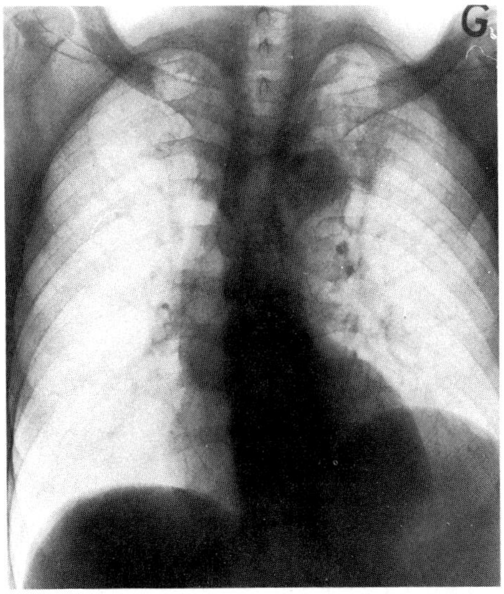

G

1131 Slight relaxation of left hemidiaphragm.

1132a

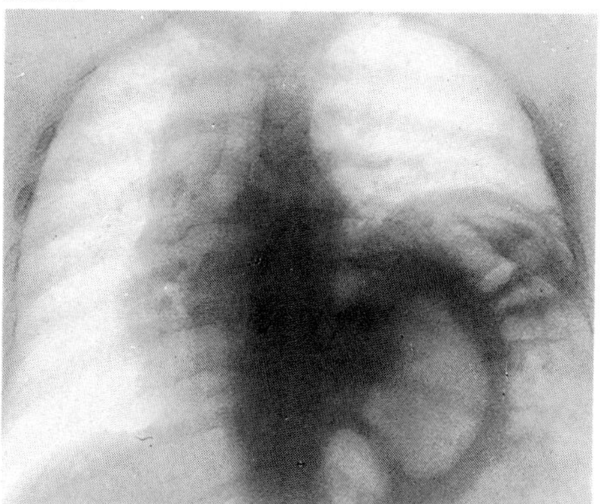

R.J. ♂ 34 yrs. 5 Dec. 1975

1132b

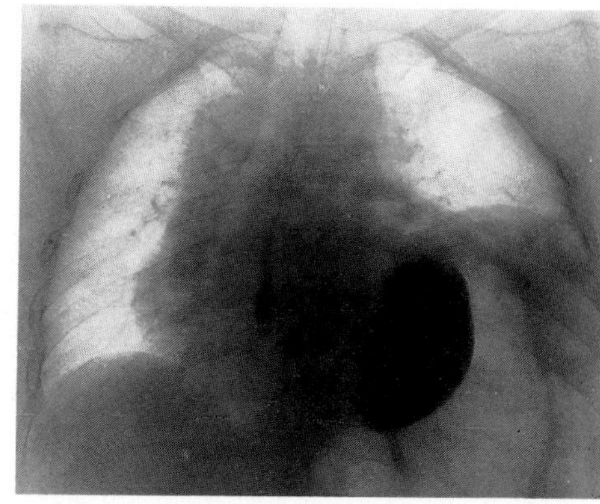

5 Dec. 1975

1132c

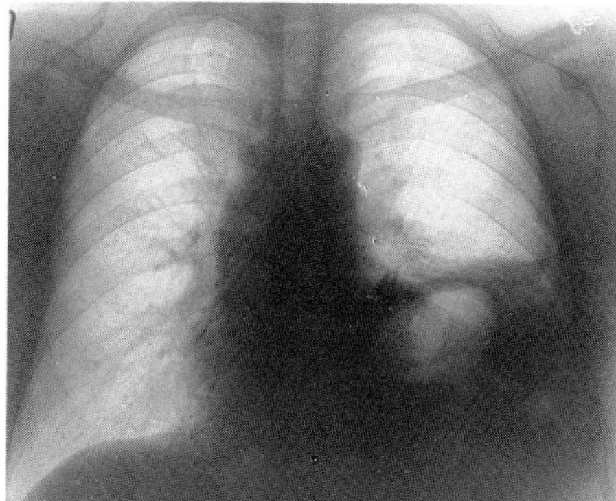

14 Dec. 1975

1132d

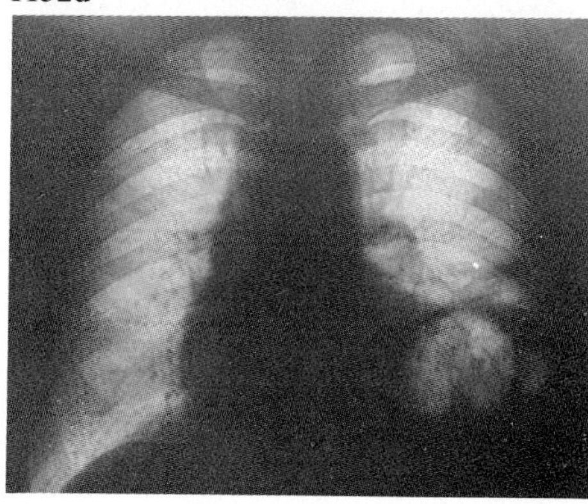

16 May 1975

1132a Large left diaphragmatic eventration. Workman squashed between 2 machines. Relaxation has the radiological appearance of rupture. The mediastinum is displaced to the right. **1132b** A barium study shows the stomach and colon to be above the normal position of the left hemidiaphragm. Laparotomy reveals a long-standing diaphragmatic relaxation with no traumatic damage. **1132c** Upright postoperative X-ray: in this position, there is no mediastinal displacement. **1132d** Subsequent research into the case produced this X-ray dating from 6 months before the accident.

1133a

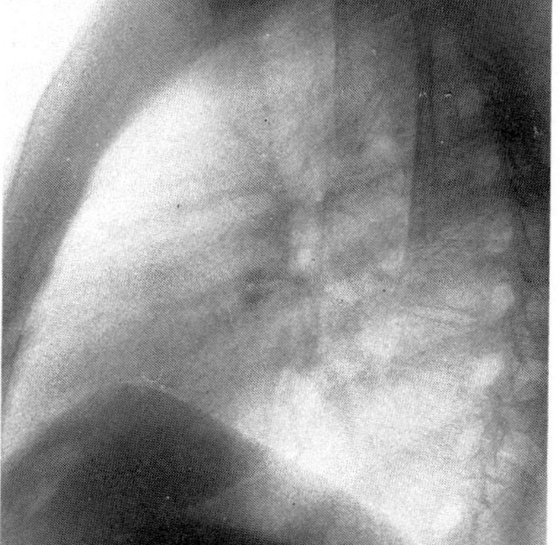

H.R. ♂ 36 yrs.

1133a Relaxation of right hemidiaphragm with Chilaiditi's syndrome. Old X-ray, obtained shortly after an injury to the right thorax and abdomen.

1133b

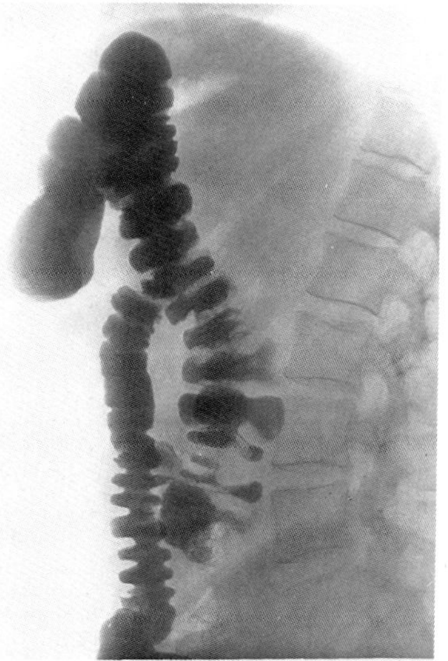

1963

1133b Barium study: lateral view . . .

1133c

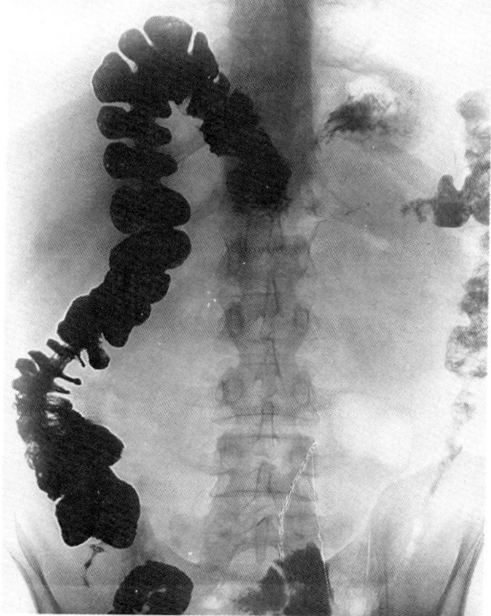

1963

1133c . . . and anterior view. Clearly, the colon could migrate through a rupture or peripheral avulsion of the right hemidiaphragm. However, this eventuality is rare (see **1097**).

Open wounds of the diaphragm

(see also Volume I, chapter 3)

The possibility of a diaphragmatic wound should be entertained seriously in any case of a penetrating or perforating wound of the chest. The following factors should be taken into consideration: (1) the patient's account of his injury, (2) the instrument used, (3) the likely path of the wound, (4) the position of the patient at the moment of impact, (5) the information provided by X-ray and sinography.

The criteria by which the likelihood of a wound to the diaphragm can be assessed are given in Volume I, chapter 3 (see page 143).

The choice between a thoracic and an abdominal approach is made usually on the basis of the sinogram. Examination of all the abdominal viscera should be routine. It should not be overlooked that peristalsis can quickly alter the position of a damaged portion of intestine.

As much of the diaphragm as possible should be examined. Sometimes there may be as many as four holes. Any fragment of foreign body measuring more than a few millimetres should be removed.

By their nature, stab wounds tend to be short and peripheral; they are usually less dangerous than gunshot wounds. These often entail either a double perforation or a large gash (caused by cartridge gas released by a point-blank shot, or by the 'tumbling' of a long-range shot). In most such cases, the subdiaphragmatic injuries are particularly life-threatening.

Whatever its length or position, no wound of the diaphragm ever cicatrizes spontaneously. Untreated, a wound is likely sooner or later to give rise to a strangulated hernia with ileus. This is a particularly common consequence of small dimension (stab) wounds. Whether or not accompanied by damage to adjacent viscera, every wound must be closed immediately with two solid layers of sutures.

The prognosis depends upon the interval between accident and treatment, and on associated intra-abdominal and intrathoracic injuries. The only risk engendered by the wound itself is intercoelomic contamination.

A pulmonary abscess sometimes signals delayed transdiaphragmatic migration of a foreign body from the abdomen. Deep impalement with a diaphragmatic wound also sometimes may have late pleuropulmonary repercussions.

Even when the elucidation of a diaphragmatic wound is delayed nevertheless it should be repaired without hesitation.

1134

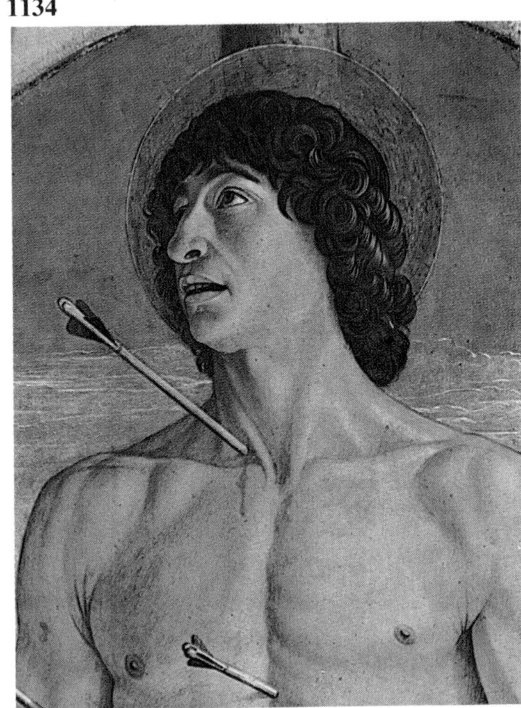

Giovanni Bellini: Saint Sebastian, martyr. Polyptych, 1464-1468, in the Chapel of Saint Vincent Ferrier, Venice.

1134 The lower arrow, entering through the 6th intercostal space on a downward trajectory, **may be thought to have traversed the diaphragm** and perforated abdominal viscera. Cardiac perforation is unlikely.

1135a

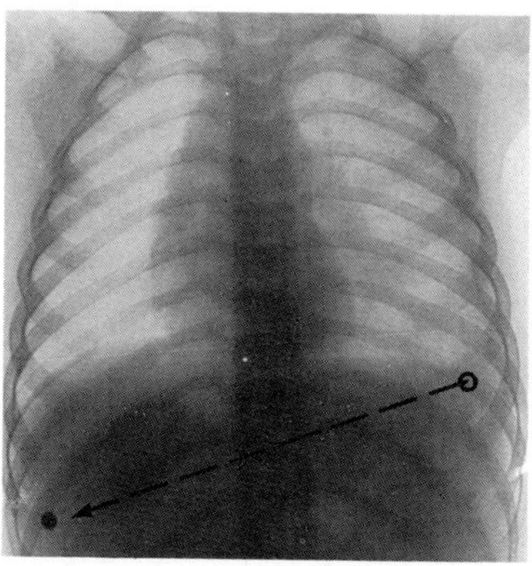

C.T. ♂ 3 yrs. 6 April 1971

1135b

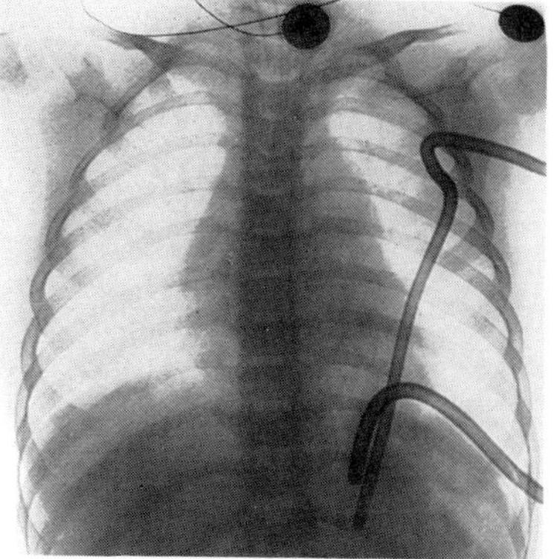

6 April 1971

1135c

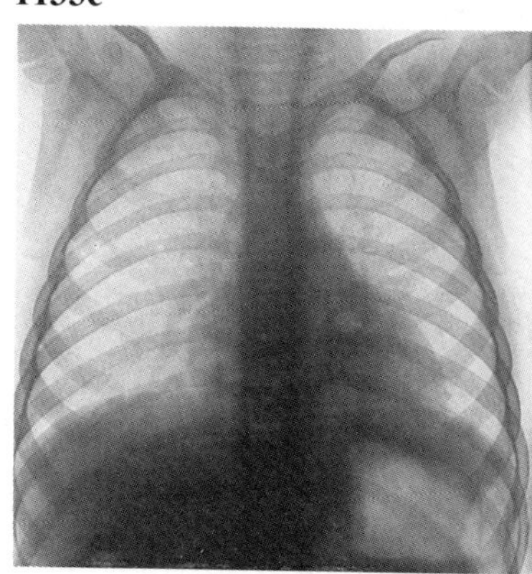

19 April 1971

1135a Single diaphragmatic wound by low velocity bullet. Thoraco-abdominal perforation inflicted by a low velocity bullet having entered in the 6th intercostal space, along the axillary line. Injuries include a tension left haemopneumothorax due to laceration of the lower lobe of the left lung, a single diaphragmatic wound, perforation of the lower oesophagus, a wound of the liver and perforation of the inferior vena cava. The bullet is lodged in the right lobe of the liver (see **1262**).

1135b A laparotomy has been performed to repair the abdominal damage, close the diaphragm and remove the bullet. Pleural aspiration brings the mediastinum back to its normal position.

1135c Recovery.

1136a

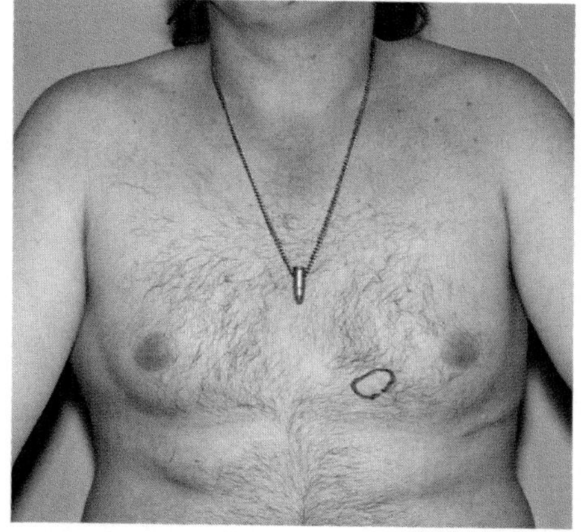

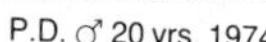

P.D. ♂ 20 yrs. 1974

1136b

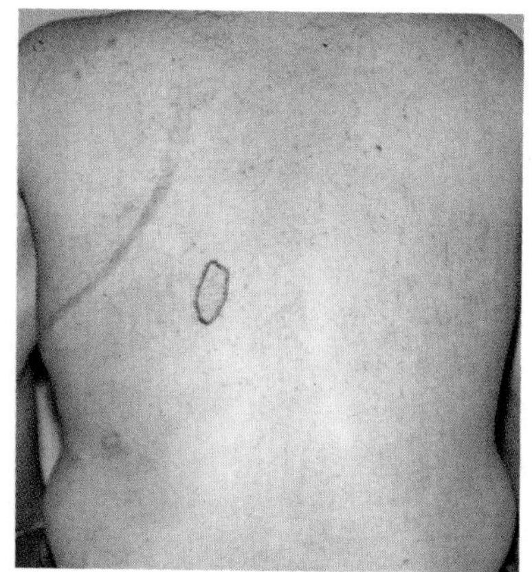

1136c

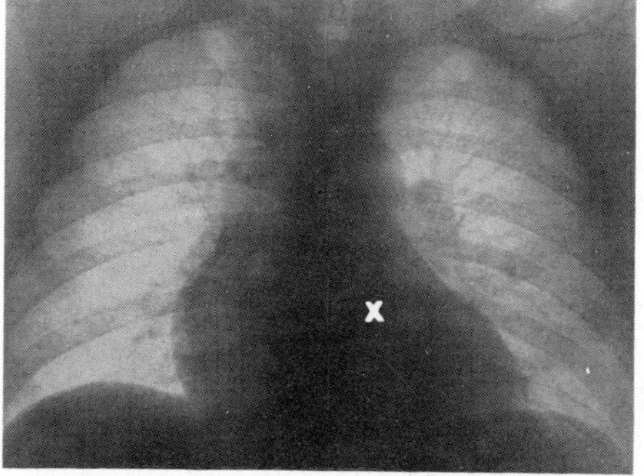

P.D. ♂ 17 yrs. 16 Oct. 1971

1136d

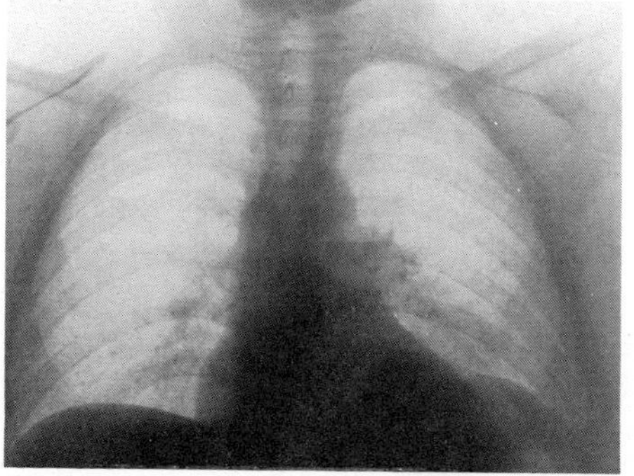

16 Oct. 1971

1136e

5th intercostal space

L

8th intercostal space

1136f

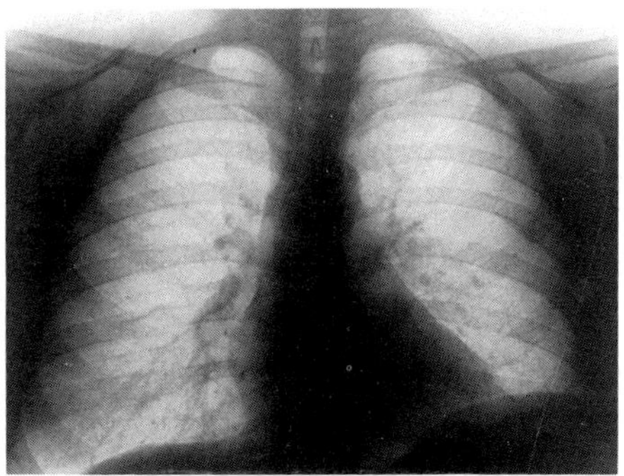

30 May 1974

1136a Double diaphragmatic wound by middle velocity bullet. Accidental short-range wound with a 7.65 bullet. Entry wound. (Photograph taken after recovery.)

1136b Exit wound.

1136c At first sight, the bullet would seem to have had an entirely intrathoracic trajectory (Ⓧ). The upper mediastinum and the right atrium appear enlarged. Clinical and radiological evidence seems to suggest cardiac tamponade. (Anteroposterior, supine X-ray.)

1136d However, on a postero-anterior film taken in the sitting position, the outlines of the mediastinum and atrium are almost normal. A left thoracotomy for delayed shock reveals only minimal intrathoracic damage. The patient's shout at the moment of the accident meant that the bullet traversed the diaphragm . . .

1136e . . . lacerating the liver, passing through the stomach and tearing the spleen. Having then re-traversed the diaphragm, it caused a minor pulmonary wound. Incision of the diaphragm: haemostasis of the liver, splenectomy, repair of the stomach and closure of the diaphragm.

1136f Three years later, left lung function is normal. Diaphragmatic sequelae are minor.

1137

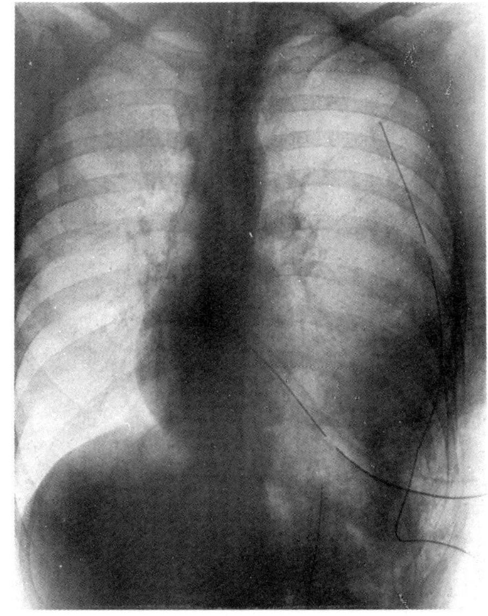

J.F. ♀ 34 yrs. 17 Mar. 1968

1137 Laceration of diaphragm by high velocity bullet. Thoraco-abdominal wounds from a point-blank shot from an assault rifle. Gas from the cartridge has caused significant emphysema of the lower thoracic wall and the left hypochondrium. Emergency exploration (thoraco-phreno-laparotomy) reveals a flail chest with paradoxical motion over 4 ribs, a pulmonary laceration-contusion with a haemothorax, a 5cm tear of the diaphragm, a ruptured spleen and injuries to the adrenal gland and liver. Repair. Recovery.

1138

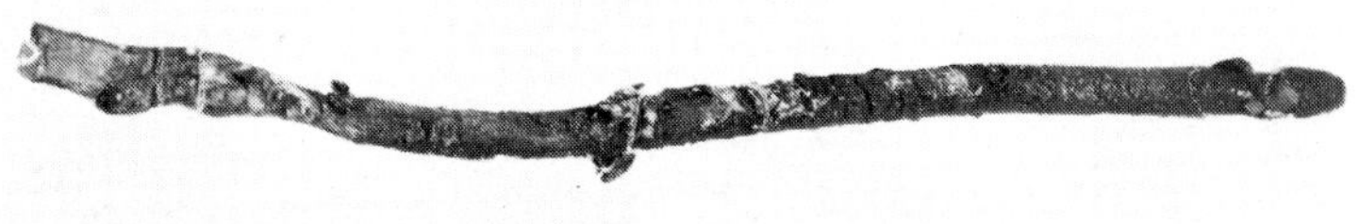

D.E. ♀ 26 yrs. 16 July 1942

1138 Gradual perforation of diaphragm. Probe found in a pulmonary abscess, 5 years after an abortive manoeuvre during which it disappeared, apparently through a posterior vaginal perforation. From the retroperitoneum, it traversed the diaphragm and entered the pulmonary parenchyma. Thoracotomy revealed a portion of the omentum blocking the diaphragmatic perforation. The perforation was sutured and the abscess drained. Death 2 months later due to infection.

1139 Repair of small wound of left hemidiaphragm.

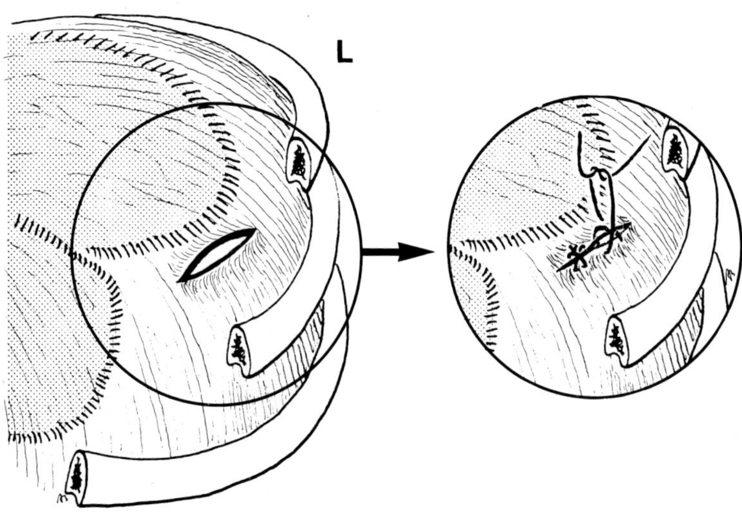

A. Evaluation of supradiaphragmatic injuries

B. Evaluation of subdiaphragmatic injuries (possibly through a diaphragmatic incision)

C. Check for possible second wound

D. Two-layer suturing

N.B. The choice between a thoracic and an abdominal approach is made according to the wound localisation and sometimes according to the fistulography.

11 Trauma of the oesophagus

(by Augustin Besson and Marcel Savary)

The five-fold increase in the incidence of oesophageal injuries in the last 30 years is attributable to various factors.

Around 1950, foreign body injuries were most frequent. Their absolute number has not decreased, but they are now less common than instrumental perforations which have tripled in number in three decades. In addition, recent developments in upper gastro-intestinal endoscopy have made oesophageal injuries easier to diagnose; injuries sustained during vomiting, in particular, are now recognised more readily.

1140

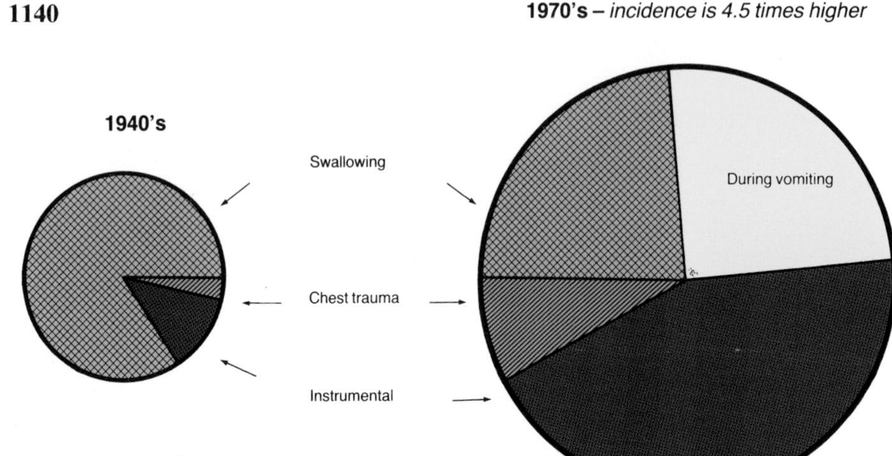

1140 Aetiopathogenesis of oesophageal injuries, **historical survey** (in our material, $n = 121$)

Any injury – whether a wound, laceration, rupture, corrosion or perforation – of the oesophagus is potentially fatal. The prognosis deteriorates by the hour as virulent oesophageal flora invades the ill vascularised surrounding tissues. The Admiral of the Dutch Fleet, Baron of Wassenaer and Lord of Rosenburg, died a few hours after an oesophageal rupture; Boerhaave's 1724 account of his demise is detailed and vivid.

About half of all transmural oesophageal injuries are diagnosed and treated late.

1141

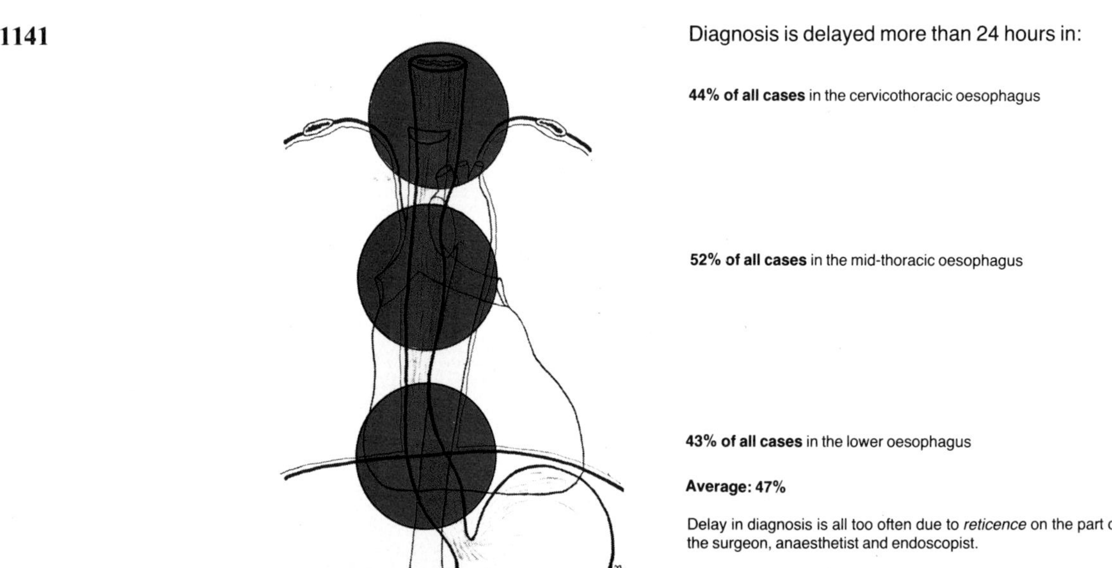

1141 Late diagnosis of oesophageal injuries treated surgically ($n = 128$).

Oesophageal perforation is the most life-threatening of all digestive perforations. If treatment is delayed, the prognosis is almost certainly fatal, whatever the age of the patient.

In the course of the chapter, we will pay particular attention to a number of severe complications collected from our own files, from the files of the ENT clinic and from those of neighbouring regional hospitals.

About half of the cases cited were transferred to the University Hospital when the patient was already in very poor condition. The incidence of complication in our own cases is relatively low.

We have included any case we consider to be instructive.

1142

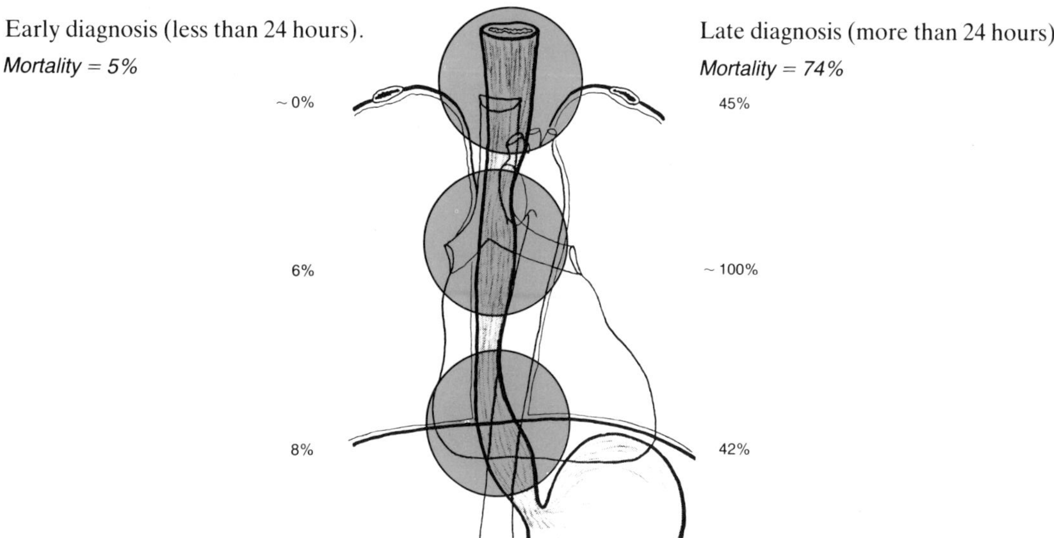

1142 Overall mortality following surgery for an oesophageal injury (n = 128).

Diagnosis of oesophageal perforation can be difficult, particularly in cases of (1) instrumental wounds (especially when inflicted during general anaesthesia), (2) emetic rupture when vomiting is not reported and (3) violent cervicothoracic trauma, blunt or open, when oesophageal damage is overshadowed by more obvious injuries.

Most other oesophageal injuries are detected early either because they are clinically evident or, because discrete symptoms or signs have indicated an emergency upper gastro-intestinal study (or endoscopy).

Aetiology

1143

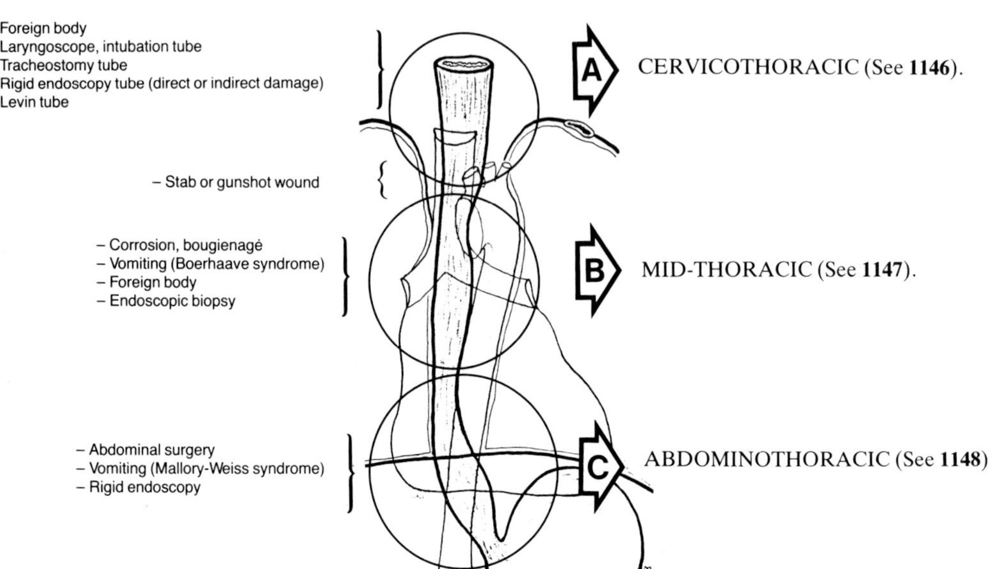

1144

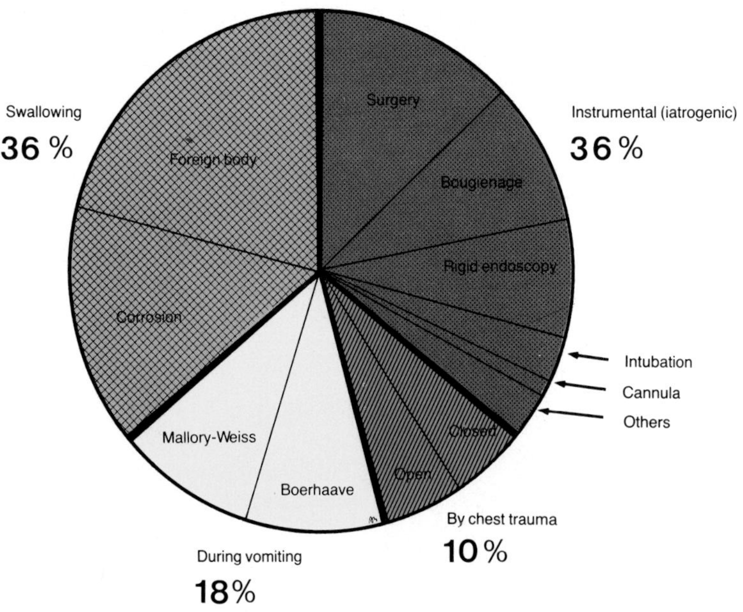

1144 Aetiopathogenesis of oesophageal injuries
Treated surgically over the last 3 decades (in our material, $n = 121$).

Perforation of the oesophagus

The incidence of perforation in different parts of the oesophagus depends upon the aetiology of injury. The diagram below gives overall incidences.

1145

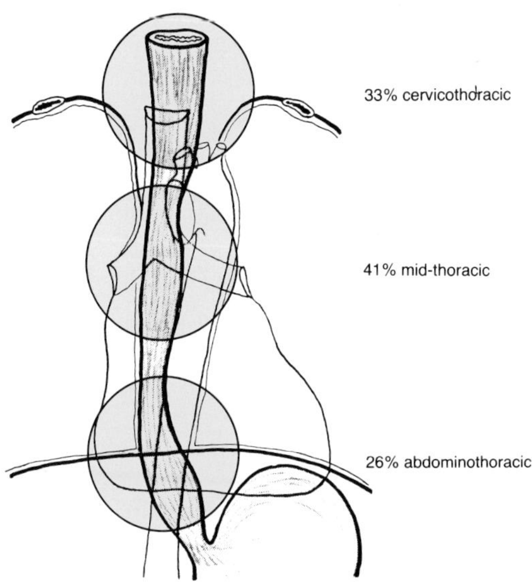

1145 Localisation of oesophageal injuries treated surgically (n = 121).

Symptoms

The patient's *history* usually clarifies the cause of injury: emetic injury, swallowing injury, intubation or endoscopy accident, etc . . . If a history is unobtainable (multiple injury patient with brain damage, unco-operative or intoxicated patient), diagnosis must be made on the basis of the patient's symptoms and signs.

The chief complaint is usually *excruciating pain* on swallowing (odynophagia); the pain is so sharp that many patients spontaneously regurgitate their saliva to avoid having to swallow. The patient's localisation of his pain gives little indication of the actual site of injury. Odynophagia is sometimes misread as a symptom of myocardial infarction or acute pancreatitis.

Haematemesis usually alarms sufficiently to be reported. The sequence of events is important; haematemesis after violent vomiting indicates emergency fibroscopy.

A *cough* on swallowing is usually a late symptom of a fistula between the oesophagus and the respiratory tract.

Clinical and radiological signs

Signs of oesophageal injury

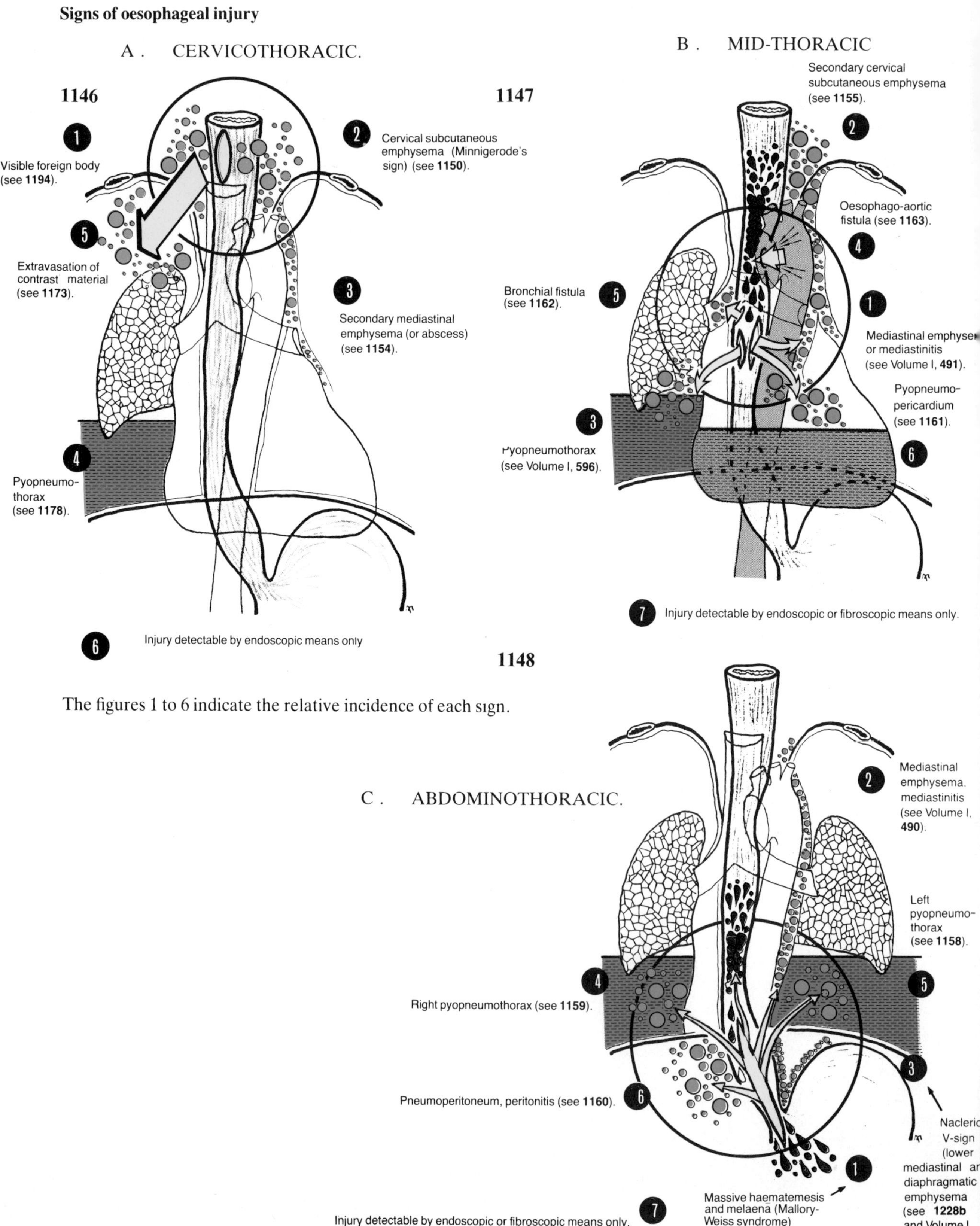

The figures 1 to 6 indicate the relative incidence of each sign.

1151a

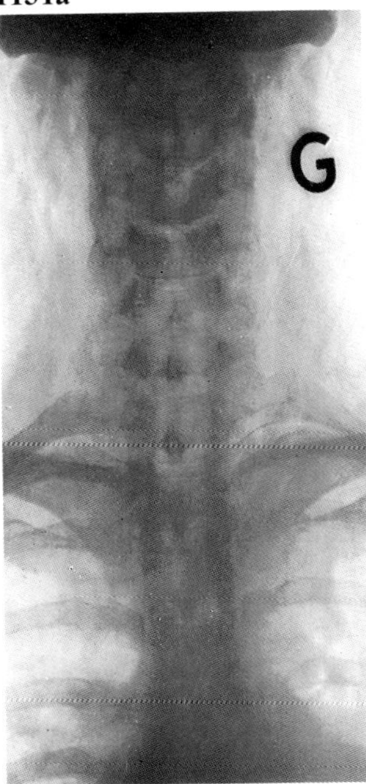

B.S. ♂ 56 yrs. 17 Sep. 1964

1151b

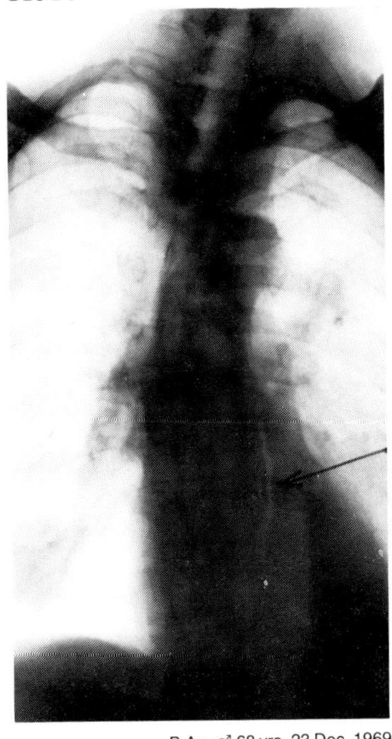

B.Au. ♂ 68 yrs. 23 Dec. 1969

1151a Mediastinal emphysema extending to cervical subcutaneous tissue, following a wound to the upper thoracic oesophagus.

1151b Periaortic emphysema. Early sign of 'spontaneous' cardio-oesophageal rupture.

1152

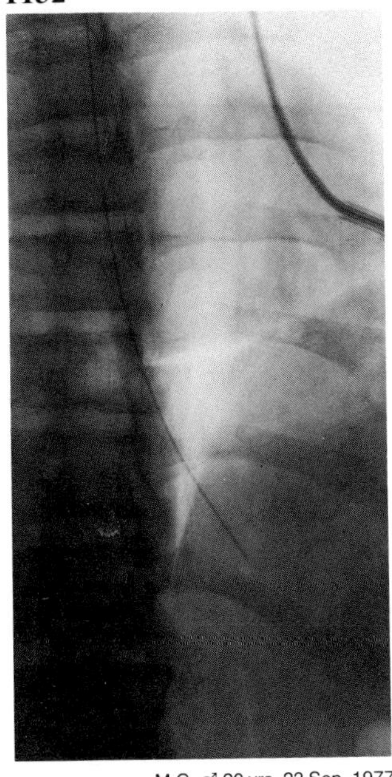

M.C. ♂ 20 yrs. 23 Sep. 1977

1152 Naclerio's 'V' sign is not pathognomic. In this case it is due to mediastinal emphysema after a barotrauma (see Volume I, **500, 504**).

MEDIASTINITIS

Mediastinitis is a frequent and severe complication of oesophageal perforation; it should be pre-supposed in every case. It develops very quickly, and should be treated urgently.

1153 Mediastinitis following oesophageal perforation is life-threatening.

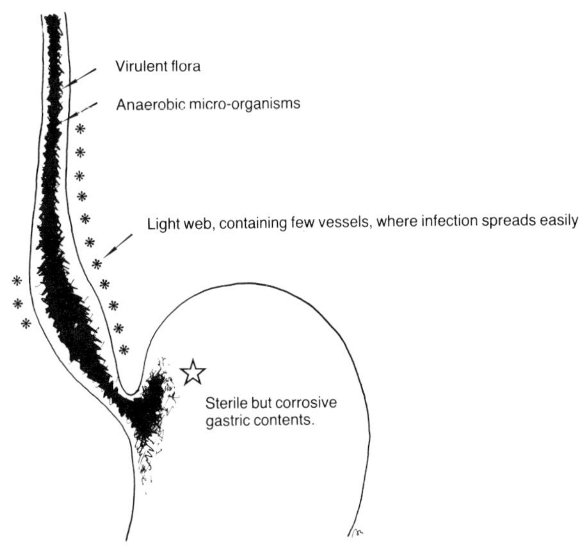

1154a

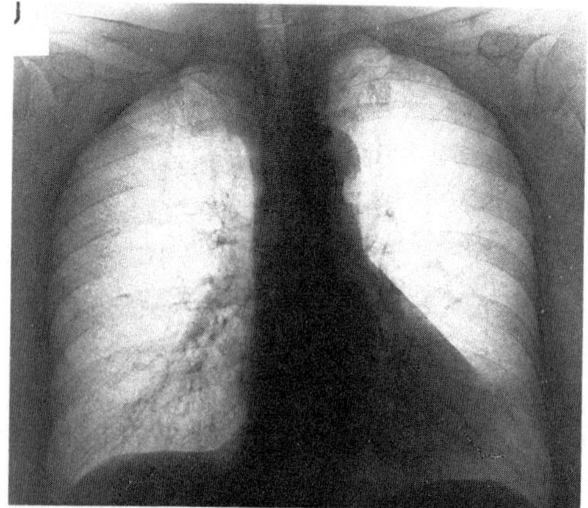

G.R.M. ♀ 67 yrs. 5 June 1973

1154b

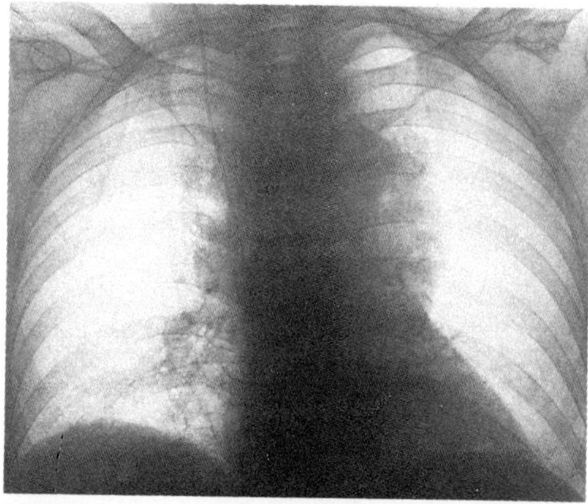

14 June 1973

1154c

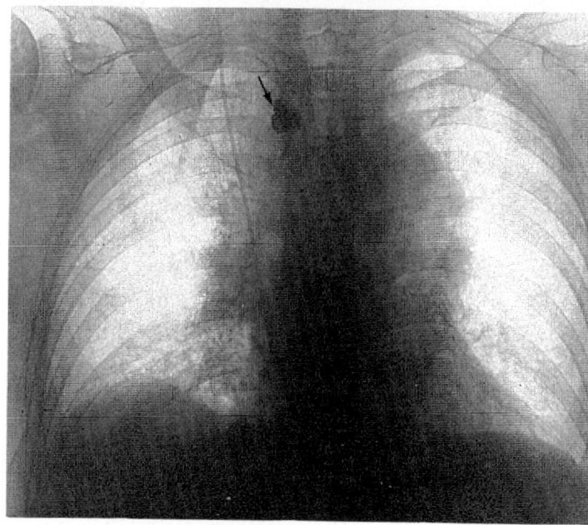

19 June 1973

1154d

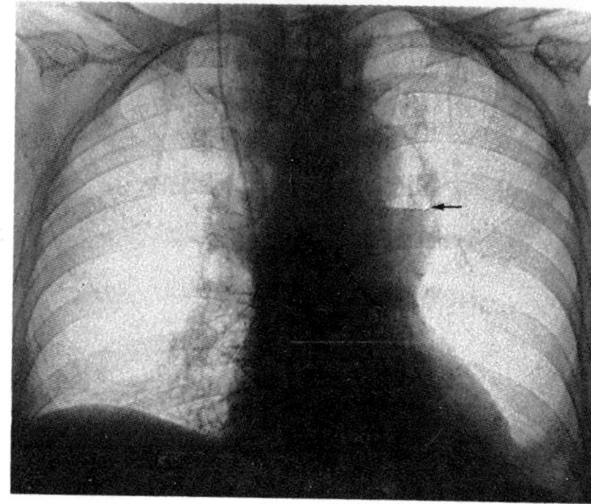

20 June 1973

1154e

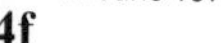

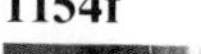

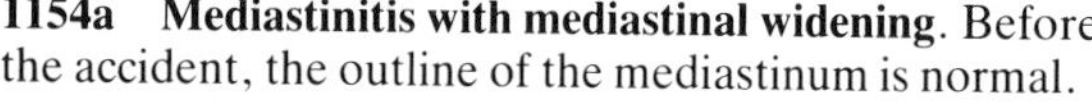

June 1973

1154f

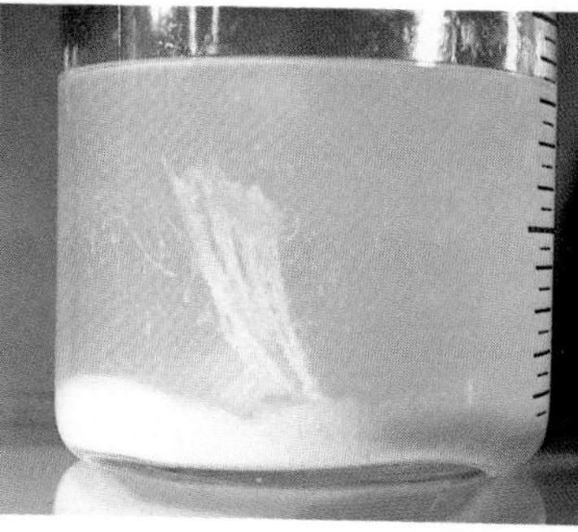

20 June 1973

1154a Mediastinitis with mediastinal widening. Before the accident, the outline of the mediastinum is normal.

1154b Nine days after repeated attempts at oro-tracheal intubation (during which an oesophageal wound was inflicted but not detected) the mediastinum is widened, especially to the left. The patient is in septic shock.

1154c Fourteen days after injury, the mediastinum is still larger. The film shows extravasation of iodine solution (→). Perforation of the oesophagus is diagnosed.

1154d Secondary mediastinal abscess evidenced by a hydro-aeric (→) level in the sitting position. Cervicotomy and Spühl-drainage.

1154e The abscess (with a hydro-aeric level) is located in the anterior mediastinum.

1154f The patient has received large doses of tetracyclines. Pyogenic germs have been replaced in the abscess by candida tropicalis. Progressive cachexia proves fatal within a month. (Prof. R. Mégevand, Hôpital Cantonal, Geneva.)

1155

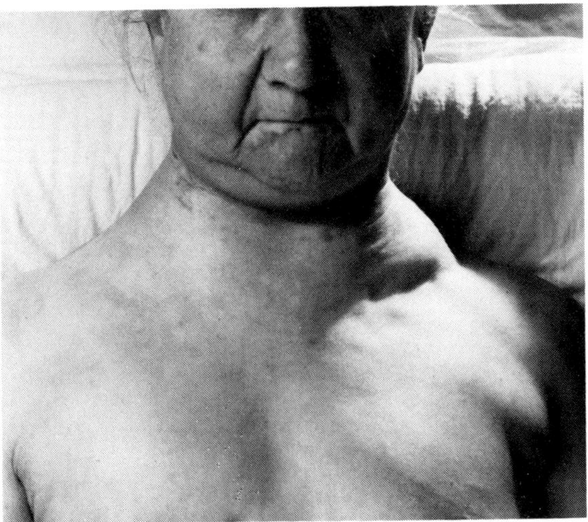

V.D. ♀ 67 yrs. 15 Jan. 1948

1155 Bilateral cervical propagation of mediastinitis. The oesophageal wound (caused by a prune-stone) lies 3cm below Killian's mouth. Crepitation can be palpated.

1156a

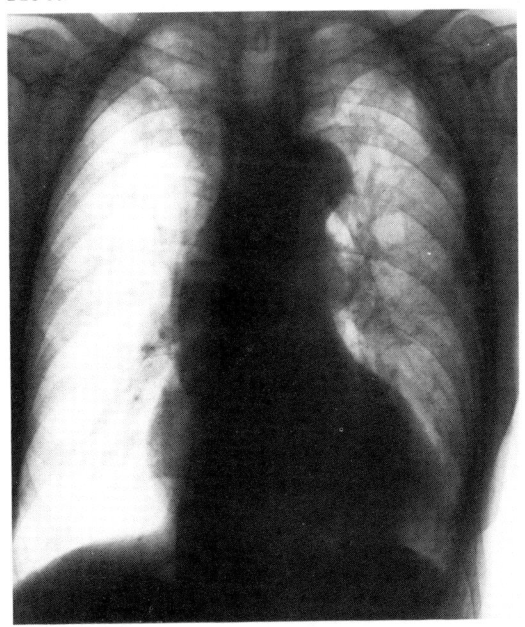

T.L. ♀ 60 yrs. 19 Sep. 1974

1156a Even if well tolerated for several days, mediastinitis after emetic rupture is usually fatal if treatment is late. The admission X-ray, taken 5 days after a traumatic episode of vomiting, shows moderate mediastinal emphysema.

1156b An upper gastro-intestinal study with **barium** (!) reveals a large rupture (1.5cm in length) 2.5cm above the cardia. Barium extravasates into the mediastinum.

1156c The extravasation in close-up. Thoracotomy and laparotomy for repair and drainage. Post-operative death.

1156b

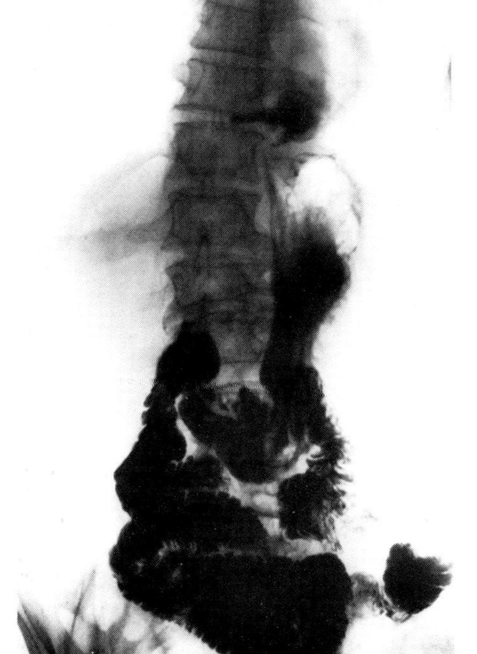

20 Sep. 1974

1156c

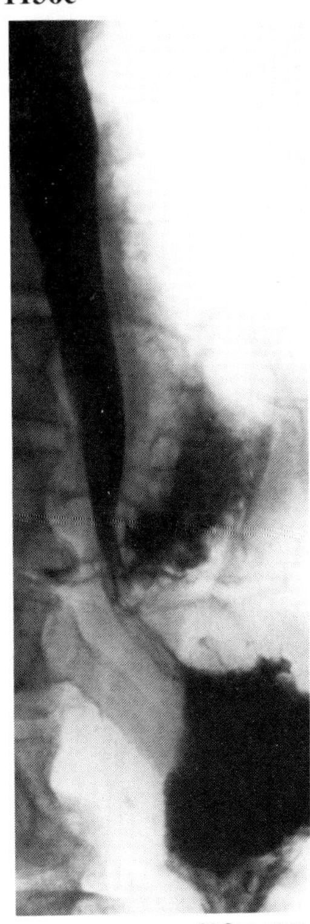

20 Sep. 1974

PLEURAL FISTULA

Regardless of its localisation, oesophageal perforation usually extends to one or other pleural cavity (see **1149, 1156, 1160, 1173, 1178, 1228, 1256**). Pleural fistulisation can be immediate or delayed. In most cases, the effusion is mixed (hydropneumothorax or pyopneumothorax). An eosophagogram with soluble contrast material is indicated to confirm and locate the oesophageal perforation.

1157

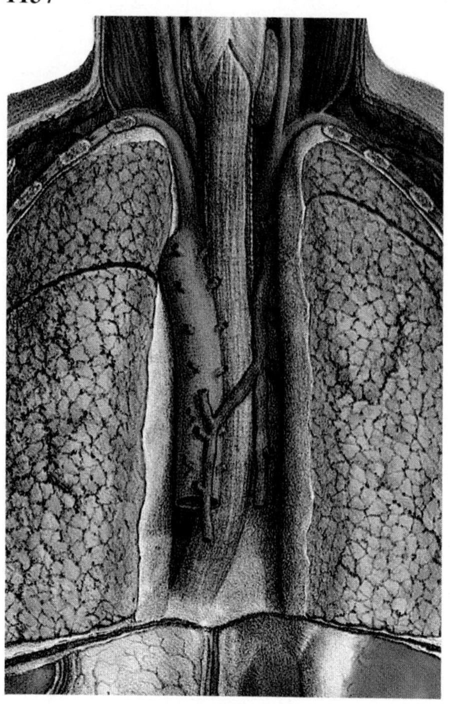

1157 It is clear from the anatomy that any rupture of the lower oesophagus (see here from behind with the vertebrae removed) is likely to extend to one or other of the pleural cavities. (Bourgery, 1867).

1158a

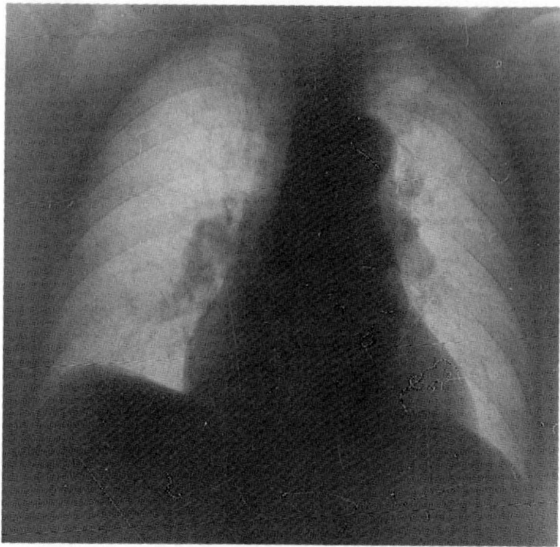

1158b A.B. ♀ 83 yrs. 8 Aug. 1973

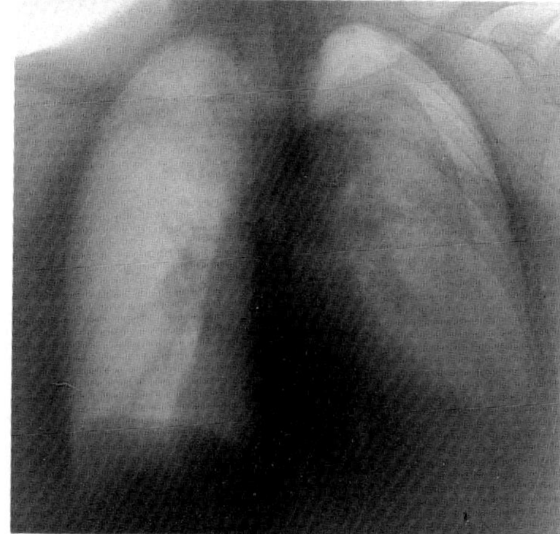

1158c

20 Aug. 1973

1158d 18 Aug. 1973

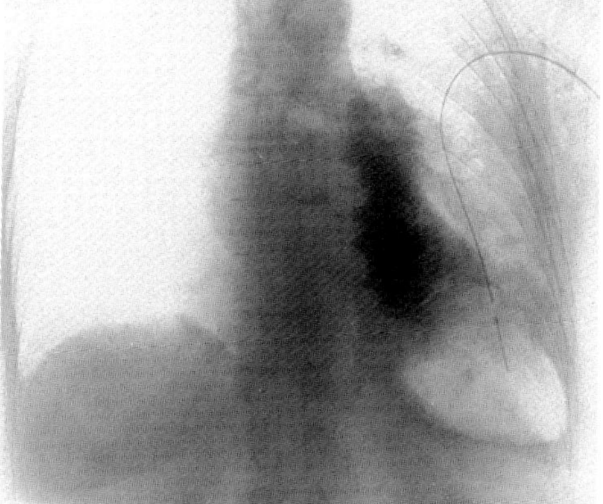

20 Aug. 1973

1158a Mid-thoracic (emetic?) rupture of oesophagus with secondary extension to left pleural cavity. Initial X-ray.

1158b Ten days after a total hip-replacement, a cryptogenetic mid-thoracic rupture suddenly provokes a left pyopneumothorax.

1158c Oesophageal rupture, is confirmed by extravasation of contrast material (→) 2cm below the main-stem bronchus (⟶), i.e. through the aortic arch.

1158d Unusually, extravasation extends to the left pleural cavity.

1159a

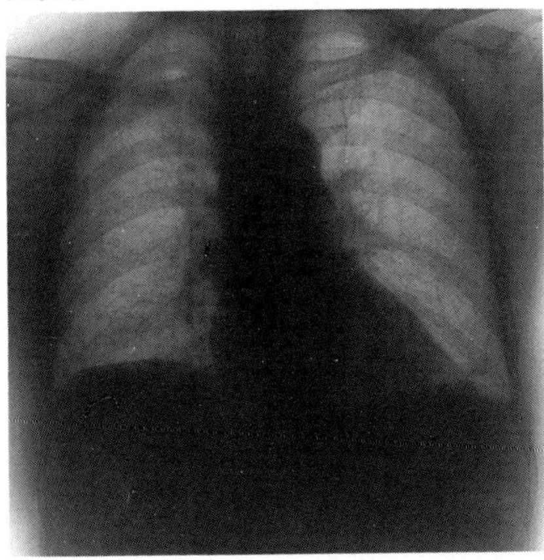

C.J. ♂ 55 yrs. 18 May 1975

1159a Unrecognised Mallory-Weiss-Boerhaave syndrome with late right pleural fiistula. For 2 days the patient has been suffering from acute abdominal pains following the perforation of a long-standing duodenal ulcer (see **1256**). During these 2 days, he has been trying to obtain some relief through self-induced vomiting. He is admitted with sudden and massive postemetic haematemesis (aggravated by his intake of anti-coagulants for coronary insufficiency). The admission X-ray is normal.

1159b Nine days after the initial episode of haematemesis and 7 days after admission, the lower gastro-oesophageal rupture extends suddenly to the right pleural cavity, causing a highly compressive pyopneumothorax. Respiratory distress, cardiac arrest. Successful resuscitation. Transfer to the Surgical Ward.

1159c Drainage. (For follow-up, see **1256**).

1159b

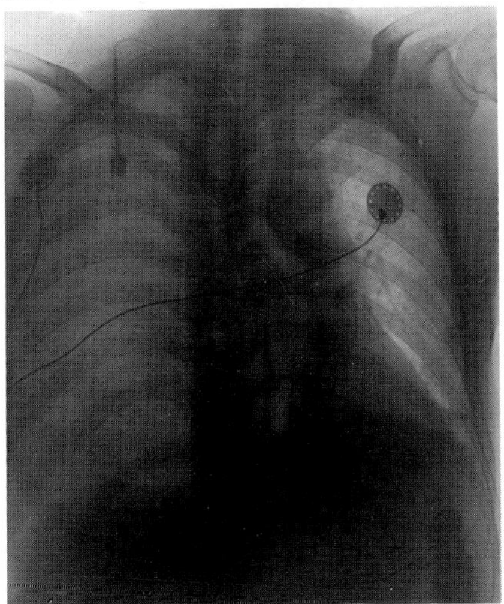

25 May 1975, 14 hrs.

1159c

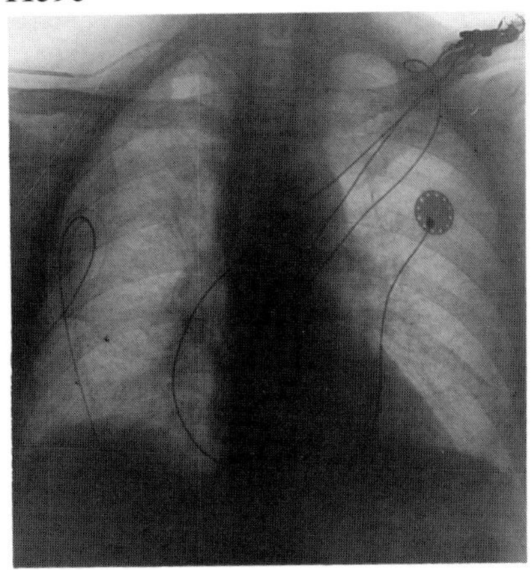

25 May 1975, 15.30 hrs.

PERITONEAL FISTULA

Peritoneal fistulisation after oesophageal perforation is less common than pleural fistulisation. When it occurs, it is usually as a result of emetic rupture. In cases of violent vomiting where the cardia ruptures when it rises momentarily into the chest, peritoneal and pleural fistulisation (or mediastinal contamination) can occur simultaneously.

Peritonitis following gastro-oesophageal rupture with peritoneal fistula is rapidly symptomatic; it is usually diagnosed and treated earlier than pleural fistula.

1160a

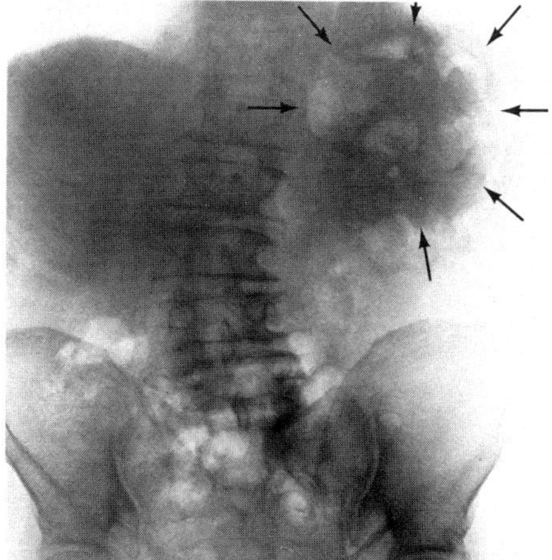

B.A1. ♂ 65 yrs. 15 May 1969

1160b

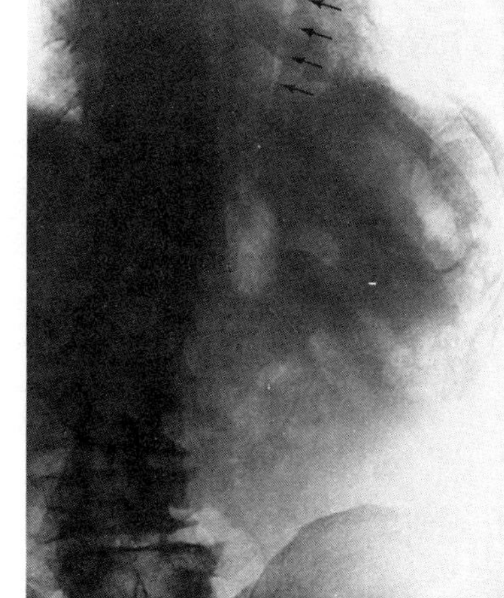

15 May 1969

1160a Extravasation of air into left hypochondrium (→) and mediastinum following a gastro-oesophageal rupture with a Mallory-Weiss-Boerhaave syndrome. The film shows a localised pneumoperitoneum . . .

1160b . . . and a lower pneumomediastinum.

1160c

15 May 1969

1160d

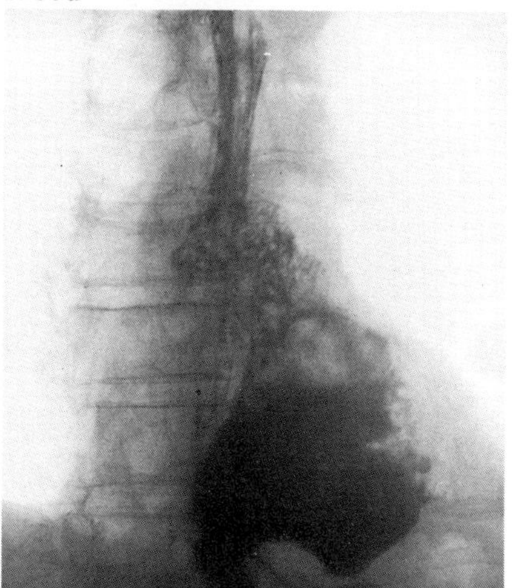

15 May 1969

1160c A contrast study with hydrosoluble material reveals a 3 cm gastro-oesophageal rupture. Extravasation can be seen above and below the left hemidiaphragm (→).

1160d Contrast material rises into the mediastinum and enters the left pleural cavity.

Pneumoperitoneum is sometimes noticed after an upper oesophageal (or tracheal) injury with significant mediastinal emphysema. Emphysema extends along the diaphragmatic crura and descending aorta (X-ray shows Naclerio's 'V' sign, see **1148**), and air then leaks into the peritoneal cavity through a small tear in the peritoneal serous membrane. Pneumoperitoneum can arise in similar fashion from compressive pneumothorax. The pneumoperitoneum can be massive even when the mediastinal emphysema is only slight (see Volume I, **692**).

In the absence of a direct oesophagoperitoneal fistula, pneumoperitoneum is usually benign, and disappears spontaneously.

PERICARDIAL FISTULA

Fistulas into the neighbouring pericardium or tracheobronchial tree are usually a late complication of corrosion. They occur after (attempted) bougienage.

1161 Oesophagopericardial fistula after repeated bougienage for cicatricial stenosis. Three months after alkaline necrosis of the oesophagus (treated conservatively), an oesophagopericardial fistula develops suddenly, causing purulent pericarditis. X-ray after pericardiocentesis shows the pericardial sac dilated with air (→). Left thoracotomy: drainage of pericardial and pleural cavities. Oesophagectomy proves impossible (see also **849, 850, 1162, 1215**).

1161

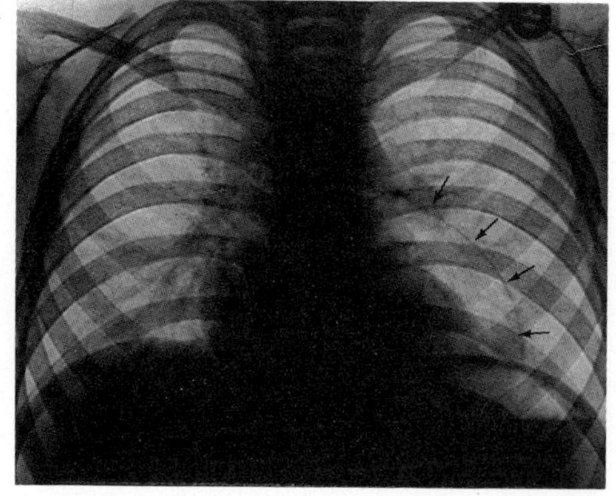

G.C. ♂ 2 yrs. 7 Nov. 1958

RESPIRATORY FISTULAS

1162

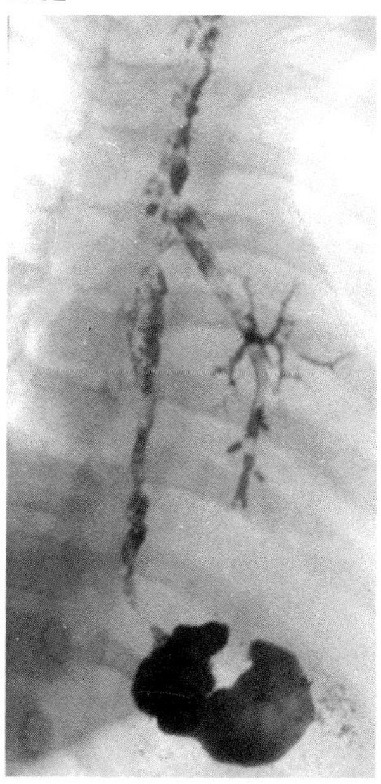

G.C. ♂ 2 yrs. 20 Jan. 1959

1162 Oesophagobronchial fistula five months after alkaline necrosis of the oesophagus. An upper gastro-intestinal study picks out the tracheobronchial tree through a fistula in the left main-stem bronchus. There are few symptoms because the patient is not being fed by mouth.

AORTIC FISTULA

Post-traumatic oesophago-aortic fistulisation is rare. It has two causes:

- an oesophageal perforation (whether iatrogenic or by a foreign body) with gradual erosion of the aortic wall (see **989**),
- a post-traumatic pseudo-aneurysm of the aorta that gradually penetrates the wall of the oesophagus (see **1163**).

In both cases, the symptoms and signs are those of upper gastro-intestinal haemorrhage. Even if haemorrhage is initially slight, it is potentially fatal at any moment.

1163a

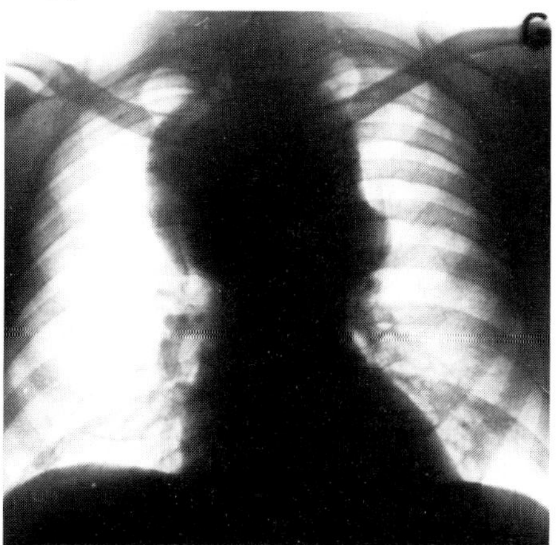

F.R. ♂ 51 yrs. 15 Dec. 1951

1163b

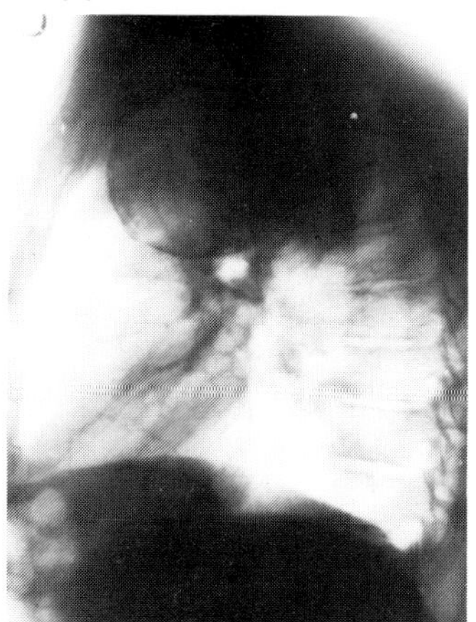

15 Dec. 1951

1163c

15 Dec. 1951

1163a Late aortic fistula. This X-ray is of a patient who sustained a partial rupture of the aortic arch in a motorcycle accident 31 years before. The rupture was not detected, and in the intervening years a pseudo-aneurysm has developed. At the time of admission, the superior vena cava is occluded by compression . . .

1163b . . . and the trachea is displaced. The principal symptom is severe dyspnoea.

1163c The oesophagus is also displaced far to the right (→). The pseudo-aneurysm suddenly ruptures into the oesophageal lumen, causing massive haematemesis and melaena. Unsuccessful attempt at repair through a sternotomy. Death during surgery.

Misleading radiological findings

1164a

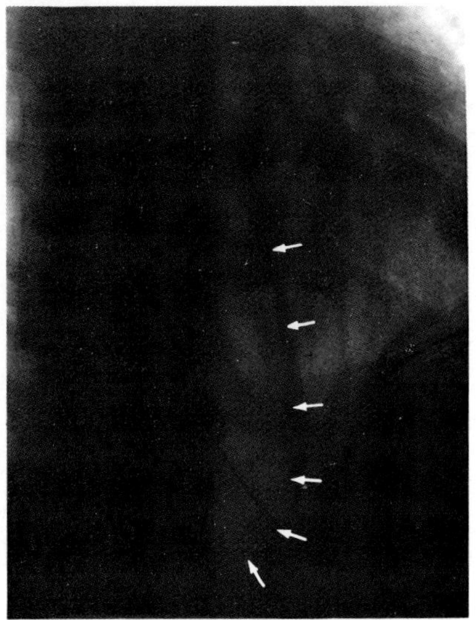

R.R. ♂ 23 yrs. 17 June 1977

1164a Pseudo-rupture of lower oesophagus: pneumatocele by barotrauma. The X-ray shows a pneumatocele caused by air in the triangular ligament of the left lung (→) An oesophageal barium study is normal.

1164b

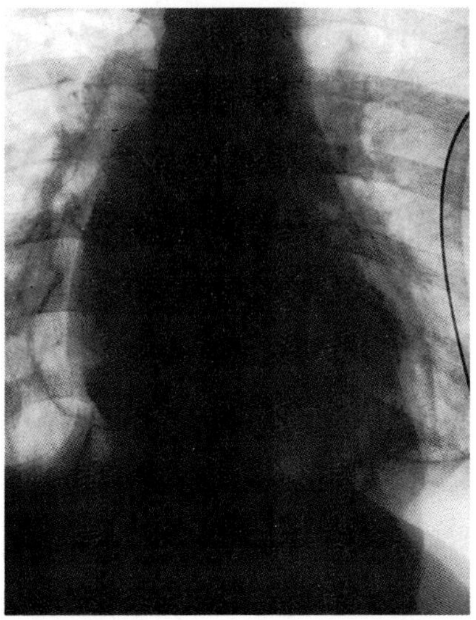

17 June 1977

1164b The symmetrical pneumatocele is the result of mechanical ventilation with positive end-expiratory pressure.

1165a

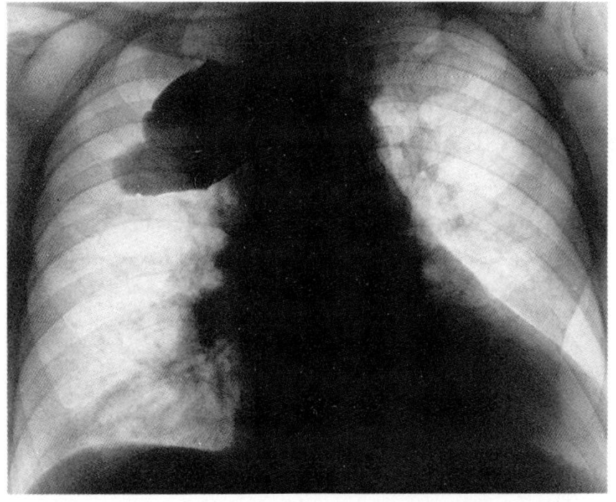

S.H. ♂ 84 yrs. 15 July 1977

1165a Pseudo-laceration of oesophagus. This standard chest X-ray obtained during a barium study suggests massive extravasation into the right pleural cavity.

1165b

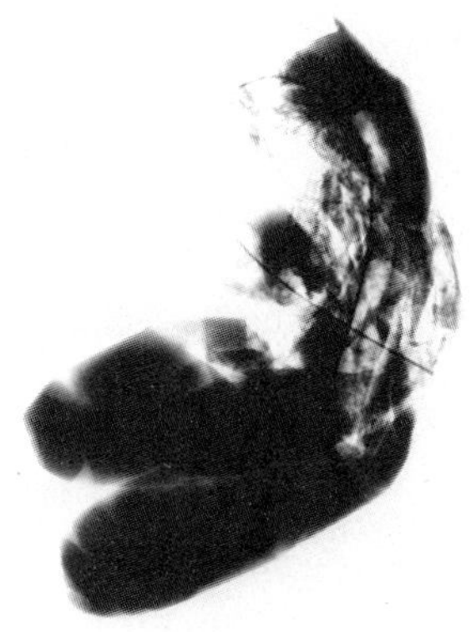

15 July 1977

1165b But, in fact, contrast material has simply flooded back through the Levin tube to fill a plastic glove secured to the patient's chest.

Endoscopy

Endoscopy is generally contra-indicated when oesophageal laceration or perforation is suspected. It is particularly dangerous in patients with major cardiorespiratory difficulties; insufflation of air into the oesophagus can aggravate mediastinal emphysema to the point of causing cardiac arrest.

If endoscopy becomes necessary as a last resort, the entire tracheobronchial tree and oesophagus should be examined. Whether a rigid or flexible tube is preferable depends upon the circumstances.

It is usually possible to examine the injury directly. Sometimes, however, indirect signs only are visible: clots, haemorrhage, air bubbles or even a view of the mediastinum through the broken oesophageal wall. It must be cautioned, too, that endoscopy gives falsely negative results more often than oesophagography – especially if the laceration is small or situated in the upper oesophagus.

1166

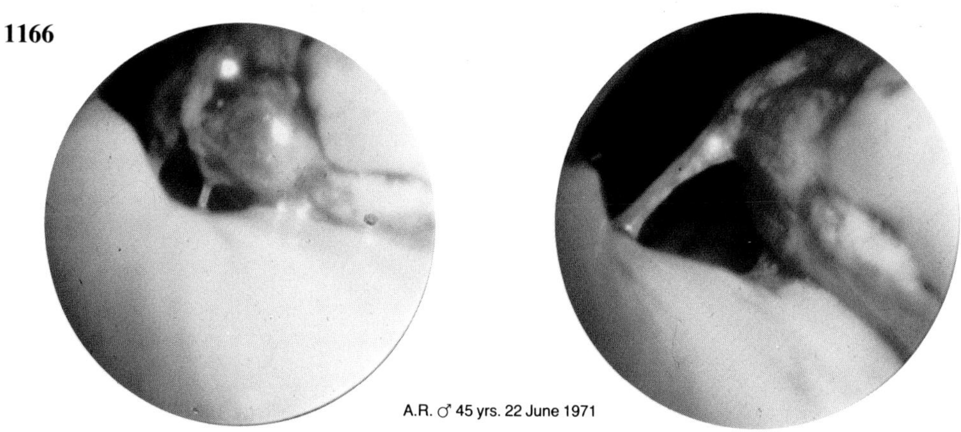

1166 Endoscopic view of an incomplete emetic laceration of the cardia.

General management

Treatment consists of (1) *repairing* the laceration, (2) *covering it*, (3) *draining* the mediastinum and neighbouring cavities, and (4) *discharging* the oesophagus of any saliva or gastric residue. On occasion, it can be necessary also (5) to *exclude*, (6) *resect*, and (7) *replace* part of the oesophagus. Steps (5), (6) and (7) are basically required in cases of corrosion, or if treatment is late.

Choice of technique depends upon:

- the aetiology of the injury,
- its localisation,
- its dimensions,
- the time-lapse,
- subsequent complications,
- the general condition of the patient.

1167 1. **REPAIR** (in 2 layers)

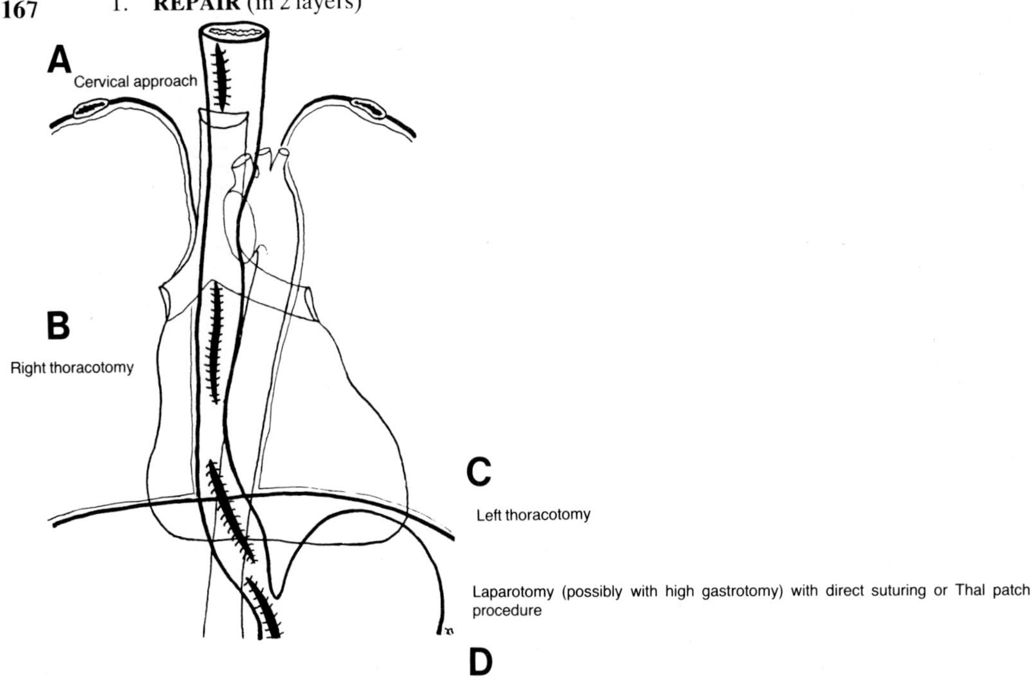

N.B. Repair is sometimes fragile, if not impossible

1168 2. **COVER** with:

1169 3. **DRAIN**

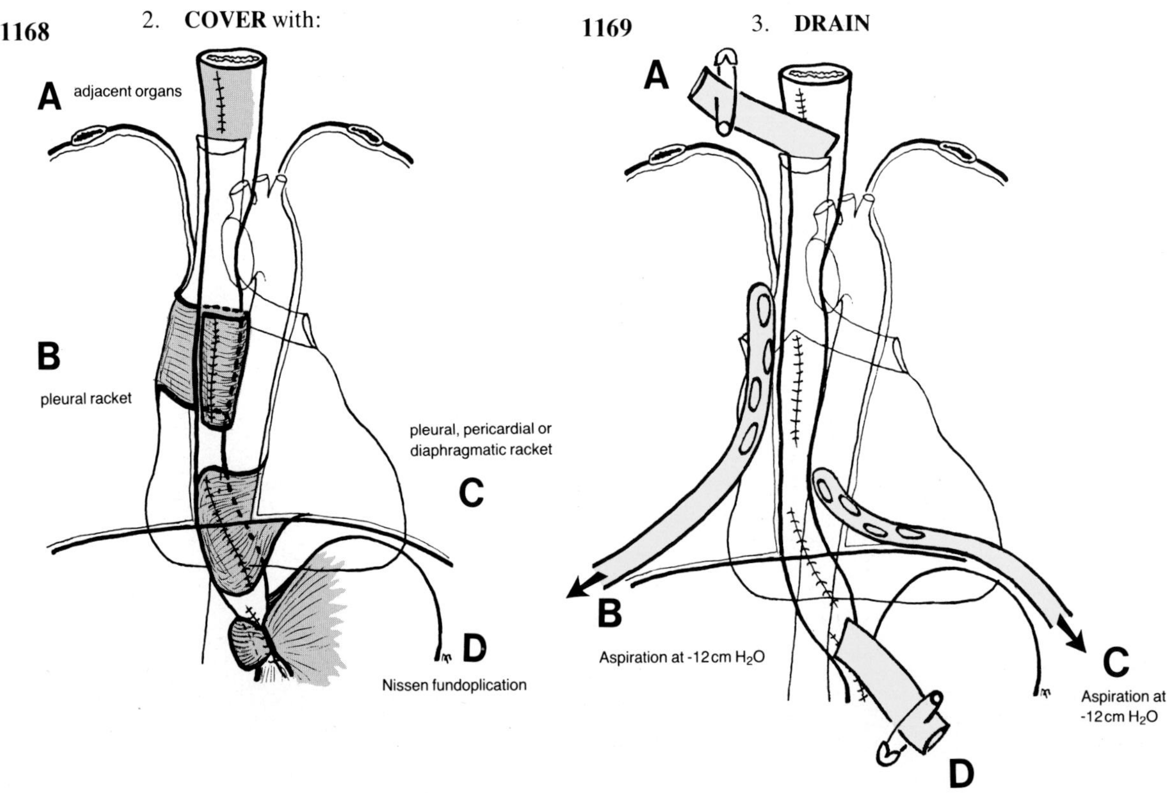

1170

4. **DISCHARGE**

1171

5. **EXCLUDE**

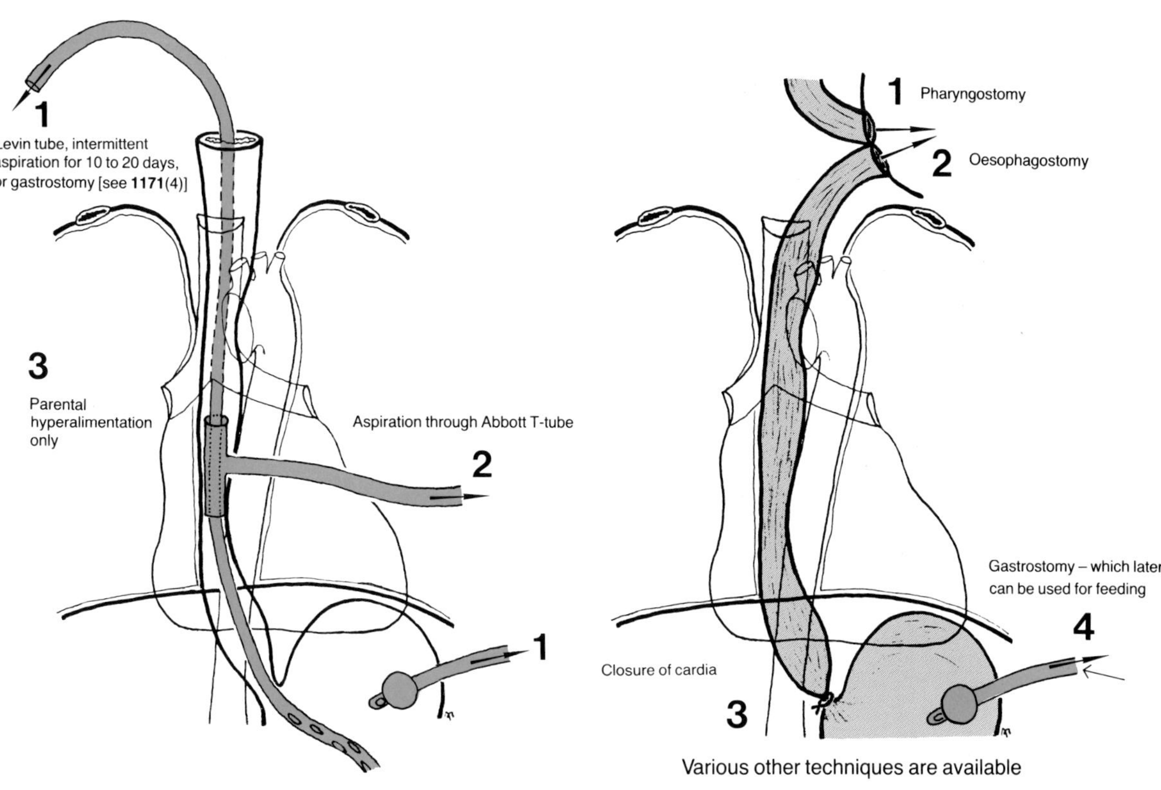

1172

6. **RESECT**

7. **REPLACE** (to re-establish continuity of digestive tract)

N.B.: Steps (6) and (7) can be done in reverse order.

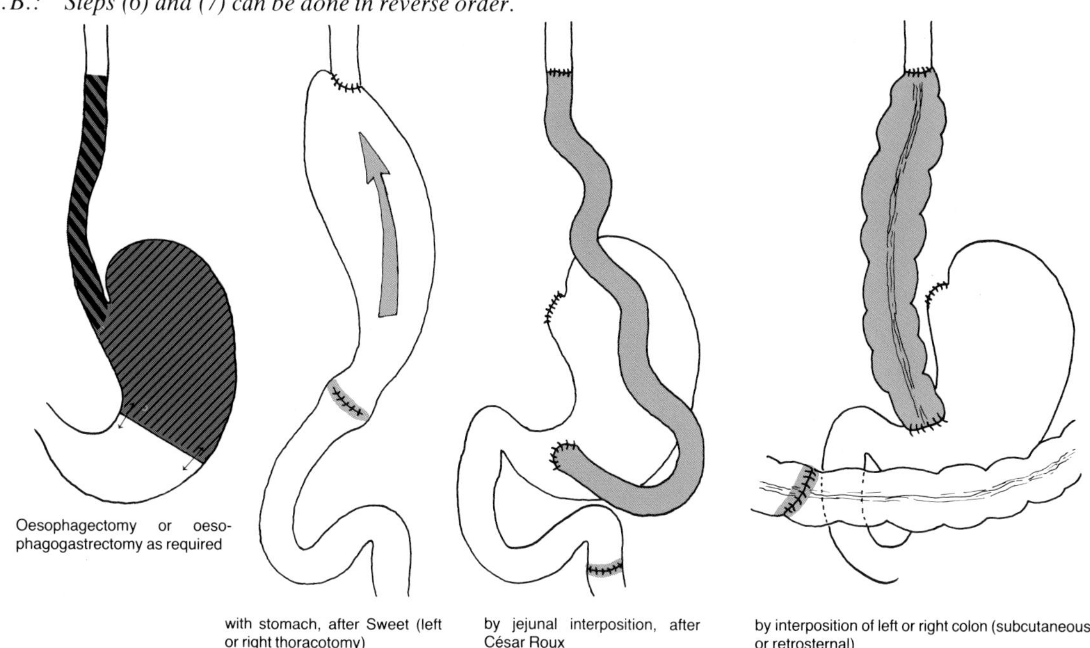

Caustic burns in the oesophagus increase the risk of cancer (in attenuated form) by 1000 (on average, 35 years later).

Instrumental perforations of the oesophagus

Instrumental perforations are currently the commonest type of oesophageal injury. Their incidence has risen as new diagnostic and therapeutic procedures have come into use.

They can be classified according to their localisation (see **1145**), their aetiology (see **1143**), or the time-lapse before diagnosis (see **1141, 1142**).

All instrumental perforations are iatrogenic. *All are of very poor prognosis if unrecognised, but are relatively insignificant if detected early and treated adequately.*

Aetiology of instrumental perforations of the oesophagus:

	Incidence (in our material)
– abdominal surgery	41%
– bougienage or probing	27%
– rigid endoscopy	22%
– endotracheal intubation	8%
– a tracheostomy tube	2%
– fibroscopy	none

Mortality in our cases is 34%. Death is directly or indirectly attributable to the oesophageal injury in over half of them.

The prognosis depends upon how early diagnosis and treatment are effected.

Only 50% of cases are treated within 24 hours.

Perforations sustained	Treated *Early*	*Late*
– during abdominal surgery	23%	18%
– during probing or bougienage	17%	10%
– during rigid endoscopy	7%	15%
– during endotracheal intubation	3%	5%
– from a tracheostomy tube	–	2%
	50%	50%

When treatment is effected within the first 24 hours, postoperative mortality is reduced to 5%.

During tracheal intubation

Oro- and nasotracheal intubation is common. It is usually a safe procedure, but an injury sometimes can be inflicted at the aerodigestive junction (see **1154**). Injury can be produced by the tip of the laryngoscope, by the tracheal tube or its introducer, by over-inflation (sudden or gradual) of the cuff (see **741, 750**), or by an accessory instrument.

Most injuries of this sort consist of a superficial, mucosal lesion of no great significance. A few, however, are transmural.

Wounds to the digestive tract are located either in the pharynx, or in the piriform sinuses, or at Killian's mouth (immediately above the cricopharyngeal muscle on the back wall, or in front and slightly below).

The complex anatomy of the region makes it difficult to assess the extent and gravity of damage. Underestimation or misdiagnosis greatly increases the threat to the patient's life. The least suspicion of a wound commands an upper gastrointestinal study with hydrosoluble contrast material or direct examination with a laryngoscope or rigid oesophagoscope.

1173a

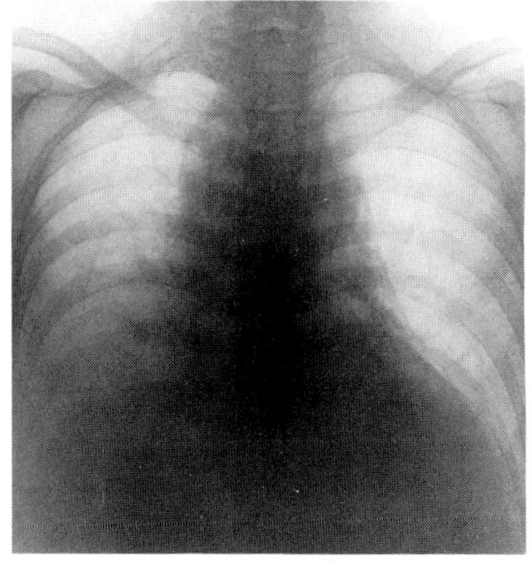

M.H. ♀ 51 yrs. 19 Oct. 1975

1173b

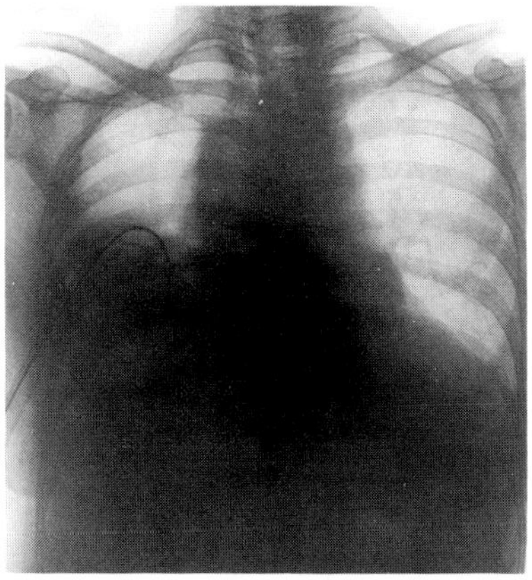

25 Oct. 1975

1173c

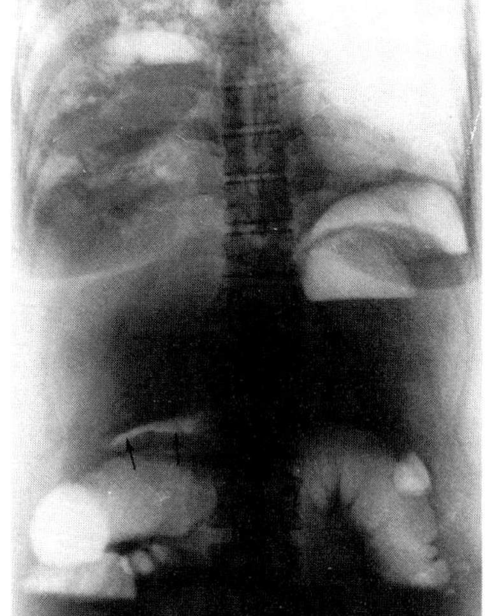

30 Oct. 1975

1173d

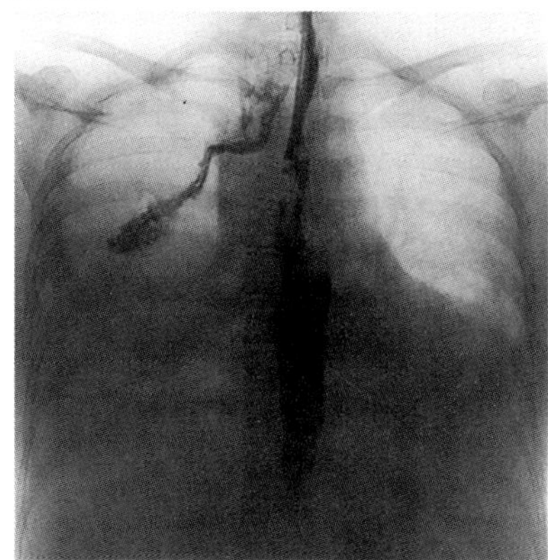

30 Oct. 1975

1173e

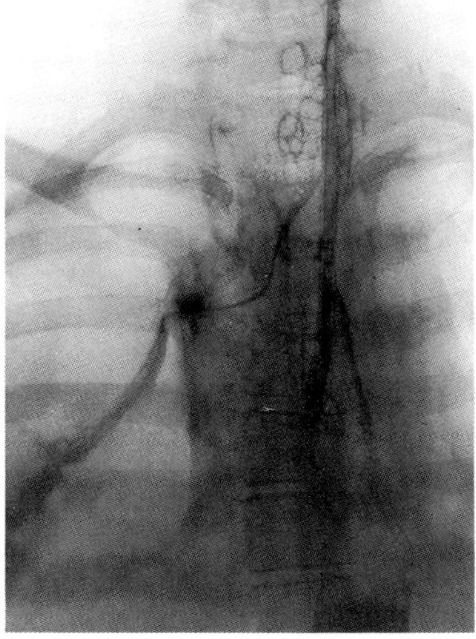

30 Oct. 1975

1173f

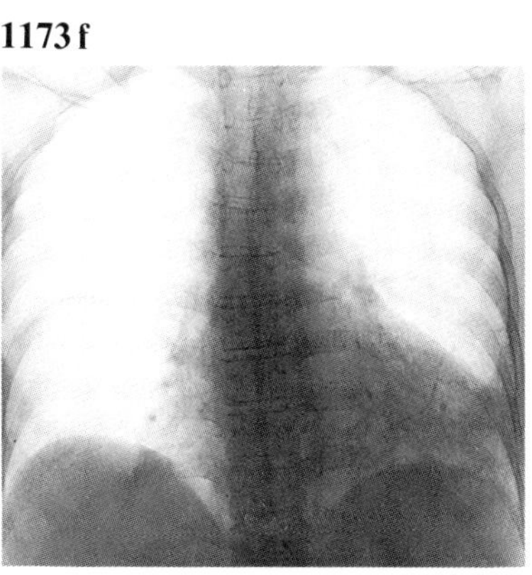

13 Feb. 1976

1173a Oesophageal wound during orotracheal intubation. Two days after several attempts at intubation (during which the tube was momentarily introduced into the oesophagus), the patient is in respiratory distress and has a right pyopneumothorax. Bronchoscopic examination is negative. An oesophageal injury is not suspected.

1173b The pyopneumothorax is drained, but to no effect.

1173c By the 13th day, the right pyopneumothorax is organised. The patient is in septic shock and extreme respiratory difficulty. A localised pneumoperitoneum (→) has arisen from a perforated duodenal ulcer. Transfer to University Hospital.

1173d The upper oesophageal perforation is finally diagnosed when contrast material extravasates into the right pleural cavity during an upper gastro-intestinal study.

1173e Close-up of the oesophagopleural fistula. The oesophageal rupture was closed through a cervical approach; the pleural cavity was cleaned and drained through a right thoracotomy; and the ulcer was treated through a laparotomy. Several re-interventions. Oesophageal and abdominal healing.

1173f Final X-ray taken after 3 months in the intensive care unit. Psychiatric sequelae.

By tracheostomy tube

Oesophageal damage during the performance of a tracheostomy is exceptional. It can occur subsequently, however, due to:

- malpositioning of the tube, aggravated by the weight of the ventilator tubings,
- ischaemia caused by the cuff (especially a high-pressure cuff),
- an over-inflated cuff that gradually erodes the membranous wall of the trachea causing an abscess and then a fistula into the oesophagus.

1174

Causes of tracheo-oesophageal fistulisation in tracheostomy patients *(see page 51)*.

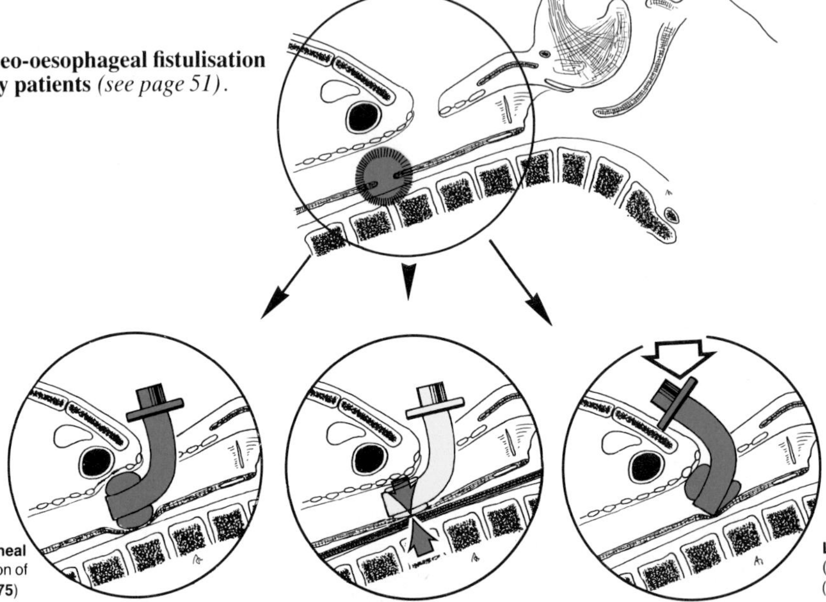

1175a

J.R. ♂ 66 yrs. 26 Jan. 1967

1175b

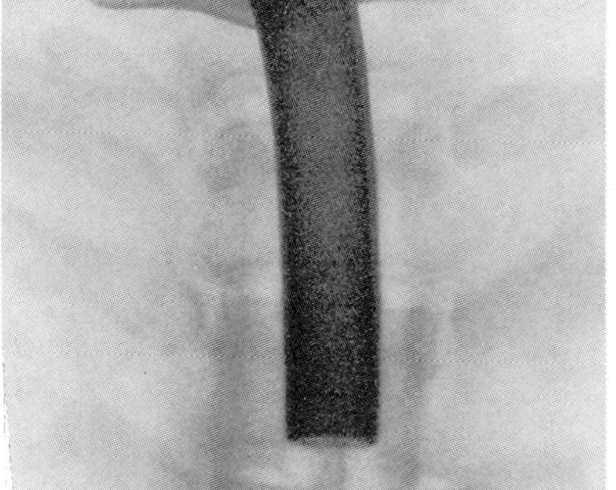

31 Jan. 1967

1175c

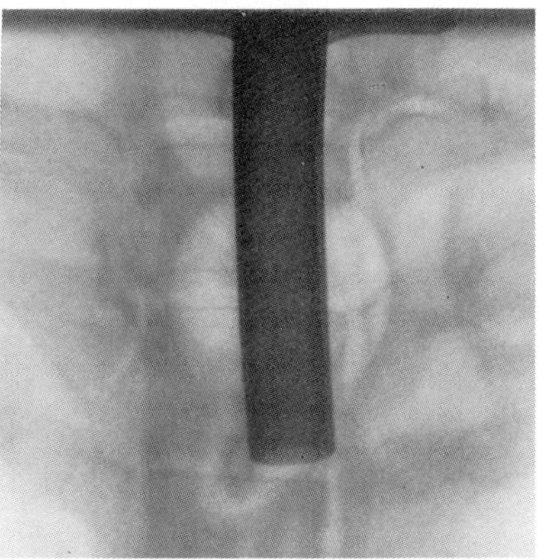

4 Feb. 1967

1175d

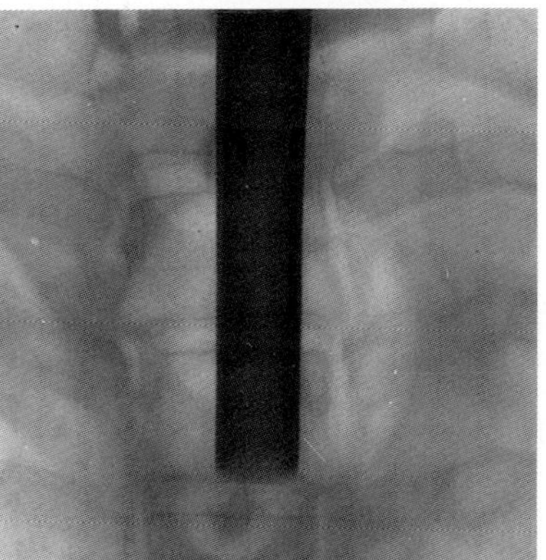

15 Feb. 1967

1175a Tracheo-oesophageal fistula by gradual over-inflation of cuff of tracheostomy tube. Severe multiple injuries sustained during a 15 m fall include a flail chest with paradoxical motion, and contusion of the heart, lungs and brain. The admission X-ray shows an endotracheal tube already in place.

1175b A tracheostomy has been performed for positive pressure ventilation and bronchial aspiration. The cuff is of normal dimension.

1175c Over the next few days, the cuff is inflated progressively in an attempt to seal an air leak due to acute tracheal necrosis. On this X-ray, the diameter of the cuff is twice that of the trachea.

1175d By the time the patient dies (from brain damage), the diameter of the cuff has reached 3.8cm. Autopsy reveals a tracheo-oesophageal fistula.

By Levin tube

The introduction of a Levin tube can result in a wound anywhere along the length of the oesophagus. The upper oesophagus is often damaged by accessory instruments (especially MacGill forceps). Lower down, injury often takes the form of a direct perforation (especially when the tube is large and rigid), or a tear produced by the deflection of the tube against an obstacle.

1176a

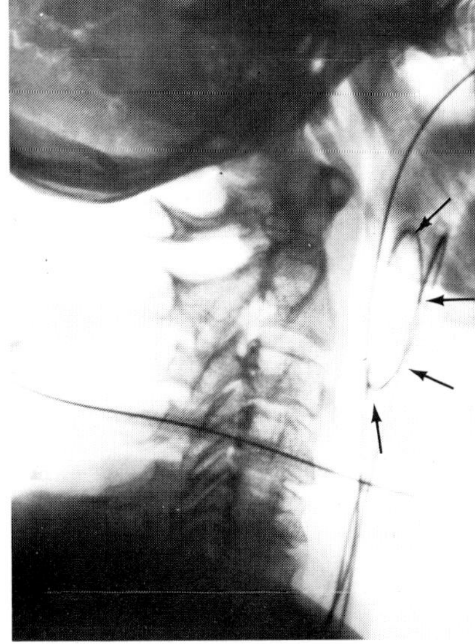

M.M. ♀ 76 yrs. 18 Dec. 1974

1176b

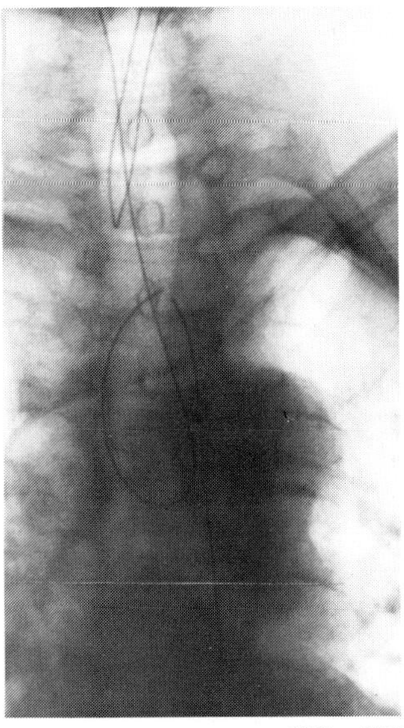

18 Dec. 1974

1176a Convolution of Levin tube. Lateral view: the superior (→) loop could lacerate the piriform sinuses.

1176b Anterior view: the lower loop is immediately above the aortic arch and could tear the mid-thoracic oesophagus.

1177a

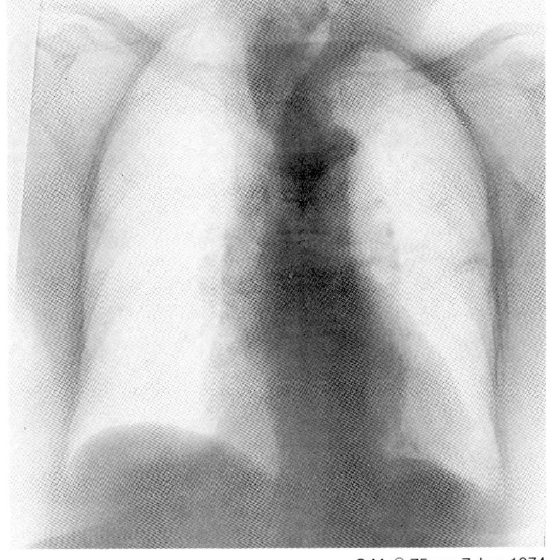

S.M. ♀ 75 yrs. 7 Jan. 1974

1177a Massive cervical and thoracic subcutaneous emphysema with mediastinal emphysema, after introduction of Levin tube. Before intubation.

1177b

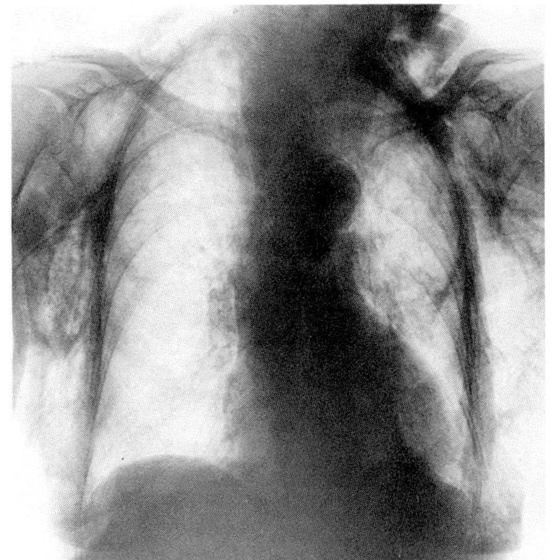

11 Jan. 1974

1177b Twelve hours after intubation.

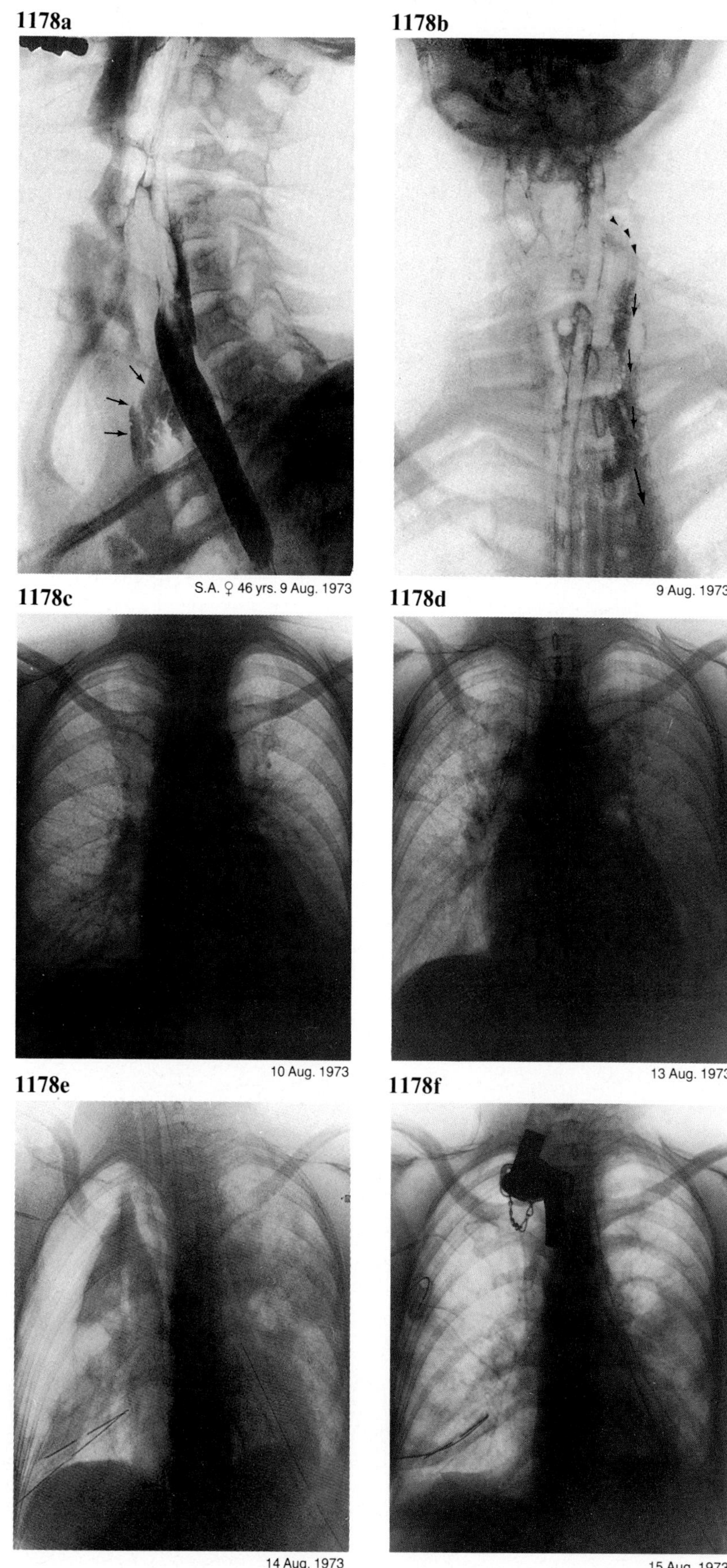

1178a S.A. ♀ 46 yrs. 9 Aug. 1973

1178b 9 Aug. 1973

1178c 10 Aug. 1973

1178d 13 Aug. 1973

1178e 14 Aug. 1973

1178f 15 Aug. 1973

1178g

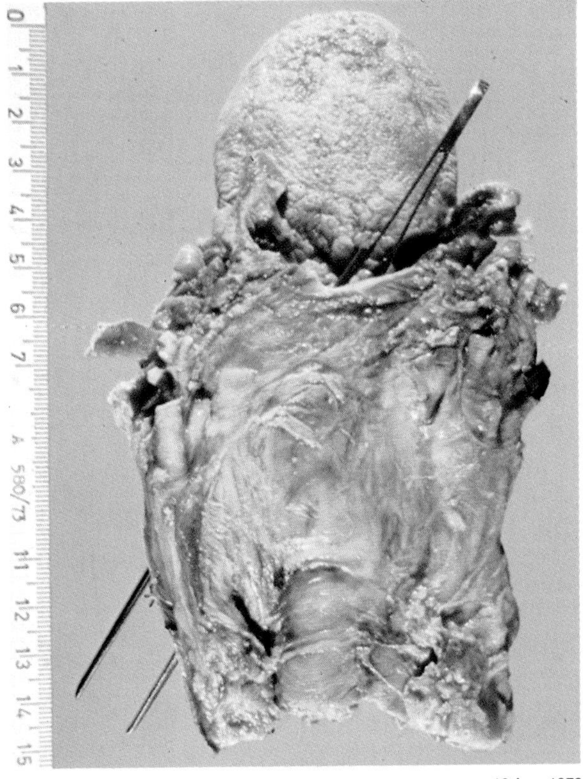

1178h

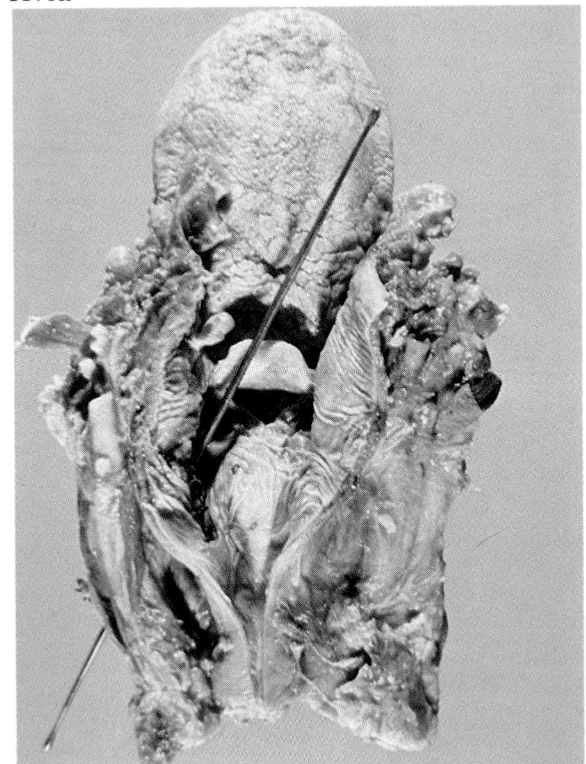

1178a Pharyngeal perforation by large gastric tube introduced during anaesthesia to facilitate repair of a hiatal hernia. The immediate postoperative lateral X-ray shows subcutaneous emphysema and extravasation of contrast material. (→).

1178b Anterior view. The oesophagus now contains a small calibre Levin tube. Contrast material can be seen to extravasate from the left piriform sinus into the upper mediastinum (→). Immediate cervical exploration reveals a 5cm laceration. Repair and drainage.

1178c A left pleural effusion develops nonetheless (upright X-ray). The right pneumoperitoneum is the result of the initial laparotomy.

1178d Infection of the pleural effusion results in empyema with septic shock. Left thoracotomy: mediastinal and pleural drainage.

1178e A sudden right pyopneumothorax develops the following day. It proves difficult to drain.

1178f The right lung finally re-expands but septic shock worsens, and a stress ulcer develops. Death 3 days later, 9 days after the repair of the pharyngeal wound.

1178g Autopsy: posterior view of the unopened pharynx. (Prof. D. Gardiol, Lausanne.)

1178h The laceration lies in the left piriform sinus. The suture line is dehiscent.

1178i Left lateral view of the pharyngomediastinal fistula.

1178i

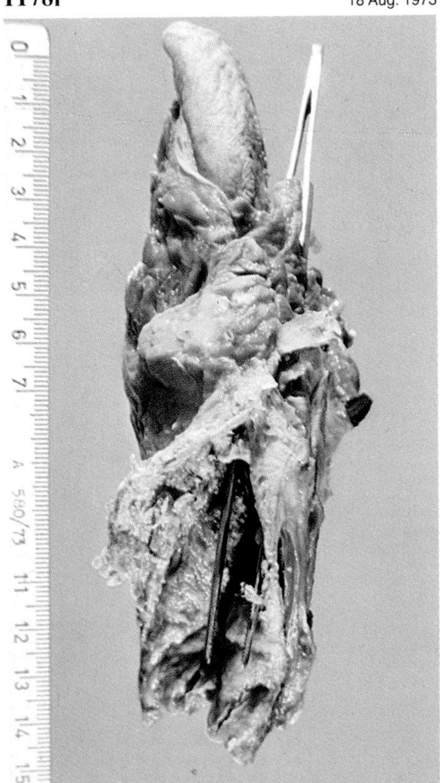

During bougienage

Tears during bougienage for cicatricial stricture usually occur in necrotic areas (the oesophageal walls remain necrotic for a long time after corrosion). Repeated tears can lead to a fistula into the tracheobronchial tree or pericardium (see **1161, 1162**). By this time, the damage is often beyond repair.

During oesophagoscopy

Injury during rigid or flexible oesophagoscopy can be direct or indirect. Incidence has risen in recent years as endoscopy of the proximal part of the digestive tract has become a common diagnostic procedure. Indirect laceration of the upper oesophagus by compression between a rigid endoscope and vertebral osteophytes is particularly dangerous. This type of injury most commonly occurs when the neck is extended to allow examination of the lower oesophagus; since it is inflicted at such a distance from the tip of the tube, it often passes undetected. A routine search should be made as the endoscope is withdrawn.

1179

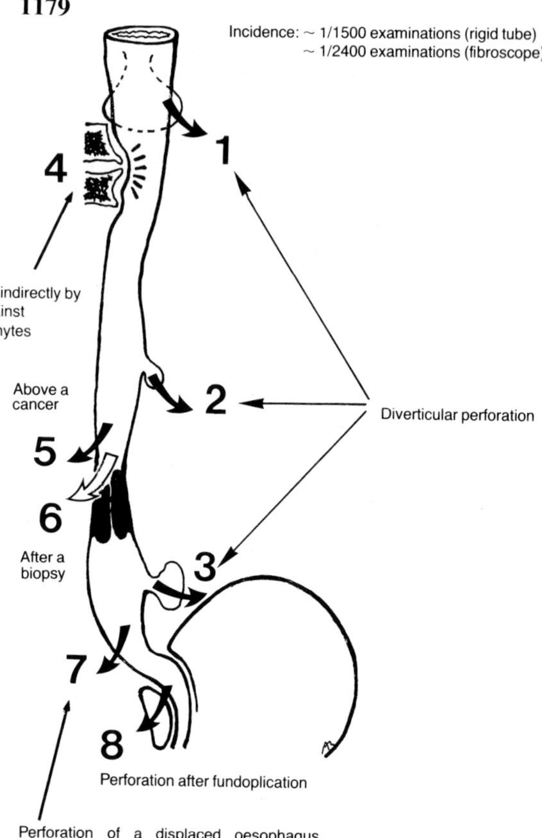

1179 Causes of oesophageal injury during rigid and flexible oesophagoscopy.

1180a

T.E. ♀ 71 yrs. 20 April 1978

1180a Rigid endoscopy can be dangerous in the presence of **vertebral osteophytes**.

1180b

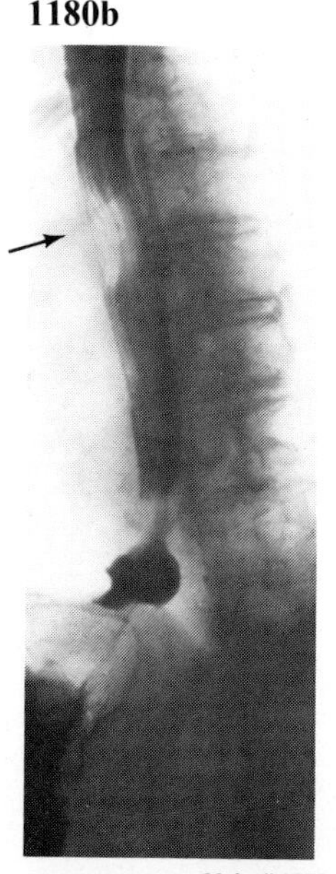

20 April 1978

1180b A barium study shows the extrinsic impression of osteophytes on the oesophageal wall.

1180c

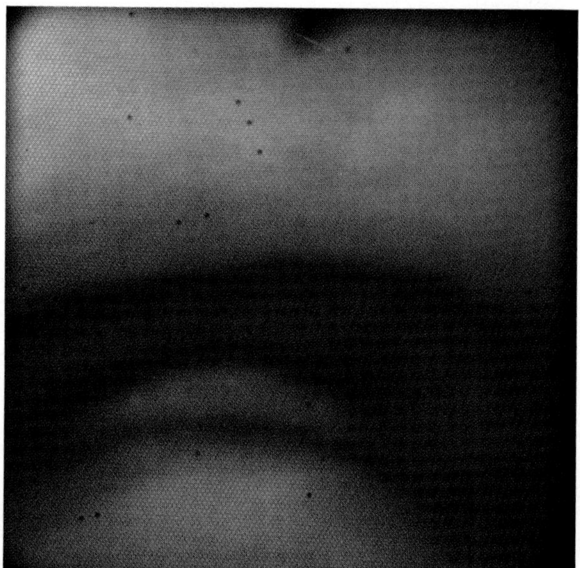

20 April 1978

1180c In this case, the osteophytes are sufficiently large to make the introduction of the fibroscope difficult.

1181

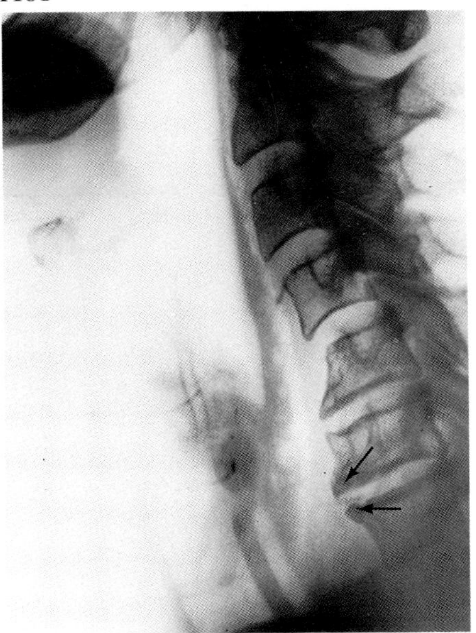

1181 Indirect perforation of cervical oesophagus by compression of a rigid endoscope against osteophytes (→). Minnigerode's sign is clearly visible.

1182a

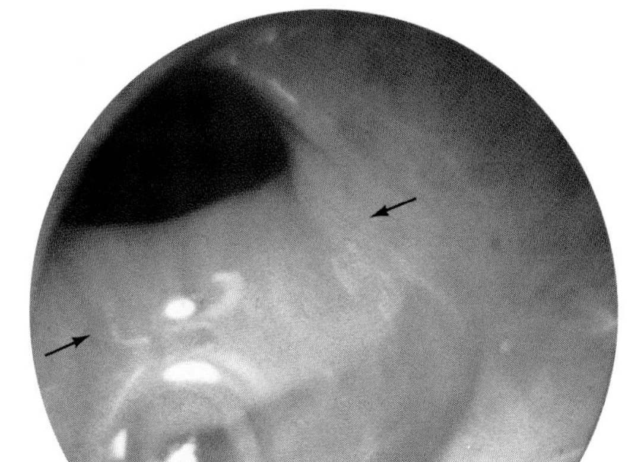

1182a The **cricopharyngeal muscle** (→) is spastic and a Zenker's diverticulum is beginning to develop. The mucosa was perforated subsequently by a Levin tube. (The same risk exists during fibroscopy, for again the area must be passed through 'blindly'.)

1182b

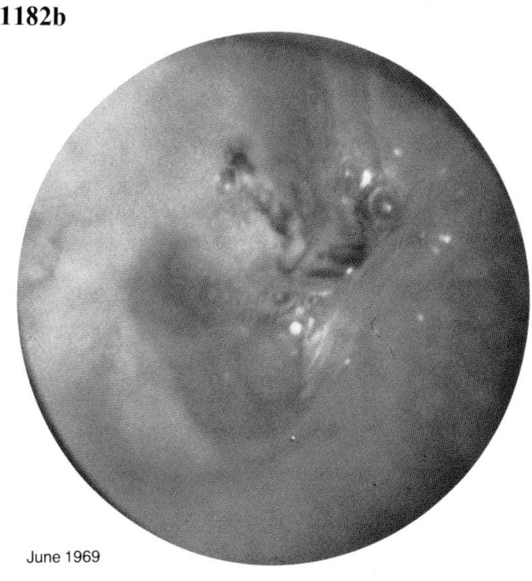

1182b The injury has been repaired. A suture is visible.

1183a

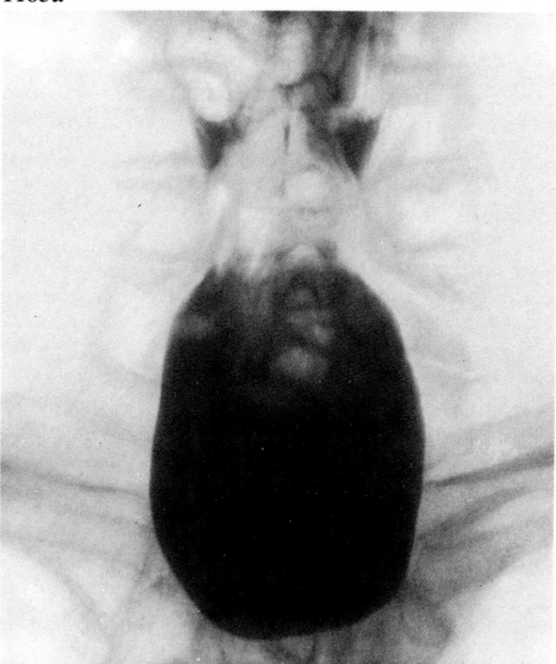

B.M. ♂ 69 yrs. Mar. 1979

1183b

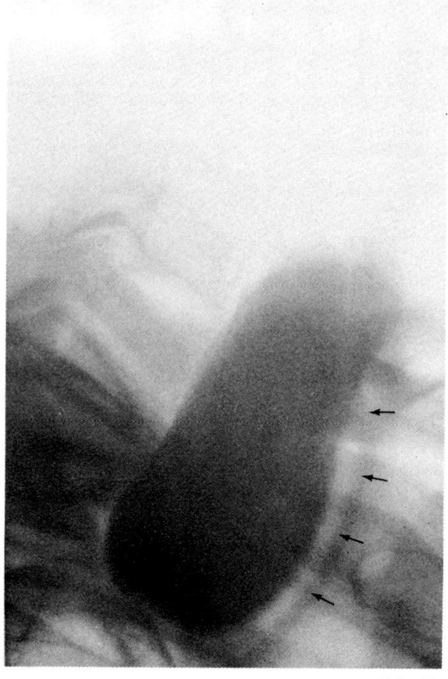

K.O. 1967

1183a A large Zenker's diverticulum can almost obliterate the oesophageal lumen (→).

1183c

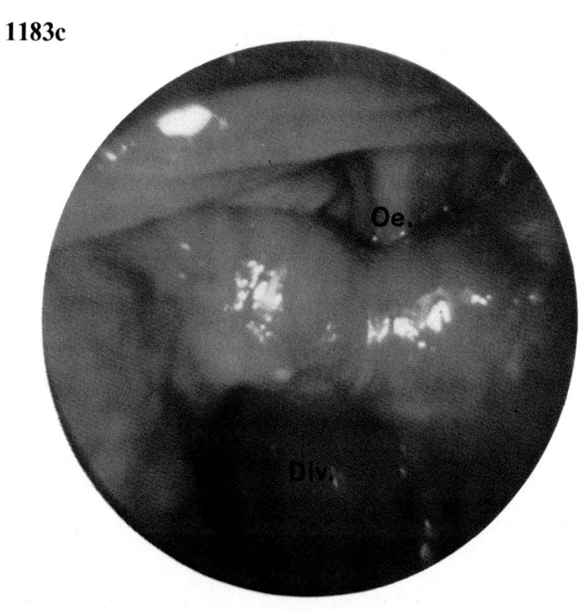

1184a 1184b 1184c

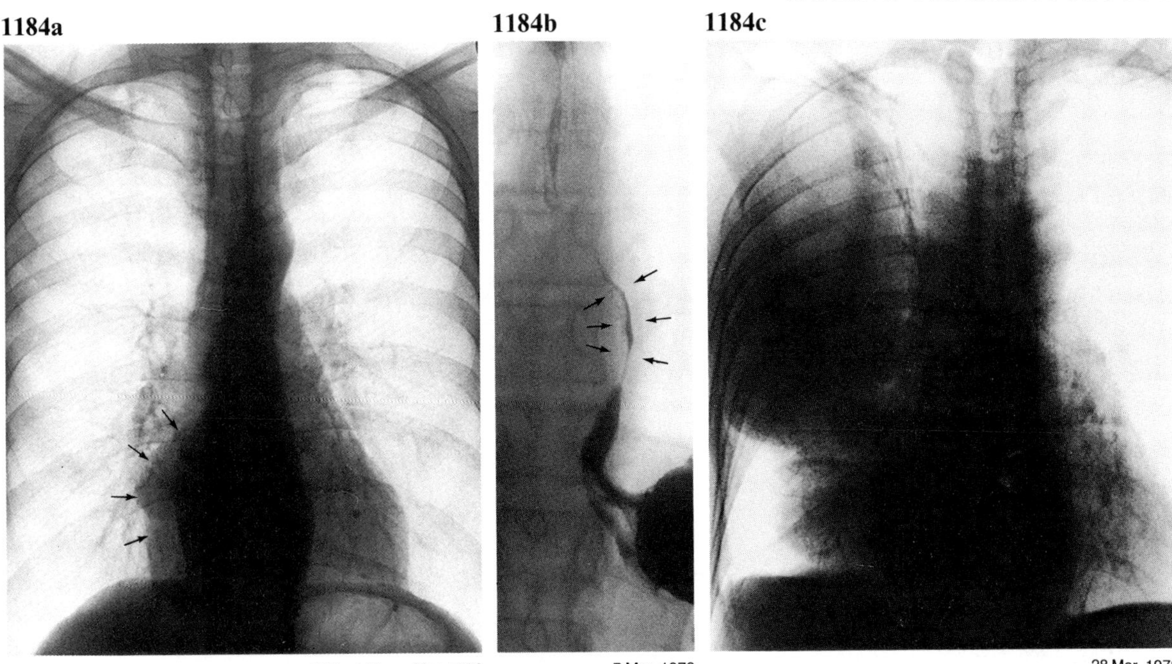

C.R. ♂ 48 yrs. Mar. 1972 7 Mar. 1972 28 Mar. 1972

1184d

28 Mar. 1972

1184e

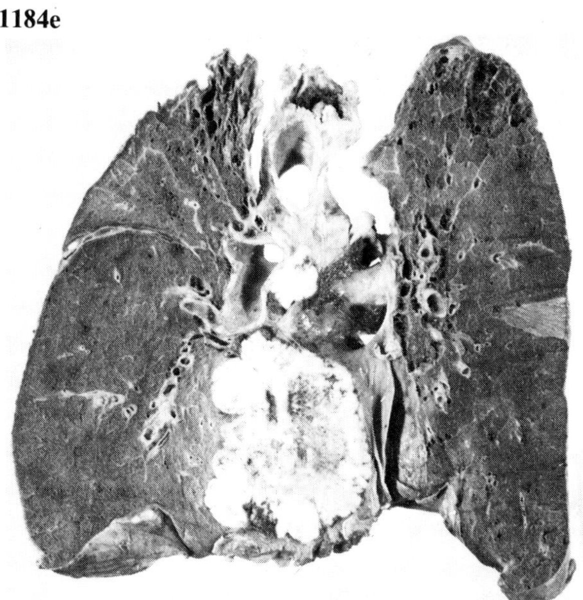

6 April 1972

1184a Perforation of oesophagus during endoscopic biopsy. The opaque region along the right cardiac border (→) corresponds to an oat cell carcinoma of the lung.

1184b Dysphagia. A barium study shows extrinsic compression of the lower oesophagus.

1184c Endoscopic biopsy of the oesophageal wall is followed by sudden and massive pleural empyema, and respiratory distress. The opaque region in the lower right lung field has increased in diameter.

1184d This upright X-ray shows a massive right pyopneumothorax. Right thoracotomy for pleural toilet and drainage. Death 9 days later due to the erosion of the descending aorta by the tumour.

1184e Autopsy shows direct invasion of the oesophagus and aorta by the oat cell carcinoma. (Institute of Pathology, Lausanne.)

During surgery

The external walls of the oesophagus are delicate; the risk of damage during surgery is high. Damage can occur:

* to the **cervical** oesophagus during
- surgery for a vertebral abscess or fracture,
- thyroid or parathyroid surgery,
- radical neck dissection,
- cervical re-intervention;

* to the **mid-thoracic** oesophagus during
- pulmonary resection, particularly when major,
- pleurectomy,
- excision of a posterior mediastinal tumour,
- thoracotomy for a hiatal hernia;

* to the **abdominothoracic** oesophagus during

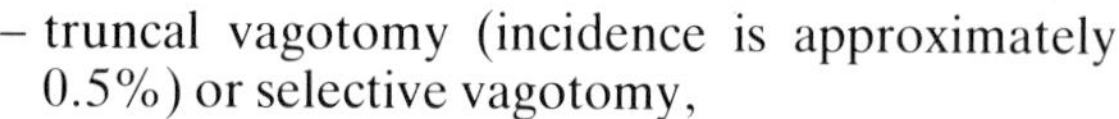

- truncal vagotomy (incidence is approximately 0.5%) or selective vagotomy,
- myotomy (according to Heller or Thorbjarnarson),
- repair of a hiatal hernia.

Oesophageal injury during surgery can be caused by a number of mechanisms: over-use of haemostatic electrocoagulation, accidental section of cicatricial tissue, digital laceration of the posterior wall (such damage often passes unnoticed), inadvertent opening of a diverticulum . . .

All of these injuries are relatively minor if detected and treated without delay.

1185a

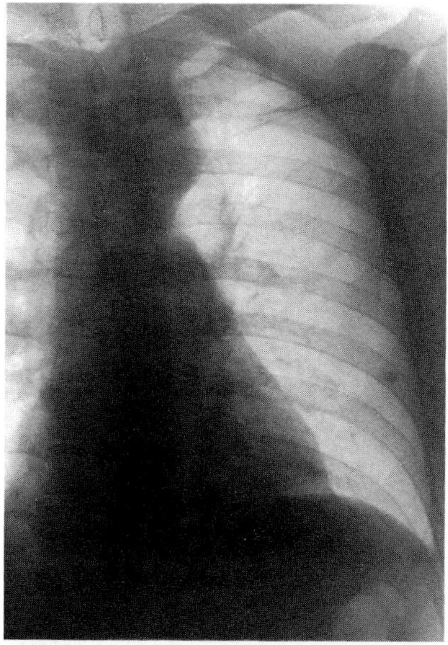

B.R. ♂ 44 yrs. 30 May 1969

1185b

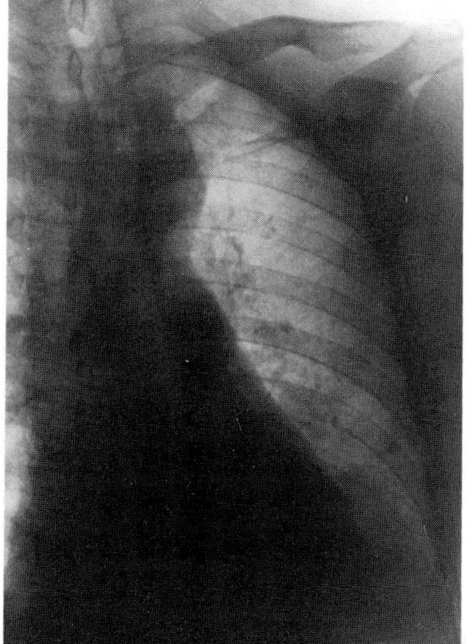

3 June 1969

1185a Digital **laceration of abdominal oesophagus during surgery** for a hiatal hernia. **Immediate repair** and Nissen fundoplication.

1185b Short-lived left pleural effusion. Recovery.

1185c Follow-up 6 years later.

1185c

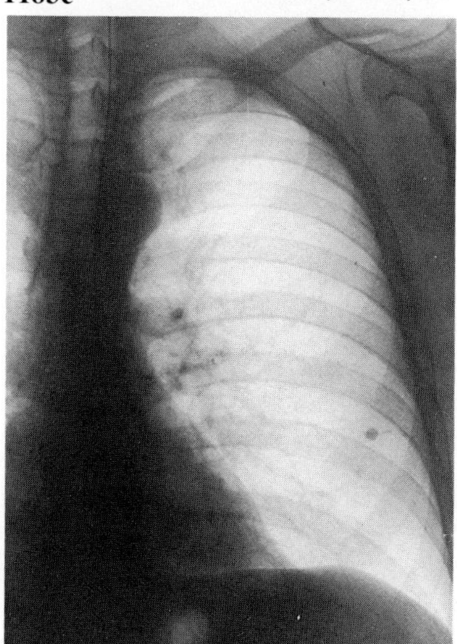

24 July 1975

1186

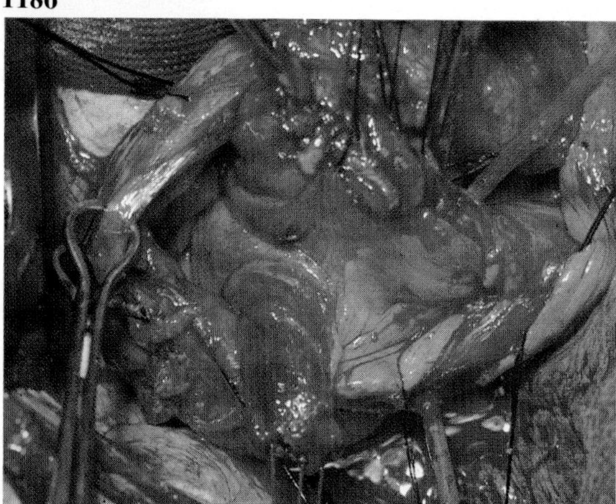

B.E. ♀ 48 yrs. 28 May 1970

1186 Large tear of abdominal oesophagus during surgery for hiatal hernia. Slow recovery. The 4cm wound was repaired and drained immediately, but 3 weeks later the suture line broke down. The photograph shows the wound through a thoracotomy immediately before re-suturing and a Nissen procedure. Subsequent stenosis was treated according to Thal. Recovery was slow.

1187a

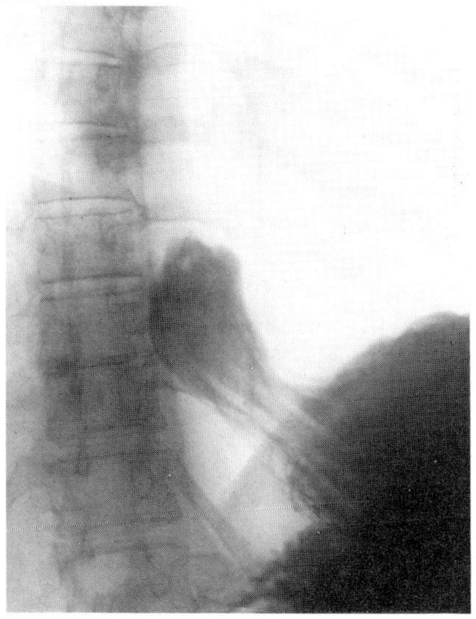

B.S. ♂ 31 yrs. 1964

1187a Tear of abdominal oesophagus. Late treatment. Death. The hiatal hernia before surgery.

1187b As the hernia was being repaired, the lower part of the oesophagus was torn but the injury was not recognised. The following day, a left pleural effusion appears.

1187c By the 4th day, there is a right pyothorax and significant mediastinal emphysema. The left pleural effusion is more pronounced.

1187d Diagnosis is established when hydrosoluble contrast material is seen to extravasate into the mediastinum. The tear is repaired 2 days later through a thoracotomy.

1187e A postoperative oesophagomediastinal fistula is treated conservatively.

1187f The fistula gradually closes but septic shock persists, leading to anuria. Death 8 days later from a massive digestive haemorrhage.

1187b

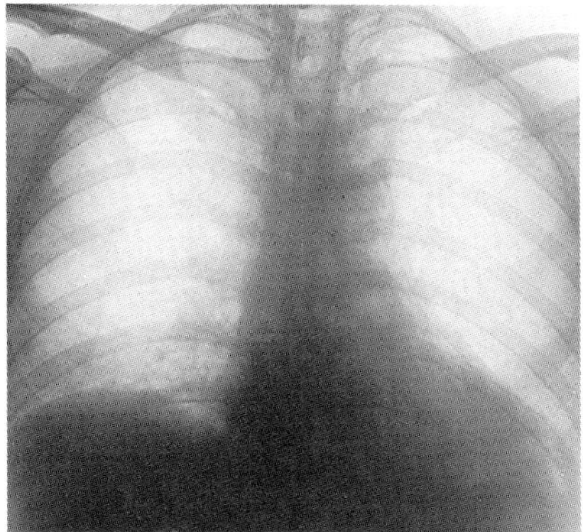

18 Sep. 1964

1187c

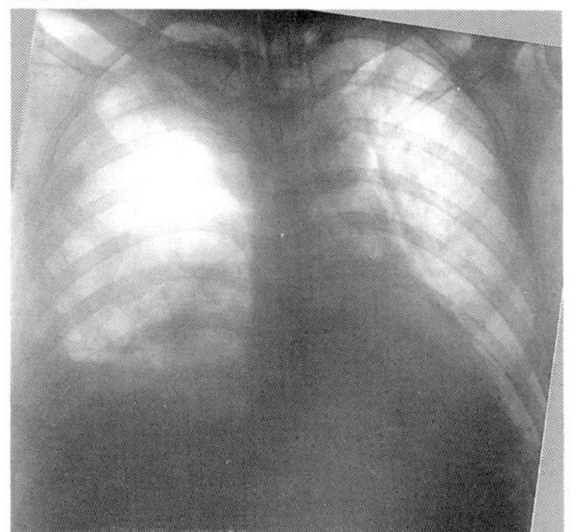

21 Sep. 1964

1187d

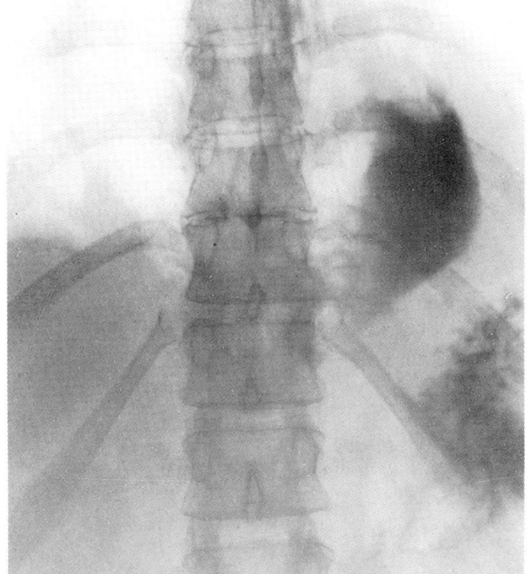

21 Sep. 1964

1187e

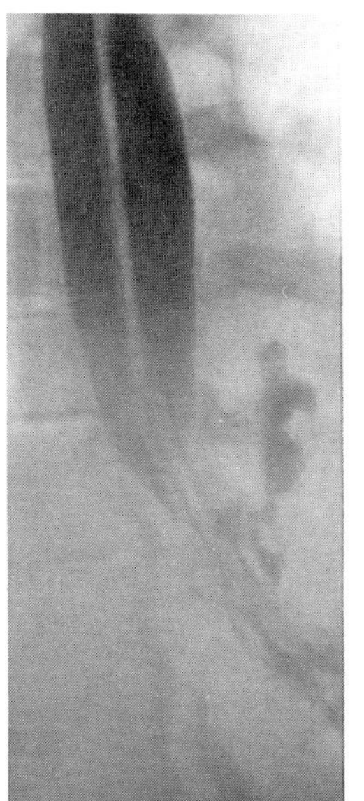

9 Oct. 1964

1187f

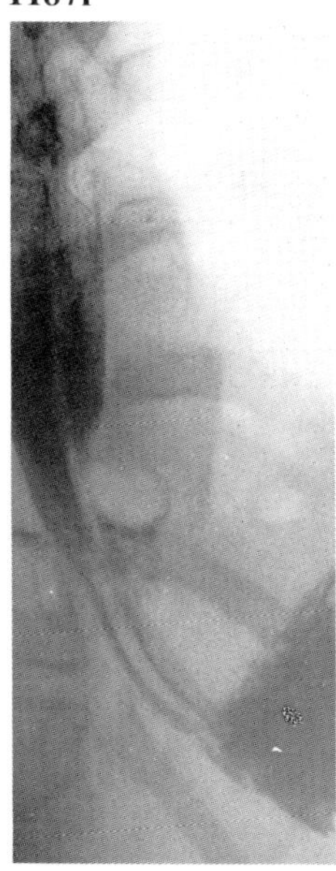

5 Nov. 1964

Swallowing injury of the oesophagus

Food, pills, foreign bodies and corrosive fluids can damage the oesophagus.

The various injuries have known effects and a stable incidence; they are now proportionally less frequent than other types of oesophageal trauma (see page 252).

When superficial, the different types of swallowing injury have different endoscopic appearances.

Food

A food bolus *swallowed whole* can produce an epithelial tear at the oesophageal mouth. Rigid endoscopy is the basic diagnostic tool: the longitudinal linear tear is usually located in the posterior wall of Killian's mouth; it can be erosive, haemorrhagic or exudate.

The resultant acute odynophagia often misleadingly suggests a foreign body injury. This aetiology usually can be ruled out by X-ray and fibroscopy of the upper oesophagus.

1188a

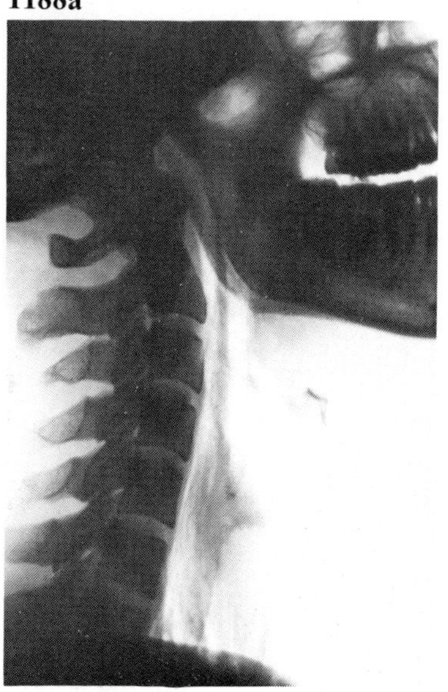

M.A. ♂ 20 yrs. 12 Oct. 1970

1188a Pharyngo-oesophageal perforation by food trauma. Peri-oesophageal emphysema . . .

1188b

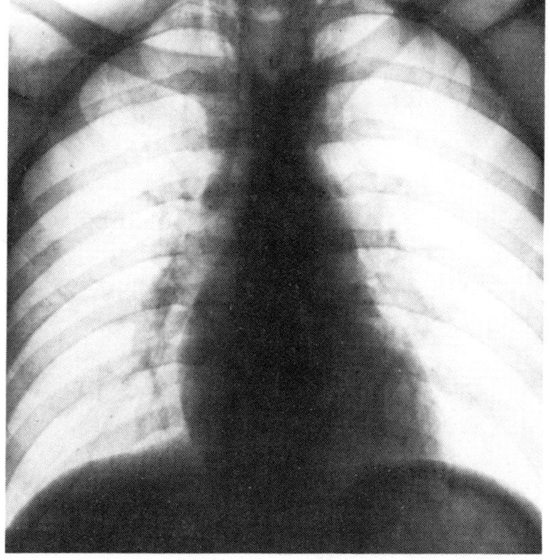

13 Oct. 1970

1188b . . . leads to mediastinal emphysema. Conservative treatment. Recovery.

1189

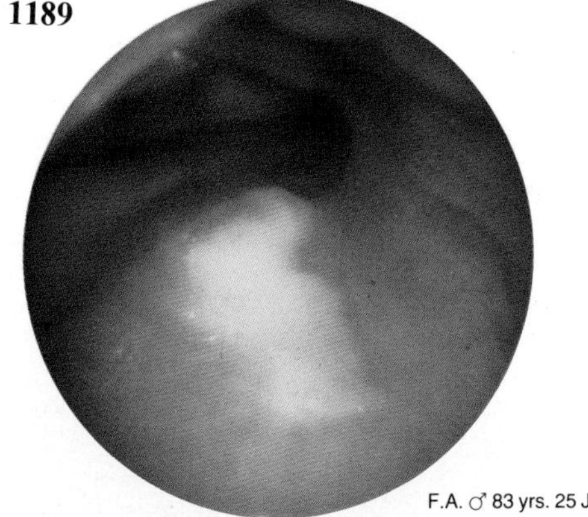

F.A. ♂ 83 yrs. 25 Jan. 1974

1189 Food trauma. Erosion at Killian's mouth.

An ordinary food bolus sometimes produces endoscopically visible subepithelial haematomas. Vascular fragility, especially when due to acute viral infection, is the main predisposing factor. Damage can be extensive.

1190

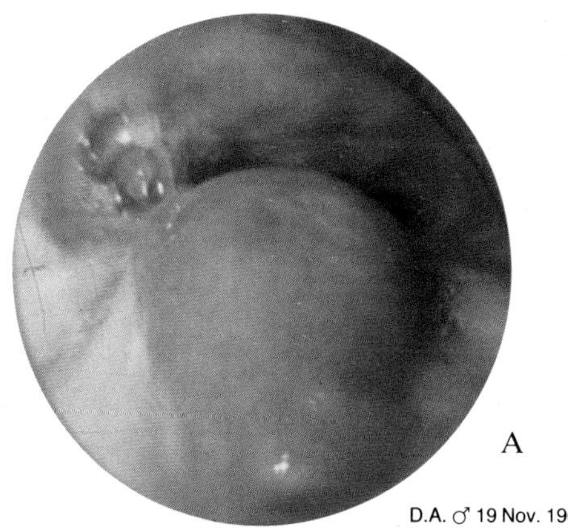

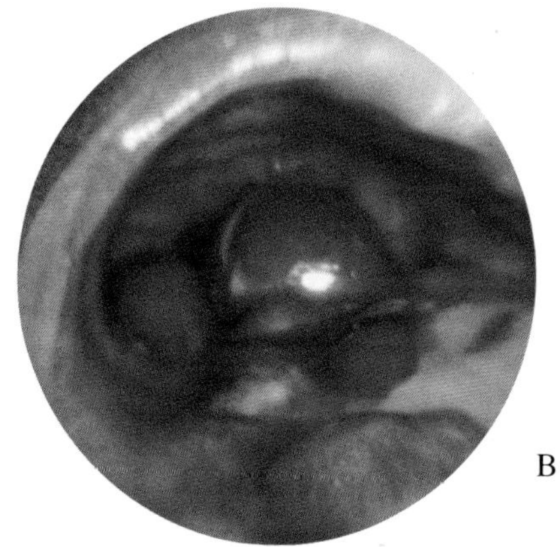

1190 Food trauma. This young man with influenza complained of acute odynophagia in the upper oesophagus after an ordinary meal. Instead of the suspected foreign body, rigid endoscopy reveals large submucosal haematomas along the entire length of the oesophagus. The most severe injuries are at the mouth of the oesophagus (A) and in the cervical oesophagus (B). Complete recovery is confirmed endoscopically a week later.

Foreign bodies

Of the many foreign bodies swallowed, very few injure the oesophagus.

Injury to a healthy oesophagus usually occurs at Killian's mouth or in the cervical oesophagus. A foreign body which passes harmlessly through the cervical oesophagus usually reaches the stomach without difficulty. Incarceration in the mid-thoracic or lower oesophagus generally implies an obstructive tumour, motility disorders or some other oesophageal disease.

Children swallow a wide variety of foreign bodies, but rarely is the oesophagus injured. In adults, the commonest causes of injury are bone splinters, fish bones and dentures.

1191 Age distribution of patients with an incarcerated foreign body in the oesophagus (in our material, $n = 288$)

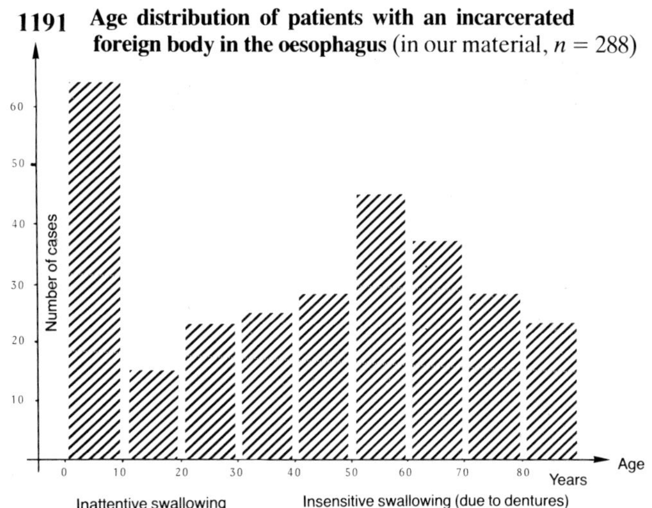

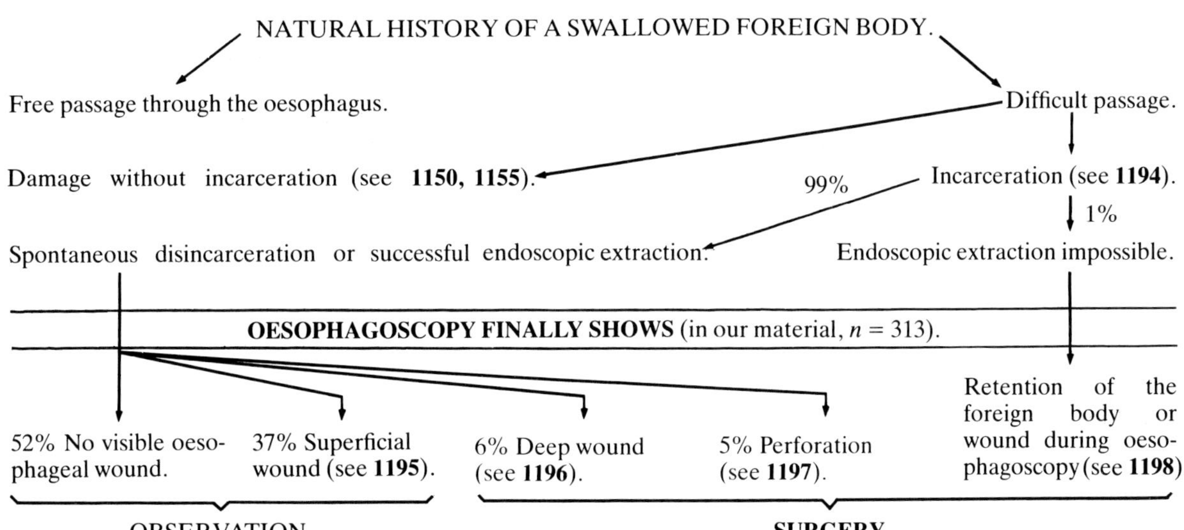

1192 **1193**

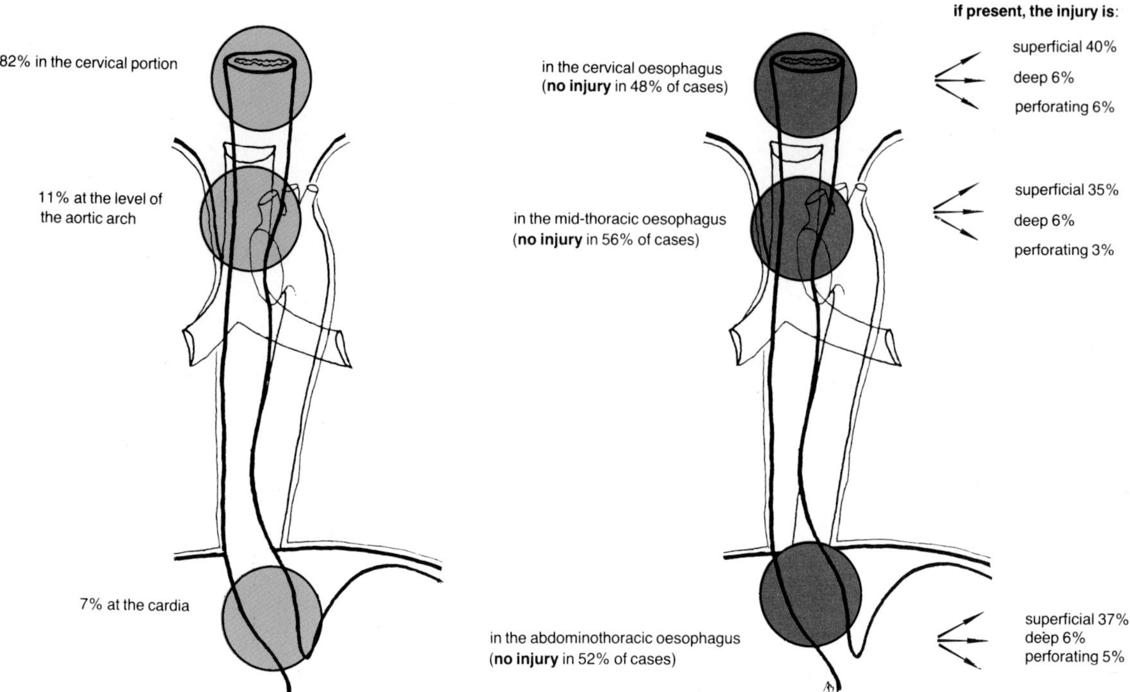

1192 Localisation of foreign bodies incarcerated in oesophagus (in our material, $n = 313$).

1193 Incidence of oesophageal injury after spontaneous disincarceration or endoscopic extraction of foreign body ($n = 313$).

1194

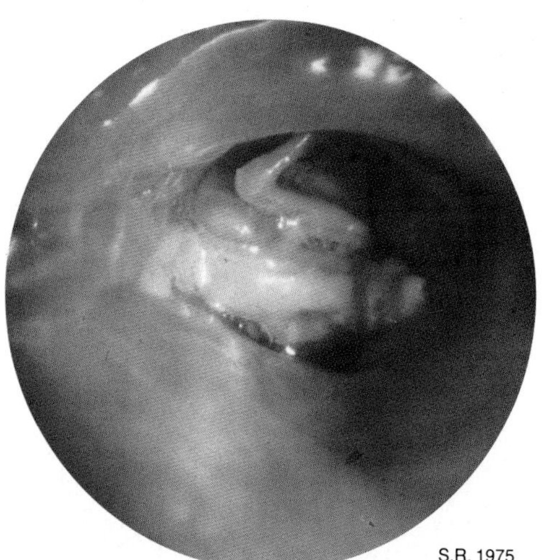

1194 Foreign body (a fragment of rabbit bone and meat) **incarcerated in cervicothoracic oesophagus**. Endoscopic extraction.

1195

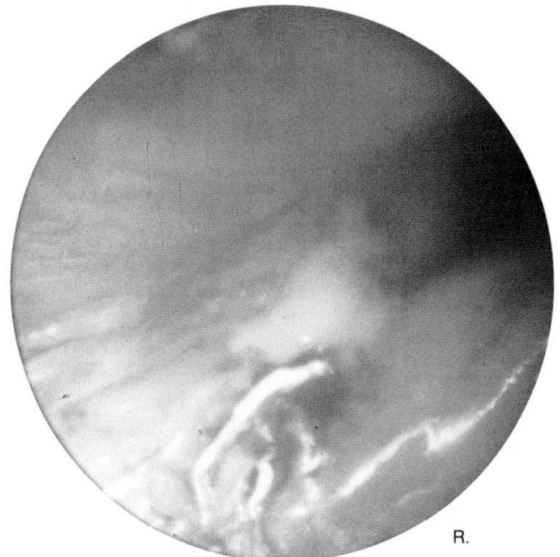

1195 Superficial mucosal injury detected after extraction of a foreign body.

1196

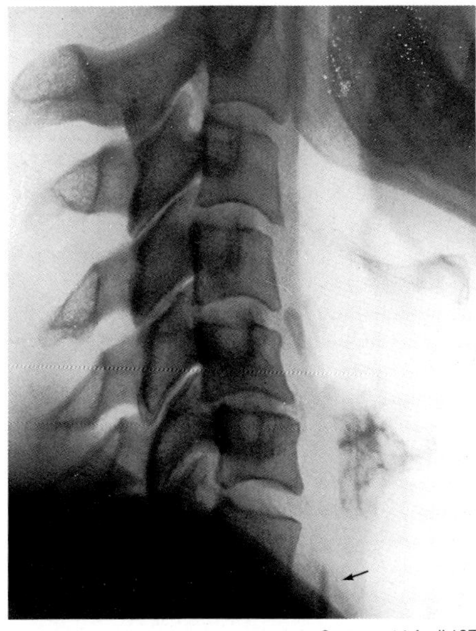

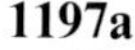

P.D. ♀ 62 yrs. 14 April 1975

1196 Foreign bodies can be difficult to see on standard X-rays. Lateral X-ray of the neck shows a splinter of lamb bone incarcerated below the Killian mouth. The rent in the oesophageal wall is 3cm long. The splinter has been incarcerated for 39 hours. There are clinical signs of mediastinitis.

1197a Injury at Killian's mouth caused by the incarceration of a partial denture. Right cervical emphysema.

1197b A lateral film clearly shows Minnigerode's sign (→). Successful endoscopic extraction of the denture; cervical drainage. Recovery.

1198a Long-term incarceration of coin in upper thoracic oesophagus of child. A coin (20 old French francs) was discovered by serendipity in a child who had been suffering from stridor and swallowing difficulties for about 6 months. Without the child having been examined, the parents had put him on a liquid diet.

1198b Inflammation around the oesophagus has caused tracheal stenosis. Endoscopic extraction proves impossible, so a cervical oesophagotomy is performed. The oesophagus heals within 2 months. Tracheal stenosis recedes gradually.

1197a

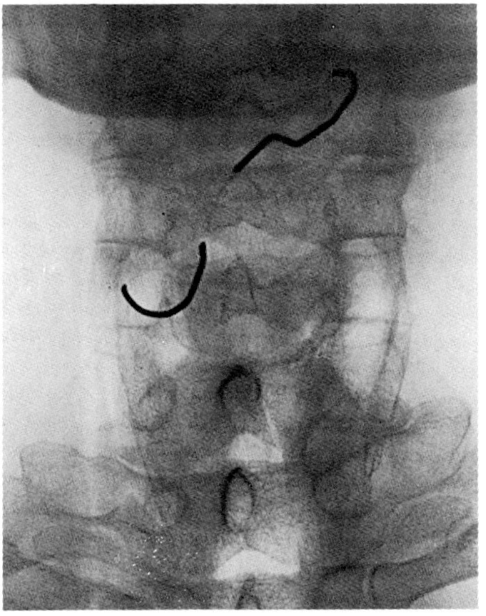

R.V. ♂ 71 yrs. 18 Sep. 1976

1197b

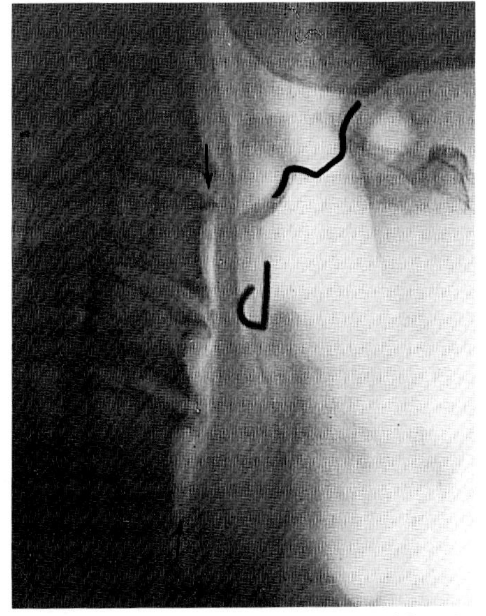

18 Sep. 1976

1198a

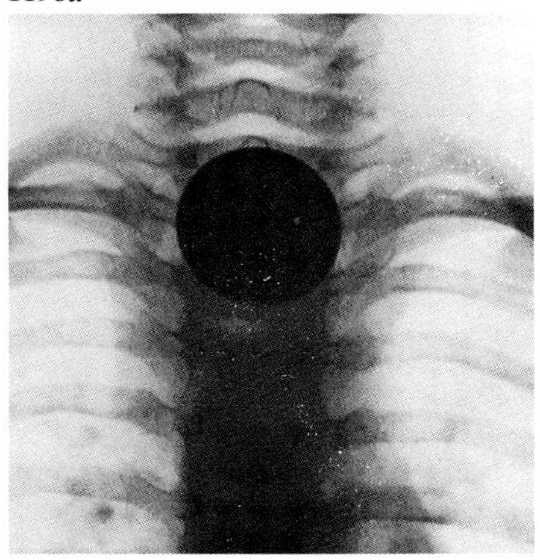

B.M.–E. ♂ 2 yrs. 28 April 1972

1198b

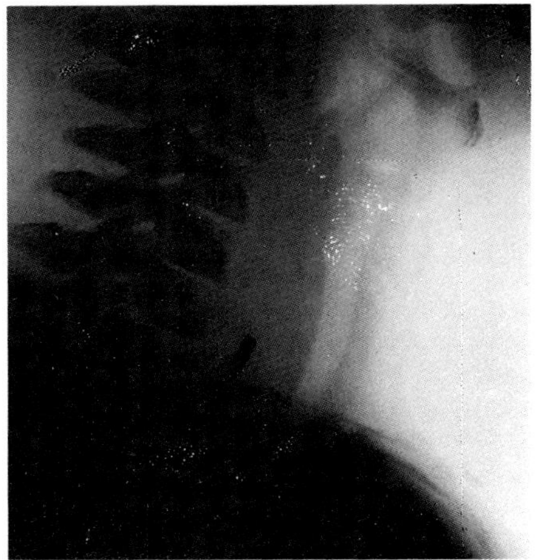

28 April 1972

Pills

Temporary incarceration of a tablet or capsule in the proximal oesophagus sometimes causes dysphagia in patients with no pre-existing oesophageal disease. Endoscopic examination then may reveal acute oesophagitis (with erosion or exudation) on a single circular segment of the oesophagus. Reported cases are few but the injury is doubtless more frequent than the literature suggests.

Potassium chloride tablets, certain anticholinergic drugs and antibiotics (especially tetracyclines) are commonly involved.

The oesophagus is usually eroded at the level of the aortic arch. Vital Lugol colouring confirms the disappearance of the epithelium and biopsy demonstrates unspecific submucosal inflammation. The epithelium heals within about 10 days.

1199a

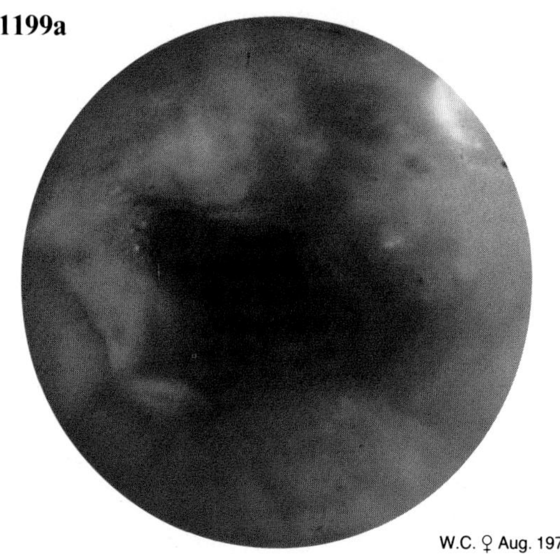

1199b

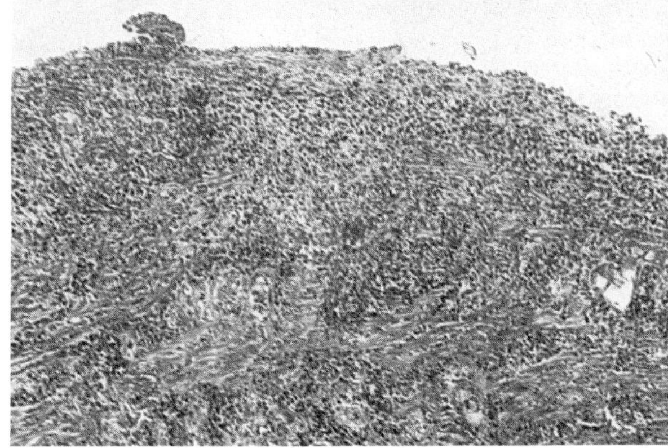

1199a Oesophagitis after a pill was incarcerated at the level of the aortic arch.

1199b Histological examination reveals sloughing of the oesophageal mucosa and an acute, unspecific inflammation of the submucosa. Recovery in 10 days.

Corrosion

Corrosion of the oesophagus has become rare. It is commonest in children who accidentally swallow caustic soda, bleach or a detergent. It also occurs in young adults who swallow concentrated acids and alkalis in suicide attempts. Respiratory burns are commonly associated.

Alkali corrosion is usually limited to the oesophagus. Most concentrated alkalis are viscous and clinging. The liquefaction of the oesophageal mucosa results in thrombosis of the submucosal vessels. Inflammatory stenosis is then followed by cicatricial stricture. Fistulisation is common in the long term.

When alkali reaches the stomach, it is partially neutralised by the gastric juice. As a result, the stomach and duodenum usually remain intact.

1200 Corrosion of upper digestive tract by concentrated **alkali**.

1201 Corrosion of upper digestive tract by concentrated **acid**.

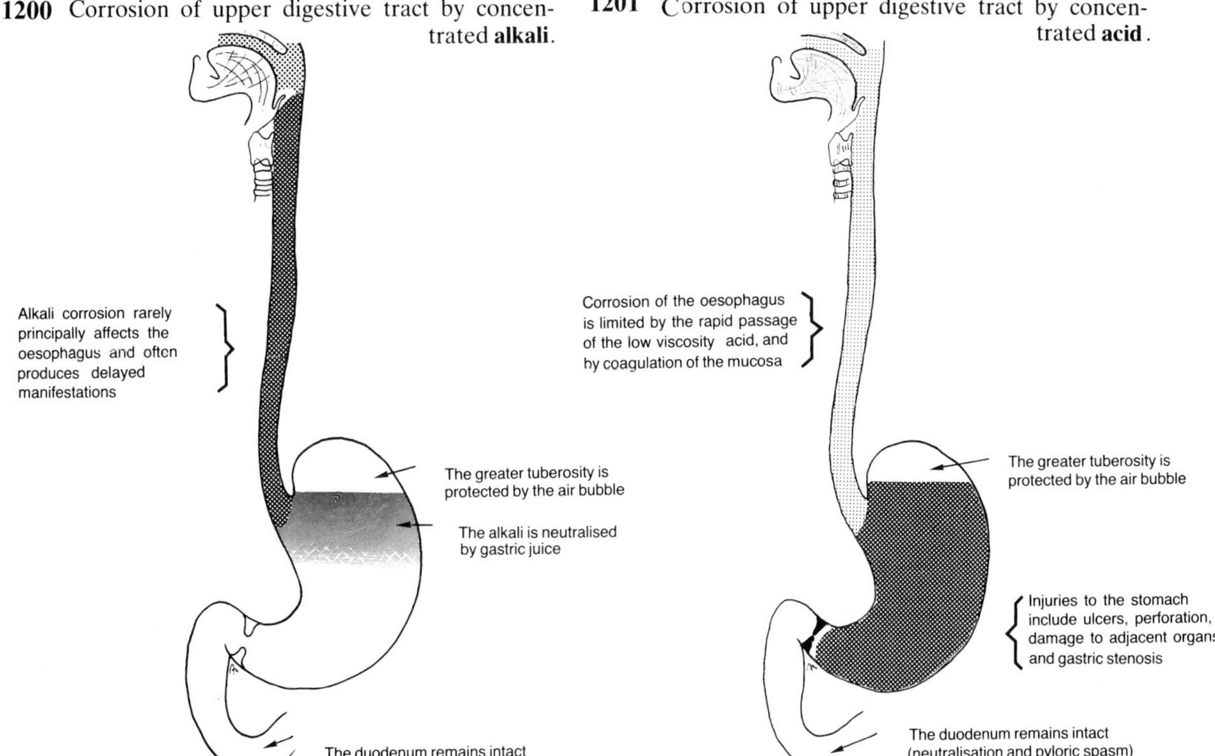

The *corrosive effect of concentrated acid* on the oesophageal wall is limited by two factors. First, most acids are of low viscosity and, therefore, pass swiftly through the oesophagus and, second, the proteins in the mucosa coagulate and protect the oesophageal wall from deep corrosion.

In the stomach, on the other hand, corrosion is often severe. It frequently takes the form of ulcers, perforations and serious intraperitoneal injuries. Gastric stenosis is common (see **1217**).

Pancreatic juice usually neutralises the acid when it reaches the duodenum. Some authorities argue further that a pyloric spasm helps to protect the intestine.

Treatment of corrosion in the upper portion of the digestive tract is difficult and prolonged. Complications are frequent. They vary with the concentration and nature of the corrosive substance.

The **early phase** of corrosion (the first 24 hours) is characterised (1) by *respiratory difficulties* – epiglottic or laryngeal oedema and tracheobronchial burns whose radiological appearance is often similar to that of a Mendelson's syndrome; (2) by a *corrosive burn of part of the digestive tract* – the burn is sometimes transmural and allows caustic material to spread into the mediastinum, peritoneum or retroperitoneum (the outcome in such cases is usually fatal); and sometimes (3) by *shock*. The therapeutic aims in this phase are to neutralise the caustic material, to treat the respiratory injuries and to resuscitate the patient.

The **intermediate phase**, the phase of cicatrization, can last from one month to three months. The common accidents in this phase are (1) *respiratory difficulties* resulting from the broncho-aspiration of food, (2) *digestive complications,* consisting of severe digestive haemorrhage or perforation with mediastinitis or peritonitis, and (3) *septic complications*, for example bronchopneumonia, or sepsis from the catheters. During this phase, oral feeding should be replaced by parenteral hyperalimentation, and prophylactic measures taken against infection. Endoluminal oesophageal manoeuvres (dilatation or the introduction of a Levin tube) are very often damaging; corticoids are nearly always ineffective. In most cases, surgery for digestive complications fails because of the fragility of the corroded tissues.

The **late phase** is the phase of the cicatricial stenosis. By this stage, oral feeding is usually impossible. Repeated dilatation often has to be supplemented by surgical resection to forestall late malignant complications. This procedure is frequently very difficult. The resected portion of oesophagus is replaced with a section of stomach, or small or large intestine (see **1167 – 1172**). The appropriate moment for surgery is not easy to determine for stenosis sometimes continues to evolve for months or years.

In addition, it has been established that the risk of oesophageal cancer after corrosion is about 1000 times greater than normal. Cancer develops after an average delay of 35 years. It should be treated in the same way as any other oesophageal neoplasm. The prognosis is poor.

1202

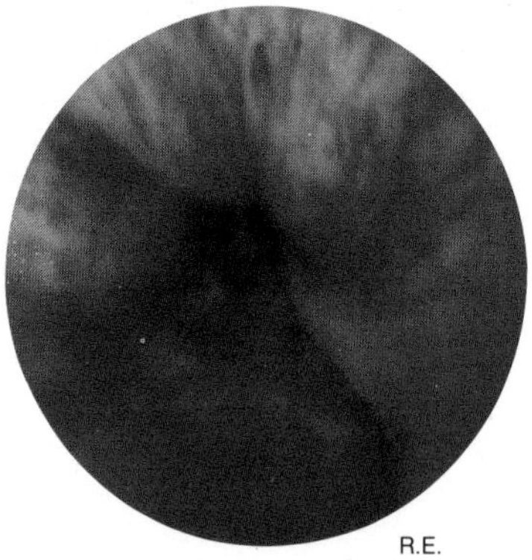

1203

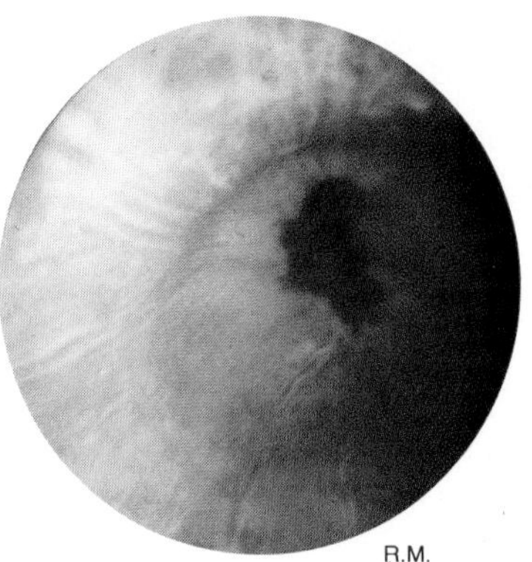

1204

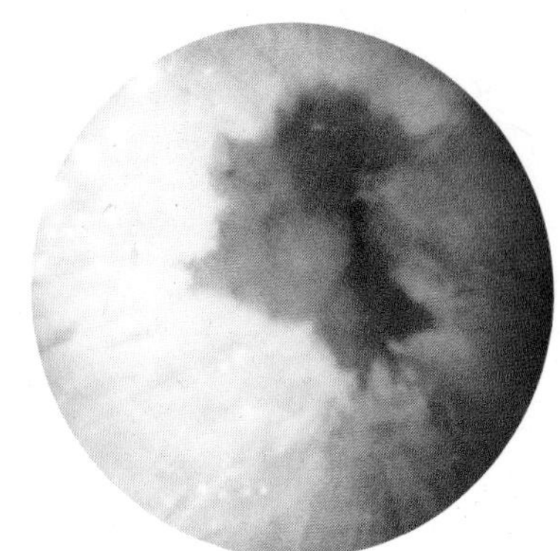

R.E.

R.M.

1202 Caustic oesophageal corrosion at the cardia. First degree: erythematous phase.

1203, 1204 First degree: papyraceous coagulation by the acid in the superficial layers of the lower oesophageal mucosa. The Z-line is well contrasted.

1205

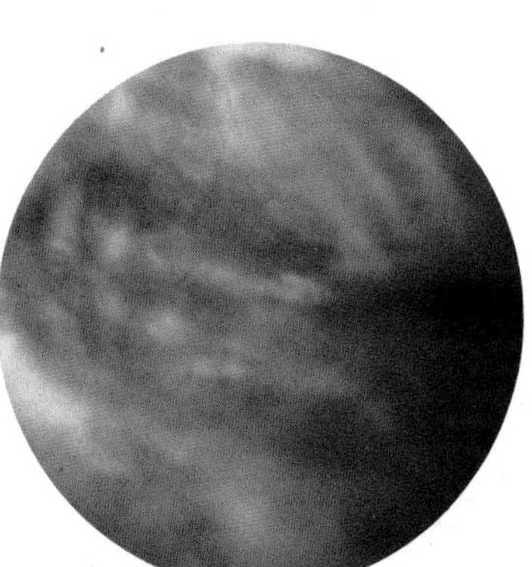

1206

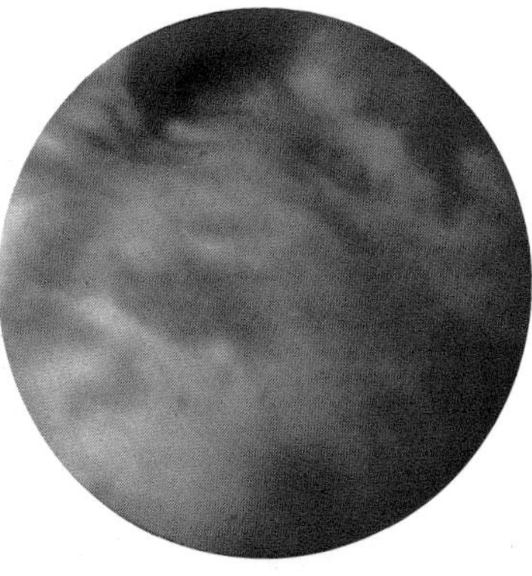

R.

1207

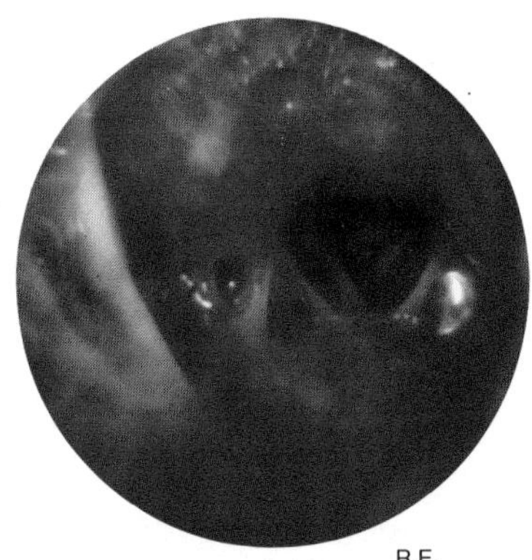

R.E.

1205, 1206 Second degree: mucosal exudation as a result of acid corrosion.

1207 Third degree: haemorrhagic necrosis as a result of acid corrosion.

1208

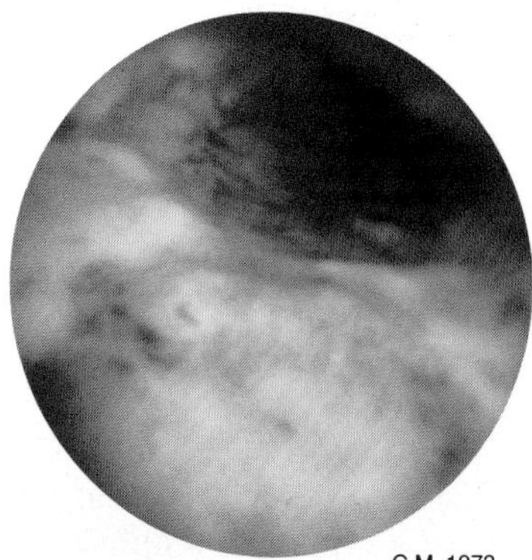

C.M. 1973

1209

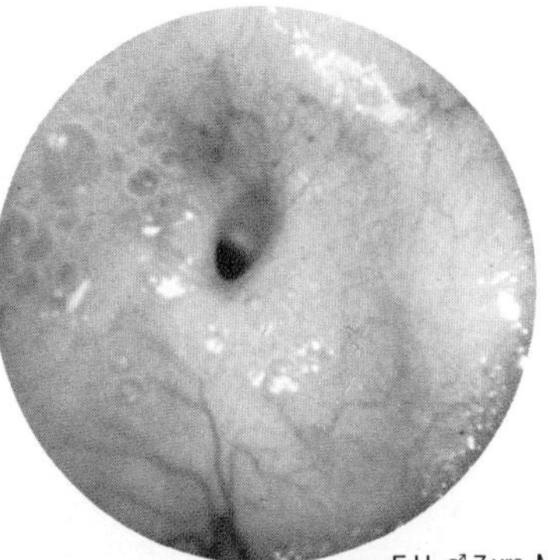

1210

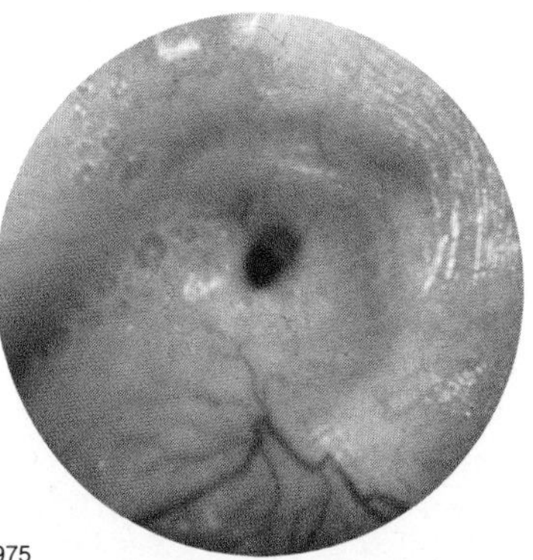

E.H. ♂ 7 yrs. Mar. 1975

1208 Third degree: 10 days after an acid burn, the lower oesophagus is coated with fibrin.

1209, 1210 Oesophageal stenosis 16 months after a bleach burn. Intraparietal inflammation and submucosal hypervascularisation are clearly in evidence. Surgery at this stage often leads to iterative stenosis.

1211

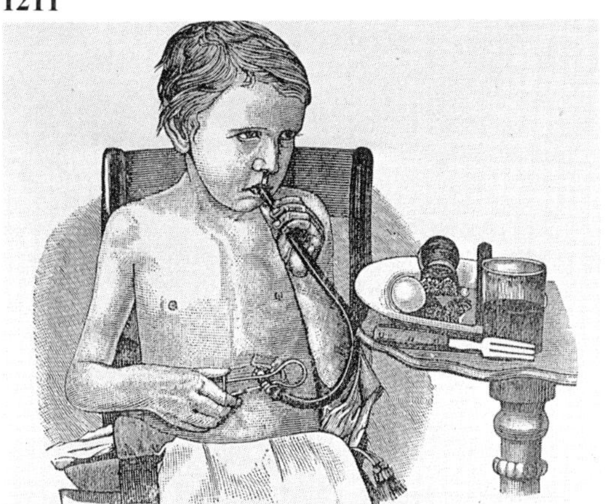

1211 Oesophageal corrosion used to be incurable. Masticated food had to be regurgitated through a permanent gastrostomy. (J. Bryant, New York, 1905.)

1212a

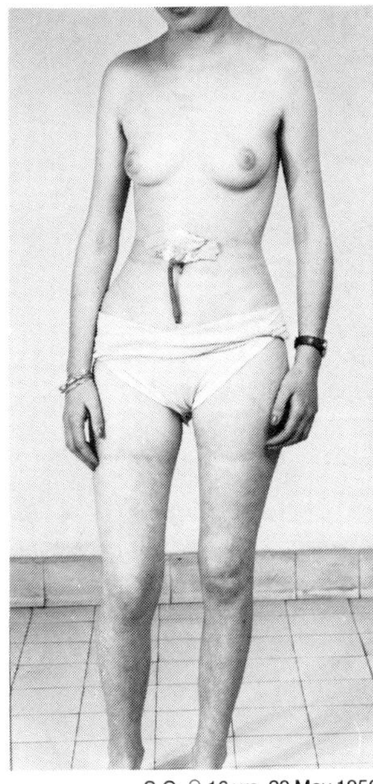

S.G. ♀ 16 yrs. 29 May 1950

1212a This girl has been feeding through a gastrostomy tube for 10 years following an alkali burn of the oesophagus with complete stenosis. **Her nutritional state is good**.

1212b A left thoracotomy with diaphragmatic incision has been performed for gastrolysis, liberation of the oesophagus at the aortic arch and closure of the gastrostoma; these manoeuvres were followed by a partial oesophagectomy and oesophagogastric anastomosis according to Sweet. An upper gastrointestinal study 10 days later is satisfactory. At late control (28 years after corrosion), the patient's health is excellent. *N.B. Today, surgery would have been performed much earlier.*

1212b

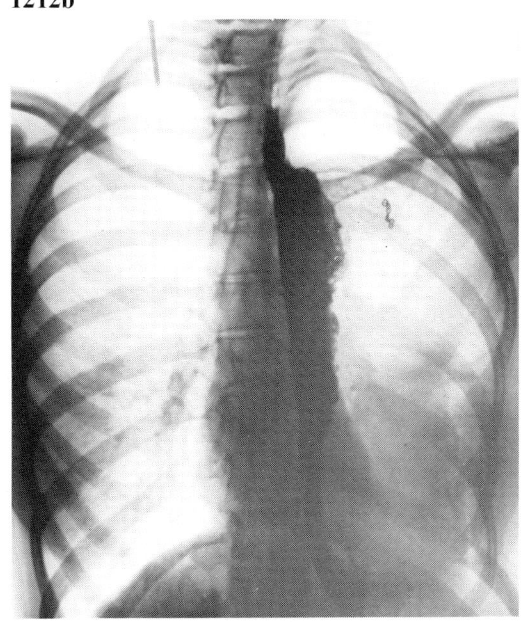

16 June 1950

1213a

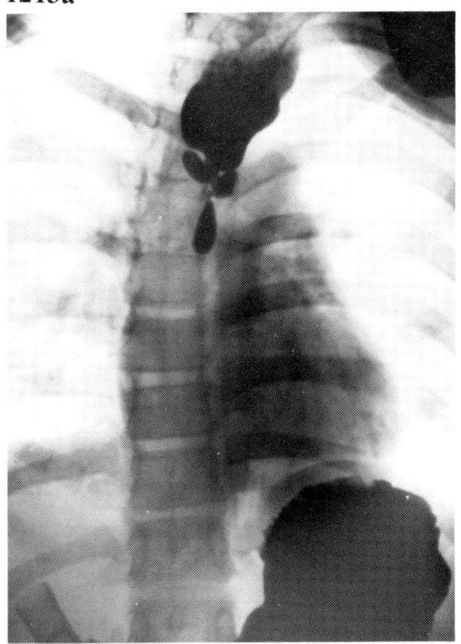

M.S. ♂ 16 yrs. 1 June 1951

1213a Nine year-old oesophageal corrosion treated by transposition of stomach into left chest. The thoracic oesophagus is completely obstructed, but the stomach is intact.

1213b Barium study taken after oesophagogastric anastomosis (without oesophagectomy) through a combined abdominal and left thoracic approach. Uneventful recovery with a weight gain of 10 kg.

1213b

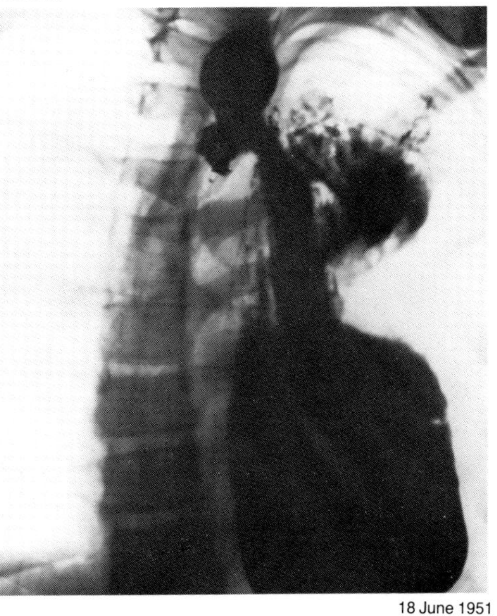

18 June 1951

1214a

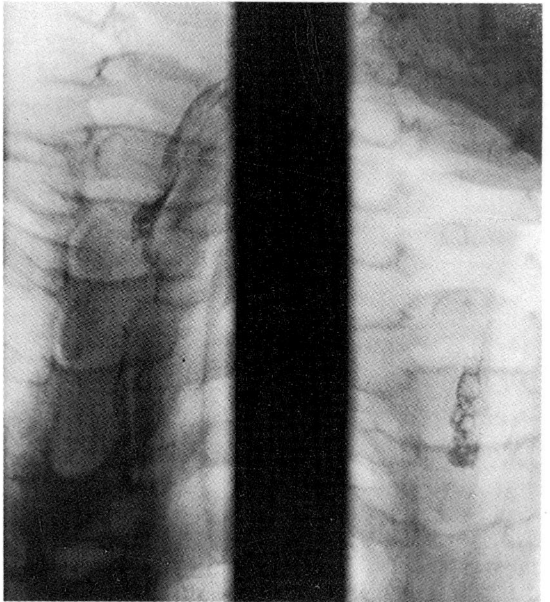

O.J. ♂ 13 yrs. 19 Mar. 1976

1214b

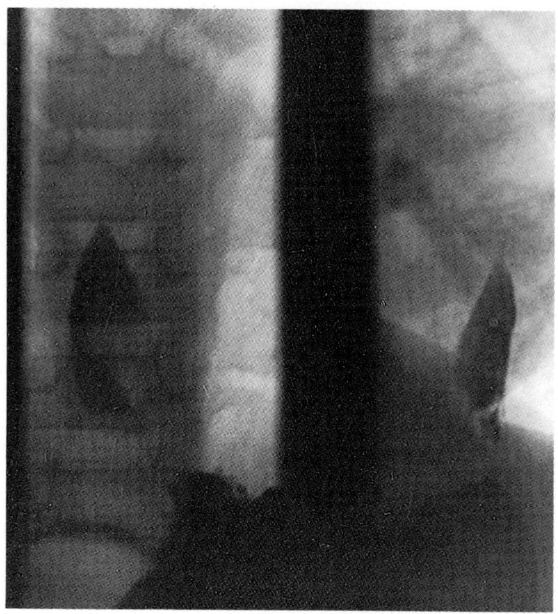

19 Mar. 1976

1214c

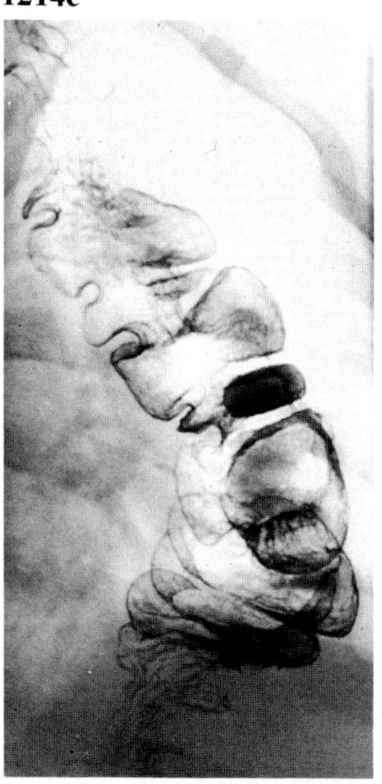

6 July 1976

1214a Total corrosive stenosis treated by retro-sternal colon interposition. Two years have elapsed since the child swallowed bleach. Bougienage was effective in the short term but a barium study shows that the oesophagus is now completely obstructed. The child is being fed through a gastrostomy. (Prof. N. Genton, Lausanne.)

1214b A barium study is performed through the gastrostomy tube. The photograph shows 2 cm of the lower oesophagus. The thoracic oesophagus is completely obstructed over 8 cm.

1214c A left thoracotomy for complete removal of the oesophageal mucosa and colon interposition is later followed by a distal oesophagectomy. Recovery. (Prof. N. Genton, Lausanne.)

1215a

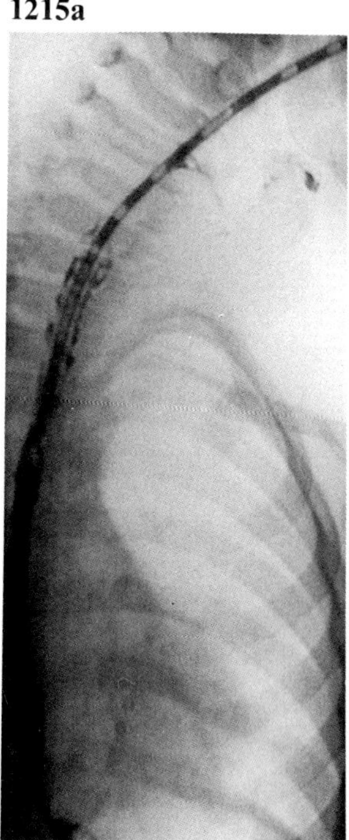

G.C. ♂ 2 yrs. 23 Aug. 1958

1215b

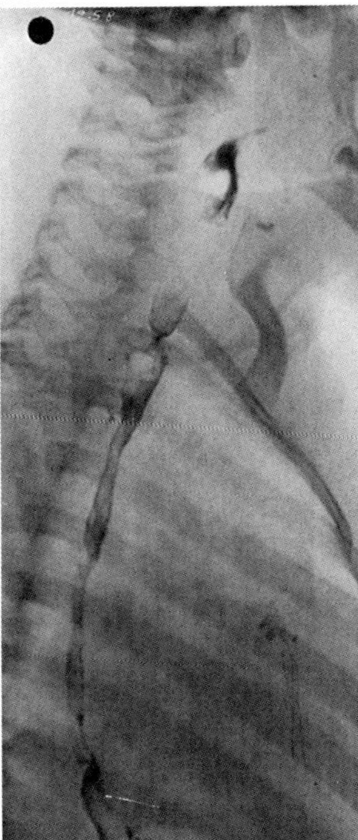

13 Dec. 1958

1215c

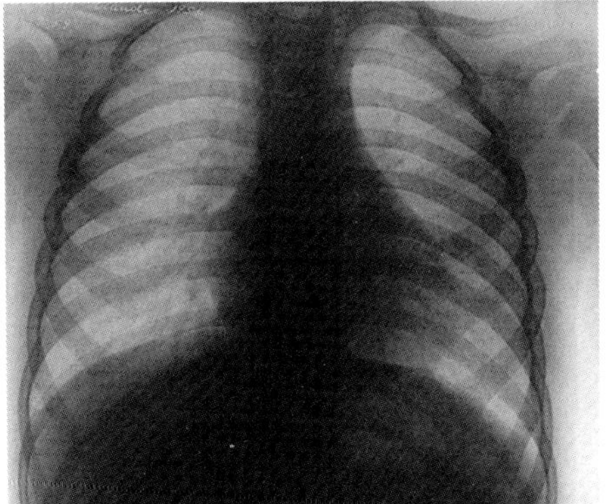

12 Feb. 1959

1215d

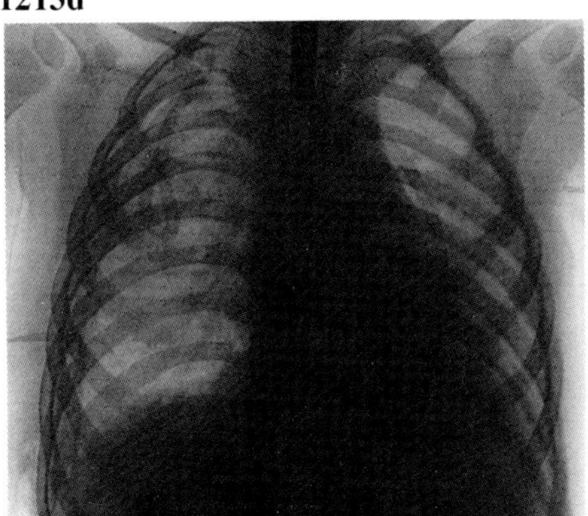

8 Mar. 1959

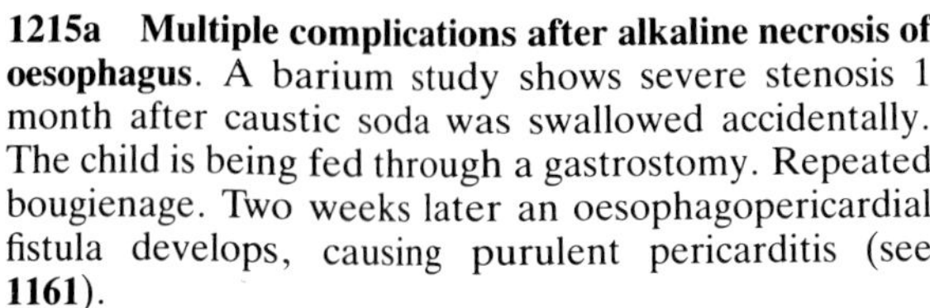

1215a Multiple complications after alkaline necrosis of oesophagus. A barium study shows severe stenosis 1 month after caustic soda was swallowed accidentally. The child is being fed through a gastrostomy. Repeated bougienage. Two weeks later an oesophagopericardial fistula develops, causing purulent pericarditis (see **1161**).

1215b Obstruction is now almost complete. A cervical approach fails. One month later, an oesophagobronchial fistula develops (see **1162**), but there are few symptoms because food is not being taken orally.

1215c X-ray immediately before a partial oesophagectomy through the right chest.

1215d The oesophagectomy could not be completed because fibrosis prevented dissection of the mediastinum. Postoperative complications include a compressive left pneumothorax. Death 4 days later.

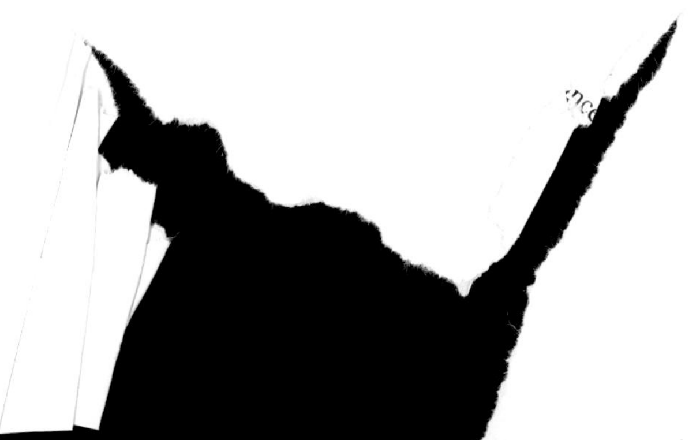

1216a

D.A.–M. ♀ 30 yrs. 6 Aug. 1971

1216b

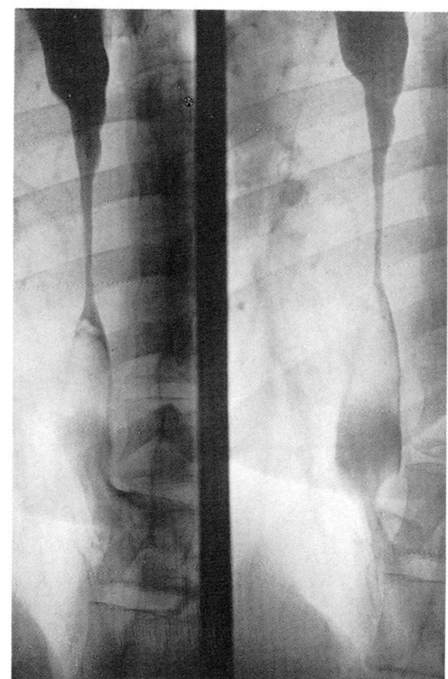

8 Oct. 1971

1216c

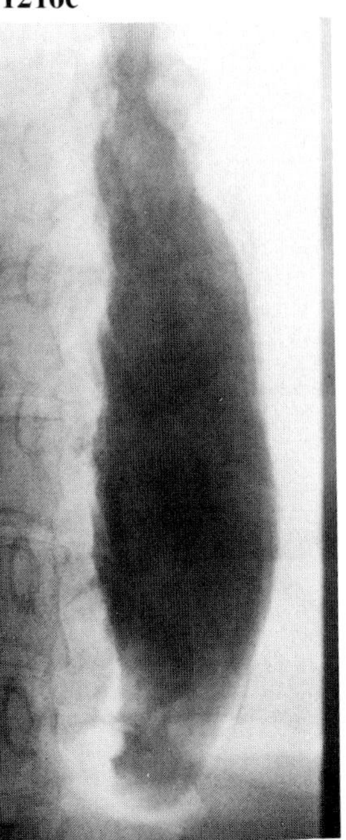

19 Nov. 1971

1216d

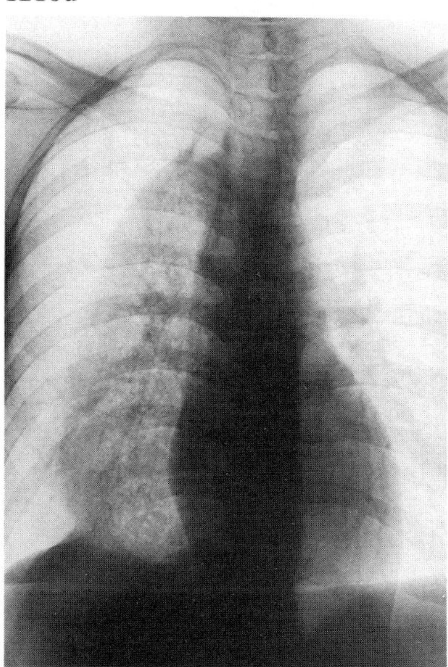

31 Dec. 1971

1216e

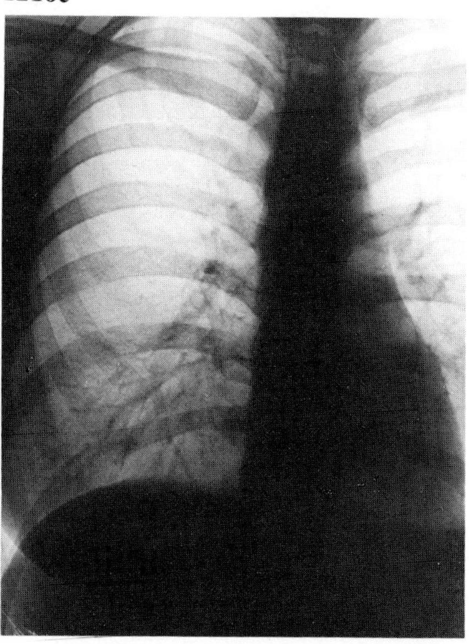

1 Oct. 1971

1216f

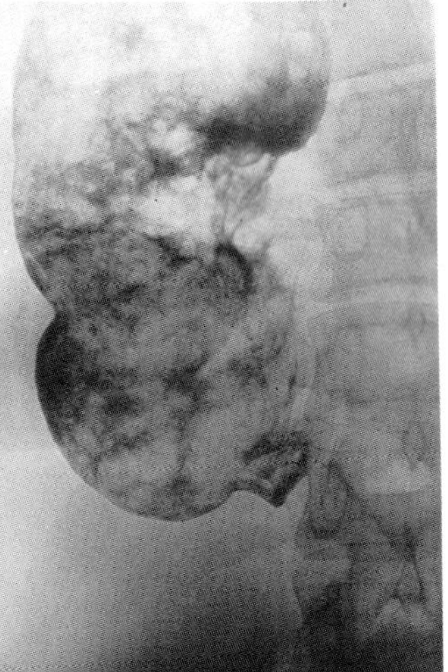

26 Jan. 1973

1216a Gradual acid stenosis treated by oesophagectomy and gastric transposition into right chest. Eight months previously the patient swallowed 100 ml of concentrated hydrochloric acid. Mid-thoracic stenosis caused dysphagia. *Unusually, the stomach is intact*.

1216b Cicatricial stricture becomes tighter, and on 30th October the stenosed area is excised (through a right thoracotomy) to forestall the risk of late cancer.

1216c Postoperative barium study.

1216d Chronic distension of the stomach 12 days later is probably due to poor passage through the pyloroplasty.

1216e The pre-operative X-ray for comparison.

1216f Despite significant gastric residue and difficulty in emptying her stomach, the patient is in good general condition and refuses further surgery. Her condition since has remained unchanged.

1217a

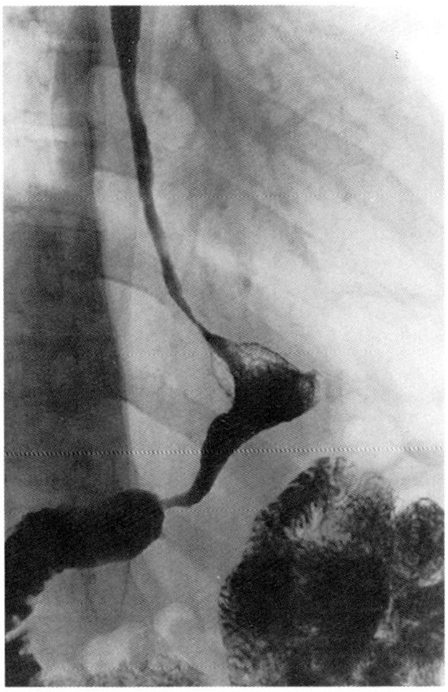

1217b

8 Nov. 1965

S.Y. ♂ 23 yrs. 15 Oct. 1965

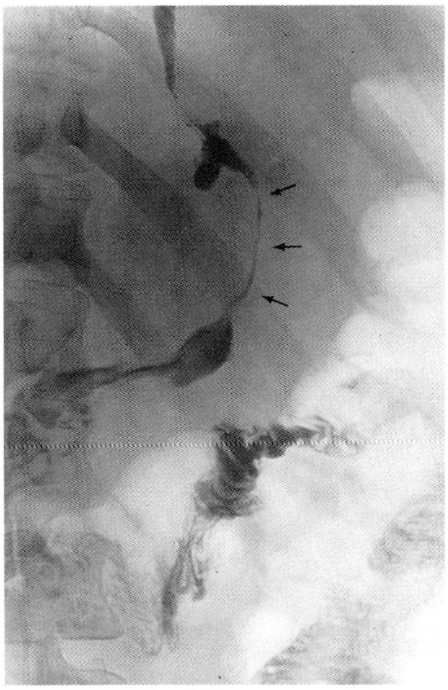

1217c

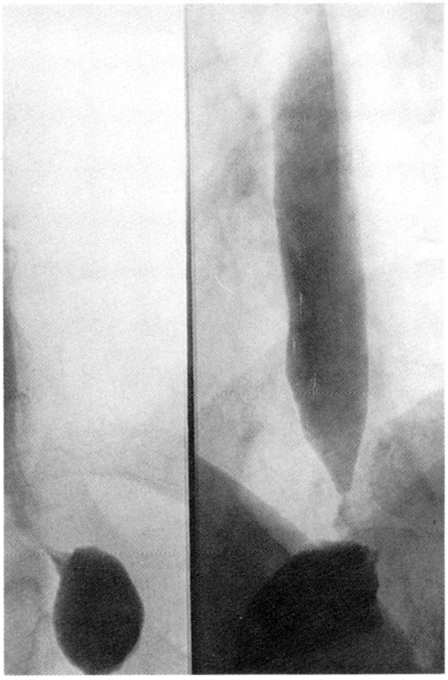

1217d

1217e

28 Jan. 1966

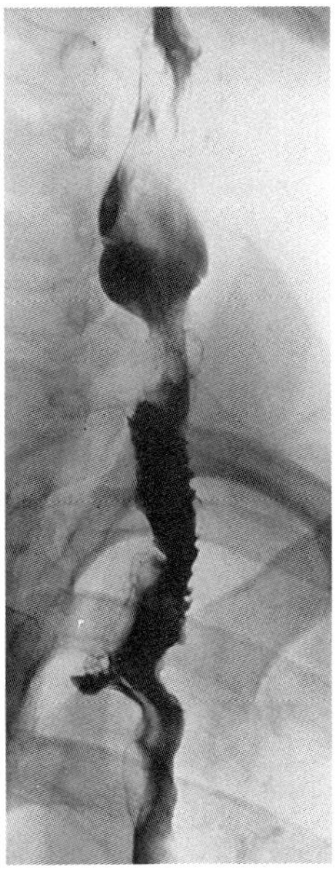

2 Dec. 1966

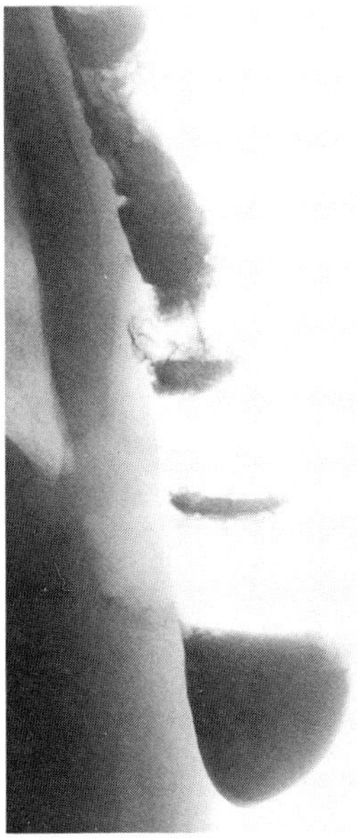

29 May 1970

1217a Acid burn of oesophagus and stomach, treated by subcutaneous presternal colon interposition. 100 ml of concentrated hydrochloric acid were swallowed about a week before this X-ray was taken. The oesophagus is intact but the stomach has contracted severely. The duodenum displays normal mobility and morphology.

1217c Stenosis almost completely obstructs the stomach; feeding is maintained through a jejunostomy.

1217b Despite the relatively sound condition of the oesophagus, oral feeding remains impossible because of the filiform gastric lumen (→). A presternal interposition is performed with the right colon and a small segment of the terminal ileum.

1217d After repeated remedial intervention, free passage is obtained through the oesophagus, ileum and colon.

1217e Four and a half years later, the patient has some difficulty emptying the subcutaneous portion of the colon. His overall condition is nevertheless stable. An oesophagectomy will be performed (3 years later) to forestall the possibility of late cancer. No post-operative complications.

1218a

M.N. ♀ 69 yrs. 28 Sep. 1978

1218b

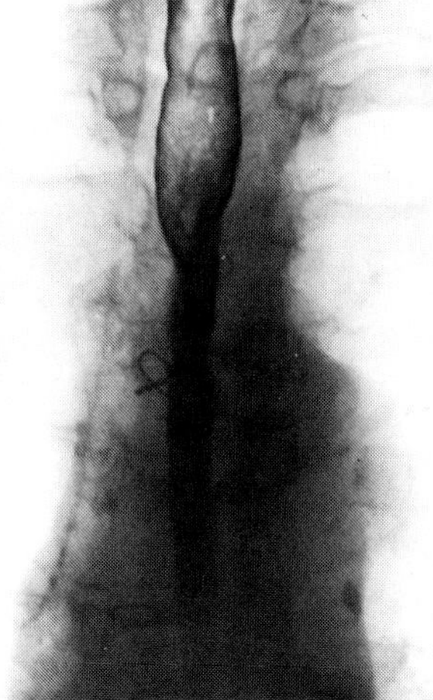

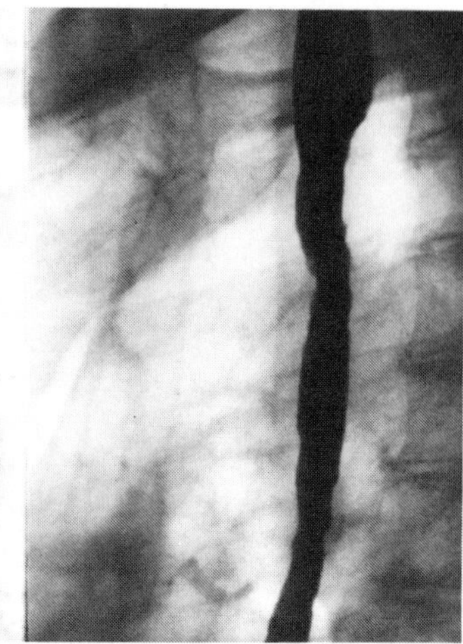

10 Nov. 1978

1218a Carcinoma of oesophagus after corrosion caused by hydrochloric acid swallowed accidentally **61 years earlier**. Upper oesophageal stenosis had been dilated periodically throughout the patient's life. A recent bout of dysphagia, therefore, was attributed initially to a new episode of stenosis. However, endoscopic biopsy reveals a squamous cell carcinoma (→) 3cm below the oesophageal mouth.

1218b Dysphagia disappears temporarily after irradiation. Death 5 months later due to recurrent cancer.

Pneumatic rupture of the oesophagus and stomach

Pneumatic rupture is rare. It is caused by a blast of compressed air or by sudden and violent over-inflation.

It can occur in the oesophagus or in the stomach when transposed into the thorax.

Primary suturing gives the best chance of survival. A third of patients die.

1219a

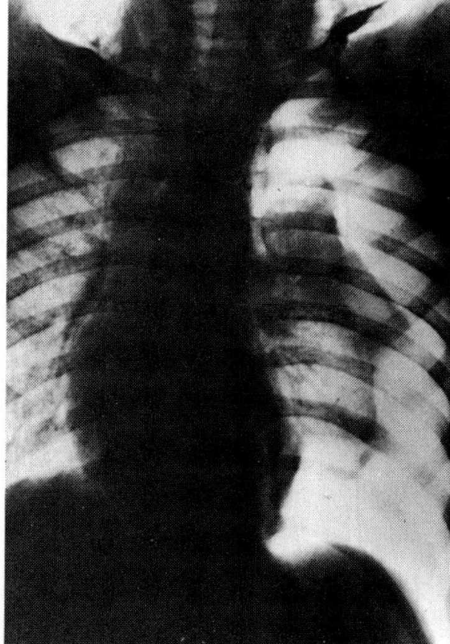

1219a Accidental pneumatic rupture. This 6-year-old child bit the inner tube of a tractor tyre. The explosion brought immediate respiratory distress with cyanosis, shock and a compressive left pneumothorax.

1219b

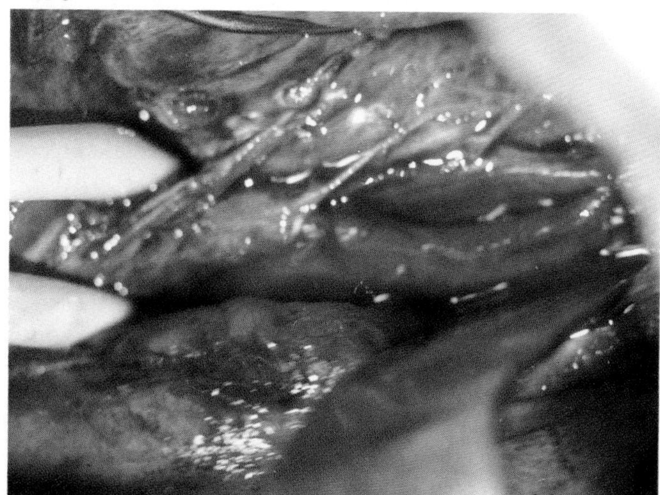

1219b An emergency left thoracotomy reveals a 6cm laceration (terminating 1cm above the cardia) in the anterolateral oesophageal wall. Respiratory difficulties continue postoperatively. A mediastinal abscess is drained, and a feeding jejunostomy performed. Recovery is slow but complete. (Dr E.T. Gelfand, Edmonton, Canada.)

1220a

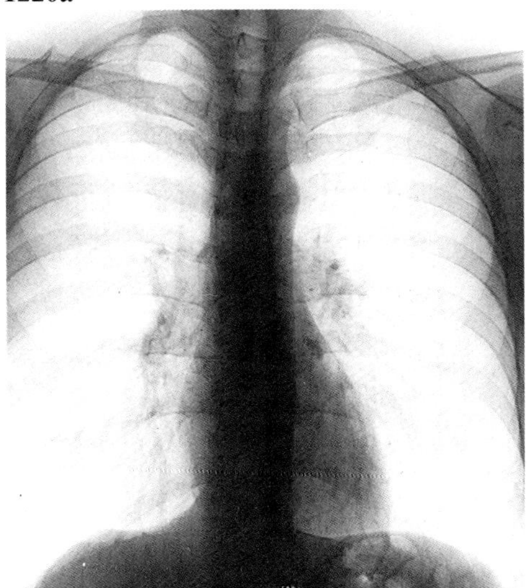

C.A. ♂ 45 yrs. 16 Mar. 1976

1220b

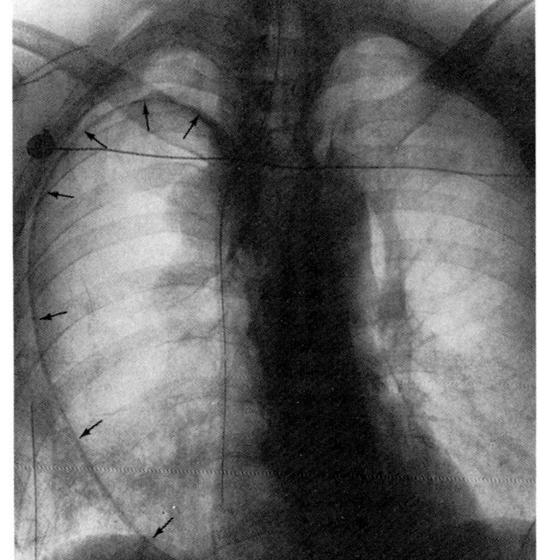

17 Mar. 1976

1220c

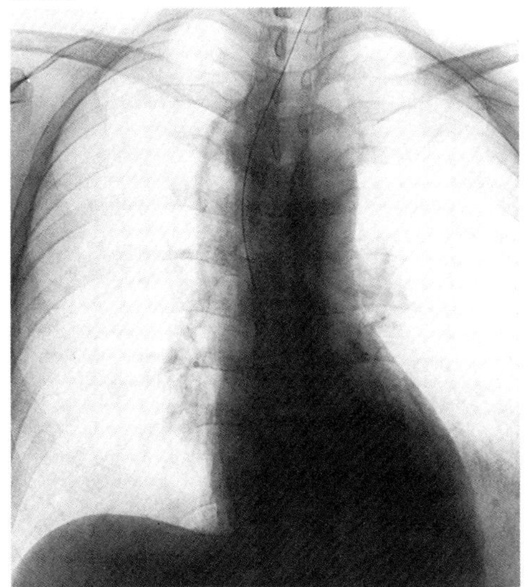

27 Mar. 1976

1220a Rupture by over-inflation of stomach transposed into chest. Pre-operative X-ray of a patient admitted for cancer of the lower oesophagus. Right thoracotomy for oesophageal resection and gastro-oesophageal anastomosis (according to Sweet).

1220b A few hours after surgery, an error in manipulating the Levin tube forces some 4000 ml of air into the stomach. Massively over-inflated (→), the stomach ruptures in 3 places.

1220c Repair. Recovery.

The Mallory-Weiss and Boerhaave syndrome

Effort rupture of the oesophagus is the result of a violent increase in pressure in the abdomen – Valsalva's manoeuvre, hiccoughing, defecation, delivery, epileptic attack, external heart massage or lifting of a heavy weight, for example. The commonest cause of all is violent emesis.

N.B. Emetic injuries are discussed in detail because, (1) they are often rather poorly described, (2) their thoracic and/or abdominal consequences are similar to other oesophageal injuries.

Predisposing factors

Gastro-oesophageal rupture during vomiting commonly occurs in patients with a hiatal hernia, a large epiphrenic diverticulum or oesophageal motility trouble (particularly in alcoholics).

It can arise also if fundoplication completely prevents gastro-oesophageal reflux, making the stomach into a closed space.

1221

In the oesophagus, the mucosal membrane is the **strongest** layer

In the stomach – and particularly around the cardia – the mucosal membrane is the most **fragile** layer

An oesophageal mucosa weakened by **oesophagitis** (particularly at stage III or IV) is particularly predisposed to rupture.

Oesophagitis is most often the result of gastro-oesophageal reflux; it is especially common in cases of hiatal hernia or prolonged Levin intubation.

1222

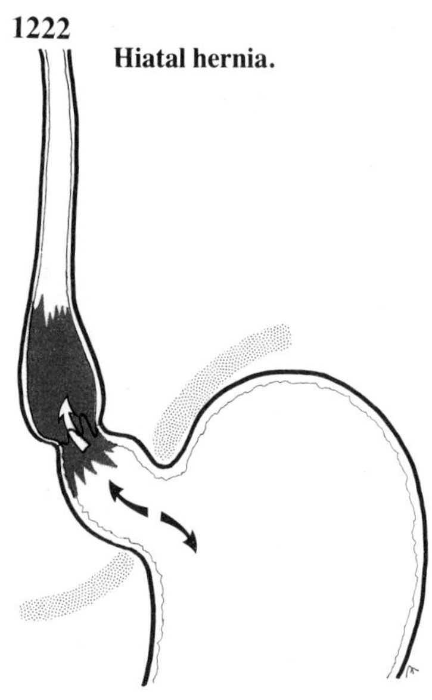

Hiatal hernia.

1223a

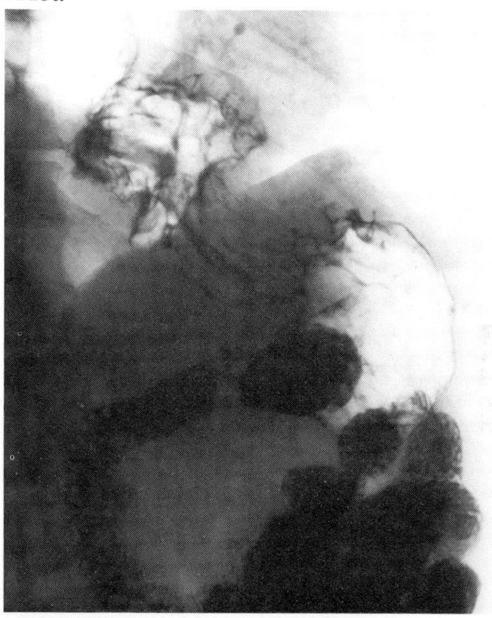

T.A. ♂ 57 yrs. 11 Aug. 1978

1223b

1223a/b More than half of all emetic gastro-oesophageal ruptures occur in patients with a hiatal hernia. In this case, several years of gastro-oesophageal reflux and infection have weakened significantly the lower oesophagus. An episode of vomiting is followed by severe haematemesis. Eight units of blood are transfused and a laparotomy performed for a Nissen fundoplication, truncal vagotomy and pyloroplasty. Recovery.

1224

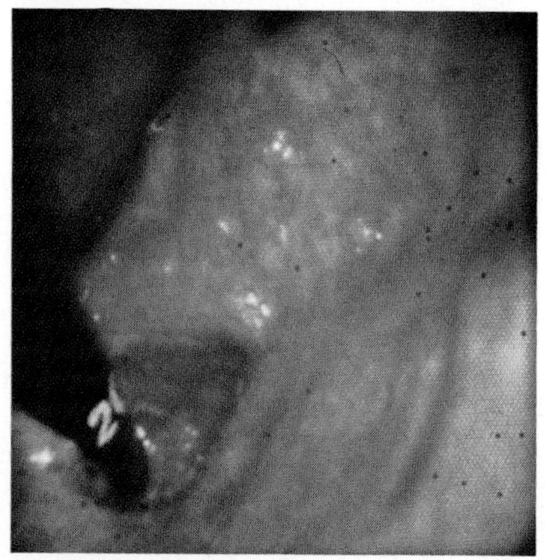

S.M. ♀ 35 yrs. 30 June 1976

1224 Large hiatal hernia observed by inversion of a fibroscope.

1225

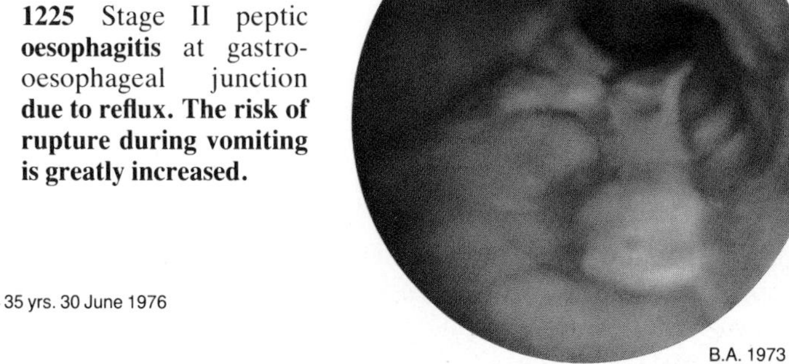

B.A. 1973

1225 Stage II peptic **oesophagitis** at gastro-oesophageal junction **due to reflux. The risk of rupture during vomiting is greatly increased.**

1226

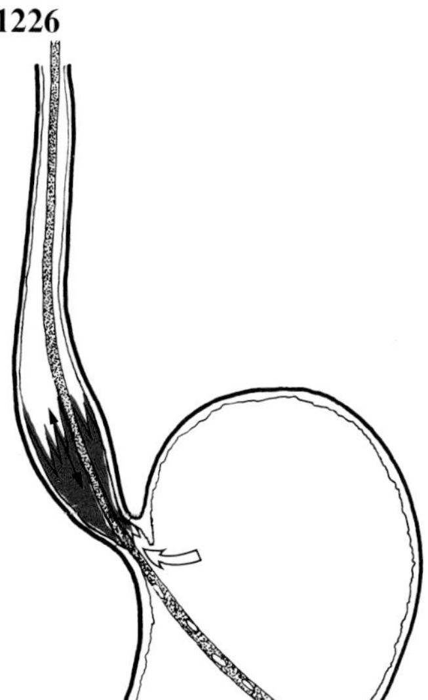

1226 **Oesophagitis caused by reflux around Levin tube**. Levin intubation should be avoided if possible. When a Levin tube is used, it should be connected to suction.

1227

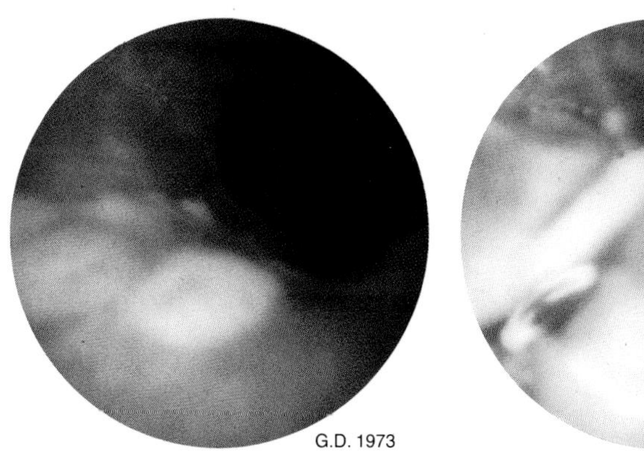

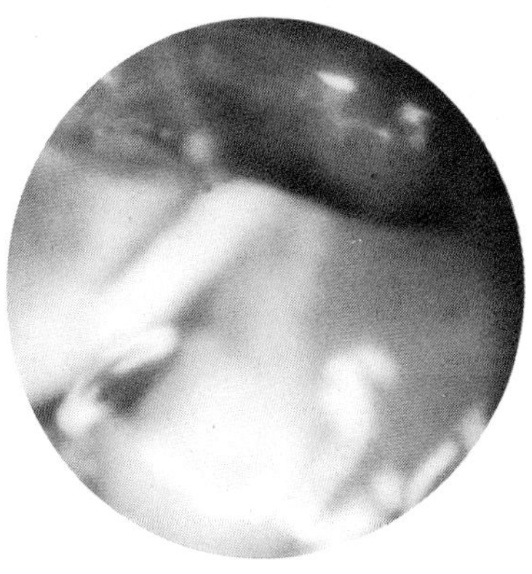

G.D. 1973

1227 **Levin intubation** exposes the oesophagus to various injuries. On the left, the mucosa has been eroded around the cricopharyngeal muscle; on the right, the lower oesophagus is inflamed as a result of passive reflux around the tube. Such conditions increase the risk of rupture.

1228a

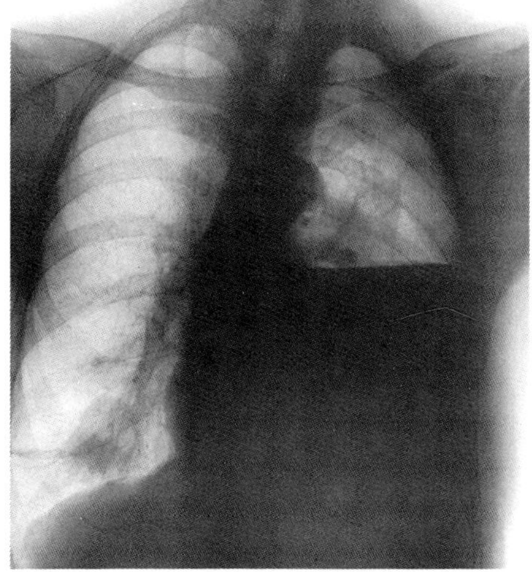

B.A. ♂ 68 yrs. 23 Dec. 1969

1228b

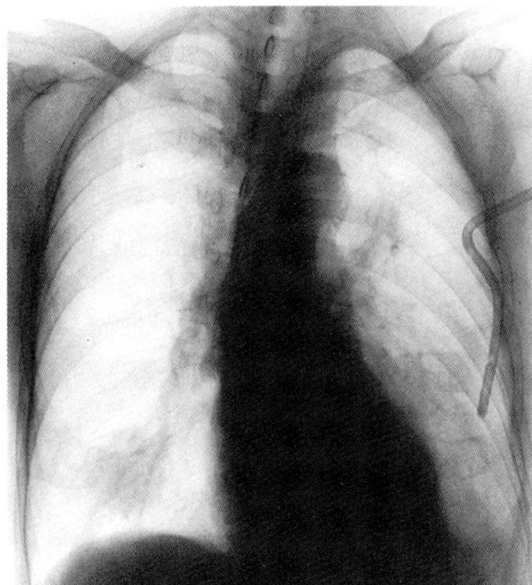

23 Dec. 1969

1228a Mallory-Weiss-Boerhaave syndrome with left pleural fistulisation in patient wearing Levin tube. This cachetic patient was admitted with a metastatic cancer of the rectum. A feeding Levin tube has been in place for several weeks, during which chronic gastro-oesophageal reflux and oesophagitis have weakened the lower oesophagus. The patient suddenly develops a pyopneumothorax and an acute abdomen after vomiting a cup of tea.

1228b Periaortic mediastinal emphysema soon appears. The pyopneumothorax has been aspirated (see **1151b** and Volume I, **490**).

1228c Oesophageal rupture is confirmed by a contrast study, but extensive metastases of the rectal cancer make surgery pointless. Death 3 days later.

1228c

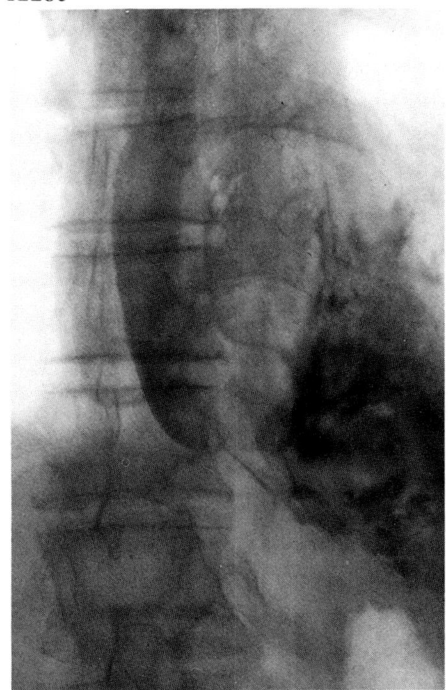

23 Dec. 1969

1229a

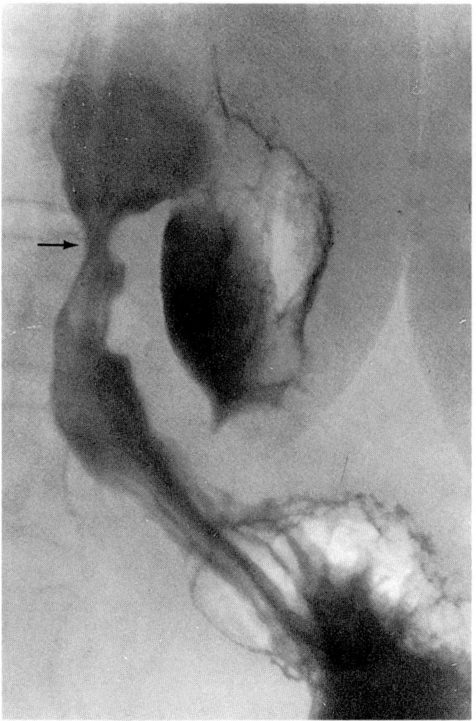

R.M. ♀ 74 yrs. 22 Aug. 1960

1229b

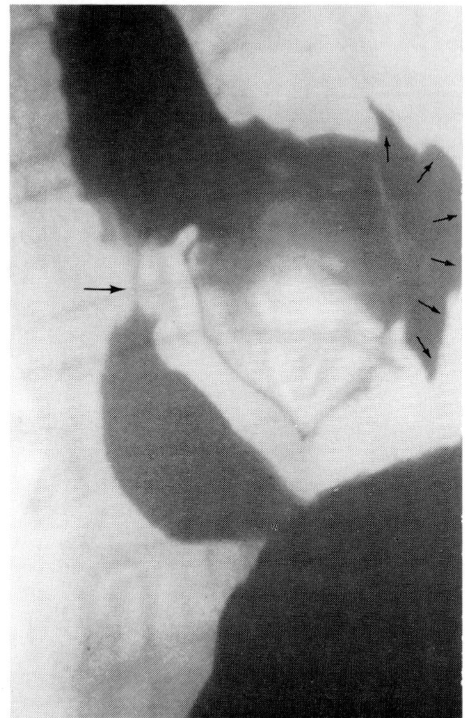

26 Aug. 1960

1229c

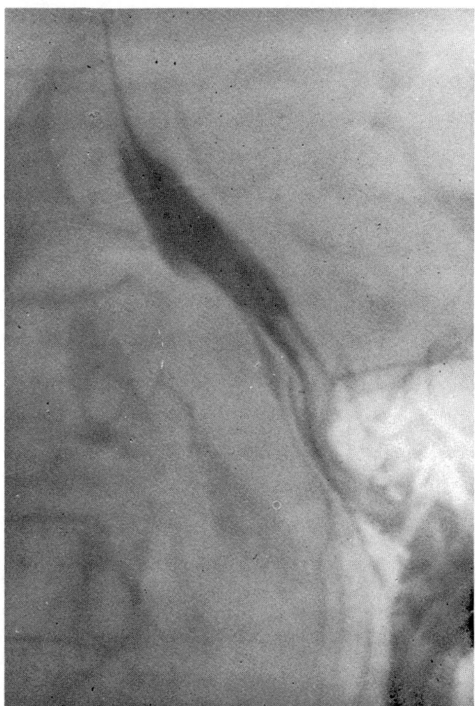

10 Nov. 1965

1229d

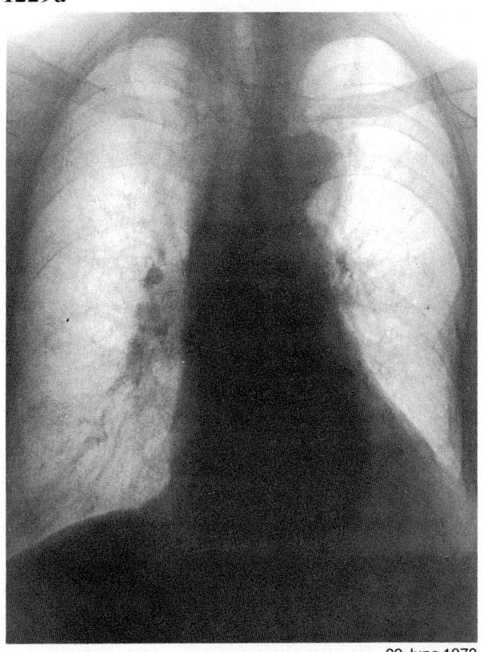

22 June 1972

1129a Rupture of epiphrenic oesophageal diverticulum during vomiting. The X-ray shows an oesophageal diverticulum 7cm above the diaphragm. In addition, the old lady has a hiatal hernia and reflux oesophagitis. The cardia (→) is 4cm above the diaphragm.

1129b The diverticulum gradually ruptures during a series of vomiting episodes; the resultant fistula is soon sealed by surrounding inflammation. Left thoracotomy to resect the diverticulum, cover the oesophagus and repair the hernia.

1129c Smooth postoperative course. Subsequent weight gain of 15kg.

1129d Recovery is well maintained 6½ years later.

1230

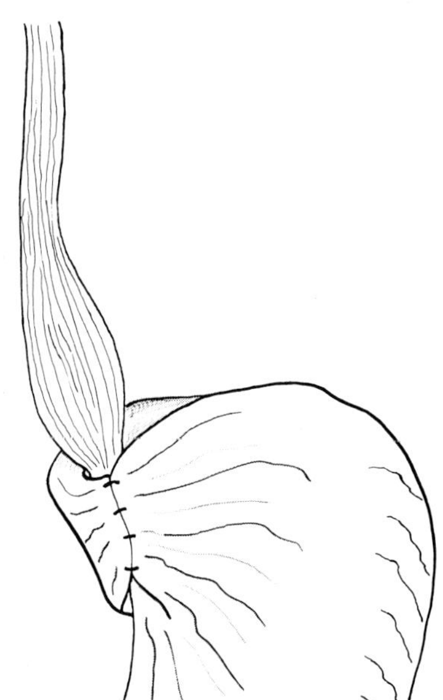

1230 **Fundoplication.**

1231

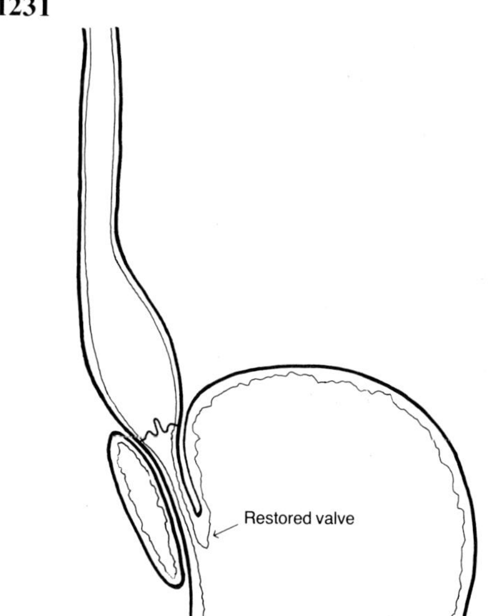

1231 **Cross-section of fundoplication.**

1232

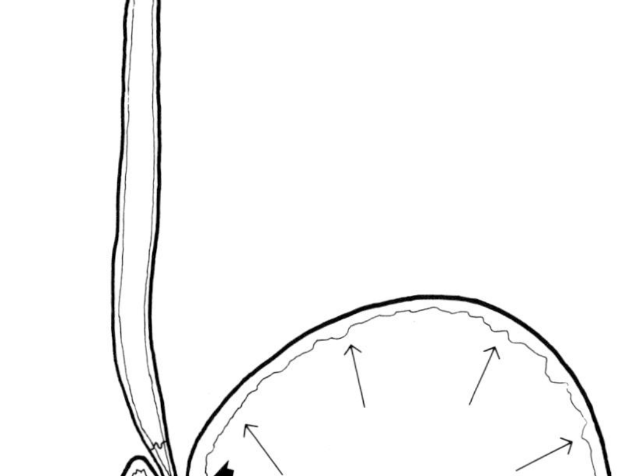

1232 **Acute gastric dilatation after fundoplication.**

1233a

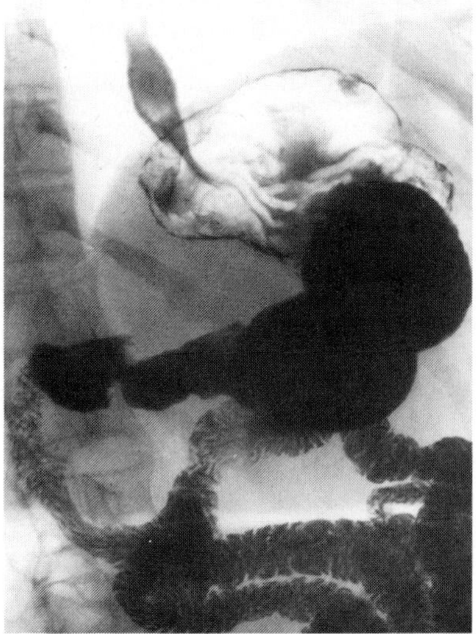

A.M. ♀ 52 yrs. 20 May 1965

1233b

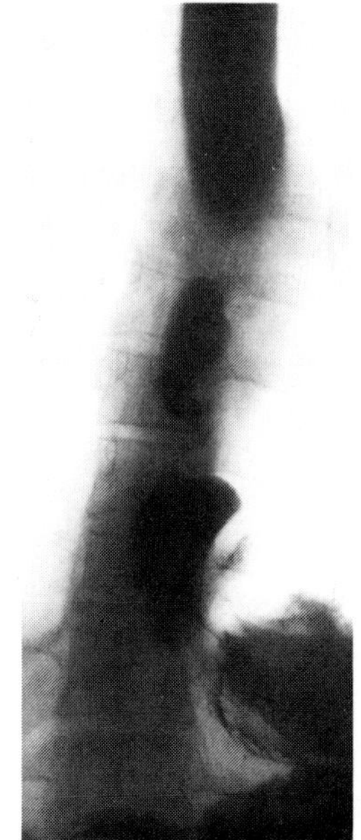

8 Oct. 1966

1233a Attempts at vomiting after fundoplication can result in gastric rupture. The patient has a hiatal hernia and oesophagitis. The stomach is of normal dimension.

1233b The close-up shows the hernia and cardia a few days before surgical restoration of the His angle.

1233c

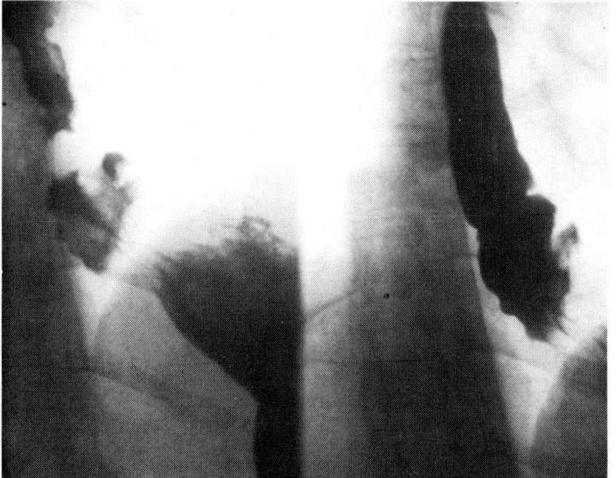

25 Nov. 1966

1233d

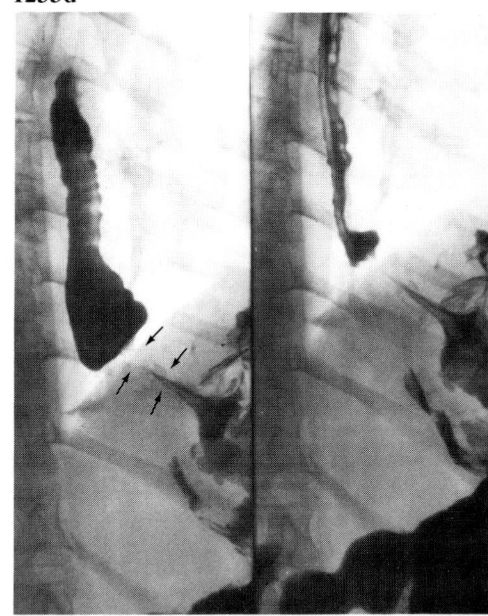

22 Dec. 1966

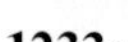

1233e

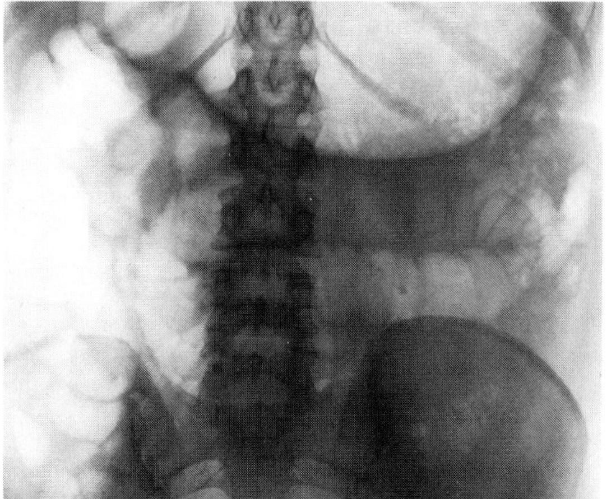

27 Dec. 1966

1233c The hiatal hernia recurs soon after the operation. X-ray shows the shadow of the cardia with significant gastro-oesophageal reflux. Endoscopy reveals severe inflammation of the lower oesophagus. Nissen fundoplication and pyloroplasty are performed.

1233d A barium study taken a few weeks later shows that the wrapping around the lower oesophagus (the anti-reflux valve) is too long and too tight. The oesophagus has healed, but swallowing is difficult.

1233e Sudden, acute dilatation of the stomach after a meal causes intense abdominal pain.

1233f

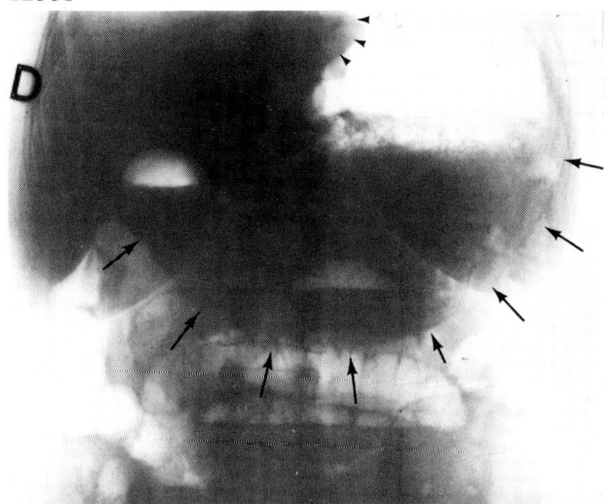

1233f The patient attempts unsuccessfully to vomit. X-ray shows the mass effect of the fundoplication (→), and the gastroduodenal limit (→).

1233g

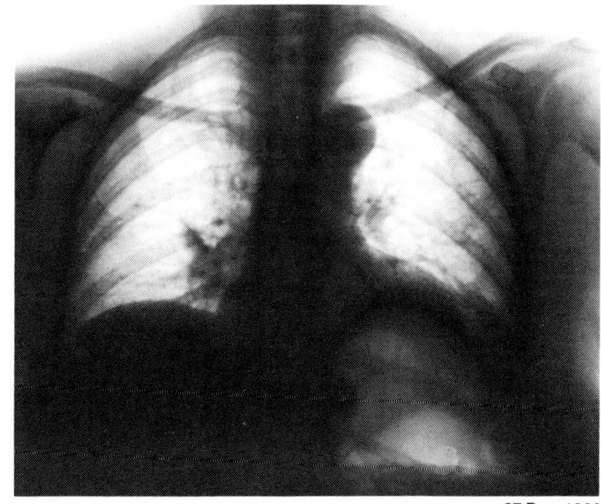

1233g Dilatation increases. Laparotomy reveals a 2 cm posterior rupture of the fundoplication with surrounding necrosis. Repair, covering. Death shortly afterwards.

Mechanism

1234

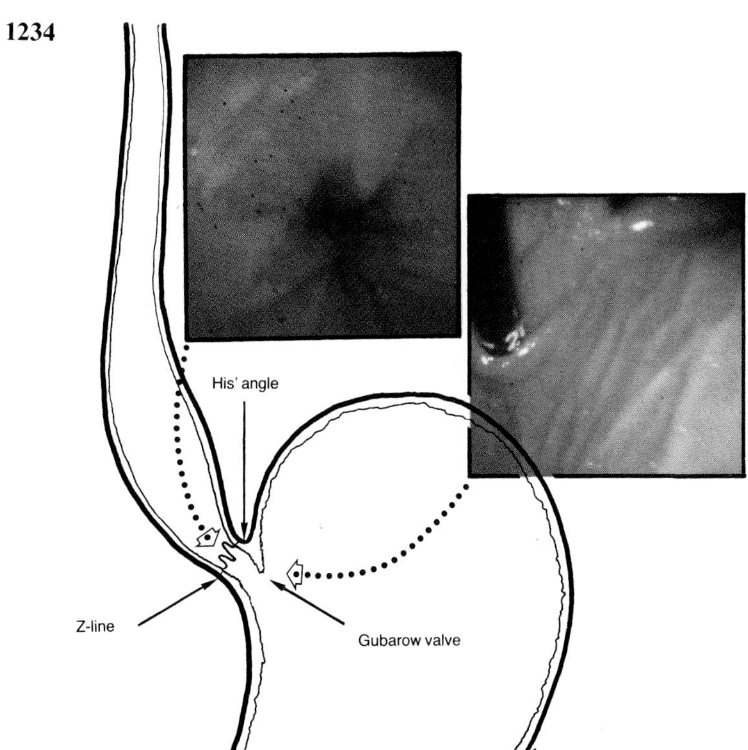

1234 Normal gastro-oesophageal junction.

Vomiting begins with a sudden rise in intra-abdominal pressure that is accentuated when the gastric antrum contracts violently to expel its contents into the oesophagus. This process almost always creates a *gastro-oesophageal mucosal prolapse*.

A fibroscope placed close to the cardia gives a clear view of the retrograde prolapse when the patient retches or vomits. Endo-oesophageal pressure at the time of vomiting (measured through the biopsy canal of the fibroscope) can reach 240 cm of water.

1235

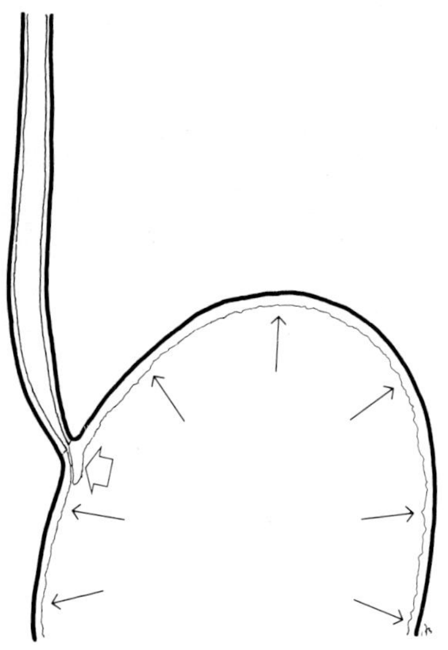

1235 **Acute gastric dilatation.**

Electromyographic studies on the diaphragm of the dog have shown two separate phases in vomiting.

(1) In the preparatory retching phase, the diaphragm and crura contract at the same time as the stomach and abdominal muscles. These brief, rhythmical contractions compress the lower oesophagus. If there is a retrograde prolapse, these contractions can cause a **superficial** intrathoracic **laceration of the gastric mucosa**. The prolapse can be observed endoscopically during retching produced by overinflation of the stomach.

(2) During actual vomiting, the crura relax while the two hemidiaphragms, the abdominal muscles and the gastric antrum all suddenly contract. This relaxation of the crura permits the free herniation of the cardia and upper stomach through the hiatus. The likelihood of a classic Mallory-Weiss-Boerhaave syndrome (**mucosal and then muscular rupture** or vice versa) is greater when vomiting is violent or unco-ordinated, especially if induced.

1236

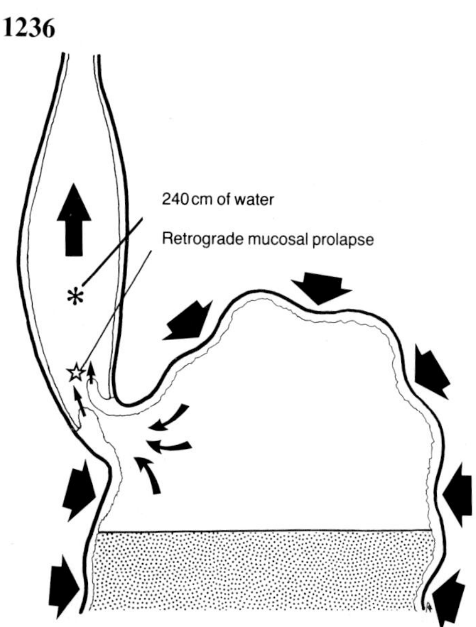

1236 **Vomiting.**

1237 **Small gastro-oesophageal retrograde mucosal prolapse**, observed endoscopically during vomiting. (Dr G. Miller, Soleure.)

1238 **Larger mucosal prolapse** seen after surgery.

1237

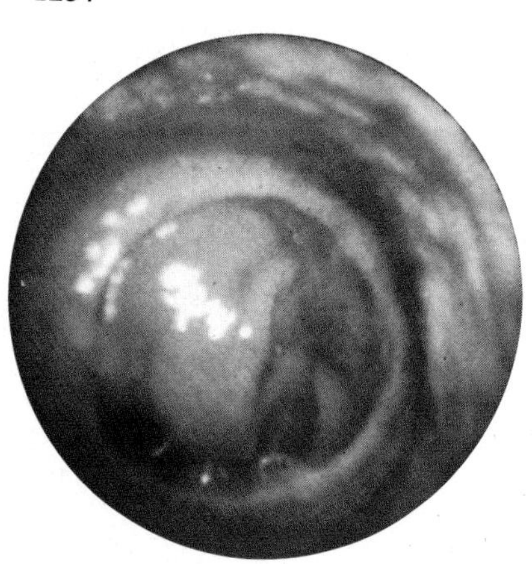

1238

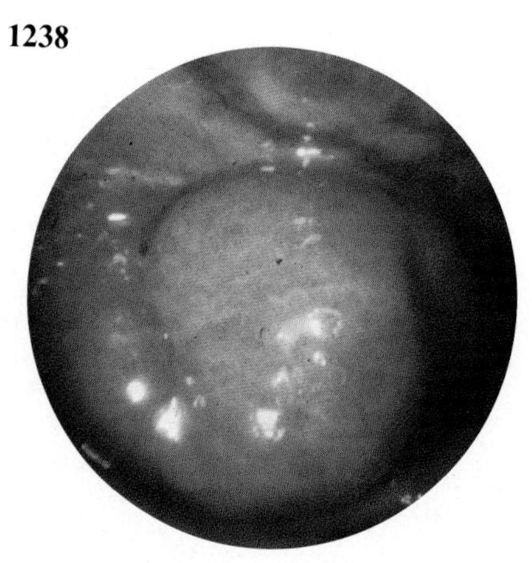

Massive gastro-oesophageal retrograde mucosal prolapse observed fibroscopically during vomiting.

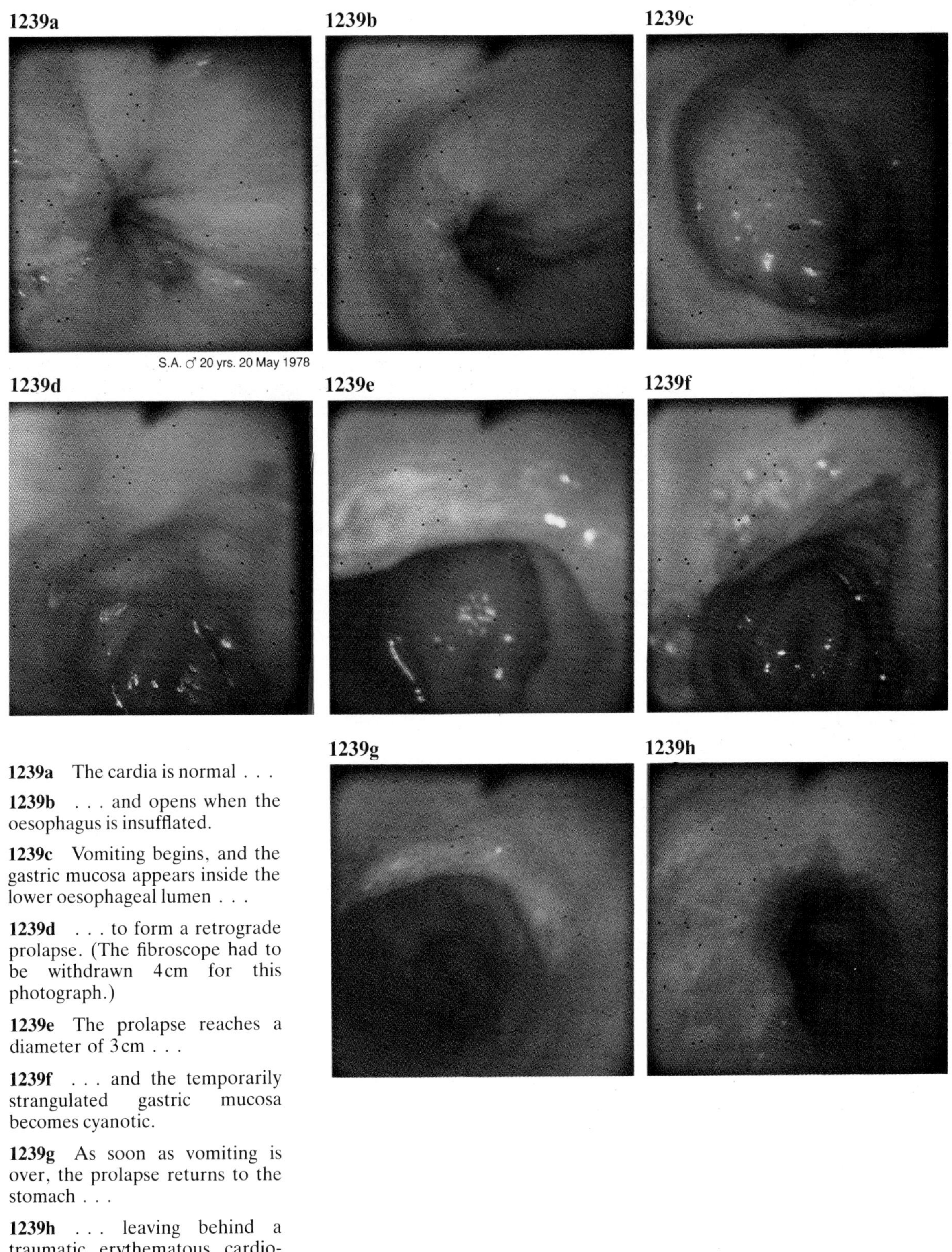

1239a The cardia is normal . . .

1239b . . . and opens when the oesophagus is insufflated.

1239c Vomiting begins, and the gastric mucosa appears inside the lower oesophageal lumen . . .

1239d . . . to form a retrograde prolapse. (The fibroscope had to be withdrawn 4cm for this photograph.)

1239e The prolapse reaches a diameter of 3cm . . .

1239f . . . and the temporarily strangulated gastric mucosa becomes cyanotic.

1239g As soon as vomiting is over, the prolapse returns to the stomach . . .

1239h . . . leaving behind a traumatic erythematous cardio-gastropathy.

1240

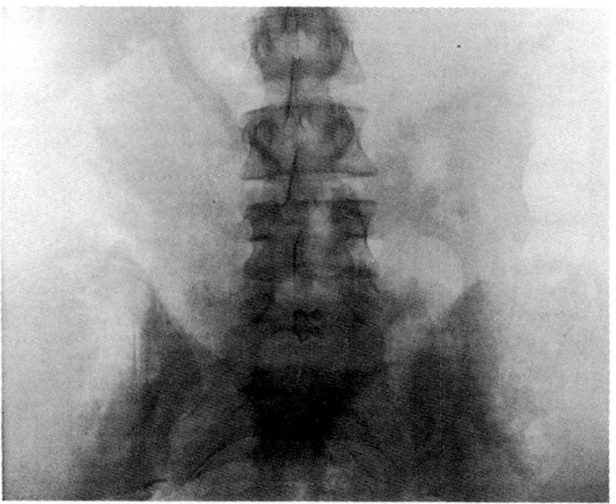

J.M. ♀ 16 yrs. 15 Sep. 1973

1240 Acute gastric dilatation predisposes to violent vomiting and to partial or complete rupture of the lower oesophagus. This patient sustained multiple injuries when knocked down by a lorry. Her stomach dilated when she cried with pain on the way to hospital.

1241

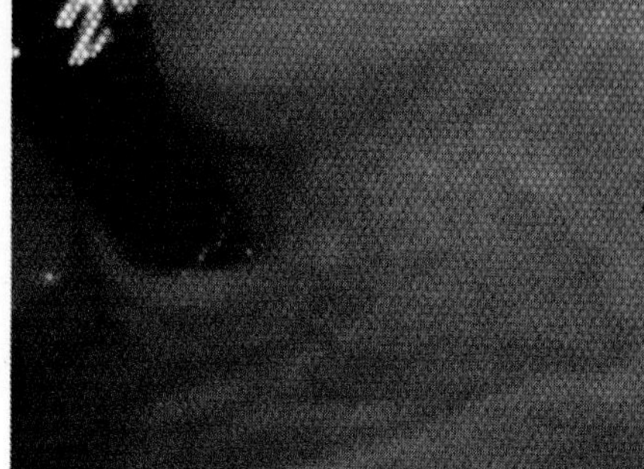

Aug. 1977

1241 Hiatal incompetence by induced gastric dilatation. Inflation of the stomach through an endoscope has forced open the cardia; the result is a small gastric hernia.

After a particularly violent episode of vomiting, the mucosal prolapse can become *incarcerated* above the cardia.

In cases where it returns spontaneously to the stomach after incarceration, histological examination of the prolapsed mucosa often reveals oedema, intramucosal haemorrhage and sometimes also epithelial rupture. Early biopsy usually forestalls inflammation.

Most injuries are located on the gastric wall of the cardia; therefore, they are generally referred to as *cardiogastropathies*.

When vomiting is even more violent, the initial mucosal *laceration* can become a transmural *rupture*.

Finally, the literature also contains reports of *subserous haematomas* due to tears of short splenic vessels.

1242

Emetic injuries.

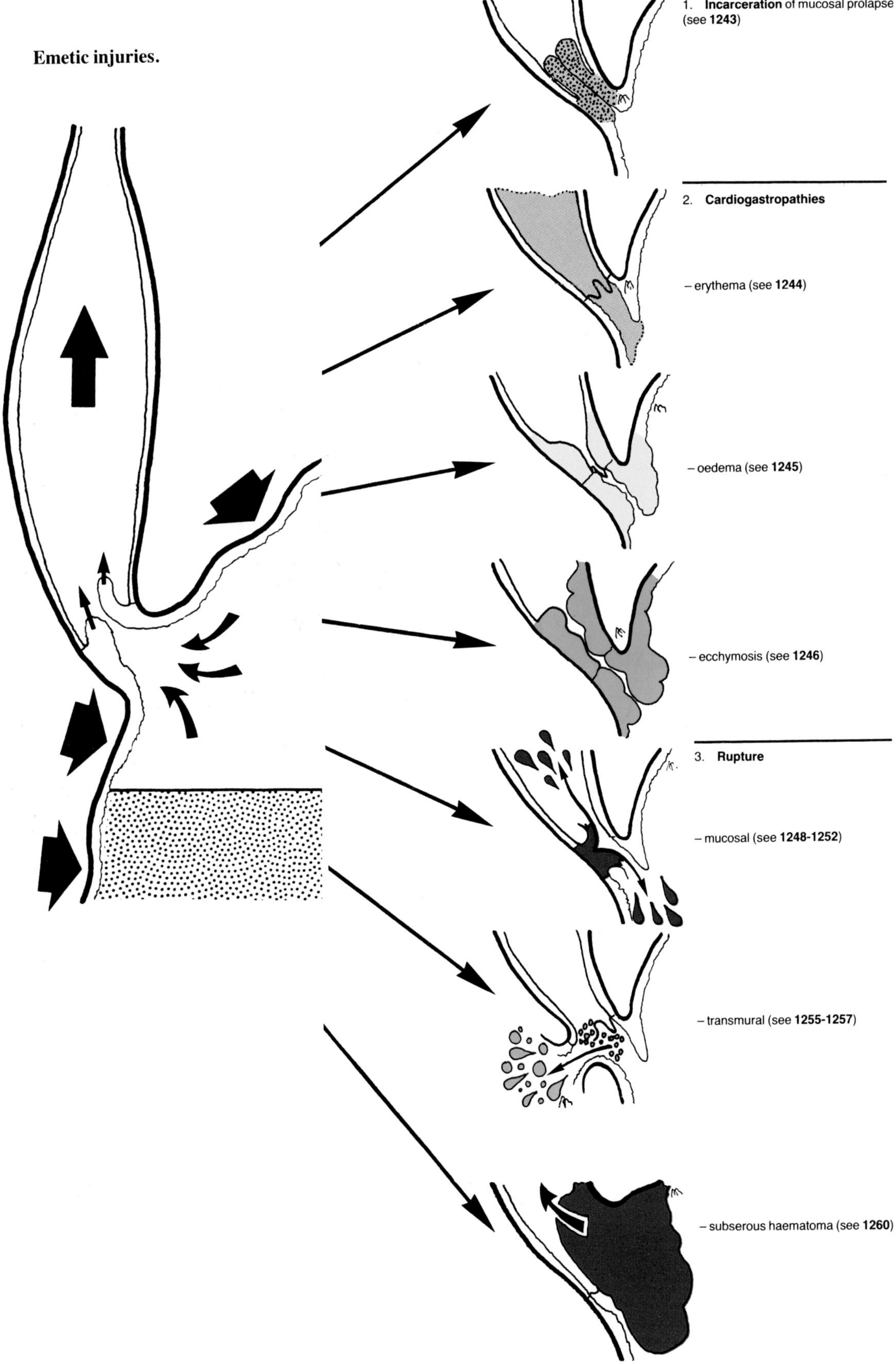

Incarceration of mucosal prolapse

1243

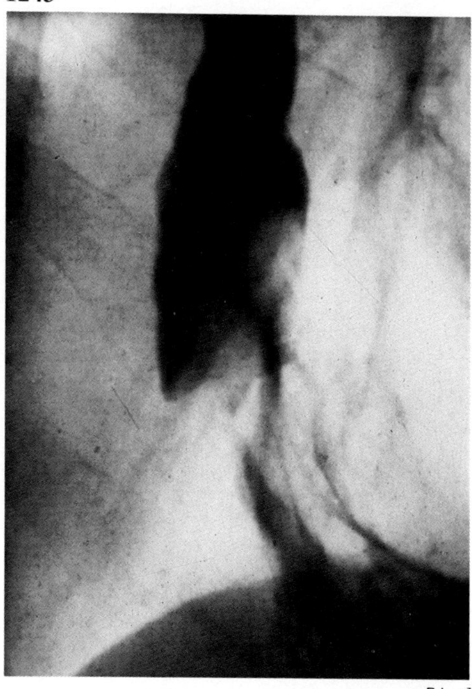

B.L. ♂

1243 X-ray of incarcerated mucosal prolapse.

Postemetic cardiogastropathy

Three different forms of postemetic cardiogastropathy can be distinguished endoscopically:
- erythema,
- oedema,
- ecchymosis.

Ecchymosis can extend upwards, in which case the oesophageal mucosa is dissected by a haematoma; however, this condition is very rare.

1244

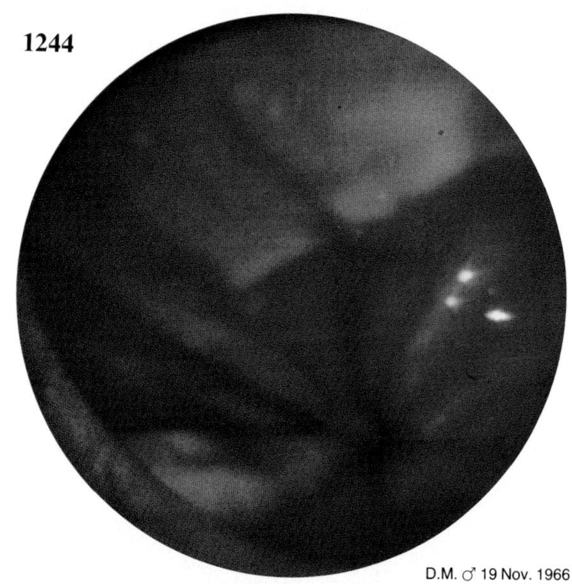

D.M. ♂ 19 Nov. 1966

1244 Postemetic cardiogastropathy: erythema.

1245a

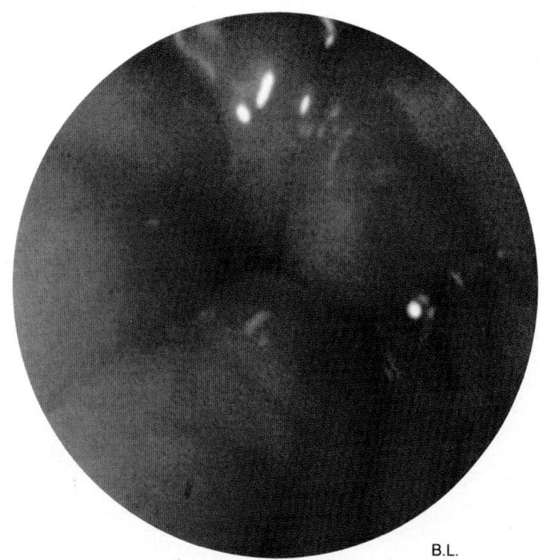

B.L.

1245a Postemetic cardiogastropathy: oedema.

1245b

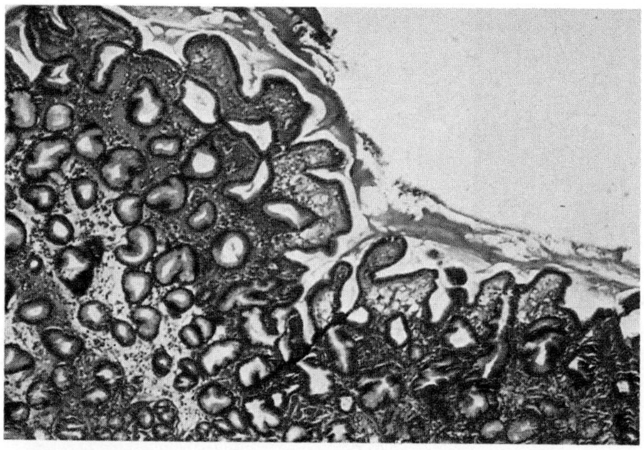

1245b Biopsy reveals significant mucosal oedema, but there is no sign of inflammation.

1246a

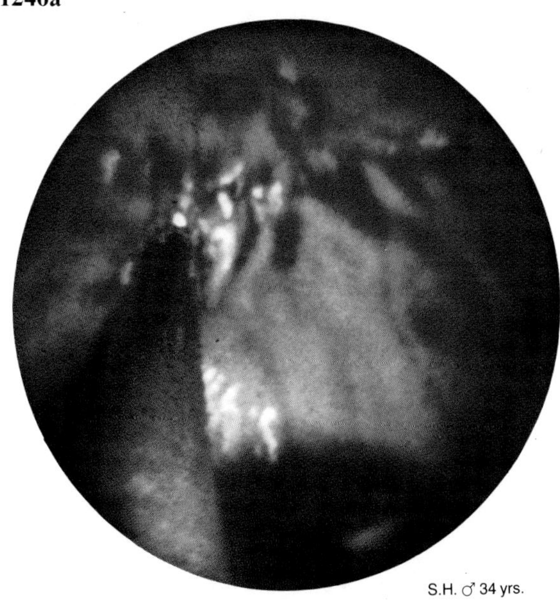

1246b

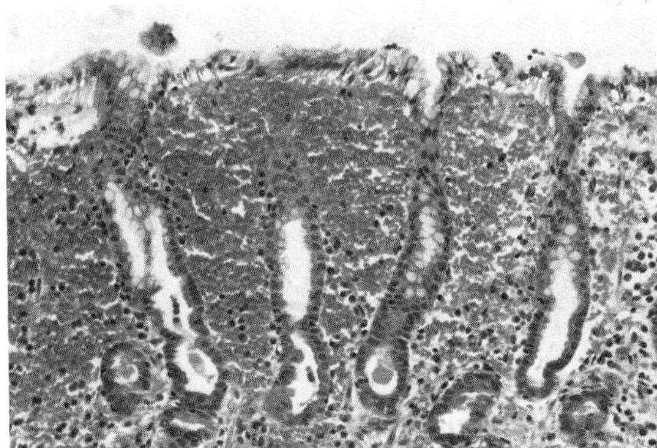

1246a Postemetic cardiogastropathy: ecchymosis. The greater tuberosity is here seen through an inverted fibroscope. (Dr G. Miller, Soleure.)

1246b Biopsy reveals bloody mucosal extravasation, but there is no sign of inflammation.

Mucosal tear

Emetic epithelial laceration of the cardia (first described by Mallory and Weiss in 1929) is produced by the same mechanism as the other traumatic cardiogastropathies already described. The difference is that it is the result of more violent vomiting. The longitudinal tear usually measures several centimetres and is located on the posterior right wall of the gastro-oesophageal junction. Cases of multiple tears (double, triple or star-shaped) are frequent.

The initial signs (haematemesis and/or melena) are sometimes only slight. 5% to 10% of all upper gastro-intestinal haemorrhages are attributable to a Mallory-Weiss syndrome.

The mucosal laceration usually cicatrizes spontaneously in 8 to 10 days; surgical repair is seldom necessary.

The prognosis remains good so long as the initial tear does not subsequently become transmural. Fortunately, this rarely happens.

1247

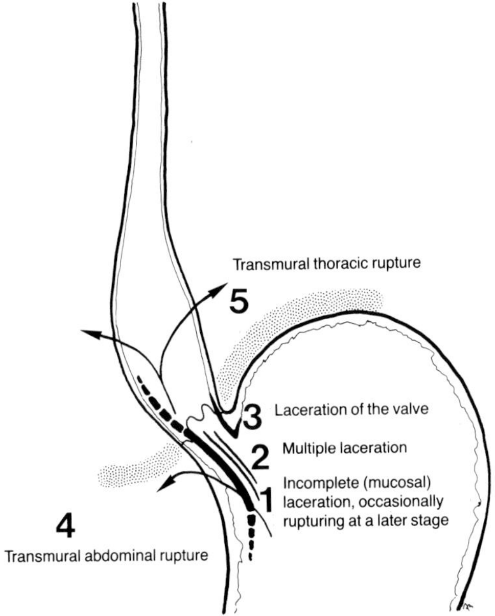

1247 Classic localisations of postemetic gastro-oesophageal laceration (Mallory-Weiss syndrome) (see also **1254**).

1248

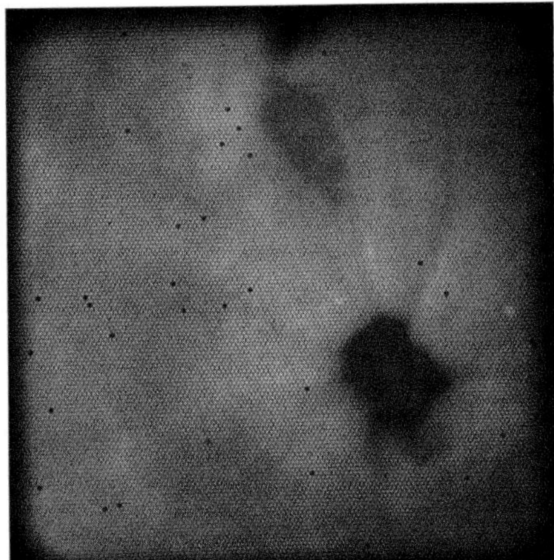

1248 Postemetic laceration of oesophageal mucosa. The laceration of the anterior wall is short and superficial; the cardia and gastric mucosa are intact.

1249a

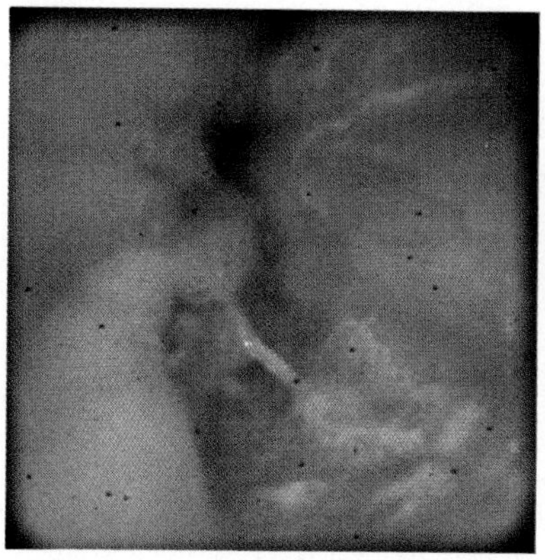

N.Y. ♂ 23 yrs. 31 Dec. 1977

1249b

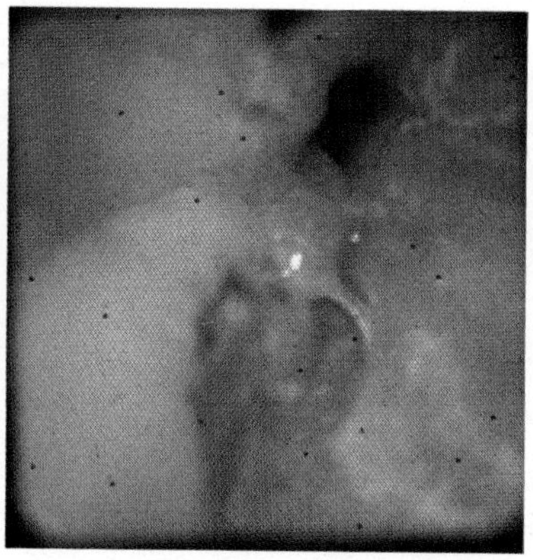

31 Dec. 1977

1249c

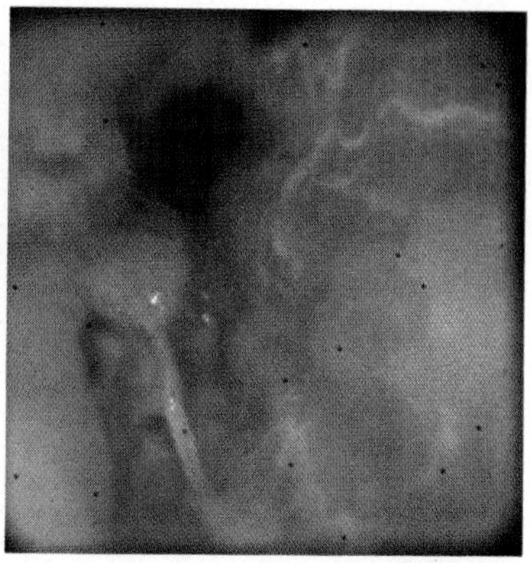

31 Dec. 1977

1249d

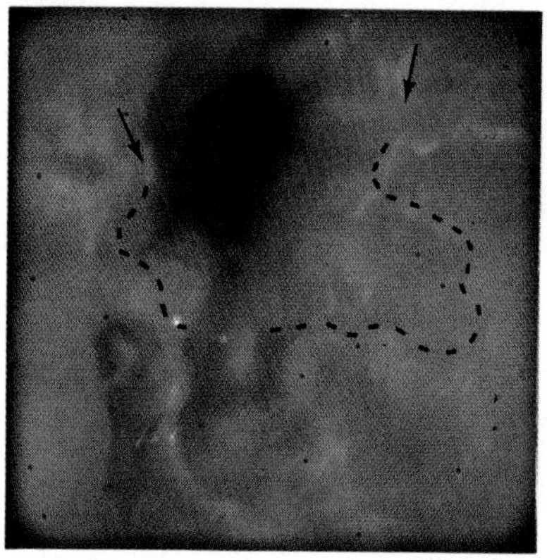

31 Dec. 1977

1249e

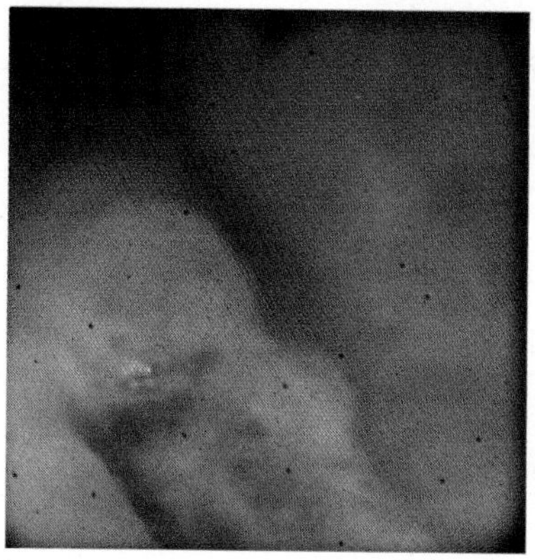

31 Dec. 1977

1249f

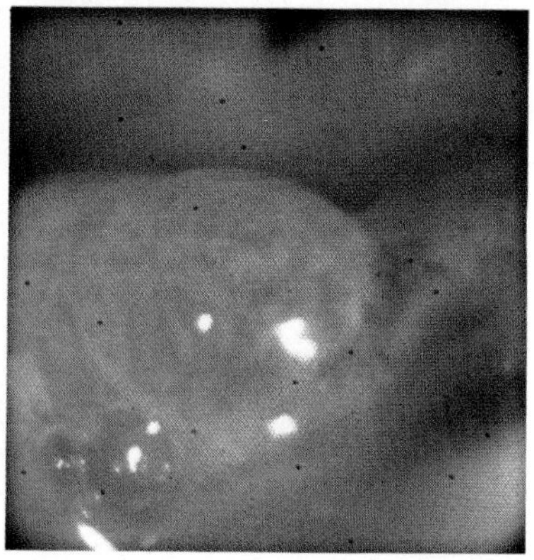

31 Dec. 1977

1249g

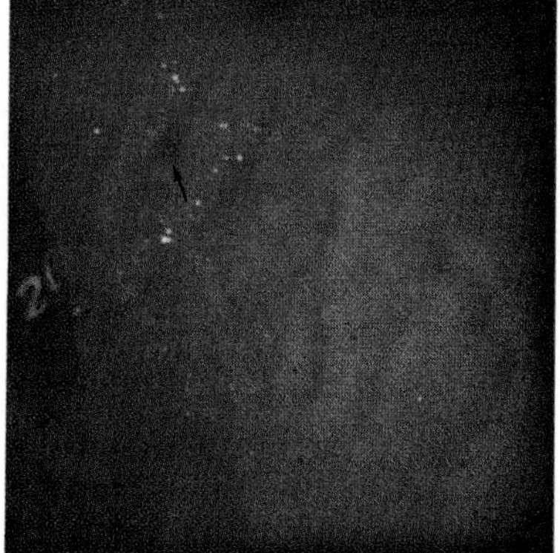

31 Dec. 1977

1249a Mallory-Weiss syndrome: 2nd day fibroscopic study. The patient suffered a single episode of haematemesis (followed by melena) after 2 beers. A longitudinal mucosal laceration of the right posterior wall begins 3.5cm above the cardia.

1249b It is deep (viewed from 3cm above the cardia which is held open by insufflation) . . .

1249c . . . and fibrinous (from 2.5cm above the cardia).

1249d It spans the gastro-oesophageal junction (from 2cm above the cardia).

1249e Its borders are oedematous (from 1.5cm above the cardia) . . .

1249f . . . and so particularly is the gastric edge (close-up view 1cm above the cardia). The lesion could be mistaken for a tumour.

1249g The Gubarow valve is intact but there is a petechia (→) on the greater tuberosity. Conservative treatment. Recovery.

1250a

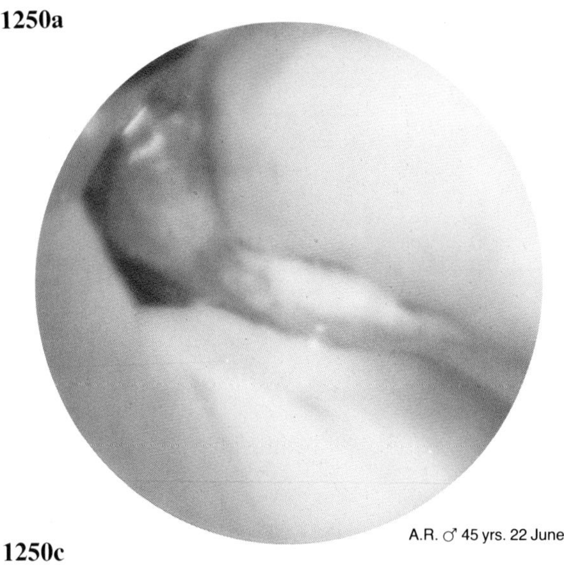

1250b

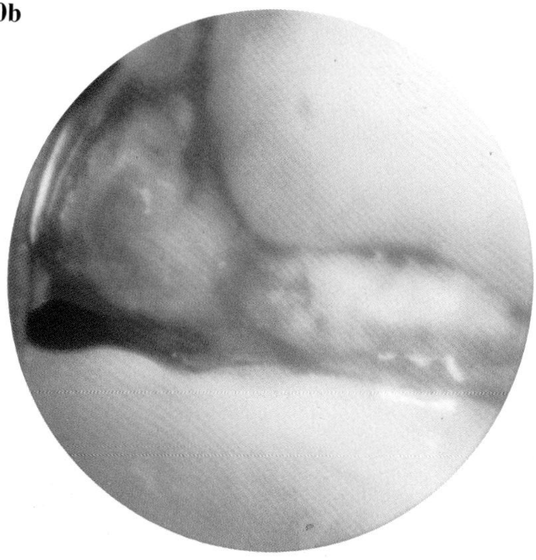

A.R. ♂ 45 yrs. 22 June 1971

1250c

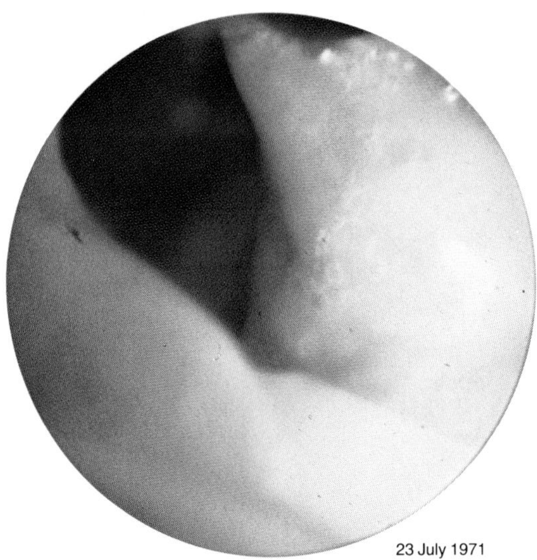

23 July 1971

1250d

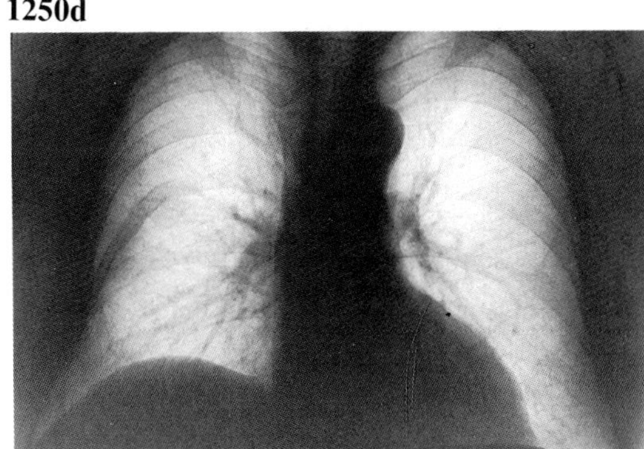

14 Sep. 1977

1250e

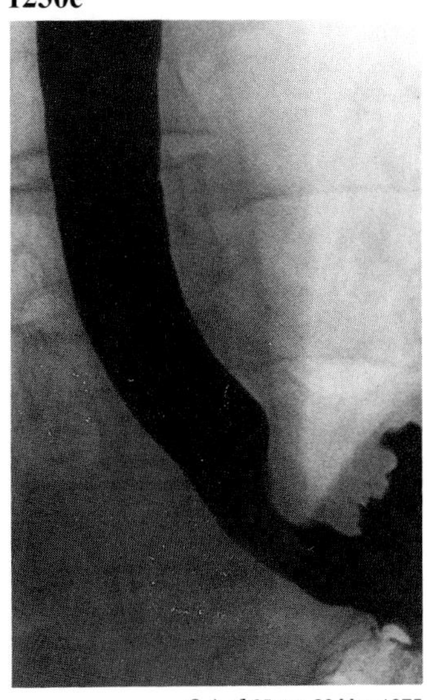

G.J. ♂ 65 yrs. 20 May 1975

1250a/b Mallory-Weiss syndrome: Rigid endoscopy. There is a 3cm longitudinal tear in the right posterior wall of the oesophagus. The tear has caused recurrent episodes of haematemesis aggravated by haemophilia. This study was carried out 4 days after the last episode of haematemesis. Conservative treatment.

1250c A month later, a second rigid endoscopic examination shows the mucosa fully healed. However, in the course of this examination the upper oesophagus is perforated against an osteophyte. The perforation is repaired through a cervical incision. A right thoracotomy and a laparatotomy are needed later for a stress ulcer (vagotomy and pyloroplasty followed by fundoplication). Recovery.

1250d/e No oesophageal or thoracic sequelae 6 years later.

1251

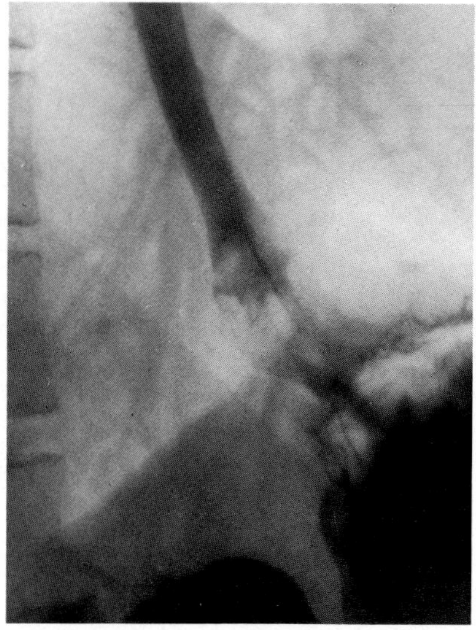

1252

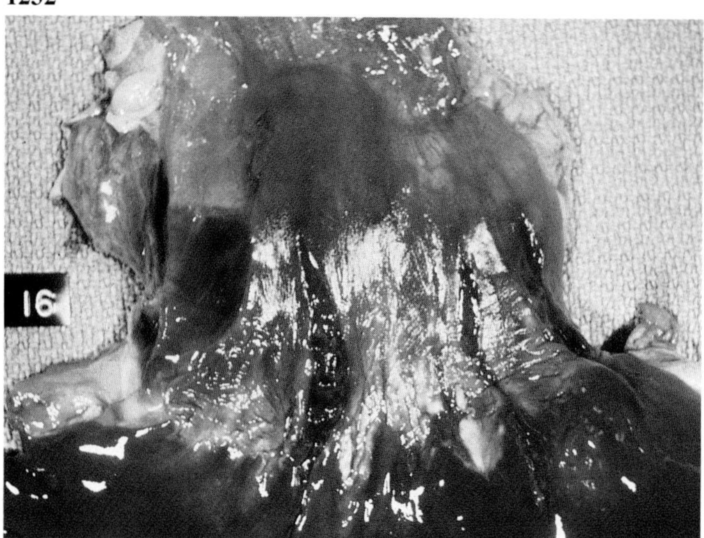

1251 Mallory-Weiss-Boerhaave syndrome: 3rd day barium study. A 4cm mucosal laceration of the right oesophageal wall and lesser gastric curvature is the result of self-induced vomiting. The mucosal folds of the cardia are oedematous. The patient describes a fierce burning sensation on swallowing ('like swallowing molten lead'). On admission, he is even regurgitating his saliva. On the 8th day, the laceration extends to the right pleural cavity (see **1256**).

1252 Mallory-Weiss syndrome. (Operative specimen.) Multiple mucosal tears span the Z-line. (Prof. M.O. Cantor, Bloomfield Hills, Michigan.)

Rupture

So-called 'spontaneous rupture' of the oesophagus was first described in 1724. The accepted mechanism is as follows: traumatising vomiting causes a muscular tear through which the mucosa herniates and then bursts. This injury usually occurs in the lower left wall of the oesophagus where it has no support from adjacent organs. The other main site (chiefly in patients who try to stifle vomiting) is higher on the right, just below the azygos vein.

Retrograde prolapse of the gastro-oesophageal mucosa probably also plays its part in the mechanism of the lower rupture. A patient may display epithelial tears of the cardia (as described by Mallory-Weiss), allied to a contiguous transmural rupture of the lower oesophagus (see **1256**).

An oesophageal rupture which extends immediately to the pleural cavity is characterised by excruciating pain, particularly on swallowing. Mediastinitis and pleural effusion (to the left in 50% of cases, and to the right in 20% of cases) soon follow.

The prognosis of oesophageal rupture is poor; mortality is about 70%.

With rare exceptions, an untreated rupture is fatal within 48 hours.

1253

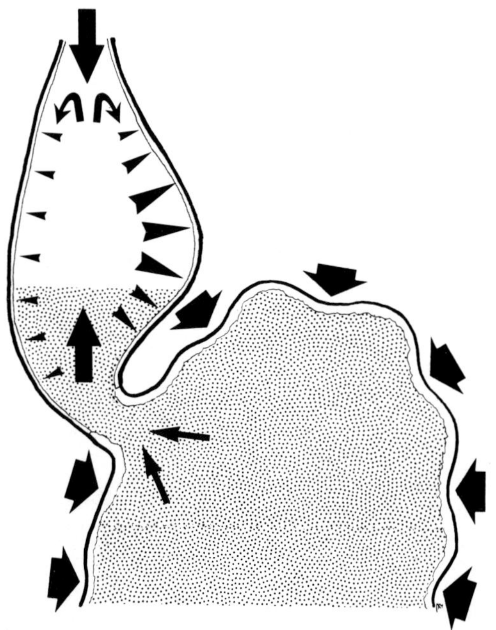

1253 Stifled vomiting (by a closed Killian's mouth, or by simultaneous swallowing).

1254

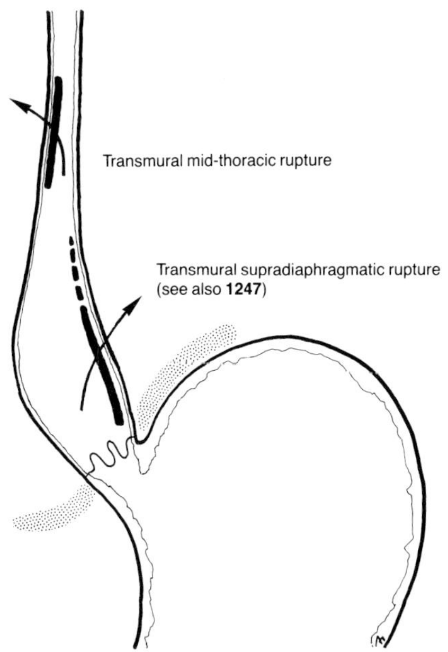

1254 Classic localisation of spontaneous post-emetic oesophageal rupture (Boerhaave syndrome).

1255a

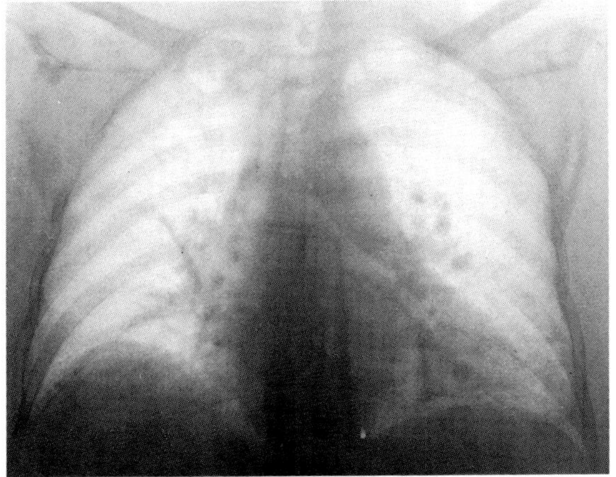
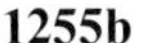

R.A. ♀ 55 yrs. 21 Oct. 1966

1255a Mallory-Weiss syndrome with peritoneal fistulisation. A massively obese patient weighing 147 kg (Broca index, 2.29) vomited violently after a lavish meal causing a 7 cm longitudinal transmural tear of the right wall of the cardia. Food erupted into the peritoneum. The mediastinum remained free of emphysema. Laparotomy, direct repair. Recovery.

1255b

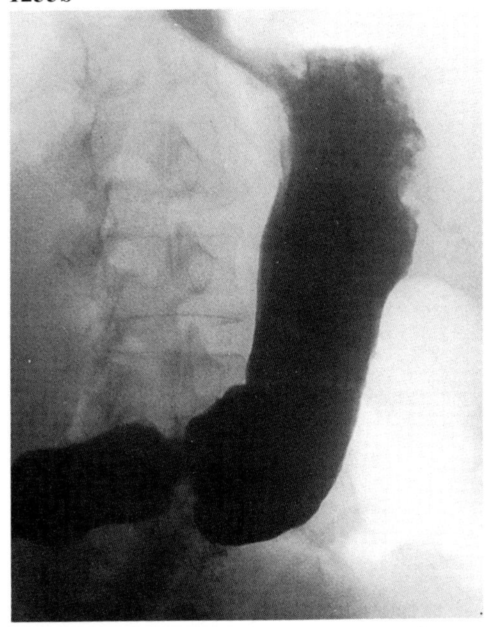

30 Oct. 1967

1255b Barium study one year later.

1256a

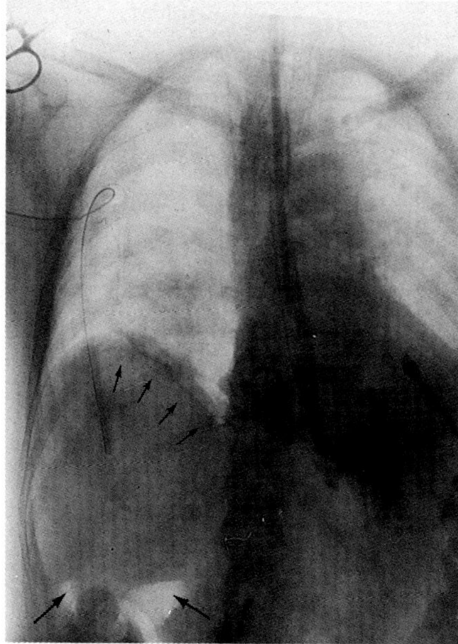

G.J. ♂ 55 yrs. 25 May 1975 16 hrs.

1256b

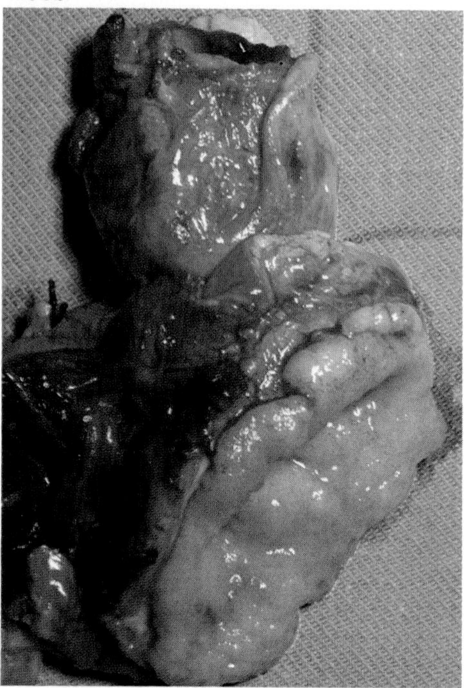

25 May 1975

1256c

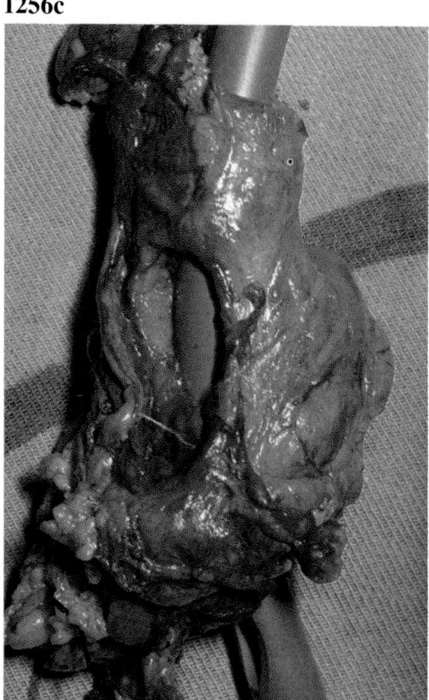

25 May 1975

1256d

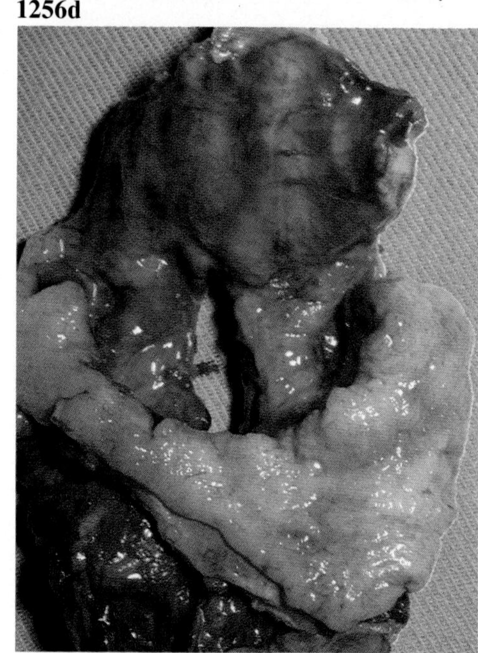

25 May 1975

1256a Unrecognised Mallory-Weiss syndrome with late right pleural fistulisation (see also **1159, 1251**). Gastro-oesophageal rupture was diagnosed fibroscopically 9 days after a traumatising episode of vomiting. The diagnosis is here confirmed by extravasation of hydrosoluble contrast material into the drained right pleural cavity (→). Note also a subhepatic pneumoperitoneum (**→**) due to perforation of a pre-existing duodenal ulcer, likewise undetected.

1256b Emergency laparotomy and right thoracotomy for excision of the damaged portion of the gastro-oesophageal junction.

1256c The transmural rupture is at the level of the diaphragmatic hiatus; it extends from the right oesophageal wall to the lesser gastric curvature. A tube has been introduced into the gastro-oesophageal lumen.

1256d Seen from within, the rupture measures 4 cm. The oesophageal mucosa and contiguous tissues have been partly digested by gastric juice.

Death from dehiscence of the gastro-oesophageal anastomosis 14 days after the operation.

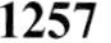

1257

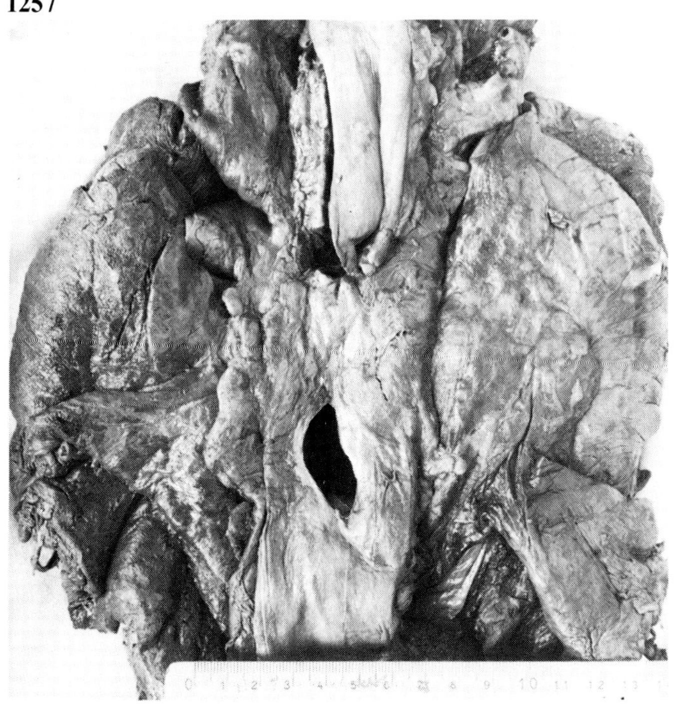

F.M. ♀ 80 yrs. 11 Dec. 1961

1257 Spontaneous rupture of oesophagus. The senile patient died 8 hours after admission and 36 hours after being overcome by sudden and unexplained weakness. Autopsy revealed a 4 cm vertical laceration of the oesophagus 15 cm below Killian's mouth and 5 cm above the cardia (for X-rays, see Volume I, **491**). Since no vomiting was noticed by members of the family, death may have been due to rupture of a retrocardial peptic ulcer. The oesophagus, however, was not inflamed.

1258a

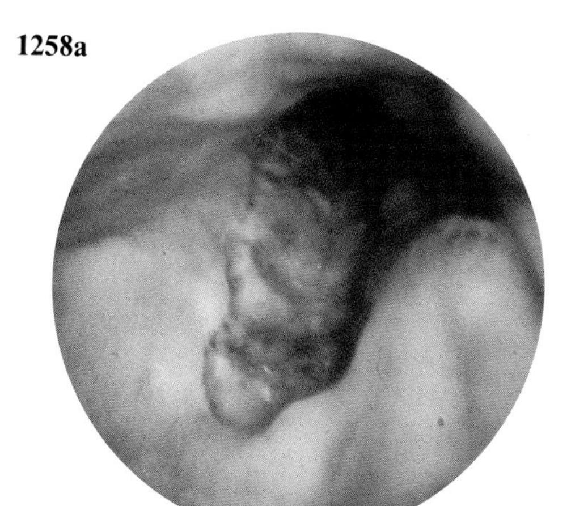

S.J. ♀ 71 yrs. 29 Mar. 1974

1258b

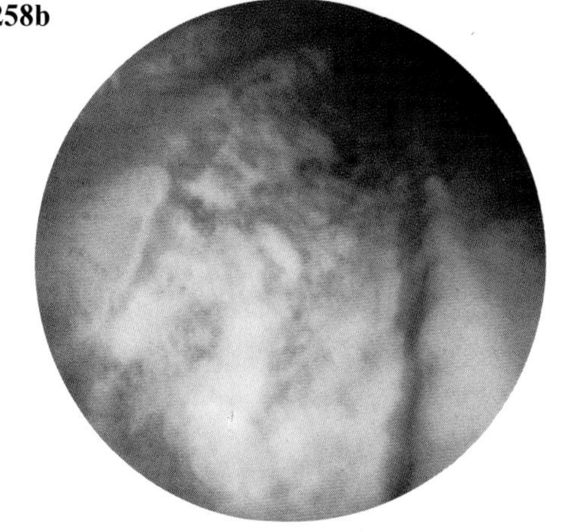

1258c

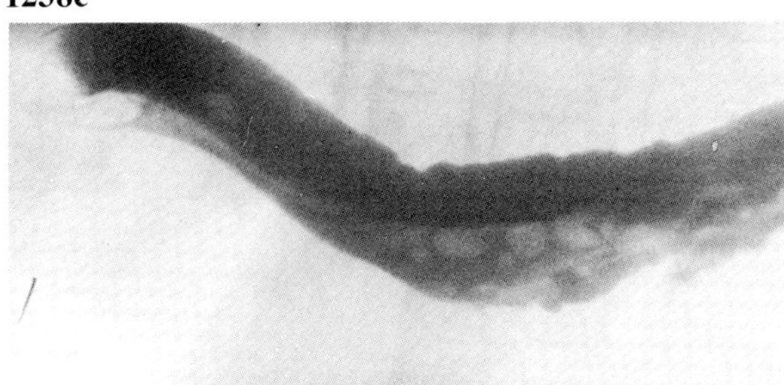

1258d

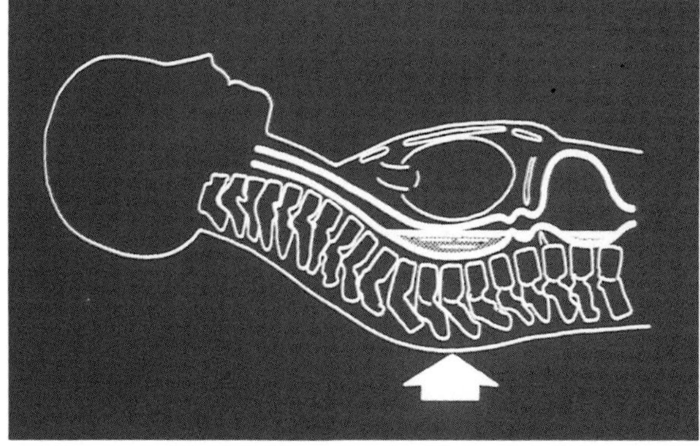

1258a/b Endoscopic view of oesophageal peptic ulcer in old kyphoscoliotic woman. Ulcers of this type can rupture into the pleural cavity.

1258c X-ray.

1258d Mechanism: massive ulceration of this type is caused by chronic oesophageal reflux through an incompetent cardial junction. In an aged bed-ridden patient, gastric juice stagnates in the lowest section of the oesophagus and creates a longitudinal retrocardiac ulcer on the rear oesophageal wall.

Intramural haematoma

In rare cases, particularly in the presence of a hiatal hernia, vomiting can push the stomach so far into the chest that the short splenic vessels are torn off the greater tuberosity. The result is an often massive intramural gastro-oesophageal haematoma.

Similarly, the victim of a high-speed car accident can sustain a blow to the abdomen (usually on the steering wheel) that is sufficiently violent to cause a seromuscular tear of the oesophagus, and so create an (often large) extramucosal haematoma. This eventuality is likewise rare.

1259

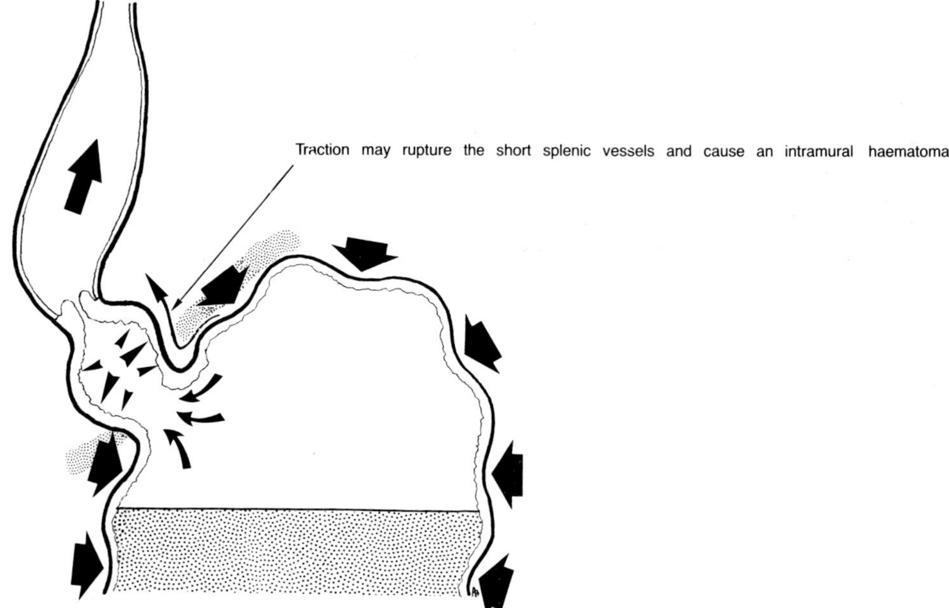

1259 Vomiting in presence of hiatal hernia (or vomiting with temporary herniation).

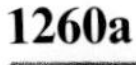

1260a

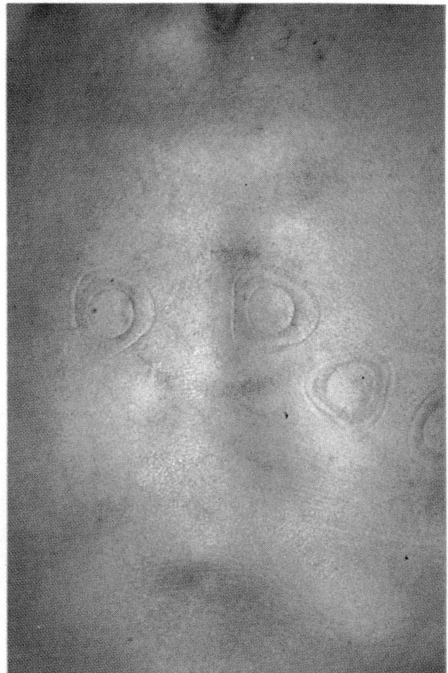

1260b

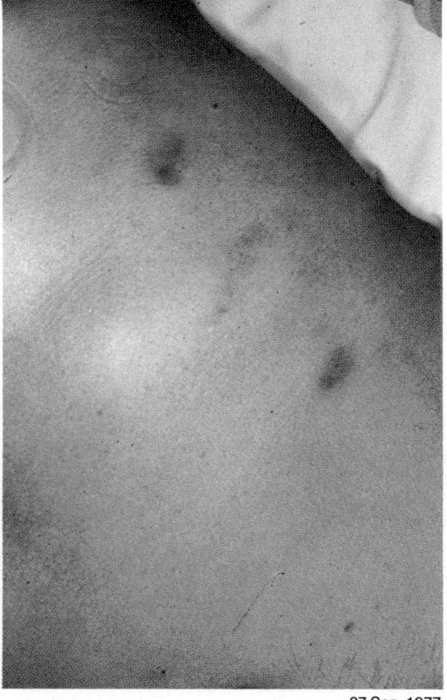

1260a Intramural gastro-oesophageal rupture after blunt chest impact. The presternal imprint of the boss of the steering wheel after a high-speed impact which also resulted in traumatic blindness and a partial scalp. (Ignore ECG leads marking.)

1260b The imprint of the lower half of the steering wheel extends along the left costal margin. The impact caused a splenic rupture and a 10 cm gastro-oesophageal laceration with an intramural haematoma of some 300 ml. Laparotomy, splenectomy and evacuation of the haematoma. Death from liver failure on the 10th day.

Oesophageal injury from external chest trauma

Cervicothoracic trauma (whether open or closed) exceptionally affects the oesophagus, which is protected by its anatomical situation and its suppleness.

In some countries, **penetrating or perforating wounds** of the chest (see Volume I, chapter 3), whether by a bullet, by some other projectile or by a knife, are the most frequent causes of oesophageal injury. In more pacific countries, such injuries are very rare (0.6% of chest trauma cases, in our experience). Wounds of the oesophagus quite often are detected only at surgery. The prognosis is poor, principally because the spinal cord, heart and great vessels are often damaged at the same time.

Injuries by **blunt trauma** are no more frequent. Blunt injury of the oesophagus implies violent deceleration and is often allied to other life-threatening damage. This explains (1) *the frequence and gravity of the injuries associated* with blunt oesophageal injuries (injuries to the trachea, lungs, large vessels, heart, spinal cord and liver); (2) *the poor prognosis* of these injuries (63% mortality within 10 days of admission); (3) the fact that *death* is more often *attributable to the associated injuries* than to the oesophageal injury; (4) the *difficulty of diagnosing the oesophageal injury*. (It is generally only noticed during surgery performed for another reason, or at autopsy). Indeed, in a complex clinical situation, signs of oesophageal perforation attract little attention; cervicomediastinal emphysema and/or pneumothorax, for instance, are attributable usually to concomitant respiratory injuries.

1261

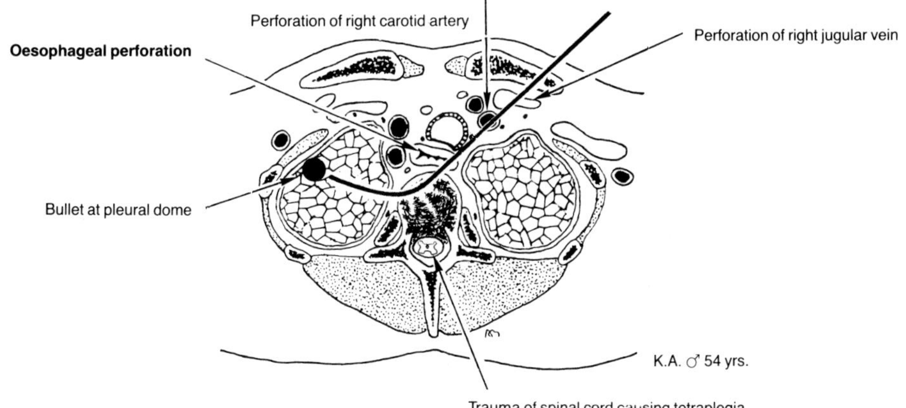

1261 Open wounds of the oesophagus always entail other serious injuries. Path of a middle velocity bullet in the cervicothoracic region, as seen from above (for X-ray, see Volume I, **256**).

1262

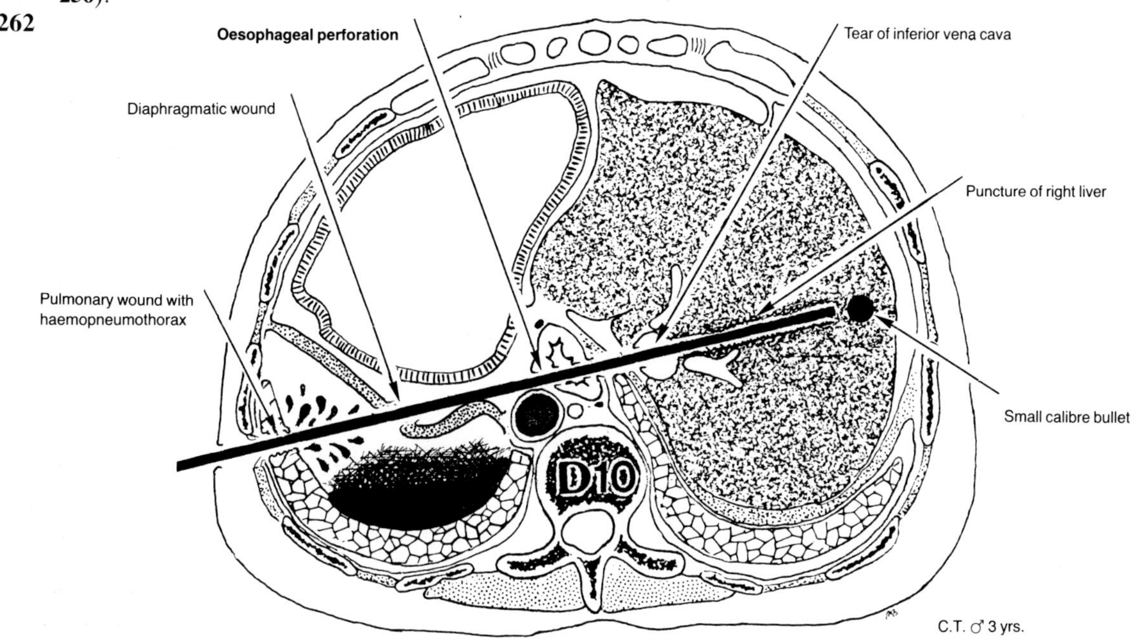

1262 Path of a low velocity .22" L.R. bullet through the abdominal oesophagus of a child, as seen from above (for X-ray, see **1135**).

1263a

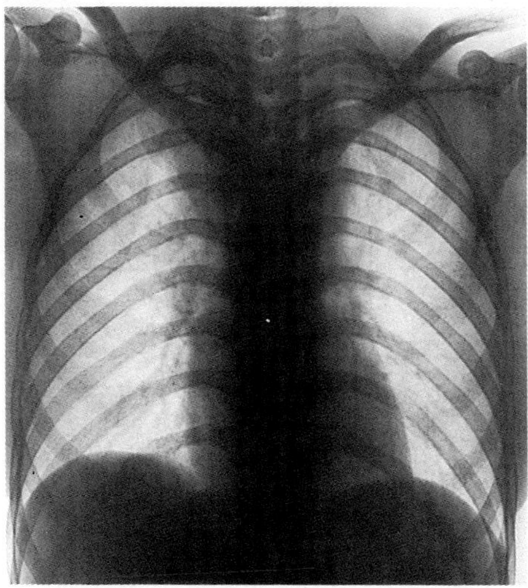

F.J. ♀ 26 yrs. 19 May 1968

1263b

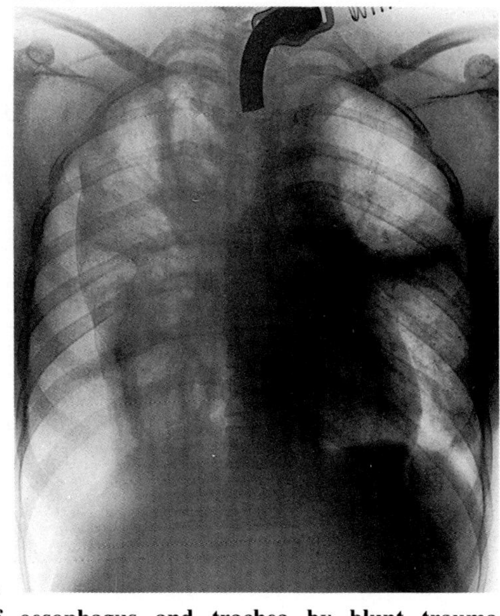

22 May 1968

1263c

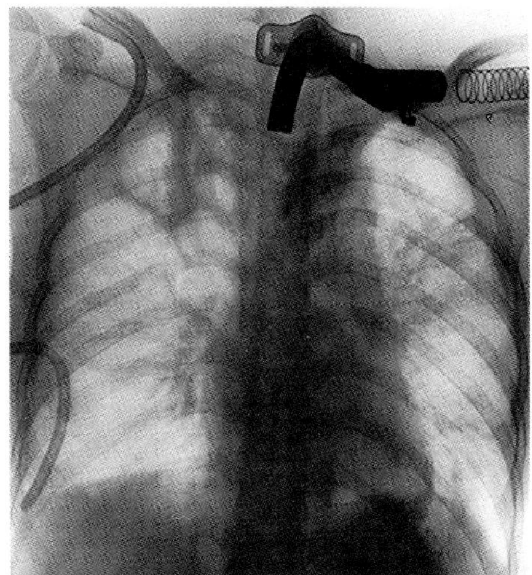

22 May 1968

1263a Rupture of oesophagus and trachea by blunt trauma sustained in a head-on car crash (front right passenger). The tracheo-oesophageal injury is not immediately recognised.

1263b The tracheal rupture is discovered during a tracheostomy performed for respiratory insufficiency. Shortly thereafter, a compressive right pneumothorax appears with inversion of the right hemidiaphragm.

1263c The right pleural cavity is drained; patient is put under controlled ventilation. Air continues to leak into the right pleural cavity.

1263d On the 5th day, extravasation of contrast material (→) shows that the upper oesophagus has ruptured into the right pleural cavity.

1263e Right thoracotomy: methylene blue flows through a 2cm oesophageal laceration surrounded by a mediastinal abscess. Repair, drainage. The tracheostomy tube erodes the innominate artery 5 days later. Massive haemorrhage. Repair is attempted. Death.

1263d

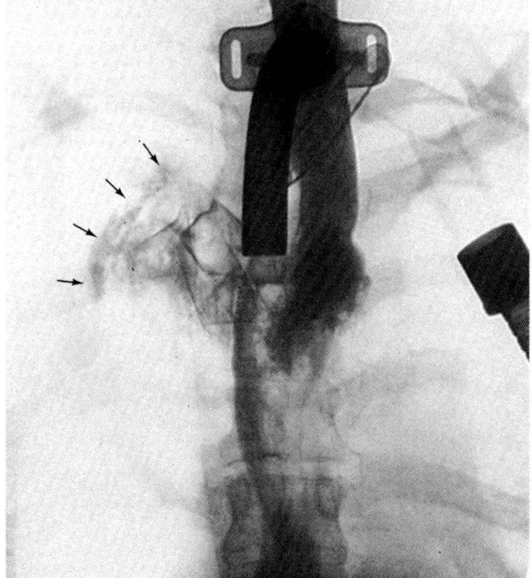

24 May 1968

1263e

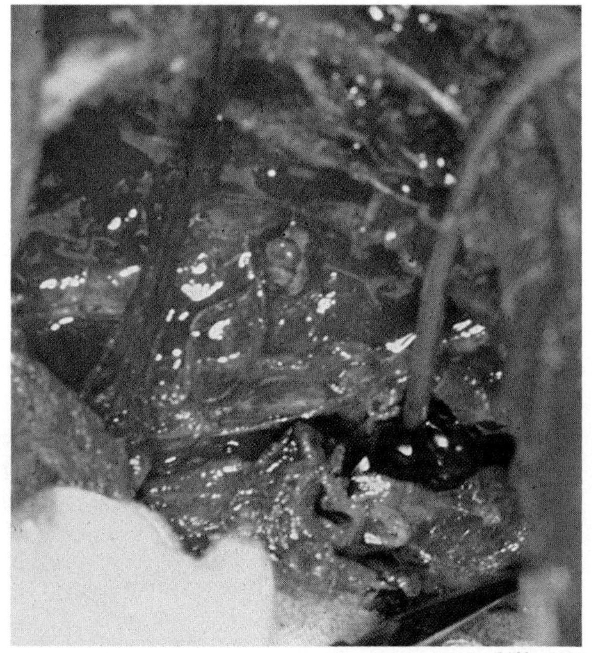

24 May 1968

Bibliography

Chapter 7: Trauma of the trachea and major bronchi

Botta, Y. and Meyer, R. (1978). Reconstruction expérimentale de la trachée par microchirurgie. *Praxis* **67**, 1588–1592.

Grover, F.L., Ellestad, C., Arom, K.V., Root, H.D., Cruz, A.B. and Trinkle, J.K. (1979). Diagnosis and management of major tracheobronchial injuries. *Ann. Thorac. Surg.* **28**, 384–391.

Orringer, M.B. and Sloan, H. (1980). Anterior mediastinal tracheostomy. Indications, techniques, and clinical experience. *J. Thorac. Cardiovasc. Surg.* **78**, 850–859.

Orringer, M.B. (1980). Endotracheal intubation and tracheostomy. Indications, techniques, and complications. *Surg. Clin. North Amer.* **60**, 1447–1464.

Pecora, D.V. and Seinige, U. (1982). Prolonged endotracheal intubation. *Chest* **82**, 130.

Taryle, D.A., Chandler, J.E., Good, J.T. Jr., Potts, D.E. and Sahn, S.A. (1979). Emergency room intubations – complications and survival. *Chest* **75**, 541–543.

Wiot, J.F. (1983). Tracheobronchial trauma. *Semin. Roentgenol.* **18**, 15–22.

a. Inhalation trauma

Agee, R.N., Long, J.M. III, Hunt, J.L., Petroff, P.A., Lull, R.J., Mason, A.D. Jr. and Pruitt, B.A. Jr. (1976). Use of 133Xenon in early diagnosis of inhalation injury. *J. Trauma* **16**, 218–224.

Bose, P. and El Mikatti, N. (1981). Foreign bodies in the respiratory tract. A review of forty-one cases. *Ann. Roy. Coll. Surg. of Eng.* **63**, 129–131.

Chu, C.-S. (1981). New concepts of pulmonary burn injury. *J. Trauma* **21**, 958–961.

Dudgeon, D.L., Parker, F.B., Frittelli, G. and Rabuzzi, D.D. (1980). Bronchiectasis in pediatric patients resulting from aspirated grass inflorescences. *Arch. Surg.* **115**, 979–983.

Essomba, R. and Nguimbous, J.F. (1982). La chirurgie des corps étrangers trachéo-bronchiques chez le nourris-son et l'enfant. A propos de six observations. *Ann. Chir. Thorac. Cardiovasc.* **36**, 126–128.

Getzen, L.C. and Pollak, E.W. (1981). Fatal respiratory distress in burned patients. *Surg. Gynec. Obstet.* **152**, 741–744.

Haury, J.-A. and Savary, M. (1978). Broncho-aspirations de corps étrangers chez l'enfant. *Méd. et Hyg.* **36**, 3417–3422.

Head, J.M. (1980). Inhalation injury in burns. *Amer. J. Surg.* **139**, 508–512.

Huber, J., Ettlin, E. and Hardmeier (1980). Tod infolge schlecht sitzenden Zahnersatzes. *Schweiz. Med. Wschr.* **110**, 1146–1148.

Majeski, J.A., Schreiber, J.T., Cotton, R. and MacMillan, B.G. (1980). Tracheoplasty for tracheal stenosis in the pediatric burned patient. *J. Trauma* **20**, 81–86.

Moskowitz, D., Gardiner, L.J. and Sasaki, T. (1982). Foreign-body aspiration. Potential misdiagnosis. *Arch. Otolaryng.* **108**, 806–807.

Moylan, J.A., Adib, K. and Birnbaum, M. (1975). Fiberoptic bronchoscopy following thermal injury. *Surg. Gynec. Obstet.* **140**, 541–543.

Moylan, J.A. and Chan, C.-K. (1978). Inhalation injury – an increasing problem. *Ann. Surg.* **188**, 34–37.

Nakao, M.A., Killam, D. and Wilson, R. (1983). Pneumothorax secondary to inadvertent nasotracheal placement of a nasoenteric tube past a cuffed endotracheal tube. *Critical Care Med.* **11**, 210–213.

Peitzman, A.B., Shires, G.T. III, Corbett, W.A., Curreri, P.W. and Shires, G.T. (1981). Measurement of lung water in inhalation injury. *Surgery* **90**, 305–312.

Petajan, J.H., Voorhees, K.J., Packham, S.C., Baldwin, R.C., Einhorn, I.N., Grunnet, M.L., Dinger, B.G. and Birky, M.M. (1975). Extreme toxicity from combustion products of a fire-retarded polyurethane foam. *Science* **187**, 742–744.

Walker, H.L., McLeod, C.G. and McManus, W.F. (1981). Experimental inhalation injury in the goat. *J. Trauma* **21**, 962–964.

b. Trauma of the trachea

Andrews, M.J. and Pearson, F.G. (1973). An analysis of 59 cases of tracheal stenosis following tracheostomy with cuffed tube and assisted ventilation, with special reference to diagnosis and treatment. *Brit. J. Surg.* **60**, 208–212.

Aubert, M., Bocca, A., Ohanessian, J. and Latreille, R. (1978). Les ruptures trachéales par sonde d'intubation. *Lyon Chir.* **74**, 355–357.

Baumann, J. and Forster, E. (1960). Chirurgie de la trachée. *Poumon Coeur,* Paris **1**, 5–104.

Bex, J.-P., Rioux, C., Louville, Y., Neveux, J.-Y., Sawa, A. and Mathey, J. (1976). Chirurgie de la trachée et de la bifurcation trachéo-bronchique. Analyse d'une expérience de 23 ans (1951–1974). *Ann. Chir. Thorac. Cardiovasc.* **15**, 47–50.

Bricard, H., Sillard, B., Leroy, G., Quesnel, J., Segol, P. and Gignoux, M. (1979). Rupture trachéale après intubation par sonde de Carlens. *Ann. Chir.* **33**, 238–241.

Cooper, J.D. (1977). Trachea-innominate artery fistula: Successful management of 3 consecutive patients. *Ann. Thorac. Surg.* **24**, 439–447.

Dellon, A.L., Wells, J.H. and Cowley, R.A. (1978). A surgical procedure to prevent tracheo-innominate artery erosion. *J. Trauma* **18**, 550–553.

Dor, J., Forster, E. and Le Brigand, H. (1964). *Ruptures traumatiques des bronches et de la trachée thoracique.* Doin, Paris.

Ekeström, S. and Bergdahl, (1983). Intrathoracic tracheal rupture following blunt chest trauma. *Acta Chir. Scand.* **149**, 221–223.

Gebauer, P.W. (1951). Reconstructive surgery of the trachea and bronchi: late results with dermal grafts. *J. Thorac. Surg.* **22**, 568.

Grillo, H.C. (1979). Surgical treatment of postintubation tracheal injuries. *J. Thorac. Cardiovasc. Surg.* **78**, 860–875.

Grillo, H.C., Cooper, J.D., Geffin, B. and Pontoppidan, H. (1971). A low-pressure cuff for tracheostomy tubes to minimise tracheal injury. A comparative clinical trial. *J. Thorac. Cardiovasc. Surg.* **62**, 898–907.

Kufaas, T. (1983). Tracheal reconstruction with free periosteal grafts. An experimental study on rabbits. *Scand. J. Thorac. Cardiovasc. Surg.* **31**.

Lawhorne, T.W., Jeyasingham, K. and Kieffer, R.F. (1978). Transection of the trachea secondary to blunt trauma. *Brit. J. Surg.* **65**, 176–178.

Layton, T.R., Di Marco, R.F. and Pellegrini, R.V. (1980). Tracheoesophageal fistula from nonpenetrating trauma. *J. Trauma* **20**, 802–805.

Levasseur, P., Dartevelle, P., Rojas-Miranda, A., Merlier, M. and Le Brigand, H. (1980). Les résections anastomoses de trachée pour sténoses trachéales non tumorales. A propos de 68 cas. *J. Chir.*, Paris **106**, 109–113.

Martyn, J.W. (1982). Traumatic tracheoesophageal fistula. *J. Thoracic. Cardiovasc. Surg.* **83**, 790–791.

Neville, W.E., Bolanowski, P.J.P. and Soltanzadeh, H. (1976). Prosthetic reconstruction of the trachea and carina. *J. Thorac. Cardiovasc. Surg.* **72**, 525–538.

Nordin, U. and Ohlsén, L. (1982). Prevention of tracheal stricture in end-to-end anastomosis. *Arch. Otolaryng.* **108**, 308–314.

Perelman, M.I. (1976). *Surgery of the trachea.* Mir Publishers, Moscow.

Snow, N., Richardson, J.D. and Flint, L.M. (1981). Management of necrotizing tracheostomy infections. *J. Thorac. Cardiovasc. Surg.* **82**, 341–344.

Stemmer, E.A., Oliver, C., Carey, J.P. and Connolly, J.E. (1976). Fatal complications of tracheotomy. *Amer. J. Surg.* **131**, 288–290.

Travis, S.P.L. and Layer, G.T. (1983). Traumatic transection of the thoracic trachea. *Ann. Roy. Coll. of Surg. Eng.* **65**, 240–241.

c. *Bronchial rupture*

Al-Omeri, M.M. (1969). Traumatic rupture of left main stem bronchus. Successful repair three months after injury. *Arch. Surg.* **99**, 346–348.

Bardford, J.L. (1906). Case of extensive rupture of the trachea with complete detachment of the left bronchus without external injury. *Lancet* **II**, 1509.

Bisson, A. and Germain, V. (1976). Rupture bronchique par un ballonnet de sonde de Carlens. *Ann. Chir. Thorac. Cardiovasc.* **15**, 51–53.

Burton, N.A., Fall, S.M., Lyons, T. and Graeber, G.M. (1983). Rupture of the left main-stem bronchus with a polyvinylchloride double-lumen tube. *Chest* **83**, 928–929.

Buytendijk, H.J., Lubbers, H.J.B.J. and Maesen, F.P.V. (1968). Rupture traumatique d'une bronche et carcinome bronchique. Un problème de médecine légale. *Presse Médicale* **14**, 664–666.

Cohn, Roy. (1972). Non-penetrating wounds of the lungs and bronchi. *Surg. Clin. North Amer.* **52**, 585–595.

Couraud, L. and Bruneteau, A. (1973). Les ruptures trachéo-bronchiques post-traumatiques. Réflexions sur leur traitement à propos d'une expérience personnelle de 12 cas. *Ann. Chir. Thorac. Cardiovasc.* **12**, 35–38.

Eastridge, C.E., Hughes, F.A. Jr., Pate, J.W., Cole, F. and Richardson, R. (1970). Tracheobronchial injury caused by blunt trauma. *Amer. Rev. Respir. Dis.* **101**, 230–237.

Ellis, F.H. Jr., Andersen, H.A. and Hayles, A.B. (1955). Complete traumatic rupture of the bronchus with successful surgical repair: Report of a case in a 3-year-old child. *Mayo Clin. Proc.* **30**, 268–276.

Foster, J.M.G., Lau, O.J. and Alimo, E.B. (1983). Ruptured bronchus following endobronchial intubation. A case report. *Brit. J. Anaesth.* **55**, 687–688.

Gomez-Engler, H.E., Barker, A.F., Klein, R., Dietl, C.A., Macmanus, Q., Torstveit, J., Knight, R., Lawrence, H. and Starr, A. (1980). Post-traumatic bronchial stenosis and acute respiratory insufficiency. *J. Thorac. Cardiovasc. Surg.* **79**, 864–867.

Guest, J.L. Jr. and Anderson, J.N. (1977). Major airway injury in closed chest trauma. *Chest* **72**, 63–66.

Kaufmann, M., Meyer, W. and Maurer, W. (1974). Funktionelle Ergebnisse nach Bronchusanastomosen. *Helv. Chir. Acta* **41**, 93–100.

Kirsch, M.M., Orringer, M.B., Behrendt, D.M. and Sloan, H. (1976). Management of tracheobronchial disruption secondary to non-penetrating trauma. *Ann. Thorac. Surg.* **22**, 93–101.

Latarjet, M. (1958). Déchirure bronchique traumatique traitée avec succès par suture immédiate. *Poumon Coeur*, Paris **14**, 147.

Leape, L.L. (1971). Bronchial avulsion. Successful repair after bilateral pneumothorax. *J. Thorac. Cardiovasc. Surg.* **62**, 470–472.

Logreais, Y., DeSaint Florent, G., Danrigal, A., Barre, E., Maurel, A., Vanetti, A., Renault, P., Galey, J.J. and Mathey, J. (1970). Traumatic rupture of the right main bronchus in an eight-year-old child successfully repaired eight years after injury. *Ann. Surg.* **172**, 1039–1047.

Lynne-Davies, P., Ganguli, P.C. and Sterns, L.P. (1972). Pulmonary function following traumatic rupture of the bronchus. *Chest* **61**, 400–402.

Mahaffey, D.E., Greech, O., Boren, H.G. and DeBakey, M.E. (1955). Traumatic rupture of the left-main bronchus successfully repaired eleven years after injury to the chest. *Amer. J. Surg.* **90**, 253.

Myers, W.O., Leape, L.L. and Holder, T.M. (1971). Bronchial rupture in a child, with subsequent stenosis, resection and anastomosis. *Ann. Thorac. Surg.* **12**, 442–445.

Neugebauer, M.K., Fine, J.B. and Hoyt, T.W. (1974). Traumatic rupture of the trachea and right main stem bronchus. *J. Trauma* **14**, 265–269.

Nonoyama, A., Masuda, A., Kasahara, K., Mogi, T. and Kagawa, T. (1976). Total rupture of the left main bronchus successfully repaired nine years after injury. *Ann. Thorac. Surg.* **21**, 445–448.

Perruchoud, A., Tschan, M., Heitz, M., Anderes, U., Henchoz, L. and Herzog, H. (1982). Komplikationen des Bronchoskopie. *Schweiz. Med. Wschr.* **112**, 784–789.

Rahbar, A., Chang, F.C. and Farha, S.J. (1978). Rupture of the bronchus: Case report of successful resection and anastomosis in a 13-month-old infant. *J. Trauma* **18**, 140–141.

Sauvage, R. (1954). Réimplantation de la branche souche droite dans la trachée trois mois après une rupture totale de la bronche par traumatisme extérieur. *Mem. Acad. Chir.*, Paris **80**, 187.

Schoenberg, S. (1912). Bronchialrupturen bei Thoraxkompression. *Klin. Wochenschr.*, Berlin **49**, 2218.

Urschel, H.C. Jr. and Razzuk, M.A. (1973). Management of acute traumatic injuries of tracheobronchial tree. *Surg. Gynec. Obstet.* **136**, 113–117.

d. *Open wounds of the trachea and major bronchi*

Sulek, M., Miller, R.H. and Mattox, K.L. (1983). The management of gunshot and stab injuries of the trachea. *Arch. Otolaryng.* **109**, 56–59.

Symbas, P.N., Hatcher, C.R. Jr. and Boehm, G.A.W. (1976). Acute penetrating tracheal trauma. *Ann. Thorac. Surg.* **22**, 473–477.

Vichard, P., Grosdidier, J., Lafon, M., Arbez Gindre, F., Suzanne, J., Boissel, P. and Watelet, F. (1976). Transfixion par balle du tronc veineux innominé, de la trachée et de l'oesophage. Considérations thérapeutiques. *Chirurgie* **102**, 235–240.

Chapter 8: Trauma of the heart and pericardium

Arom, K.V., Richardson, J.D., Webb, G., Grover, F.L. and Trinkle, J.K. (1977). Subxiphoid pericardial window in patients with suspected traumatic pericardial tamponade. *Ann. Thorac. Surg.* **23**, 545–549.

Balakrishnan, S., Hartman, C.W., Grinnan, G.L.B., Bartel, A.G., Crisler, C. and Brickman, D. (1979). Pericardial fluid gas analysis in hemorrhagic pericardial tamponade. *Ann. Thorac. Surg.* **27**, 55–58.

Buechner, H.A. (1980). Pneumopericardium following laparoscopy. *Chest* **77**, 811.

Elkin, D.C. and Campbell, R.E. (1951). Cardiac tamponade: treatment by aspiration. *Ann. Surg.* **133**, 623–630.

Friedman, H.S., Sakurai, H., Choe, S.-S., Lajam, F. and Celis, A. (1980). Pulsus Paradoxus: A manifestation of a marked reduction of left ventricular end-diastolic volume in cardiac tamponade. *J. Thorac. Cardiovasc. Surg.* **79**, 74–82.

Galmiche, J.M. and Pinsard, M. (1982). Pyo-pneumo-péricarde compliquant une perforation d'ulcère sur une hernie hiatale. *J. Radiol.* **63**, 203–206.

Higgins, C.B., Broderick, T.W., Edwards, D.K. and Shumaker, A. (1979). The hemodynamic significance of massive pneumopericardium in preterm infants with respiratory distress syndrome. Clinical and experimental observations. *Radiology* **133**, 363–368.

Khan, R.M.A. (1974). Air tamponade and tension pneumopericardium. An unusual complication of subtotal pericardiectomy. *J. Thorac. Cardiovasc. Surg.* **68**, 328–330.

Morgan, B.C., Guntheroth, W.G. and Dillard, D.H. (1965). Relationship of pericardial to pleural pressure during quiet respiration and cardiac tamponade. *Circ. Research* **XVI**, 493–498.

Pollard, W.M., Schuchmann, G.F. and Bowen, T.E. (1981). Isolated chylopericardium after cardiac operations. *J. Thorac. Cardiovasc. Surg.* **81**, 943–946.

Posthumus, D.L. and Peirce, T.H. (1978). Fatal tension pneumopericardium complicating tracheostomy. *Chest* **73**, 107–108.

a. Pericardial injuries

Arndt, R.D., Frank, C.G., Schmitz, A.L. and Haveson, S.B. (1978). Cardiac herniation with volvulus after pneumonectomy. *Amer. J. Roentgenol.* **130**, 155–156.

Beck, H.I., Laursen, S.Ø. and Darling, K. (1982). Pneumopericardium as a complication of a benign gastric ulcer. A case report. *Scand. J. Thorac. Cardiovasc. Surg.* **16**, 63–64.

Christides, C., Laskar, M., Kim, M., Grousseau Renaudie, D. and Pouget, X. (1981). Rupture péricardique avec luxation du coeur associée à un infarctus du myocarde et à une rupture de l'isthme de l'aorte post-traumatique. *J. Chir.*, Paris **118**, 505–508.

Clark, D.E., Wiles, C.S. III, Lim, M.K., Dunham, C.M. and Rodriguez, A. (1983). Traumatic rupture of the pericardium. *Surgery* **93**, 495–503.

Duveau, D., Michaud, J.L., Letenneur, J., Arnaud, J. and Cornet, E. (1979). La luxation extrapéricardique du coeur dans les traumatismes fermés du thorax. Une nouvelle observation. Revue de la littérature. *Ann. Chir.* **33**, 597–600.

Ebel, T.A., Goldman, A.L. and Molina, J.E. (1980). Post-pneumonectomy shock: heart dislocation. *Chest* **77**, 787–788.

Guest, J.J. (1965). Late manifestations of trauma of the pericardium. *Surg. Gynec. Obstet.* **120**, 787.

Larrieu, A.J., Wiener, I., Alexander, R. and Wolma, F.J. (1980). Pericardiodiaphragmatic hernia. *Amer. J. Surg.* **139**, 436–440.

Roebuck, E.J. and Minford, J. (1983). Traumatic rupture of the pericardium with herniation of the heart. *Brit. J. Radiol.* **56**, 585–588.

Sbokos, C.G., Karayannacos, P.E., Kontaxis, A., Kambylafkas, J. and Skalkeas, G.D. (1977). Traumatic hemopericardium and chronic constrictive pericarditis. *Ann. Thorac. Surg.* **23**, 225–229.

Wetstein, L., Ergin, M.A. and Griepp, R.B. (1982). Colopericardial fistula: complication of colonic interposition. *Tex. Instit. J.* **9**, 373–376.

Zenker, R. (1954). Résultats du traitement chirurgical de la péricardite calcifiante (Panzerherz). *Méd. et Hyg.* **18**, 722–726.

b. Blunt heart injuries

Allen, R.P. and Liedtke, A.J. (1979). The role of coronary artery injury and perfusion in the development of cardiac contusion secondary to non-penetrating chest trauma. *J. Trauma* **19**, 153–156.

Atcheson, S.G., Petersen, G.V. and Fred, H.L. (1975). Ill-effects of cardiac resuscitation. Report of two unusual cases. *Chest* **67**, 615–618.

Brantigan, C.O., Burdick, D., Hopeman, A.R. and Eiseman, B. (1978). Evaluation of technetium scanning for myocardial contusion. *J. Trauma* **18**, 460–463.

Brennan, J.A., Field, J.M. and Liedtke, A.J. (1979). Reversible heart block following non-penetrating chest trauma. *J. Trauma* **19**, 784–788.

Desforges, G., Ridder, W.P. and Lenoir, R.J. (1955). Successful suture of ruptured myocardium after non-penetrating injury. *N. Eng. J. Med.* **252**, 567–569.

Dow, R.W. (1982). Myocardial rupture caused by trauma. *Surgery* **91**, 246–247.

Dupon, H., Godin, J.F., Duveau, D., Pelleray, C., Train, M. and Rozo, L. (1979). Insuffisance mitrale d'origine traumatique par ischémie d'un pilier chez un sujet de vingt ans. *Ann. Chir.* **33**, 582–586.

Fesani, F. (1983). L'insuffisance tricuspidienne post-traumatique isolée. Description d'un cas contrôlé dix années après l'intervention chirurgicale. *Coeur* **14**, 199–202.

Goltz, F. (1863). Vagus und Herz. *Virchows Archiv.* **26/1**, 1–33.

Hendel, P.N. and Grant, A.F. (1981). Blunt traumatic rupture of the heart. Successful repair of simultaneous rupture of the right atrium and left ventricle. *J. Thorac. Cardiovasc. Surg.* **81**, 574–576.

Le Treut, Y.P., Herve, L., Boutboul, R., Cardon, J.M. and Bricot, R. (1980). Ruptures du ventricule droit et du plancher péricardique à thorax fermé. Guérison chirurgicale. *J. Chir.*, Paris **117**, 699–700.

McIlduff, J.B. and Foster, E.D. (1978). Disruption of a normal aortic valve as a result of blunt chest trauma. *J. Trauma* **18**, 373–375.

Naccarelli, G.V., Haisty, W.K. and Kahl, F.R. (1980). Left ventricular to right atrial defect and tricuspid insufficiency secondary to non-penetrating cardiac trauma. *J. Trauma* **20**, 887–891.

Parr, G.V.S., Pae, W.E., Pierce, W.S. and Zelis, R. (1981). Cardiogenic shock due to ventricular rupture. A surgical approach. *J. Thorac. Cardiovasc. Surg.* **82**, 889–891.

Pifarré, R., Grieco, J., Garibaldi, A., Sullivan, H.J., Montoya, A. and Bakhos, M. (1982). Acute coronary artery occlusion secondary to blunt chest trauma. *J. Thorac. Cardiovasc. Surg.* **83**, 122–125.

Rheuban, K.S., Tompkins, D.G., Nolan, S.P., Berger, B., Martin, R. and Schneider, J.A. (1981). Myocardial necrosis and ventricular aneurysm following closed chest injury in a child. *J. Trauma* **21**, 170–173.

Sklar, J., Clarke, D., Campbell, D., Pearce, B., Appareti, K. and Johnson, M. (1982). Traumatic ventricular septal defect and lacerated mitral leaflet. Two-dimensional echocardiographic demonstration. *Chest* **81**, 247–249.

Snow, N., Richardson, J.D. and Flint, L.M. Jr. (1982). Myocardial contusion: implications for patients with multiple traumatic injuries. *Surgery* **92**, 744–750.

Stein, P.D., Sabbah, H.N., Viano, D.C. and Vostal, J.J. (1982). Response of the heart to non-penetrating cardiac trauma. *J. Trauma* **22**, 364–373.

Stelter, W.J., Walter, P., Ernst, R. and Werdan, K. (1982). Successful closure of a traumatic pulmonary arteriovenous fistula of the main pulmonary artery. *World J. Surg.* **6**, 484–489.

Symbas, P.N. (1972). *Traumatic injuries of the heart and great vessels.* Charles C. Thomas, Springfield.

Turina, M. and Kugelmeier, J. (1983). Herzverletzungen und ihre Spätfolgen. *Chirurgie* **54**, 129–134.

Watanabe, T., Katsume, H., Matsukubo, H., Furukawa, K. and Ijichi, H. (1981). Ruptured chordae tendineae of the tricuspid valve due to non-penetrating trauma. Echocardiographic findings. *Chest* **80**, 751–753.

c. *Open wounds of the heart*

Abbott, J.A., Cousineau, M., Cheitlin, M., Thomas, A.N. and Lim, R.C. Jr. (1978). Late sequelae of penetrating cardiac wounds. *J. Thorac. Cardiovasc. Surg.* **75**, 510–518.

Arbulu, A. and Thoms, N.W. (1972). Control of bleeding from a gunshot wound of the inferior vena cava at its junction with the right atrium by means of a Foley catheter. *J. Thorac. Cardiovasc. Surg.* **63**, 427–429.

Beck, C.S. (1926). Wounds of the heart: the technique of suture. *Arch. Surg.* **13**, 205.

DeGennaro, V.A., Bonfils-Roberts, E.A., Ching, N. and Nealon, T.F. (1980). Aggressive management of potential penetrating cardiac injuries. *J. Thorac. Cardiovasc. Surg.* **79**, 833–837.

Del Vecchio, S. (1895). Sutura del cuore. *Reforma Med.* **11**, 38.

Dubost, H., Salvestrini, J., Dubernet, A., Lucchini, J., Saavedva, C., Wilson and Cachera, J.P. (1965). Communication inter-ventriculaire traumatique. Fermeture chirurgicale sans circulation extracorporelle. *Ann. Chir. Thorac. Cardiovasc.* **4**, 448–456.

Enders, G.C., Graeber, G.M. and Poirier, R.A. (1978). Wounds traversing two or more cardiac chambers. Case presentation of two survivors and review of the literature. *J. Thorac. Cardiovasc. Surg.* **76**, 83–89.

Evans, J., Gray, L.A. Jr., Abi Rayner, M.D. and Fulton, R.L. (1979). Principles for the management of penetrating cardiac wounds. *Ann. Surg.* **189**, 777–784.

Fallahnejad, M., Kutty, A.C.K. and Wallace, H.W. (1980). Secondary lesions of penetrating cardiac injuries. A frequent complication. *Ann. Surg.* **191**, 228–233.

Jones, E.W. and Helmsworth, J. (1968). Penetrating wounds of the heart: Thirty years' experience. *Arch. Surg.* **96**, 671–682.

Kucharczyk, W., Weisbrod, G.L., Cooper, J.D. and Todd, T. (1982). Cardiac tamponade as a complication of thin-needle aspiration lung biopsy. *Chest* **82**, 120–121.

Lau, V.-K. and Viano, D.C. (1981). Experimental cardiac trauma – ballistics of a captive bolt pistol. *J. Trauma* **21**, 39–41.

Midell, A.I., Replogle, R. and Bermudez, G. (1975). Spontaneous closure of a traumatic ventricular septal defect following a penetrating injury. *Ann. Thorac. Surg.* **20**, 339–342.

Pantano, J.A., Singleton, R.T. and Turney, S.Z. (1977). Traumatic ventricular septal defect and delayed post-pericardiotomy ventricular herniation. *J. Trauma* **17**, 161–163.

Parmley, J.F., Mattingly, T.W. and Manion, W.C. (1958). Penetrating wounds of the heart and aorta. *Circulation* **17**, 953–973.

Pearce, C.W., MacCool, E. and Schmidt, F.E. (1966). Control of bleeding from cardiovascular wounds: balloon catheter tamponade. *Ann. Surg.* **163**, 257–259.

Reece, I. (1983). Penetrating cardiac injuries in the United Kingdom. *Thorax* **38**, 81–83.

Steichen, F.M., Dargan, E.L., Efron, G., Pearlman, D.M. and Weil, P.H. (1971). A graded approach to the management of penetrating wounds of the heart. *Arch. Surg.* **103**, 574–580.

Symbas, P.N. (1982). *Penetrating wounds to the heart.* Curr. Probl. Cardiol., Yearbook, Chicago.

Symbas, P.N., Harlaftis, N. and Waldo, W.J. (1976). Penetrating cardiac wounds: A comparison of different therapeutic methods. *Ann. Surg.* **183**, 377–381.

Thandroyen, F.T. and Matisonn, R.E. (1981). Penetrating thoracic trauma producing cardiac shunts. *J. Thorac. Cardiovasc. Surg.* **81**, 569–573.

Trinkle, J.K., Toon, R.S., Franz, J.L., Arom, K.V. and Grover, F.L. (1979). Affairs of the wounded heart: Penetrating cardiac wounds. *J. Trauma* **19**, 467–472.

d. *Electric injury of the heart*

Fouchard, J., Duval-Arnould, G., Simon, J.C., Chapuis, Y. (1979). Thrombose artérielle par électro-traumatisme. *J. Chir.,* Paris **116**, 27–30.

Halpérin, D.S., Oberhänsli, I. and Rouge, J.C. (1982). Accidents électriques chez l'enfant. *Rev. Méd. Suisse Romande* **102**, 1055–1060.

Kirchmer, J.T. Jr., Larson, D.L. and Tyson, K.R.T. (1977). Cardiac rupture following electrical injury. *J. Trauma* **17**, 389–391.

Sances, A. Jr., Larson, S.J., Myklebust, J. and Cusick, J.F. (1979). Electrical injuries. *Surg. Gynec. Obstet.* **149**, 97–107.

Wilkinson, C. and Wood, M.D. (1978). High voltage electric injury. *Amer. J. Surg.* **136**, 693–696.

e. *Foreign body injury to the heart*

Adar, R., Bass, A. and Walden, R. (1982). Iatrogenic complications in surgery. Five years' experience in general and vascular surgery in a University Hospital. *Ann. Surg.* **196**, 725–729.

Bassan, M.M. and Merin, G. (1977). Pericardial tamponade due to perforation with a permanent endocardial pacing catheter. *J. Thorac. Cardiovasc. Surg.* **74**, 51–54.

David, M., Brenot, R., Weiller, M., Coulon, C., Jabeuf, R. and Viard, H. (1981). Tamponade par perforation myocardique iatrogène à propos de 5 observations, à propos de la communication de J. Descotes, séance du 11.3.81. *J. Chir.,* Paris **107**, 387–388.

Duerr, S. and Cocco, T. (1977). Gunshot wound of the abdomen with cerebral embolisation. *J. Trauma* **17**, 155–157.

Fisk, R.L., Addetio, A., Gelfand, E.T., Brooks, C.H. and Dvorkin, J. (1977). Missile migration from lung to heart with delayed systemic embolisation. *Chest* **72**, 534–535.

Gilsanz, F., Burgos, R., Rufilanchas, J.J., Agosti, J. and Avello, F. (1981). Extraction of fragments of intracardiac catheters with the dormia urological catheter. *Scand. J. Thorac. Cardiovasc. Surg.* **15**, 301–303.

Hasse, J., Burkart, F. and Grädel, E. (1978). Behandlung der iatrogenen transvenösen Fremdkörperembolie. *Schweiz. Med. Wschr.* **108**, 1470–1474.

Krog, M., Berggren, L., Brodin, M. and Wickbom, G. (1982). Pericardial tamponade caused by central venous catheters. *World J. Surg.* **6**, 138–143.

Lee, M.E. and Chaux, A. (1980). Unusual complications of endocardial pacing. *J. Thorac. Cardiovasc. Surg.* **80**, 934–940.

Levin, A.R., Spach, M.S., Anderson, P.A. and Capp, M.P. (1965). Cardiac perforation following left ventricular cineangiocardiography. *Circulation* **32**, 593–595.

Lindgren, K.M., McShane, K. and Roberts, W.C. (1982). Acute rupture of the pulmonic valve by a balloon-tipped catheter producing a musical diastolic murmur. *Chest* **81**, 251–253.

Mautner, R.K. and Giles, T.D. (1979). Angina pectoris associated with a metallic fragment in the heart. *Chest* **75**, 605–606.

Nehme, A.E. (1980). Intracranial bullet migrating to pulmonary artery. *J. Trauma* **20**, 344–346.

Rich, N.M., Collins, G.J. Jr., Andersen, C.A., McDonald, P.T., Kozloff, L. and Ricotta, J.J. (1978). Missile emboli. *J. Trauma* **18**, 236–239.

San Filippo, J.A., Cohn, J., Gupte, P., Barbato, J., Feldman, M. and Del Guercio, R.M. (1981). Noninvasive cardiopulmonary monitoring. *Surgery* **90**, 313–318.

Chapter 9: Trauma of the thoracic aorta and great vessels

Besson, A., Saegesser, F. and Blanc, D. (1978). Rupture traumatique de l'aorta et des gros vaisseaux intrathoraciques. Revue collective et description de 67 observations dont une exemplaire. *Praxis* **67**, 266–285.

Cohen, D., Johansen, K., Cottingham, K., Clayson, K. and Simonowitz, D. (1980). Trauma to major visceral veins: an underemphasised cause of accident mortality. *J. Trauma* **20**, 928–932.

Hewes, R.C., Smith, D.C. and Lavine, M.H. (1979). Iatrogenic dehydromediastinum simulating aortic laceration. *AJR* **133**, 817–820.

Kirshner, R., Seltzer, S., D'Orsi, C. and DeWeese, J.A. (1983). Upper rib fractures and mediastinal widening: indications for aortography. *Ann. Thorac. Surg.* **35**, 450–454.

Lazrove, S., Harley, D.P., Grinnell, V.S., White, R.A. and Nelson, R.J. (1982). Should all patients with first rib fracture undergo arteriography? *J. Thorac. Cardiovasc. Surg.* **83**, 532–537.

Livoni, J.P. and Barcia, T.C. (1982). Fracture of the first and second rib: incidence of vascular injury relative to type of fracture. *Radiology* **145**, 31–33.

McConnell, B.J., McConnell, R.W. and Guiberteau, M.J. (1981). Radionuclide imaging in blunt trauma. *Radiol. Clin. North Amer.* **19**, 37–50.

Sloan, T.J. and Burch, B.H. (1983). Large mediastinal hematomas not associated with aortic rupture. Case presentations and surgical approach. *Chest* **83**, 109–111.

Stallone, R.J. (1979). Peripheral embolisation following blunt thoracic trauma. *J. Trauma* **19**, 72.

Wilson, R.F., Arbulu, A., Bassett, J.S. and Walt, A.J. (1972). Acute mediastinal widening following blunt chest trauma. *Arch. Surg.* **104**, 551–558.

a. Rupture of the aorta

Atkins, C.W., Buckley, M.J., Daggett, W., McIlduff, J.B. and Austen, W.G. (1981). Acute traumatic disruption of the thoracic aorta: a ten-year experience. *Ann. Thorac. Surg.* **31**, 305–309.

Allmendinger, P.D., Takata, H., Ellison, L.H. and Humphrey, C.B. (1982). Report of 37 patients with traumatic rupture of the thoracic aorta. *Tex. Heart Instit. J.* **9**, 71–73.

Aubert, M., letoublon, C., Rambaud, J.J., Alibeu, J.P., Jacquot, C., Terraube, R. and Contamin, C. (1980). Rupture traumatique de l'isthme aortique compliquée d'ischémie mésentérique. *J. Chir.*, Paris **117**, 183–187.

Ayella, R.J., Hankins, J.R., Turney, S.Z. and Cowley, R.A. (1977). Ruptured thoracic aorta due to blunt trauma. *J. Trauma* **17**, 199–205.

Bodily, K., Perry, J.F. Jr., Strate, R.G. and Fischer, R.P. (1977). The salvageability of patients with post-traumatic rupture of the descending thoracic aorta in a primary trauma center. *J. Trauma* **17**, 754–760.

Bolvig, L. and Andresen, J. (1981). Haemoptysis associated with traumatic rupture of the thoracic aorta. *Scand. J. Thor. Cardiovasc. Surg.* **15**, 221–222.

Charles, K.P., Davidson, K.G., Miller, H. and Caves, P.K. (1977). Traumatic rupture of the ascending aorta and aortic valve following blunt chest trauma. *J. Thorac. Cardiovasc. Surg.* **73**, 208–211.

Donzeau-Gouge, G.P., Bical, O., Blondeau, P., Piwnica, A., Carpentier, A., D'Allaines, C., Soyer, R., Brunet, A., Nottin, R., Chauvaud, S., Fabiani, J.N., Deloche, A., Petit, J. and Dubost, C. (1983). Rupture traumatique de l'aorte thoracique. A propos de 30 cas. *Arch. Mal. Coeur* **76**, 269–276.

Dreyfus, G., Dhainaut, J.F., Bachet, J., Goudot, B., Bical, O., Liebeaux, M., Brodaty, D. and Guilmet, D. (1979). Ruptures traumatiques de l'aorte thoracique. A propos de 20 observations. *J. Chir.*, Paris **116**, 699–704.

Fleming, A.W. and Green, D.C. (1974). Traumatic aneurysms of the thoracic aorta. Report of 43 patients. *Ann. Thorac. Surg.* **18**, 91–101.

Fontan, F., Chauve, A., Deville, C. and Baudet, E. (1978). Ruptures traumatiques de l'isthme aortique: Réparation chirurgicale. Résultats. *Chirurgie* **104**, 38–43.

Gundry, S.R., Williams, S., Burney, R.E., MacKenzie, J.R. and Cho, K.J. (1983). Indications for aortography. Radiography after blunt chest trauma: a reassessment of the radiographic findings associated with traumatic rupture of the aorta. *Invest. Radiol.* **18**, 230–237.

Harrington, D.P., Barth, K.H., White, R.I. and Brawley, R.K. (1980). Traumatic pseudoaneurysm of the thoracic aorta in close proximity to the anterior spinal artery: a therapeutic dilemma. *Surgery* **87**, 153–156.

Heiberg, E., Wolverson, M.K., Sundaram, M. and Shields, J.B. (1983). CT in Aortic Trauma. *Amer. J. Roentgenol.* **140**, 1119–1124.

Hilgenberg, A.D., Rainer, W.G. and Sadler, T.R. (1981). Aneurysm of the descending thoracic aorta. Replacement with the use of a shunt or bypass. *J. Thorac. Cardiovasc. Surg.* **81**, 818–824.

Hirsch, J.H., Carter, S.J. and Chikos, P.M. (1978). Traumatic pseudoaneurysms of the thoracic aorta: two unusual cases. *Amer. J. Roentgenol.* **130**, 157–160.

Katz, N.M., Blackstone, E.H., Kirklin, J.W. and Karp, R.B. (1981). Incremental risk factors for spinal cord injury following operation for acute traumatic aortic transection. *J. Thorac. Cardiovasc. Surg.* **81**, 669–674.

Katz, S., Mullin, R. and Berger, R.J. (1974). Traumatic transection associated with retrograde dissection and rupture of the aorta. *Ann. Thorac. Surg.* **17**, 273–276.

McCollum, C.H., Graham, J.M., Noon, G.P. and DeBakey, M.E. (1979). Chronic traumatic aneurysms of the thoracic aorta: an analysis of 50 patients. *J. Trauma* **19**, 248–252.

Maurage, C., Marchand, M., Lacombe, A., Gold, F., Autret, E., Chantepie, A. and Laugier, J. (1983). Rupture traumatique de l'aorte chez un enfant. *Arch. Franç. Pédiat.* **40**, 113–114.

Merin, G., Bitran, D., Donchin, Y., Weinshtein, D. and Borman, J.B. (1981). Traumatic rupture of the thoracic aorta during pregnancy. Surgical considerations. *Chest* **79**, 99–100.

Meyer, J.A., Neville, J.F. Jr. and Hansen, W.G. (1969). Traumatic rupture of the aorta in a child. *JAMA*, Chicago **208**, 527–529.

Mitchell, R.L. and Enright, L.P. (1983). The surgical management of acute and chronic injuries of the thoracic aorta. *Surg. Gynec. Obstet.* **157**, 1–4.

Nelson, A.R. (1970). Chronic hemothorax from contained aortic rupture. *Ann. Thorac. Surg.* **9**, 186–188.

Ouchi, H., Ohara, I. and Kijima, M. (1965). Intraluminal protrusion of completely disrupted intima: an unusual form of acute arterial injury. *Surgery* **57**, 220–224.

Parmley, L.F. (1958). Non-penetrating traumatic rupture of the aorta. *Circulation* **17**, 1086.

Patterson, R.H., Burns, W.A. and Jannotta, F.S. (1973). Rupture of the thoracic aorta: complication of resuscitation. *JAMA*, Chicago **226**, 197.

Pezzella, A.T., Effler, D.B. and Levy, I. (1982). Nonoperative management of unusual blunt traumatic rupture of the thoracic aorta. *Tex. Heart Instit. J.* **9**, 359–362.

Pinet, F., Vuilliez, J.G., Gourdol, Y., Celard, P., Villard, J. and Cognet, J.B. (1983). La radiologie d'urgence dans les ruptures traumatiques aiguës de l'aorta thoracique. Dépistage des formes atypiques. A propos de cinquante-deux observations. *Ann. Radiol.* **26**, 284–289.

Rauber, K. and Kollath, J. (1983). Die Diagnose der aortenruptur durch digitale Subtraktionsangiographie (DSA). *Fortschr. Röntgenstr.* **139**, 167–170.

Schechter, L.S. and Held, B.T. (1974). Right-sided extrapleural hematoma: an unusual presentation of ruptured aortic aneurysm. *Chest* **65**, 355–357.

Sevitt, S. (1977). The mechanisms of traumatic rupture of the thoracic aorta. *Brit. J. Surg.* **64**, 166–173.

Simeone, J.F., Minagi, H. and Putman, C.E. (1975). Traumatic disruption of the thoracic aorta: significance of the left apical extrapleural cap. *Radiology* **117**, 265–268.

Stelter, W.J., Becker, H.M. and Heberer, G. (1983). Rupturen und traumatische Aneurysmen der Aorta. *Chirurgie* **54**, 135–142.

Sturm, J.T., Marsh, D.G. and Bodily, K.C. (1979). Ruptured thoracic aorta: evolving radiological concepts. *Surgery* **85**, 363–367.

Symbas, P.N., Tyras, D.H., Ware, R.E. and Diorio, D.A. (1973). Traumatic rupture of the aorta. *Ann. Surg.* **178**, 6–12.

Thévenet, A. and Mary, H. (1975). Ruptures traumatiques de l'aorta isthmique. Problèmes de réparation d'urgence. *Ann. Chir. Thorac. Cardiovasc.* **14**, 81–90.

Tissot, E., Lomessy, A., Karo, G. and Motin, J. (1982). Rupture traumatique de l'isthme aortique et ischémique mésentérique. *J. Chir.*, Paris **119**, 679–680.

Tobis, J.M., Nalcioglu, O. and Henry, W.L. (1983). Digital subtraction angiography. *Chest* **84**, 68–75.

Voigt, G.E. (1968). Die Biomechanik stumpfer Brustverletzungen besonders von Thorax, Aorta und Herz. *Hefte Unfallheilkd.* **96**, 115.

b. Open type of aortic trauma

Also from, D.J., Marcus, N.H., Seigel, R.S., Talbot, W.A., Akl, B.F., Schiller, W.R. and Sklar, D.P. (1982). Shotgun pellet embolisation from the chest to the middle cerebral arteries. *J. Trauma* **22**, 155–157.

Carter, R., Mulder, G.A., Snyder, E.N. Jr. and Brewer, L.A. III (1978). Aorta-oesophageal fistula. *Amer. J. Surg.* **136**, 26–30.

Ctercteko, G. and Mok, C.K. (1980). Aorta-oesophageal fistula induced by a foreign body. The first recorded survival. *J. Thorac. Cardiovasc. Surg.* **80**, 233–235.

Cysne, E., Souza, E.G., Freitas, E., Machado, E., Giameroni, R., Alves, L.P.R., Teixeira, A.S. and La Brunie, P. (1982). Bullet embolism into the cardiovascular system. *Tex. Heart Instit. J.* **9**, 75–80.

Dupas, J.-L., Capron, J.-P., Delamarre, J., Bove, N. and Lorriaux, A. (1977). Anévrisme de l'aorte fissuré dans l'oesophage: aspects endoscopiques. *Endosc. Dig.* **2**, 41–44.

Fein, D., Godwin, J.D., Moore, A.V., Moran, J.F. and Young, W.G. Jr. (1983). Systemic artery-to-pulmonary vascular shunt: a complication of closed-tube thoracostomy. *Amer. J. Roentgenol.* **140**, 917–919.

Halpern, N.B. and Aldrete, J.S. (1979). Factors influencing mortality and morbidity from injuries to the abdominal aorta and inferior vena cava. *Amer. J. Surg.* **137**, 384–386.

Kirsh, M.M., Orringer, M.B., Behrendt, D.M., Mills, L.J., Tashian, J. and Sloan, H. (1978). Management of unusual traumatic ruptures of the aorta. *Surg. Gynec. Obstet.* **146**, 365–370.

Pickard, L.R., Mattox, K.L., Espada, R., Beall, A.C. Jr. and DeBakey, M.E. (1977). Transection of the descending thoracic aorta secondary to blunt trauma. *J. Trauma* **17**, 749–753.

Tector, A.J., Worman, L.W., Romer, J.F., De Cock, D.G. and Lepley, D. (1974). Unusual injury to the aortic arch. A case report. *J. Thorac. Cardiovasc. Surg.* **67**, 547–552.

c. Injuries to the supra-aortic vessels

Balique, J.G., Heynen, Y.G., Robert, M.C., Espalieur, P., Allard, D., Dufraisse, G., Mangin, M., Bayon, M.C. and Cuilleret, J. (1983). Rupture de l'artère sous-clavière gauche associée à une fracture de la première côte. *J. Chir.*, Paris **120**, 265–269.

Beattie, E.J. Jr., Martini, N., Choudhry, K.U., Wright, W. and Howland, W.S. (1970). Emergency reconstruction of the superior vena cava. *Surg. Clin. North Amer.* **50**, 959–967.

Bloss, R.S. and Ward, R.E. (1980). Survival after tracheo-innominate artery fistula. *Amer. J. Surg.* **139**, 251–253.

Castagna, J. and Nelson, R.J. (1975). Blunt injuries to branches of the aortic arch. *J. Thorac. Cardiovasc. Surg.* **69**, 521–532.

Deslauriers, J., Ginsberg, R.J., Nelems, J.M. and Pearson, F.G. (1975). Innominate artery rupture. A major complication of tracheal surgery. *Ann. Thorac. Surg.* **20**, 671–677.

Fisher, R.G., Hadlock, F. and Ben-Menachem, Y. (1981). Laceration of the thoracic aorta and brachiocephalic arteries by blunt trauma. Report of 54 cases and review of the literature. *Radiol. Clin. North Amer.* **19**, 91–110.

Gangahar, D.M. and Flogaites, T. (1978). Retrosternal dislocation of the clavicle producing thoracic outlet syndrome. *J. Trauma* **18**, 369–372.

Keller, F.S., Rösch, J., Banner, R.L. and Dotter, C.T. (1982). Iatrogenic internal mammary artery-to-innominate vein fistula. Percutaneous nonsurgical closure. *Chest* **81**, 255–257.

Kieffer, E., Tricot, J.-F., Maraval, M. and Natali, J. (1979). Traumatismes fermés des troncs supra-aortiques. *J. Chir.*, Paris **116**, 333–342.

Lane, E.E., Temes, G.D. and Anderson, W.H. (1975). Tracheal-innominate artery fistula due to tracheostomy. *Chest* **68**, 678–683.

Lim, L.T., Saletta, J.D. and Flanigan, D.P. (1979). Subclavian and innominate artery trauma. A five-year experience with 17 patients. *Surgery* **86**, 890–897.

Livesay, J.J., Michals, A.A. and Dainki, E.C. (1982). Anomalous right subclavian arterial oesophageal fistula: an unusual complication of tracheostomy. *Tex. Heart Instit. J.* **9**, 105–108.

Mavroudis, C., Roon, A.J., Baker, C.C. and Thomas, A.N. (1980). Management of acute cervicothoracic vascular injuries. *J. Thorac. Cardiovasc. Surg.* **80**, 342–349.

Mehigan, J.T., Buch, W.S., Pipkin, R.D. and Fogarty, T.J. (1978). Subclavian-carotid transposition for the subclavian steal syndrome. *Amer. J. Surg.* **136**, 15–20.

Myers, W.O., Lawton, B.R., Ray, J.F. III, Kuehner, M.E. and Sautter, R. (1979). Axillo-axillary bypass for subclavian steal syndrome. *Arch. Surg.* **114**, 394–399.

O'Neill, M.J., Myers, J.L., Brown, G.R., Harrison, J.L. and De Muth, W.E. (1982). Avulsion of the innominate artery from the aortic arch associate with a posterior tracheal tear. *J. Trauma* **22**, 56–59.

Robbs, J.V., Baker, L.W., Human, R.R., Vawda, I.S., Duncan, H. and Rajaruthnam, P. (1981). Cervico-mediastinal arterial injuries. A surgical challenge. *Arch. Surg.* **116**, 663–668.

Sodal, G. and Nornes, H. (1979). Surgical correction of subclavian steal syndrome. *Scand. J. Thorac. Cardiovasc. Surg.* **13**, 315–320.

Solheim, K. (1981). Closed subclavian artery injuries. *Scand. J. Thorac. Cardiovasc. Surg.* **15**, 283–287.

Solheim, K. (1981). Closed subclavian artery injuries. *Scand. J. Thorac. Cardiovasc. Surg.* **15**, 283–287.

Thomas, A.N., Goodman, P.C. and Roon, A.J. (1978). Role of angiography in cervicothoracic trauma. *J. Thorac. Cardiovasc. Surg.* **78**, 633–638.

d. Open wounds of the thoracic vessels

Adams, P. and Walker, W.E. (1983). Gunshot wound of the aortic arch and oesophagus: unusual indication for ascending-to-abdominal aortic bypass graft. *Tex. Heart Instit. J.* **10**, 415–418.

Anyanwu, C.H., Umeh, B.U.O. and Swarup, A.S. (1982). Experience with civilian vascular injuries in Eastern Nigeria. *Angiology* **33**, 90–97.

Chang, J., Katzen, B.T. and Sullivan, K.P. (1978). Transcatheter gelfoam embolisation of post-traumatic bleeding pseudoaneurysms. *Amer. J. Roentgenol.* **131**, 645–650.

Cheek, R.C., Pope, J.C., Smith, H.F., Britt, L.G. and Pate, J.W. (1975). Diagnosis and management of major vascular injuries: a review of 200 operative cases. *Amer. Surg.* **41**, 755–760.

Eichenhorn, M.S., Pensler, M.I. and Lewis, J.W. (1980). Pulmonary arterial laceration secondary to subclavian vein catheterisation. *Chest* **78**, 120.

Elerding, S.C., Manart, F.D. and Moore, E.E. (1980). A reappraisal of penetrating neck injury management. *J. Trauma* **20**, 695–697.

Fromm, S.H., Carrasquilla, C. and Lucas, C. (1970). The management of gunshot wounds of the aorta. The use of dracon grafts to replace the injured aorta. *Arch. Surg.* **101**, 388–390.

Graham, J.M., Feliciano, D.V., Mattox, K.L., Beall, A.C. and De Bakey, M.E. (1980). Management of subclavian vascular injuries. *J. Trauma* **20**, 537–544.

Lefrak, E.A. and Noon, G.P. (1972). Management of arterial injury secondary to attempted subclavian vein catheterisation. *Ann. Thorac. Surg.* **14**, 294–298.

Quast, D.C., Shirkey, A.L., Fitzgerald, J.B., Beall, A.C. Jr. and De Bakey, M.E. (1965). Surgical correction of injuries of the vena cava. An analysis of 61 cases. *J. Trauma* **5**, 3.

Rich, N.M., Baugh, J.H. and Hughes, C.W. (1970). Acute arterial injuries in Vietnam: 1,000 cases. *J. Trauma* **10**, 359–369.

Rudich, M.D., Rowland, M.C., Seibel, R.W. and Border, J. (1978). Survival following a gunshot wound of the abdominal aorta and inferior vena cava. *J. Trauma* **18**, 548–549.

Schaff, H.V. and Brawley, R.K. (1977). Operative management of penetrating vascular injuries of the thoracic outlet. *Surgery* **82**, 182–191.

Starzl, T.E., Kampp, H.H., Beheler, E.M. and Freeark, R.J. (1963). Penetrating injuries of the inferior vena cava. *Surg. Clin. North Amer.* **43**, 387.

Stroud, W.H. and Yarbrough, D.R. (1980). Penetrating neck wounds. *Amer. J. Surg.* **140**, 323–326.

Symbas, P.N., Kourias, E., Tyras, D.H. and Hatcher, C.R. Jr. (1974). Penetrating wounds of great vessels. *Ann. Surg.* **179**, 757–762.

Turpin, I., State, D. and Schwartz, A. (1977). Injuries to the inferior vena cava and their management. *Amer. J. Surg.* **134**, 25–32.

Vichard, P.H., Grosdidier, J., Arbez-Gindre, F., Suzanne, J., Boissel, P. and Watelet, F. (1976). Transfixion par balle du tronc veineux innominé de la trachée et de l'oesophage. Considérations thérapeutiques. *Chirurgie* **102**, 235–240.

Weissberg, D. and Herczeg, E. (1980). Perforation of thoracic aortic aneurysm. A complication of mediastinoscopy. *Chest* **78**, 119–120.

Chapter 10: Trauma of the diaphragm

a. Rupture of the diaphragm

Ammann, A.M., Brewer, W.H., Maull, K.I. and Walsh, J.W. (1983). Traumatic rupture of the diaphragm: real-time sonographic diagnosis. *Amer. J. Roentgenol.* **140**, 915–916.

Aubert, M., Parent, B., Ohanessian, J., Pilichowski, P. and Latreille, R. (1980). Les hernias diaphragmatiques traumatiques droites. *Lyon Chir.* **76**, 284–288.

Bekassy, S.M., Dave, K.S., Wooler, G.H. and Ionescu, M.I. (1973). 'Spontaneous' and traumatic rupture of the diaphragm: long-term results. *Ann. Surg.* **177**, 320–324.

Besson, A. and Saegesser, F. (1979). *Traumatismos Toraco-abdominales.* Chap. 20 dans Abdomen Agudo, Avances en Cirugià par C, Perà Ed., Salvat, Barcelone, 241–273.

Besson, A. and Saegesser, F. (1981). Traumas du diaphragme, Mémoire portant sur 150 observations. *Urg. Chir. Comment.* **4**, 121–138.

Bryant, L.R., Schechter, F.G., Rees, R. and Albert, H.M. (1978). Bilateral diaphragmatic rupture due to blunt trauma. A rare injury. *J. Trauma* **18**, 280–282.

Christophi, C. (1983). Diagnosis of traumatic diaphragmatic hernia: analysis of 63 cases. *World J. Surg.* **7**, 277–280.

Clay, M.G. and Munro, A.I. (1971). Bilateral diaphragmatic hernia from blunt injury causing a Budd-Chiari syndrome: use of a liver and spleen scan in demonstrating the defects. *Amer. J. Surg.* 321–324.

Couraud, L., Barandon, E., Desplantez, J. and Zimmermann, J.-M. (1978). Les hernies diaphragmatiques étranglées ou engouées. Considérations thérapeutiques à propos de six cas. *Ann. Chir.* **32**, 295–299.

Dajee, A., Schepps, D. and Hurley, E.J. (1981). Diaphragmatic injuries. *Surg. Gynec. Obstet.* **153**, 31–32.

Düx, A. (1982). Zwerchfellhernien und -Prolapse. *Radiologe* **22**, 7–21.

Estrera, A.S., Platt, M.R., Mills, L.J. and Urschel, H.C. (1980). Rupture of the right hemidiaphragm with liver herniation: report of a case with extension of a tear of a previously undiagnosed ruptured right hemidiaphragm. *J. Trauma* **20**, 174–176.

Estrera, A.S., Platt, M.R. and Mills, L.J. (1979). Traumatic injuries of the diaphragm. *Chest* **75**, 306–313.

Freeman, T. and Fischer, R.P. (1976). The inadequacy of peritoneal lavage in diagnosing acute diaphragmatic rupture. *J. Trauma* **16**, 538–542.

Garcia-Bianch de Benito, G., Landa Garcia, J.I., Moreno Azcoita, M., Moreno Gonzale, E., De la Caille Santiuste, A., Figueroa Andollo, J. and Perez Mota, A. (1978). Rupturas traumaticas del diafragma. *Rev. Esp. Enf. Ap. Digest.* **LIV**, 115–130.

Hall, J.C., Douglas, M.C. and Burke, D. (1981). Rupture of diaphragm associated with spinal cord injury. *Aust. N.Z. J. Surg.* **51**, 594–597.

Harman, P.K., Mentzer, R.M., Weinberg, A.C., Caldwell, P.C. and Minor, G.R. (1981). Early diagnosis by liver scan of a right-sided traumatic diaphragmatic hernia. *J. Trauma* **21**, 489–490.

Hood, R.M. (1971). Traumatic diaphragmatic hernia. Collective review. *Ann. Thorac. Surg.* **12**, 311–324.

Hussain, S.A. (1980). Delayed rupture of the diaphragm following blunt trauma. *Inter. Surg.* **65**, 269–270.

Jarrett, F. and Bernhardt, L.C. (1978). Right-sided diaphragmatic injury. Rarity or overlooked diagnosis? *Arch. Surg.* **113**, 737–739.

Jensen, B.S. and Arendrup, H.C. (1981). Rupture of diaphragm. An unusual case of traumatic diaphragmatic hernia, treated in the obstructive phase. *Acta Chir. Scand.* **147**, 729–730.

Mansour, K.A. (1974). Strangulated traumatic diaphragmatic hernia: A case report. *Amer. J. Surg.* 431–433.

Meads, G.E., Carroll, S.E. and Pitt, D.F. (1977). Traumatic rupture of the right hemidiaphragm. *J. Trauma* **17**, 797–801.

Melzig, E.P., Swank, M. and Salzberg, A.M. (1976). Acute blunt traumatic rupture of the diaphragm in children. *Arch. Surg.* **111**, 1009–1011.

Nano, M., Dei Poli, M., Mossetti, C. and Maggi, G. (1980). Traumatic diaphragmatic hernias. *Surg. Gynec. Obstet.* **151**, 191–192.

Payne, J.H. and Yellin, A.E. (1982). Traumatic diaphragmatic hernia. *Arch. Surg.* **117**, 18–24.

Popovici, Z. (1971). Les lésions traumatiques du diaphragme et leurs conséquences. (A propos de 181 cas.) *J. Chir.*, Paris **102**, 343–360.

Proye, C. (1980). Rupture de coupole diaphragmatique et péricardotomie. *Ann. Chir.* **34**, 512.

Pupello, D.F., Mark, J.B.D. and Iben, A.B. (1970). Surgical treatment of traumatic rupture of the thoracic aorta and diaphragm. *Calif. Med.* **112**, 27–29.

Rebagliati, M. (1973). *Traitement des lésions traumatiques du diaphragme, aspect anesthésiologique.* Thèse, Lausanne.

Saegesser, F. and Besson, A. (1977). 493 traumatismes thoraco-abdominaux ou abdomino-thoraciques, ouverts ou fermés, avec 114 atteintes du diaphragme. 1956–1975. *Helv. Chir. Acta* **44**, 7–48.

Saur, K. and Lutz, W. (1976). Die traumatische zwerchfellruptur: Diagnostik, behandlung, spätergebnisse. *Unfallheilkunde* **79**, 349–357.

Schneider, S. and Saegesser, F. (1960). Les traumatismes thoraciques. *Helv. Chir. Acta* **27/1**, 34–116.

Shuck, J.M. and Schiller, W.R. (1980). Median sternotomy: extension of laparotomy for ruptured right hemidiaphragm. *J. Trauma* **20**, 806–808.

Stark, P. (1982). Die traumatische Zwerchfellruptur. Ein radiologisch-diagnostisches Problem. *Radiologe* **22**, 22–25.

Symbas, P.N. (1978). Blunt traumatic rupture of the diaphragm. *Ann. Thorac. Surg.* **26**, 193–194.

Tan, G.C., Hamilton, S.G.L., Gibson, P. and Simpson, J.A. (1973). Ruptured diaphragm: experience in a major accident centre over a ten-year period. *Aust. N.Z. J. Surg.* **43**, 163–168.

Visset, J., Le Neel, J.C., Duveau, D., Paineau, J. and Hingrat, J.Y. (1983). Ruptures traumatiques du diaphragme. Soixante-sept observations. *Press Méd.* **12**, 1211–1214.

Waldschmidt, M.L. and Laws, H.L. (1980). Injuries of the diaphragm. *J. Trauma* **20**, 587–592.

Ward, R.E., Flynn, T.C. and Clark, W.P. (1981). Diaphragmatic disruption secondary to blunt abdominal trauma. *J. Trauma* **21**, 35–38.

Waridel, D. (1970). Les ruptures traumatiques fermés du diaphragme. *Helv. Chir. Acta* **37**, 111–121.

Wynne, J.M. and Gough, I.R. (1979). Diagnostic pneumoperitoneum in traumatic rupture of the right diaphragm. *Aust. N.Z. J. Surg.* **49**, 473–476.

b. *Special diaphragmatic injuries*

Adamthwaite, D.N., Snyders, D.C. and Mirwis, J. (1983). Traumatic pericardiophrenic hernia: a report of 3 cases. *Brit. J. Surg.* **70**, 117–119.

Bérard, P. and Philibert, M. (1981). Occlusion du grêle par bride dans une hernie diaphragmatique post-opératoire après fundoplicature par voie thoracique. *Lyon Chir.* **77**, 180–181.

Besson, A., Macarone-Palmieri, R. and Saegesser, F. (1979). Rupture du centre tendineux du diaphragme par traumatisme thoraco-abdominal fermé, avec tamponnade par éviscération intrapéricardique secondaire du côlon. Revue de 13 cas de la littérature. *Ann. Chir.* **33**, 591–596.

Besson, A., Saegesser, F. and Sandblom, P. (1977). Traumatismes du foie accompagnant les ruptures coupolaires du diaphragme, les embrochages costaux phréno-hépatiques et les désinsertions phréno-costales. Incidence et mortalité. *Méd. et Hyg.* **35**, 2779–2782.

Dave, K.S., Bekassy, S.M., Wooler, G.H. and Ionescu, M.I. (1973). 'Spontaneous' rupture of the diaphragm during delivery. *Brit. J. Surg.* **60**, 666–668.

Hocking, M.A. and Bolton, P.M. (1978). Intrathoracic rupture of the spleen. *Brit. J. Surg.* **65**, 546–548.

Meng, R.L., Straus, A., Milloy, F., Kittle, C.F. and Langston, H. (1979). Intrapericardial diaphragmatic hernia in adults. *Ann. Surg.* **189**, 359–366.

Murchison, W.G., Harper, W.K. and Putman, J.S. (1974). Traumatic diaphragmatic hernia: late presentation as bloody pleural effusion. *Chest* **66**, 734–736.

Oparah, S.S. and Mandal, A.K. (1978). Traumatic thoracobiliary (pleurobiliary and bronchobiliary) fistulas: clinical and review study. *J. Trauma* **18**, 539–544.

Rubio-Alvarez, J., Fuster-Siebert, M. Calzadilla-Martin, G., Ledo-Andion, R. and Garcia-Bengochea, J.B. (1983). Traumatic rupture of the pericardium: report of two cases with unusual features. *Tex. Heart Instit. J.* **10**, 77–79.

Salomon, J., Feller, N. and Levy, M.J. (1969). A case of spontaneous rupture of the diaphragm. *J. Thorac. Cardiovasc. Surg.* **58**, 221–224.

Stone, A.M., Pearson, W.T., Lansdown, F.S. and Tice, D.A. (1970). Spontaneous rupture of the right diaphragm. *Ann. Thorac. Surg.* **9**, 479–482.

c. *Post traumatic relaxation*

Brouillette, R.T., Ilbawi, M.N. and Hunt, C.E. (1983). Phrenic nerve pacing in infants and children: a review of experience and report on the usefulness of phrenic nerve stimulation studies. *J. Pediat.* **102**, 32–39.

Donzeau-Gouge, G.P., Personne, C., Lechien, J., Colchen, A., Leroy, M., Seigneur, F., Hertzog, P. and Toty, L. (1982). Eventrations diaphragmatiques de l'adulte. A propos de vingt cas. *Ann. Chir. Cardiovasc.* **36**, 87–90.

Ellis, F.H. Jr. (1964). Eventration (unilateral elevation) of the diaphragm. *Hernia* **35**, 554–565. Philadelphia, J.B. Lippincott.

Huault, G., Checoury, A. and Binet, J.P. (1982). Paralysie et éventration diaphragmatique. *Ann. Chir. Cardiovasc.* **36**, 79–83.

Iverson, L.I.G., Mittal, A., Dugan, D.J. and Samson, P.C. (1976). Injuries to the phrenic nerve resulting in diaphragmatic paralysis with special reference to stretch trauma. *Amer. J. Surg.* **132**, 263–268.

Kim, J.H., Manuelidis, E.E., Glenn, W.W.L. and Kaneyuki, T. (1976). Diaphragm pacing. Histopathological changes in the phrenic nerve following long-term electrical stimulation. *J. Thorac. Cardiovasc. Surg.* **72**, 602–608.

Mickell, J.J., Sang, Oh K., Siewers, R.D., Galvis, A.G., Fricker, F.J., Mathews, R.A. and Bahnson, H.T. (1978). Clinical implications of postoperative unilateral phrenic nerve paralysis. *J. Thorac. Cardiovasc. Surg.* **76**, 297–304.

Pastor, J., Blasco, E., Garcia Zarza, A., Padilla, J., Tarazona, V., Guijarro, R. and Paris, F. (1982). Eventrations diaphragmatiques de l'adulte traitées par plicature. Résultats post-opératoires à long terme. *Ann. Chir. Cardiovasc.* **36**, 84–85.

Perrotin, J. and Moreaux, J. (1965). *Chirurgie du diaphragme. Paralysies diaphragmatiques.* Masson, Paris.

Phadke, J.G. (1979). Ehlers-Danlos syndrome with surgical repair of eventration of diaphragm and torsion of stomach. *Roy. Soc. of Med.* **72**, 781–783.

Witz, J.P., Jesel, M., Roeslin, N., Morand, G. and Wihlm, J.M. (1982). Les éventrations diaphragmatiques de l'adulte Apport de l'électromyographie. *Ann. Chir. Cardiovasc.* **36**, 91–94.

d. Open wounds of the diaphragm

Dartevelle, P., Yger, M., Gharbi, N., Vayre, P. and Merlier, M. (1981). Abcès inter-hépato-diaphragmatique avec fistule bronchique par migration tardive trans-diaphragmatique d'un corps étranger abdominal post-opératoire. *J. Chir.*, Paris **118**, 413–416.

Glinz, W. (1976). Abdominelle Komplikationen beim nicht abdominellen Trauma. *Helv. Chir. Acta* **43**, 573–578.

Grimsehl, H. and Blencke, B. (1970). Thorax- und Abdominalverletzungen im Kindesalter. *Langenbecks Arch. Chir.* **326**, 216–238.

Hopson, W.B., Sherman, R.T. and Sanders, J.W. (1966). Stab wounds of the abdomen: 5 year review of 297 cases. *Amer. Surg.* **32**, 213.

Kessler, E. and Stein, A. (1976). Diaphragmatic hernia as a long-term complication of stab wounds of the chest. *Amer. J. Surg.* **132**, 34–39.

Key, G.F. and Nance, F.C. (1976). A time-management study of 25 patients with penetrating wounds of the chest and abdomen. *J. Trauma* **16**, 524–530.

Latarjet, M., Ollagnier, Ch. and Barbe, Ch. (1975). Pleurésie purulente chronique enkystée gauche par empalement méconnu. *Chirurgie* **101**, 527–532.

Lombard-Platet, R., Vincent, B. and Maurin, T. (1981). Plaie méconnue du diaphragme gauche par coup de couteau. *Lyon Chir.* **77**, 119–120.

Sandrasagra, F.A. (1977). Penetrating thoracoabdominal injuries. *Brit. J. Surg.* **64**, 638–640.

Streichen, F.M. (1967). *Penetrating wounds of the chest and the abdomen.* Curr. Probl. Surg.

Chapter 11: Trauma of the oesophagus

Andersen, O.S. and Giustra, P.E. (1981). Nonoperative management of contained oesophageal perforation. Two case reports. *Arch. Surg.* **116**, 1214–1217.

Banks, J.G. and Bancewicz, J. (1981). Perforation of the oesophagus: experience in a general hospital. *Brit. J. Surg.* **68**, 580–584.

Barrett, N.R. (1952). *Oesophageal Trauma.* Butterworths, London. 221–241.

Berry, B.E. and Ochsner, J.L. (1973). Perforation of the oesophagus. A 30-year review. *J. Thorac. Cardiovasc. Surg.* **65**, 1–7.

Besson, A., Meyer, A., Savary, M. and Saegesser, F. (1981). Etude de 58 complications thoraciques parmi 166 traumatismes accidentels ou iatrogènes de l'oesophage. *Schweiz. Med. Wschr.* **111**, 1602–1607.

Duchatelle, J.P., Parrot, A.M., Parmentier, G. and Andreassian, B. (1980). Traumatismes de l'oesophage cervical. *J. Chir.*, Paris **117**, 365–368.

Ginsberg, R.J. and Cooper, J.D. (1983). Oesophageal fistula. *World J. Surg.* **7**, 455–462.

Goldstein, L.A. and Thompson, W.R. (1982). Oesophageal perforation: A 15-year experience. *Amer. J. Surg.* **143**, 495–503.

Harrison, M.W., Lindell, T.D. and Brant, B. (1976). Surgical treatment of late oesophageal perforations. *Amer. J. Surg.* **42**, 488–491.

Hessler, C. and Huber, O. (1977). Kystes aériques paramédiastinaux traumatiques. *Schweiz. Med. Wschr.* **107**, 816–817.

Hinder, R.A., Baskind, A.F. and Le Grange, F. (1981). A tube system for the management of ruptured oesophagus. *Brit. J. Surg.* **68**, 182–184.

Keszler, P. and Buzna, E. (1981). Surgical and conservative management of oesophageal perforation. *Chest* **80**, 158–162.

Lyons, W.S., Seremetis, M.G., deGuzman, V.C. and Peabody, J.W. Jr. (1978). Ruptures and perforations of the oesophagus: the case for conservative supportive management. *Ann. Thorac. Surg.* **25**, 346–350.

Majeski, J.A. and MacMillan, B.G. (1979). Acute oesophageal perforation in an adolescent burn patient. *J. Trauma* **19**, 288–289.

Naclerio, E.A. (1957). The 'V sign' in the diagnosis of spontaneous rupture of the oesophagus. (An early roentgen clue.) *Amer. J. Surg.* **93**, 291–298.

Payne, W.S. (1975). Management of oesophageal perforation. *Ann. Thorac. Surg.* **20**, 486–487.

Pettersson, G., Larsson, S., Gatzinsky, P. and Düdow, G. (1981). Differentiated treatment of intrathoracic oesophageal perforations. *Scand. J. Thorac. Cardiovasc. Surg.* **15**, 321–324.

Savary, M. and Besson, A. (1978). Les traumatismes de l'oesophage. *Proc. Soc. Oto-Rh-Laryngol. Lat. XXII Congress,* Montpellier, 379–383.

Savary, M. and Miller, G. (1977). *L'oesophage. Manuel et atlas d'endoscopie.* Soleure, Gassmann.

Vessal, K., Montali, R.J., Larson, S.M., Chaffee, V. and Everette-James, A. Jr. (1975). Evaluation of barium and gastrografin as contrast mediums for diagnosis of oesophageal ruptures or perforations. *J. Roentgenol. Radium Ther. Nucl. Med.* **123**, 307–319.

a. Instrumental perforation of the oesophagus

Beuret, D., Besson, A. and Saegesser, F. (1981). Perforation iatrogène de l'oesophage sus-diaphragmatique avec abcès médiastinal et empyème pleural droit. A propos d'un cas reconnue et traité au 16e jour. *Rev. Méd. Suisse Romande* **101**, 469–473.

Bugge-Asperheim, B., Birkeland, S. and Støren, G. (1981). Tracheo-oesophageal fistula caused by cuffed tracheal tubes. *Scand. J. Thorac. Cardiovasc. Surg.* **15**, 315–319.

Clifford, P.C. (1980). An unusual oesophageal perforation during intercostal drainage for empyema. *Brit. J. Surg.* **67**, 451–452.

Cornet, A., Grivaux, M., Debesse, B. and Carnot, F. (1971). Rupture gastrique. Fragilité pariétale au cours de la gastroscopie. *Sem. Hôp. Paris* **47**, 2933–2940.

Grillo, H.C., Moncure, A.C. and MacEnany, M.T. (1976). Repair of inflammatory tracheoesophageal fistula. *Ann. Thorac. Surg.* **22**, 112–119.

McDonald, H.F. (1978). Right pneumothorax following fibreoptic oesophageal dilatation. *Endoscopy* **10**, 130–132.

Mellbring, G., Domellöf, L. and Osterman, G. (1980). Fiberendoscopic intramural lesion of the oesophagus. *Acta Chir. Scand.* **146**, 527–528.

Nagaraj, H.S., Mullen, P., Groff, D.B., Shearer, L.T. and Cook, L.N. (1979). Iatrogenic perforation of the oesophagus in premature infants. *Surgery* **86**, 583–589.

Ottoni, J.C., Morand, G., Tempe, J.D., Miech, G. and Witz, J.P. (1967). Complications de la trachéotomie: les fistules trachéo-oesophagiennes. *Ann. Chir. Thorac. Cardiovasc.* **6**, 465–466.

Robinson, F.W. (1979). Prevention of oesophageal perforation. *Amer. J. Surg.* **137**, 824–828.

Sanderson, C.J. and Trotter, G.A. (1980). Eder-Puestow oesophageal dilation: a new hazard. *Brit. J. Surg.* **67**, 300–301.

Sandrasagra, F.A. and Milstein, B.B. (1978). Oesophageal intubation in the management of perforated oesophagus with stricture. *Ann. Thorac. Surg.* **25**, 399–401.

Santos, G.H., Nordberg, R.E., Stamford, W.P., Efron, G. (1977). Operative complications of abdominal vagotomy. *Amer. J. Surg.* **133**, 662–664.

Savary, M. and Miller, G. (1977). Perforations oesophagiennes à l'oesophagoscopie. (L'oesophage. Manuel et atlas d'endoscopie.) Ed. Gassmann, S.A., Soleure. 15–17.

Scholl, D.G. and Tsai, S.H. (1977). Oesophageal perforation following the use of the oesophageal obturator airway. *Radiology* **122**, 315–316.

Schulze, S., Pedersen, V.M. and Høer-Madsen, K. (1982). Iatrogenic perforation of the oesophagus. Causes and management. *Acta Chir. Scand.* **148**, 679–682.

Slater, G. and Sicular, A.A. (1982). Oesophageal perforations after forceful dilatation in achalasia. *Ann. Surg.* **195**, 186–188.

Starlinger, M., Dinstl, K. and Schiessel, R. (1978). Perforation of the oesophagus with an oblique-viewing endoscope in a patient with caustic stenosis. *Endoscopy* **10**, 209–210.

Utley, J.R., Dillon, M.L., Todd, E.P., Griffen, W.O. and Zeok, J.V. (1978). Giant tracheoesophageal fistula. Management by oesophageal diversion. *J. Thorac. Cardiovasc. Surg.* **75**, 373–377.

Wechsler, R.J., Steiner, R.M., Goodman, L.R., Teplick, S.K., Mapp, E. and Laufer, I. (1982). Iatrogenic oesophageal-pleural fistula: subtlety of diagnosis in the absence of mediastinitis. *Radiology* **144**, 239–243.

b. *Swallowing injury of the oesophagus*

Appelqvist, P. and Salmo, M. (1980). Lye corrosion carcinoma of the oesophagus. A review of 63 cases. *Cancer* **45**, 2655–2658.

Balasegaram, M. (1975). Early management of corrosive burns of the oesophagus. *Brit. J. Surg.* **62**, 444–447.

Boujibar, M., Chevret, R., Jouhari-Ouaraini, A. and Rahhali, R. (1980). Notre expérience de la correction chirurgicale des rétrécissements cicatriciels de l'oesophage (R.C.O.). *J. Chir.*, Paris **106**, 644–653.

Campbell, J.R., Webber, B.R., Harrison, M.W. and Campbell, T.J. (1982). Oesophageal replacement in infants and children by colon interposition. *Amer. J. Surg.* **144**, 29–34.

Celerier, M. and Noirclerc, M., coordinateurs (1982). Les brûlures de tractus digestif supérieur. *Forum Chir.* **28**, 36–40.

Chien, K.Y., Wang, P.Y. and Lu K.S. (1974). Oesophagoplasty for corrosive stricture of the oesophagus: an analysis of 60 cases. *Ann. Surg.* **179**, 510–515.

Cyrlak, D., Cohen, A.J. and Dana, E.R. (1983). Oesophago-pericardial fistula: causes and radiographic features. *Amer. J. Roentgenol.* **141**, 177–179.

Delpre, G. and Kadish, U. (1981). Pathogenèse des ulcères induits par la prise de doxycycline. *Gastroenterol. Clin. Biol.* **5**, 813–814.

Di Costanzo, J., Devèze, J.-L., Jouglard, J., Noirclerc, M., Ohresser, Ph. (1979). Problèmes de réanimation posés par les brûlures par caustiques du tractus digestif supérieur. *Revue du Prat.* **29**, 1267–1269.

Dubost, C., Célérier, M., Leclerc, J.P., Kaswin, R. and Choquart, P. (1976). Les grandes brûlures caustiques oeso-gastriques de l'adulte. *J. Chir.*, Paris **112**, 385–408.

Gimmon, Z. and Durst, A.L. (1981). Acid corrosive gastritis. A plea for delayed surgical approach. *Amer. J. Surg.* **141**, 381–383.

Giordano, A., Adams, G., Boies, L. Jr. and Meyerhoff, W. (1981). Current management of oesophageal foreign bodies. *Arch. Otolaryng.* **107**, 249–251.

Handler, S.D., Beaugard, M.E., Canalis, R.F. and Fee, W.E. (1981). Unsuspected oesophageal foreign bodies in adults with upper airway obstruction. *Chest* **80**, 234–237.

Hopkins, R.A. and Postlethwait, R.W. (1981). Caustic burns and carcinoma of the oesophagus. *Ann. Surg.* **194**, 146–148.

James, A.H. and Allen-Mersh, T.G. (1982). Recognition and management of patients who repeatedly swallow foreign bodies. *J. Roy. Soc. Med.* **75**, 107–110.

Kirsh, M.M., Peterson, A., Brown, J.W., Orringer, M.B., Ritter, F. and Sloan, H. (1978). Treatment of caustic injuries of the oesophagus: a ten years experience. *Ann. Surg.* **188**, 675–678.

Kobler, E., Nüesch, H.J., Bühler, H., Jenny, S. and Deyhle, P. (1979). Medikamentös bedingte Oesophagusulzera. *Schweiz. Med. Wschr.* **109**, 1180–1182.

Lamouliatte, H., Plane, D. and Quinton, A. (1981). Ulcère oesophagien après prise orale de bromure de pinaverium. *Gastroenterol. Clin. Biol.* **5**, 812–813.

Nandi, P. and Ong, G.B. (1978). Foreign body in the oesophagus: review of 2394 cases. *Brit. J. Surg.* **65**, 5–9.

Popovici, Z., Dimitriu, A.V., Cerchez, E., Georgescu, M. and Pironcof, M. (1980). L'abord chirurgical des corps étrangers de l'oesophage. *J. Chir.*, Paris **117**, 481–484.

Pouyet, M., Bouletreau, P. and Morel, J.J. (1980). Plaidoyer pour une chirurgie d'éradication d'urgence dans certaines brûlures caustiques majeures du tractus digestif supérieur. *Lyon Chir.* **76**, 389–392.

Roethlisberger, B. and Savary, M. (1976). Les corps étrangers de l'oesophage. *Praxis* **65**, 777–782.

Roux, C. (1910). Oesophago-jejuno-gastrostomose et rétrécissements cicatriciels de l'oesophage. *La Grèce médicale* **7**, 97–102.

Shaw, A. (1979). Tracheoesophageal fistula following caustic ingestion. *Surgery* **85**, 360.

Singh, A.K., Kothawla, L.K. and Karlson, K.E. (1976). Tracheoesophageal and aortoesophageal fistulae complicating corrosive oesophagitis. *Chest* **70**, 549–551.

Sugawa, C., Mullins, R.J., Lucas, C.E. and Leibold, W.C. (1981). The value of early endoscopy following caustic ingestion. *Surg. Gynec. Obstet.* **153**, 553–556.

Symbas, P.N., Vlasis, S.E. and Hatcher, C.R. Jr. (1983). Oesophagitis secondary to ingestion of caustic material. *Ann. Thorac. Surg.* 73–77.

c. *Pneumatic rupture of the oesophagus and stomach*

Badruddoja, M. and MacGregor, J.K. (1971). Rupture of the intrathoracic oesophagus by compressed air blast. *Arch. Surg.* **103**, 417–419.

Buntain, W.L. and Lynn, H.B. (1972). Traumatic pneumatic disruption of the oesophagus. *J. Thorac. Cardiovasc. Surg.* **63**, 553–560.

Canarelli, J.P., Degroote, D., Bernard, F., Krim, G. and Lenaerts, C. (1983). Rupture barotraumatique de l'oesophage thoracique chez l'enfant. A propos d'un cas. *Chir. Pédiat.* **24**, 113–136.

Cramer, F.S. and Heimbach, R.D. (1982). Stomach rupture as a result of gastrointestinal barotrauma in a scuba diver. *J. Trauma* **22**, 238–240.

Eichenhorn, M.S. (1979). Gastric rupture complicating post-extubation laryngeal oedema and the use of a manual resuscitation bag. *Chest* **76**, 324–325.

Gelfand, E.T., Fisk, R.L. and Callaghan, J.C. (1977). Accidental pneumatic rupture of the oesophagus. *J. Thorac. Cardiovasc. Surg.* **74**, 142–144.

Geroulanus. S. (1972). Magenruptur nach Sauerstoffinsuflation mit einem Nasen-Rachen-Katheter. *Schweiz. Med. Wschr.* **102**, 205–208.

Hendricks, G.L. Jr. and Barnes, W.T. (1971). Accidental rupture of the oesophagus by compressed air. *Ann. Thorac. Surg.* **12**, 437–441.

Letoquart, J.P., Saudreau, F., Loisance, C., Kerdiles, Y. and Mambrini, A. (1981). Rupture barotraumatique de l'oesophage. A propos d'un cas. *J. Chir.*, Paris **118**, 483–486.

Millat, B., Gayral, F., Simonneau, G., Alasseur, F. and Larrieu, H. (1981). Rupture de l'estomac sain par distension gazeuse. A propos de 4 observations d'évolution favorable. *Gastroenterol. Clin. Biol.* **5**, 640–645.

Pailler, J.L., Rignault, D., Millet, H. and Marhic, C. (1981). Les ruptures gastriques iatrogènes post-anesthésiques. *J. Chir.*, Paris **107**, 745–748.

d. The Mallory-Weiss-Boerhaave syndrome

Abbott, O.A., Mansour, K.A., Logan, W.D., Hatcher, C.R. and Symbas, P.N. (1970). Atraumatic so-called 'spontaneous' rupture of the oesophagus. *J. Thorac. Cardiovasc. Surg.* **59**, 67–83.

Aldrich, C.A. and Auspach, W.E. (1939). Rupture of the oesophagus from blow on abdomen. *Radiology* **32**, 93–95.

Aguilar, J.C. (1981). Fatal gastric haemorrhage: a complication of cardiorespiratory resuscitation. *J. Trauma* **21**, 573–575.

Barrett, N.R. (1947). Report of a case of spontaneous perforation of the oesophagus successfully treated by operation. *Brit. J. Surg.* **35**, 216–218.

Baulieux, J., Balique, J.G., Boulez, J., Peix, J.L. and Maillet, P. (1979). Possibilité d'un traitement chirurgical conservateur des ruptures spontanées de l'oesophage vues à un stade tardif. *Lyon Chir.* **75**, 358–362.

Biagi, G., Cappelli, G., Propersi, L. and Grossi, A. (1983). Spontaneous intramural haematoma of the oesophagus. *Thorax* **38**, 394–395.

Boerhaave, H. (1724). Atrocis, nec descripti prius, Morbi Historia, Secundum Artis Legis conscripta. *Ludg. Batav.* (Opuscula omnia 1738, 10, p.98)

Boyer, J., Mario, A., Fresneau, M. and Joubaud, F. (1978). Un cas de rupture imcomplète de l'oesophage. *Endoscopie digestive* **3**, 29–32.

de Braquilanges, E., Ratajczak, A., Yver, B., Camuzet, J.P., Lavalou, J.F., Launois, B. and Bourdinière, J. (1983). Les ruptures spontanées de l'oesophage. *Ann. Oto-laryng.*, Paris **100**, 441–445.

Brown, R. and Cohen, P. (1978). Nonsurgical management of spontaneous oesophageal perforation. *J. Amer. Med. Ass.* **240**, 140–142.

Cameron, J.L., Kieffer, R.F., Hendrix, T.R., Mehigan, D.G. and Baker, R.R. (1979). Selective nonoperative management of contained intrathoracic oesophageal disruptions. *Ann. Thorac. Surg.* **27**, 404–408.

Dooling, J.A. and Zick, H.R. (1967). Closure of an oesophagopleural fistula using onlay intercostal pedicle graft. *Ann. Thorac. Surg.* **I**, 553–557.

Finley, R.J., Pearson, F.G., Weisel, R.D., Todd, T.R.J., Ilves, R. and Cooper, J. (1980). The management of nonmaligant intrathoracic oesophageal perforations. *Ann. Thorac. Surg.* **30**, 575–583.

Frech, R.S., Roper, C. and MacAlister, W.H. (1970). Oesophageal rupture secondary to pyloric obstruction by a gastrostomy Foley catheter balloon. *J. Can. Assoc. Radiol.* **21**, 263–265.

Giuli, R., Estenne, B., Colletas, J. and Lortat-Jacob, J.-L. (1977). Les traumatismes de l'oesophage. Etude clinique et résultats thérapeutiques. A propos de 83 cas. *Ann. Chir.* **31**, 193–199.

Hastings, P.R., Peters, K.W. and Cohn, I. (1981). Mallory-Weiss syndrome. Review of 69 cases. *Amer. J. Surg.* **142**, 560–562.

Hess, B. and Kaech, F. (1982). Spontanperforation des Osophagus (Boerhaave-Syndrom) bei diffuser idiopathischer Muskelhypertrophie. *Schweiz. Med. Wschr.* **112**, 272–276.

Hight, D.W. and Philippart, A.I. (1970). Ruptured short gastric vein associated with protracted vomiting. *Arch. Surg.* **100**, 321–322.

Houck, W.S. and Griffin, J.A. (1981). Spontaneous linear tears of the stomach in the newborn infant. *Ann. Surg.* **193**, 763–768.

Hureaux, J., Da Cunha, E.X., Pereira, B., Avci, C., Delavierre, P. and Vayre, P. (1979). Nécrose par dilatation aigüe de l'estomac chez l'adulte. Cinq nouvelles observations. *Chirurgie* **105**, 412–422.

Ivey, T.D., Simonowitz, D.A., Dillard, D.H. and Miller, D.W. (1981). Boerhaave syndrome. Successful conservative management in three patients with late presentation. *Amer. J. Surg.* **141**, 531–533.

Jara, F.M. (1979). Diaphragmatic pedicle flap for treatment of Boerhaave's syndrome (1979). *J. Thorac. Cardiovasc. Surg.* **78**, 931–933.

Joffe, N. and Millan, V.G. (1970). Postemetic dissecting intramural hematoma of the oesophagus. *Radiology* **95**, 379–380.

Kostiainen, S., Kukkonen, L., Merikoski, Y. and Närhinen, M. (1981). Spontaneous rupture of the middle third of the oesophagus. *Scand. J. Thorac. Cardiovasc. Surg.* **15**, 325–328.

MacVay, C.B. (1970). Treatment of a case of combined Mallory-Weiss and Boerhaave's syndromes. *Surg. Clin. North Amer.* **50**, 1111–1117.

McLaughlin, S.J. and Buxton, B. (1982). Secondary repair of oesophagus following spontaneous rupture with the use of a celestin tube. *Aust. N.Z. J. Surg.* **52**, 83–86.

Mallory, G.K. and Weiss, S. (1929). Hémorrhages from lacerations of the cardiac orifice of the stomach due to vomiting. *Amer. J. Med. Sci.* **178**, 506–515.

Matikainen, M. (1978). Rupture of the stomach: a rare complication of resuscitation. Case report. *Acta Chir. Scand.* **144**, 61–62.

Mayer, J.E. Jr., Murray, C.A. III and Varco, R.L. (1977). The treatment of oesophageal perforation with delayed recognition and continuing sepsis. *Ann. Thorac. Surg.* **23**, 568–573.

Meyer, A., Besson, A. and Saegesser, F. (1981). Complications intrathoraciques des traumas oeso-gastriques par vomissement ou à l'effort. *Ann. Chir. Thorac. Cardiovasc.* **35**, 232–236.

Sugawa, C., Benishek, D. and Walt, A.J. (1983). Mallory-Weiss syndrome. A study of 224 patients. *Amer. J. Surg.* **145**, 30–33.

Symbas, P.N., Hatcher, C.R. Jr. and Harlaftis, N. (1978). Spontaneous rupture of the oesophagus. *Ann. Surg.* **187**, 634–640.

Thornley, P.E. and Wallwork, J. (1978). Spontaneous rupture of the oesophagus and massive pneumoperitoneum. *Brit. J. Surg.* **65**, 633–636.

Vernon, S.E. and Carmichael, G.P. (1978). Unsuspected oesophageal perforation. *J. Amer. Med. Assoc.* **240**, 2568–2569.

Watts, H.D. (1976). Postemetic hematomas: a variant of the Mallory-Weiss syndrome. *Amer. J. Surg.* **132**, 320–321.

Yeh, T.J. and Humphries, A.L. Jr. (1963). Spontaneous rupture of oesophagus associated with epiphrenic diverticulum. *J. Thorac. Cardiovasc. Surg.* **46**, 271–275.

e. Oesophageal injury from external trauma

Andreassian, B., Lacombe, M., Nussaume, O., Homareau, C., Roger, W., Coquillaud, J.-P., Dazza, F. and Baumann, J. (1973). Ruptures de l'oesophage par traumatisme fermé. *Ann. Chir. Thorac. Cardiovasc.* **12**, 409–415.

Antkowiak, J.G., Cohen, M.L. and Kyllonen, A.S. (1974). Tracheo-oesophageal fistula following blunt trauma. *Arch. Surg.* **109**, 529–531.

Debakey, M.E. and Heaney, J.P. (1953). Tracheo-oesophageal fistula due to non-penetrating injury. *Amer. Surg.* **19**, 97–106.

Defore, W.W., Mattox, K.L., Hansen, H.A., Garcia-Rinaldi, R., Beal, A.C. Jr. and DeBakey, M.E. (1977). Surgical management of penetrating injuries of the oesophagus. *Amer. J. Surg.* **134**, 734–738.

Holmes, T.W. and Netterville, R.E. (1956). Complication of first rib fracture, including one case each of tracheo-oesophageal fistula and aortic arch aneurysm. *J. Thorac. Surg.* **32**, 74–91.

Stothert, J.C., Buttorff, J. and Kaminski, D.L. (1980). Thoracic oesophageal and tracheal injury following blunt trauma. *J. Trauma* **20**, 992–995.

Symbas, P.N., Hatcher, C.R. and Vlasis, S.E. (1980). Oesophageal gunshot injuries. *Ann. Surg.* **191**, 703–707.

Index

Figures in light type refer to pages; those in **bold** type refer to illustrations. * = see Volume I.